AF333727

1996
YEAR BOOK OF
ONCOLOGY®

Statement of Purpose

The YEAR BOOK Service

The YEAR BOOK series was devised in 1901 by practicing health professionals who observed that the literature of medicine and related disciplines had become so voluminous that no one individual could read and place in perspective every potential advance in a major specialty. In the final decade of the 20th century, this recognition is more acutely true than it was in 1901.

More than merely a series of books, YEAR BOOK volumes are the tangible results of a unique service designed to accomplish the following:

- to *survey* a wide range of journals of proven value
- to *select* from those journals papers representing significant advances and statements of important clinical principles
- to provide *abstracts* of those articles that are readable, convenient summaries of their key points
- to provide *commentary* about those articles to place them in perspective

These publications grow out of a unique process that calls on the talents of outstanding authorities in clinical and fundamental disciplines, trained literature specialists, and professional writers, all supported by the resources of Mosby, the world's preeminent publisher for the health professions.

The Literature Base

Mosby and its editors survey more than 1,000 journals published worldwide, covering the full range of the health professions. On an annual basis, the publisher examines usage patterns and polls its expert authorities to add new journals to the literature base and to delete journals that are no longer useful as potential YEAR BOOK sources.

The Literature Survey

The publisher's team of literature specialists, all of whom are trained and experienced health professionals, examines every original, peer-reviewed article in each journal issue. More than 250,000 articles per year are scanned systematically, including title, text, illustrations, tables, and references. Each scan is compared, article by article, to the search strategies that the publisher has developed in consultation with the 270 outside experts who form the pool of YEAR BOOK editors. A given article may be reviewed by any number of editors, from one to a dozen or more, regardless of the discipline for which the paper was originally published. In turn, each editor who receives the article reviews it to determine whether or not the article should be included in the YEAR BOOK. This decision is based on the article's inherent quality, its probable usefulness to readers of that YEAR BOOK, and the editor's goal to represent a balanced picture of a given field in each volume of the YEAR BOOK. In addition, the editor indicates when to include figures and tables from the article to help the YEAR BOOK reader better understand the information.

Of the quarter million articles scanned each year, only 5% are selected for detailed analysis within the YEAR BOOK series, thereby assuring readers of the high value of every selection.

The Abstract

The publisher's abstracting staff is headed by a seasoned medical professional and includes individuals with training in the life sciences, medicine, and other areas, plus extensive experience in writing for the health professions and related industries. Each selected article is assigned to a specific writer on this abstracting staff. The abstracter, guided in many cases by notations supplied by the expert editor, writes a structured, condensed summary designed so that the reader can rapidly acquire the essential information contained in the article.

The Commentary

The YEAR BOOK editorial boards, sometimes assisted by guest commentators, write comments that place each article in perspective for the reader. This provides the reader with the equivalent of a personal consultation with a leading international authority—an opportunity to better understand the value of the article and to benefit from the authority's thought processes in assessing the article.

Additional Editorial Features

The editorial boards of each YEAR BOOK organize the abstracts and comments to provide a logical and satisfying sequence of information. To enhance the organization, editors also provide introductions to sections or individual chapters, comments linking a number of abstracts, citations to additional literature, and other features.

The published YEAR BOOK contains enhanced bibliographic citations for each selected article, including extended listings of multiple authors and identification of author affiliations. Each YEAR BOOK contains a Table of Contents specific to that year's volume. From year to year, the Table of Contents for a given YEAR BOOK will vary depending on developments within the field.

Every YEAR BOOK contains a list of the journals from which papers have been selected. This list represents a subset of the more than 1,000 journals surveyed by the publisher and occasionally reflects a particularly pertinent article from a journal that is not surveyed on a routine basis.

Finally, each volume contains a comprehensive subject index and an index to authors of each selected paper.

The 1996 Year Book Series

Year Book of Allergy, Asthma, and Clinical Immunology: Drs. Rosenwasser, Borish, Gelfand, Leung, Nelson, and Szefler

Year Book of Anesthesiology and Pain Management: Drs. Tinker, Abram, Chestnut, Roizen, Rothenberg, and Wood

Year Book of Cardiology®: Drs. Schlant, Collins, Engle, Gersh, Kaplan, and Waldo

Year Book of Chiropractic®: Dr. Lawrence

Year Book of Critical Care Medicine®: Drs. Parrillo, Balk, Calvin, Franklin, and Shapiro

Year Book of Dentistry®: Drs. Meskin, Berry, Kennedy, Leinfelder, Roser, Summitt, and Zakariasen

Year Book of Dermatologic Surgery®: Drs. Swanson, Glogau, and Salasche

Year Book of Dermatology®: Drs. Sober and Fitzpatrick

Year Book of Diagnostic Radiology®: Drs. Federle, Clark, Gross, Latchaw, Madewell, Maynard, and Young

Year Book of Digestive Diseases®: Drs. Greenberger and Moody

Year Book of Drug Therapy®: Drs. Lasagna and Weintraub

Year Book of Emergency Medicine®: Drs. Wagner, Dronen, Davidson, King, Niemann, and Roberts

Year Book of Endocrinology®: Drs. Bagdade, Braverman, Horton, Kannan, Landsberg, Molitch, Morley, Nathan, Odell, Poehlman, Rogol, and Ryan

Year Book of Family Practice®: Drs. Berg, Bowman, Davidson, Dexter, and Scherger

Year Book of Geriatrics and Gerontology®: Drs. Beck, Burton, Rabins, Reuben, Roth, Shapiro, and Whitehouse

Year Book of Hand Surgery®: Drs. Amadio and Hentz

Year Book of Hematology®: Drs. Spivak, Bell, Ness, Quesenberry, Wiernik, and Blume

Year Book of Infectious Diseases®: Drs. Keusch, Barza, Bennish, Klempner, Skolnik, and Snydman

Year Book of Infertility and Reproductive Endocrinology: Drs. Mishell, Lobo, and Sokol

Year Book of Medicine®: Drs. Bone, Cline, Epstein, Greenberger, Malawista, Mandell, O'Rourke, and Utiger

Year Book of Neonatal and Perinatal Medicine®: Drs. Fanaroff and Klaus

Year Book of Nephrology, Hypertension, and Mineral Metabolism: Drs. Coe, Curtis, Favus, Henderson, Kashgarian, Luke, and Myers

Year Book of Neurology and Neurosurgery®: Drs. Bradley and Wilkins

Year Book of Neuroradiology: Drs. Osborn, Eskridge, Grossman, Hudgins, and Ross

Year Book of Nuclear Medicine®: Drs. Gottschalk, Blaufox, McAfee, Wackers, and Zubal

Year Book of Obstetrics and Gynecology®: Drs. Mishell, Herbst, and Kirschbaum

Year Book of Occupational and Environmental Medicine®: Drs. Emmett, Frank, Gochfeld, and Hessl

Year Book of Oncology®: Drs. Simone, Bosl, Cohen, Glatstein, Ozols, and Tallman

Year Book of Ophthalmology®: Drs. Cohen, Augsburger, Eagle, Flanagan, Grossman, Laibson, Maguire, Nelson, Rapuano, Sergott, Tasman, Tipperman, and Wilson

Year Book of Orthopedics®: Drs. Sledge, Cofield, Dobyns, Griffin, Poss, Springfield, Swiontkowski, Wiesel, and Wilson

Year Book of Otolaryngology–Head and Neck Surgery®: Drs. Paparella, and Holt

Year Book of Pain: Drs. Gebhart, Haddox, Jacox, Janjan, Marcus, Rudy, and Shapiro

Year Book of Pathology and Laboratory Medicine: Drs. Mills, Bruns, Gaffey, and Stoler

Year Book of Pediatrics®: Dr. Stockman

Year Book of Plastic, Reconstructive, and Aesthetic Surgery®: Drs. Miller, Cohen, McKinney, Robson, Ruberg, and Whitaker

Year Book of Podiatric Medicine and Surgery®: Dr. Kominsky

Year Book of Psychiatry and Applied Mental Health®: Drs. Talbott, Ballenger, Breier, Frances, Meltzer, Schowalter, and Tasman

Year Book of Pulmonary Disease®: Drs. Bone and Petty

Year Book of Rheumatology®: Drs. Sergent, LeRoy, Meenan, Panush, and Reichlin

Year Book of Sports Medicine®: Drs. Shephard, Drinkwater, Eichner, Torg, Col. Anderson, and Mr. George

Year Book of Surgery®: Drs. Copeland, Bland, Deitch, Eberlein, Howard, Luce, Seeger, Souba, and Sugarbaker

Year Book of Thoracic and Cardiovascular Surgery®: Drs. Ginsberg, Wechsler, and Williams

Year Book of Ultrasound®: Drs. Merritt, Carroll, and Fleischer

Year Book of Urology®: Drs. DeKernion and Howards

Year Book of Vascular Surgery®: Dr. Porter

1996

The Year Book of ONCOLOGY®

Editor-in-Chief
Joseph V. Simone, M.D.
Physician-in-Chief, Memorial Sloan-Kettering Cancer Center, New York

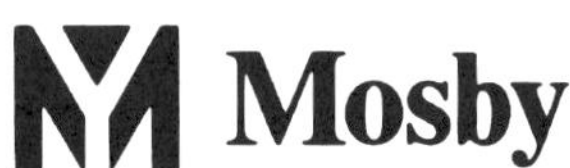 Mosby

St. Louis   Baltimore   Boston   Carlsbad   Chicago   Naples   New York   Philadelphia   Portland
London   Madrid   Mexico City   Singapore   Sydney   Tokyo   Toronto   Wiesbaden

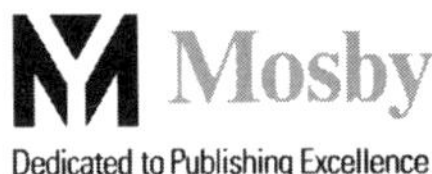 Mosby

Dedicated to Publishing Excellence

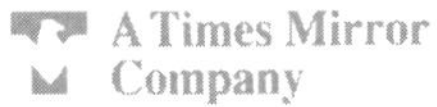 A Times Mirror
Company

Vice President and Publisher, Continuity Publishing: Kenneth H. Killion
Director, Editorial Development: Gretchen C. Murphy
Developmental Editor, Continuity: Kelly Poirier
Acquisitions Editor: Linda Sheehan
Illustrations and Permissions Coordinator: Steven J. Ramay
Manager, Continuity–EDP: Maria Nevinger
Project Supervisor, Editing: Rebecca Nordbrock
Senior Project Manager, Production: Max F. Perez
Freelance Staff Supervisor: Barbara M. Kelly
Director, Editorial Services: Edith M. Podrazik, B.S.N., R.N.
Information Specialist: Kathleen Moss, R.N.
Senior Marketing Manager: Eileen M. Lynch
Circulation Manager: Lynn D. Stevenson

Printed in the United States of America
Composition by Reed Technology and Information Services, Inc.
Printing/binding by Maple-Vail

Mosby–Year Book, Inc.
11830 Westline Industrial Drive
St. Louis, MO 63146

Editorial Office:
Mosby–Year Book, Inc.
161 North Clark Street
Chicago, IL 60601

International Standard Serial Number: 1040-1741
International Standard Book Number: 0-8151-9758-6

Associate Editors

George J. Bosl, M.D.
Professor of Medicine, Cornell University Medical College; Head, Division of Solid Tumor Oncology, Department of Medicine, Memorial Sloan-Kettering Cancer Center, New York

Alfred M. Cohen, M.D.
Professor of Surgery, Cornell University Medical College; Chief, Colorectal Service, Department of Surgery, Memorial Sloan-Kettering Cancer Center, New York

Eli Glatstein, M.D.
Professor and Chair, Department of Radiation Oncology, University of Texas Southwestern Medical Center, Dallas

Robert F. Ozols, M.D., Ph.D.
Senior Vice President of Medical Science, Fox Chase Cancer Center, Philadelphia

Martin S. Tallman, M.D.
Assistant Professor, Division of Hematology/Oncology, Northwestern University Medical School; Director, Clinical Leukemia Research Program of Robert H. Lurie Cancer Center of Northwestern University, Chicago

Contributing Editors

Richard Burt, M.D.
Director of Allogeneic Bone Marrow Transplants, Northwestern University/ Northwestern Memorial Hospital, Chicago

W.J. Gradishar, M.D.
Assistant Professor of Medicine, Northwestern University Medical School, Chicago

W.G. Finn, M.D.
Assistant Professor of Pathology, Northwestern University Medical School, Chicago

Morris Kletzel, M.D.
Associate Professor of Pediatrics, Northwestern University Medical School, Chicago

Jane N. Winter, M.D.
Associate Professor of Medicine, Northwestern University Medical School, Chicago

Table of Contents

Journals Represented

Mosby and its editors survey more than 1,000 journals for its abstract and commentary publications. From these journals, the Editors select the articles to be abstracted. Journals represented in this YEAR BOOK are listed below.

Acta Oto-Laryngologica
American Journal of Clinical Pathology
American Journal of Hematology
American Journal of Industrial Medicine
American Journal of Neuroradiology
American Journal of Obstetrics and Gynecology
American Journal of Pediatric Hematology/Oncology
American Journal of Surgery
American Journal of Surgical Pathology
Annals of Internal Medicine
Annals of Oncology
Annals of Surgery
Annals of Surgical Oncology
Annals of Thoracic Surgery
Archives of Disease in Childhood
Archives of Pathology and Laboratory Medicine
Australasian Radiology
Blood
Bone Marrow Transplantation
British Journal of Cancer
British Journal of Haematology
British Journal of Radiology
British Journal of Surgery
British Journal of Urology
British Medical Journal
Canadian Family Physician
Cancer
Cancer Research
Chest
Clinical Cancer Research
Clinical Infectious Diseases
Clinical Nuclear Medicine
Diseases of the Colon and Rectum
European Journal of Cancer
European Journal of Obstetrics, Gynecology and Reproductive Biology
European Journal of Pediatric Surgery
Gastroenterology
Gynecologic Oncology
Head and Neck
Hepatology
Infection Control and Hospital Epidemiology
International Journal of Cancer
International Journal of Gynecological Cancer
International Journal of Radiation, Oncology, Biology, and Physics
Journal of Cardiovascular Surgery
Journal of Clinical Endocrinology and Metabolism
Journal of Clinical Epidemiology

Journal of Clinical Investigation
Journal of Clinical Oncology
Journal of Developmental and Behavioral Pediatrics
Journal of Pain and Symptom Management
Journal of Pediatric Surgery
Journal of Urology
Journal of the American College of Surgeons
Journal of the American Medical Association
Journal of the National Cancer Institute
Lancet
Laryngoscope
Leukemia
Nature
Neurology
Neurosurgery
New England Journal of Medicine
Obstetrics and Gynecology
Orbit
Pediatric Pulmonology
Pediatric Research
Pediatrics
Radiology
Radiotherapy and Oncology
Seminars in Diagnostic Pathology
Southern Medical Journal
Transplantation Proceedings
Urology
Western Journal of Medicine
World Journal of Surgery

STANDARD ABBREVIATIONS

The following terms are abbreviated in this edition: acquired immunodeficiency syndrome (AIDS), cardiopulmonary resuscitation (CPR), central nervous system (CNS), cerebrospinal fluid (CSF), computed tomography (CT), deoxyribonucleic acid (DNA), electrocardiography (ECG), health maintenance organization (HMO), human immunodeficiency virus (HIV), intensive care unit (ICU), intramuscular (IM), intravenous (IV), magnetic resonance (MR) imaging (MRI), and ribonucleic acid (RNA).

NOTE

The YEAR BOOK OF ONCOLOGY is a literature survey service providing abstracts of articles published in the professional literature. Every effort is made to assure the accuracy of the information presented in these pages. Neither the editors nor the publisher of the YEAR BOOK OF ONCOLOGY can be responsible for errors in the original materials. The editors' comments are their own opinions. Mention of specific products within this publication does not constitute endorsement.

To facilitate the use of the YEAR BOOK OF ONCOLOGY as a reference tool, all illustrations and tables included in this publication are now identified as they appear in the original article. This change is meant to help the reader recognize that any illustration or table appearing in the YEAR BOOK OF ONCOLOGY may be only one of many in the original article. For this reason, figure and table numbers will often appear to be out of sequence within the YEAR BOOK OF ONCOLOGY.

Publisher's Preface

With this edition of the YEAR BOOK OF ONCOLOGY, we say goodbye to our esteemed colleague, Joseph V. Simone, M.D., with whom we have worked for the past 8 years. Throughout this time, he has provided readers with insightful and thought-provoking commentary of the highest caliber. Moreover, we at Mosby–Year Book, Inc., have been treated to an enjoyable and rewarding association. We extend our deepest appreciation to Dr. Simone for the service he has provided and for his unending support, leadership, and enthusiasm for this publication. He will be missed by all of us here, and we wish him the very best in all his future endeavors.

We are pleased that Robert F. Ozols, M.D., Ph.D., who has also been an editor for this publication during the past 8 years, has agreed to take the helm as our new Editor-in-Chief. Please join us in welcoming him to his new role.

Mosby–Year Book, Inc.

1 Cancer Etiology and Epidemiology

What Does it Mean to Be a Cancer Gene Carrier? Problems in Establishing Causality From the Molecular Genetics of Cancer
Schatzkin A, Goldstein A, Freedman LS (Natl Cancer Inst, Bethesda, Md)
J Natl Cancer Inst 87:1126–1130, 1995   1–1

Objective.—The existence of families with high incidences of various types of cancer has led to an intense search for predisposing, heritable gene mutations. It is often implicitly assumed that the mutant gene is the sole cause of the cancer, but knowledge of other genes suggests this is not necessarily true. Current knowledge of the molecular genetics of cancer was reviewed in an attempt to determine what it means to carry a cancer gene.

The Causality of Cancer Genes.—The hypothetical case of a single mutation of a gene for a cancer site, designated MUTGENE1, that is associated with cancer in affected families was considered. Four inferences might be made about this gene, the first being that it is a necessary and sufficient cause of cancer in the affected families. However, other pathways are possible. It might be inferred that MUTGENE1 causes cancer only in the presence of one or more other genes, designated GENE2, which might act either at the cellular level or at the level of gross pathology.

A third possibility is that of gene-environment interaction, in which MUTGENE1 leads to malignancies only in the presence of one or more environmental factors. In the final inference, MUTGENE1 may cause cancer only in conjunction with one or more additional genes and with one or more environmental factors. A number of other issues must be considered as well. For example, it is possible that even though an individual carrier of the mutant gene is at increased risk of cancer, some nutritional, pharmacologic, or other intervention could still be protective. Further problems arise in attempts to extrapolate from cancer-prone families to the general population, because the excess risk of cancer for individuals with mutant genes who are not members of cancer-prone families is unknown.

Discussion.—The relationships between gene mutations and cancer can be very complex, even in families documented as cancer prone. It may still be relevant to target these families for interventions against environmental risk factors. Also, large-scale epidemiologic studies will be needed before the findings from studies of cancer-prone families can be extrapolated to the general population. Such studies should be planned now to take full advantage of the advances in molecular genetics.

▶ The identification of gene mutations in families with heritable cancer has opened the possibility of genetic tests for cancer predisposition. This timely article from the *Journal of the National Cancer Institute* raises important questions and concerns regarding what it really means for members of the general population to be carriers of a cancer gene. It is emphasized repeatedly in this article that a strong association between the presence of a mutated gene and the incidence of cancer within families does not necessarily mean that a positive carrier in the general population is destined to have cancer develop. It may be that the identified mutated gene must interact with another gene present in a family for the cancer to develop, or that this gene may have to interact with environmental factors that then lead to the development of cancer. It may even be necessary for the mutated gene to interact with another gene present in the family, as well as with specific environmental factors, for the tumors to develop.

Consequently, in the general population, the presence of a mutated gene that has a much lower frequency of carrying the second obligatory gene or the same environmental factors may not lead to a markedly increased risk for cancer. This article is important to place in perspective the limitations of current genetic screening tests for the general population. At present, genetic screening has its greatest value in identifying members of cancer-prone families who are at risk for the development of disease.

R.F. Ozols, M.D., Ph.D.

Lymphoma-Associated Translocation t(14;18) in Blood B Cells of Normal Individuals
Limpens J, Stad R, Vos C, de Vlaam C, de Jong D, van Ommen G-JB, Schuuring E, Kluin PM (Univ of Leiden, The Netherlands)
Blood 85:2528–2536, 1995   1–2

Introduction.—There is considerable evidence that chromosomal translocations play a central role in the pathogenesis of B-cell lymphomas. The sporadic occurrence of precursor B-cell leukemia in patients with follicular lymphoma supports the view that t(14;18) breakpoints occur early in the process and result in deregulation of the *BCL2* proto-oncogene. However, these occurrences alone seem to be insufficient for establishing the malignant phenotype. It was hypothesized that the blood B cells of healthy individuals might have the t(14;18) translocation. The hypothesis was tested, using a highly sensitive, seminested polymerase chain reaction (PCR).

Methods.—Deoxyribonucleic acid from mononuclear cells, granulocytes, B cells, and T cells was isolated from the mononuclear cell fractions of blood samples from 9 donors obtained from a blood bank. Seminested PCR was performed using primers for *BCL2* breakpoints at JH1-5 on 14q32 and the major breakpoint region on 18q21. Amplification products were then sequenced if they hybridized with the probes.

Results.—There were t(14;18) breakpoints in the blood of 6 of the 9 donors, which were found almost exclusively in the purified B cells. Positive results for the translocation were obtained in 23 of 48 PCR experiments on B cells, in 4 of 47 experiments on mononuclear cells, in 1 of the 48 experiments on T cells, and in 1 of the 47 experiments on granulocytes. Sequence analysis detected breakpoints localized within the recognized areas of the major breakpoint region on *BCL2* and at the 5' side of the JH or DH segments of the immunoglobulin heavy chain locus. The ubiquitous detection of N-regions suggested an origin from terminal transferase-positive bone marrow precursor B cells. Contiguous JH gene segments downstream from the *BCL2*/JH breakpoint were found in 2 samples. Follicular lymphoma is characterized by similar breakpoint configurations.

Discussion.—The t(14;18) translocation occurred in approximately 1 cell per 10^5 B cells in normal, healthy individuals. These findings suggest that this translocation is generated regularly in the bone marrow precursor B cells of healthy individuals and that daughter cells carrying the translocation enter the bloodstream and travel to lymphoid tissues. Because *BCL2* is deregulated in these cells, they may be long-living cells and may selectively accumulate additional genetic damage, eventually leading to the malignant phenotype of follicular lymphoma. However, cells with only the t(14;18) breakpoint are harmless precursor tumor cells, requiring other oncogenic events for development of follicular lymphoma.

▶ The t(14;18) chromosomal translocation is frequently observed in patients with follicular lymphomas. This specific translocation involves a rearrangement of the *BCL2* oncogene. Perturbations in the *BCL2* proto-oncogene permit a survival advantage of the clonal cells by preventing apoptotic death. In this provocative report, the authors used a sensitive semi-nested PCR to examine the peripheral blood cells of healthy individuals and found that circulating B cells with t(14;18) chromosomal translocation can be identified in such patients. Six of 9 healthy individuals harbored t(14;18) breakpoints. The estimated frequency of such breakpoints in healthy individuals was approximately 1 in 10^5 or fewer circulating B cells.

The authors speculate that such a translocation is regularly generated in bone marrow precursor B cells in healthy individuals. Such cells may then sustain a sufficient amount of additional genetic damage, leading to high expression of the *BCL2* proto-oncogene, which prevents apoptosis and which may prevent apoptosis leading to follicular lymphomas. These observations are provocative and important because they imply that sophisticated techniques to detect minimal residual disease in patients with follicular lymphomas after treatment may be more complicated than was previously thought. In addition, the identification of a malignant clone in the peripheral blood may not be sufficient to establish the clonality of lymphocytosis and to establish a diagnosis of malignancy. Most importantly, these observations suggest that in healthy individuals, expansion of a potentially malignant clone may develop, but other events are required within this clone to establish malignant disease. These observations have broad implications with respect to oncogenesis.

M.S. Tallman, M.D.

The Impact of Genetic Counselling on Risk Perception in Women With a Family History of Breast Cancer
Evans DGR, Blair V, Greenhalgh R, Hopwood P, Howell A (Paterson Inst for Cancer Research, Manchester, England; Christie Hosp, Manchester, England)
Br J Cancer 70:934–938, 1994   1–3

Background.—Women with a family history of breast cancer generally seek medical attention because they believe they are at high risk. Although such women are probably helped by genetic counseling and, when the risk is substantial, by annual mammography, the psychological effect of assigning true risk and the value of mammography both need to be assessed.

Methods and Findings.—A questionnaire was used to determine risk in 517 patients newly referred to a family history clinic and in 200 women returning to the clinic at least 1 year after counseling. The uninformed, precounsel group had a correct assignment of a population lifetime risk of breast cancer of 16%. In the postcounsel group, this value was 33%. Personal risk was correct in 11% of the former group and in 41% of the latter group. After counseling, women were significantly more likely to retain information when they were sent a letter or when they thought their personal risk initially was too high.

Conclusions.—Women with a family history of breast cancer benefit from the opportunity to discuss their risk and from regular surveillance. Adherence to screening was very good in the high-risk group. Such adherence was unaffected by a change in the perceived risk in this group. For women who initially expressed a low perceived risk, counseling did not appear to change knowledge or screening behavior.

▶ I have included this paper to alert the reader to the increasing complexity and potential dangers of genetic counseling. For those of us who do not do such counseling on a regular basis, it may seem fairly straightforward, i.e., a matter of informing the patient of the risks of a particular disease based on the data as we know it. However, even more than many other transmissions of medical information, the perception of the individuals counseled, their psychological preparation, the intrafamily relationships, and their personal experience with a family member who had the disease create an intricate web for the counselor to negotiate. In addition to trying to convey an accurate picture for the individual, a counselor is often trying to motivate the patient to grasp the risk accurately and behave in an appropriate manner subsequently, e.g., by undergoing regular screening. Another issue of great concern to genetic counselors is not mentioned in this paper, i.e., the ethical and legal ramifications of providing information to family members who do not come forward for genetic counseling.

The power of the new and sophisticated methods of genetic testing, like all new technology, raises new and difficult questions about privacy and the distribution of the knowledge so gained.

J.V. Simone, M.D.

The Use of Estrogens and Progestins and the Risk of Breast Cancer in Postmenopausal Women

Colditz GA, Hankinson SE, Hunter DJ, Willett WC, Manson JE, Stampfer MJ, Hennekens C, Rosner B, Speizer FE (Harvard Med School, Boston)
N Engl J Med 332:1589–1593, 1995   1–4

Background.—Although several studies and meta-analyses have examined the relationship between postmenopausal hormone replacement therapy (HRT) and the risk of breast cancer, the findings have been inconclusive overall. The effect of combining progestins with estrogen therapy and the influence of age on the risk of breast cancer are particularly in question. These questions were examined in analysis of 1992 data from the Nurses' Health Study.

Methods.—The Nurses' Health Study, established in 1976, periodically collected prospective data on known or suspected risk factors for cardiovascular disease and cancer. Data from the 1992 follow-up questionnaire

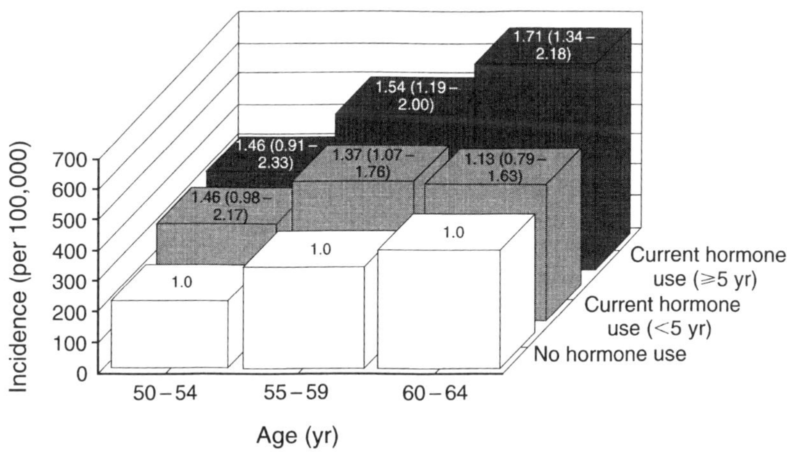

FIGURE 1.—Incidence and relative risk of breast cancer according to age and duration of current postmenopausal hormone therapy. Relative risks and 95% confidence intervals are shown on the *top of the bars;* relative risks are expressed in comparison with the risk among women in each age group who never received hormone therapy. Data have been adjusted for age at menopause, type of menopause, and family history of breast cancer in a proportional-hazards analysis. (Reprinted by permission of *The New England Journal of Medicine,* Colditz GA, Hankinson SE, Hunter DJ, et al: The use of estrogens and progestins and the risk of breast cancer in postmenopausal women. 332:1589–1593, Copyright 1995, Massachusetts Medical Society.)

TABLE 2.—Duration of Current and Past Postmenopausal Hormone Therapy and Relative Risk of Breast Cancer in the Nurses' Health Study, 1976–1992

Hormone Use	Cases of Breast Cancer	Person-Years of Follow-up	Adjusted Relative Risk (95% CI)*
None	972	374,197	1.0
Current			
1–23 Mo	82	31,966	1.14 (0.91–1.45)
24–59 Mo	140	49,672	1.20 (0.99–1.44)
60–119 Mo	150	44,112	1.46 (1.22–174)
≥ 120 Mo	141	37,454	1.46 (1.20–1.76)
Past			
1–23 Mo	193	81,047	0.90 (0.77–1.05)
24–59 Mo	120	54,046	0.86 (0.71–1.05)
60–119 Mo	89	34,952	1.00 (0.80–1.26)
≥ 120 Mo	48	18,104	1.03 (0.76–1.41)

* Adjusted for age, type of menopause, age at menopuase, parity, age at first delivery, age at menarche, family history of breast cancer, history of benign breast disease, and time period.

(Reprinted by permission of *The New England Journal of Medicine*, Colditz GA, Hankinson SE, Hunter DJ, et al: The use of estrogens and progestins and the risk of breast cancer in postmenopausal women. 332:1589–1593, Copyright 1995, Massachusetts Medical Society.)

were examined with regard to the diagnosis of breast cancer and the use of postmenopausal HRT, and the association was analyzed.

Results.—Between 1978 and 1992, the relative risk of breast cancer increased to 1.32 among women treated with estrogens alone, 1.41 among women treated with estrogen plus progestin, and 2.24 among women treated with progestins alone. There were no significant differences in the relative risk of breast cancer among the 3 groups. The risk of breast cancer also increased with age. After adjustment for age, risk increased significantly only among women who had used HRT for 5 years or more (Fig 1 and Table 2).

Conclusion.—The risk of breast cancer is increased among postmenopausal women currently treated with estrogen alone or estrogen and progestin in combination. Therefore, the addition of progestin does not reduce the risk of breast cancer associated with estrogen treatment, suggesting that ductal cells in the breast do not respond to progestin in the same way as does the endometrium, where progestin has a protective effect. Postmenopausal HRT may be a particularly strong risk factor with advancing age. The benefits and risks of HRT should be carefully weighed for each individual.

Combined Estrogen and Progestin Hormone Replacement Therapy in Relation to Risk of Breast Cancer in Middle-Aged Women

Stanford JL, Weiss NS, Voigt LF, Daling JR, Habel LA, Rossing MA (Fred Hutchinson Cancer Research Ctr, Seattle)
JAMA 274:137–142, 1995

1–5

Background.—The use of combined progestin and estrogen for hormone replacement therapy (HRT) has increased among women in the

United States. Although this combination may, in theory, alter the incidence of breast cancer, few epidemiologic data are available on the association of combined estrogen-progestin HRT and breast cancer.

Methods.—Five hundred thirty-seven 50- to 64-year-old women with breast cancer and 492 randomly selected women with no history of breast cancer were included in a case-control study. All were residents of one county in western Washington State.

Findings.—Sixty-one percent of the control group and 57.6% of the patients had used some type of menopausal hormone. The 21.5% of patients and 21.3% of control subjects who had ever used combined estrogen-progestin HRT had no increased risk of breast cancer. Compared with hormone nonusers, women who had used estrogen-progestin for 8 years or more had, if anything, a decreased risk of breast cancer risk.

Conclusion.—The use of combination estrogen-progestin HRT apparently is unrelated to an increased risk of breast cancer in middle-aged women. Further research is needed to determine whether the incidence of breast cancer is altered many years after estrogen-progestin HRT is begun, especially among long-term users.

Hormone Replacement Treatment and Breast Cancer Risk: A Cooperative Italian Study
La Vecchia C, Negri E, Franceschi S, Favero A, Nanni O, Filiberti R, Conti E, Montella M, Veronesi A, Ferraroni M, Decarli A (Istituto di Recerche Farmacologiche "Mario Negri," Milan, Italy; Centro di Riferimento Oncologico, Pordenone, Italy; Ospedale Pierantoni, Forli, Italy; et al)
Br J Cancer 72:244–248, 1995   1–6

Background.—Many epidemiologic studies have been done on the possible relationship between hormone replacement therapy (HRT) and the risk of breast cancer. Although ever using HRT apparently is not consistently related to the subsequent risk of breast cancer, several questions remain unanswered. For example, increased risks have been documented among long-term users, although no consistent risk pattern has been identified for other time factors. One study reported that HRT may have a late-stage effect on breast carcinogenesis. However, the issue of time-related factors in the possible effects of HRT on breast cancer is still open to debate. The relationship between HRT and the risk of breast cancer was further investigated using case-control data.

Methods.—Six Italian centers contributed data on 2,569 patients seen between June 1991 and February 1994 with histologically confirmed breast cancer and on 2,588 control subjects hospitalized for a wide range of acute, nonneoplastic, non–hormone-related diseases. All patients were younger than 75 years.

Findings.—Seven and a half percent of subjects from both groups reported ever using HRT. The risk of breast cancer increased as the duration of use increased. The odds ratios were 1.0 for using HRT less than 1 year,

1.3 for using it for 1 to 4 years, and 1.5 for using it for 5 years or more. Although no clear pattern of risk associated with time since beginning HRT could be identified, the odds ratio was significantly increased for women who had stopped using HRT in the preceding 10 years. Women who had quit use of HRT more than 10 years previously showed no association. The increased odds ratio for women who had quit HRT within the preceding 10 years was consistent across strata of covariates identified and was significantly associated with duration of use.

Conclusion.—Although there is no strong association between HRT and the risk of breast cancer, the risk estimate was greater than unity for women who had used HRT for 5 years or more. However, in the short to medium term after use, the risk was significantly increased, especially for long-term users. The finding of a short-term increased risk supports the notion that HRT affects one of the later stages of the breast carcinogenesis process. The flattening of risk with the passage of time since stopping HRT and, hence, the absence of a long-term cumulative excess in the risk of breast cancer after stopping exposure to HRT has important implications for the evaluation of individual risk and public health.

▶ There continues to be much debate about the relative value of HRT in postmenopausal women. The data indicate that continued hormone use reduces the risk of heart disease and protects against osteoporotic fractures; however, considerable evidence implicates endogenous estrogens in the risk of breast cancer. Early age at menarche, late menopause, parity, and obesity are all associated with an increase in the incidence of breast cancer. Some data have suggested that the concurrent use of progestins with estrogen would abrogate the increased risk of breast cancer.

The 3 previous articles address this issue. Colditz et al. (Abstract 1–4) report that the incidence and risk of breast cancer increase with both age and the length of hormone use (see Fig 1). Furthermore, this risk is greatest in women older than 60 years of age who have used hormones for 5 or more years. The relative risk of breast cancer was increased with estrogens alone, estrogen plus progestins, progestins alone, and estrogen plus testosterone. Although the latter 2 groups had the least person-years of follow-up, the relative risks were still high. La Vecchia et al. (Abstract 1–6) report generally similar findings but indicate in accompanying tables that the risk appears to decrease more than 10 years after cessation of HRT. Stanford et al. (Abstract 1–5) failed to identify the same risks in women taking both estrogen and progestins. However, they caution that greater follow-up is necessary. Both La Vecchia and Colditz identified higher risk when both drugs are taken. The discrepancies among the results of these 3 reports are probably the result of sample size differences and longer follow-up of the studies with larger numbers of patients.

Estrogens with or without progestins probably increase the risk of breast cancer in postmenopausal women. This risk must be balanced against any benefit in recommending HRT to postmenopausal women.

G.J. Bosl, M.D.

Prevalence of Human Papillomavirus in Cervical Cancer: A Worldwide Perspective
Bosch FX, Manos MM, Muñoz N, Sherman M, Jansen AM, Peto J, Schiffman MH, Moreno V, Kurman R, Shah KV, and the International Biological Study on Cervical Cancer (IBSCC) Study Group (Institut Catala d'Oncologia, Barcelona; Johns Hopkins Univ, Baltimore, Md; Internatl Agency for Research on Cancer, Lyon, France; et al)
J Natl Cancer Inst 87:796–802, 1995   1–7

Background.—Cervical cancer is the second most common cancer among women in all countries. International studies have shown that human papillomavirus (HPV) is strongly associated with cervical neoplasia. There are 35 known distinct HPV types, of which at least 20 are associated with cervical cancer. The worldwide consistency of the association between HPV types and cervical cancer was investigated.

Methods.—Stained histologic slides and biopsy specimens were obtained from 1,050 patients with invasive cervical cancer treated at 32 hospitals in 22 countries. The histologic slides were reviewed to determine the histologic type and grade of differentiation for each case. Samples of DNA were prepared from the biopsy specimens and analyzed by polymerase chain reaction (PCR), using 26 probes for specific types of HPV.

Results.—Human papillomavirus was detected in 92.9% of the specimens tested with PCR amplification. The prevalence of HPV ranged from 75% to 100% in the various countries. Twenty types of HPV were detected, and 36 specimens had 2 types of HPV. The most common type was HPV 16, occurring in 51.5% of the HPV-positive patients. Of the viruses detected, 66.5% were of the HPV 16 phylogenetic group (HPV 16, 31, 33, 35, 52, and 58) and 27.3% were of the HPV 18 phylogenetic group (HPV 18, 39, 45, 59, and 68). Human papillomavirus 16 or HPV 16–related viruses were most common in squamous cell tumors, whereas HPV 18 and HPV 18–related viruses were most common in adenocarcinomas and in adenosquamous carcinomas. Tumors associated with HPV 18 and its related viruses tended to have less differentiation than tumors associated with HPV 16 and its related viruses.

There was some geographic variance in HPV type prevalences. Human papillomavirus 16 was most common everywhere except in Indonesia, where HPV 18 was most common, even in patients with squamous cell tumors. There was an increased prevalence of HPV 45 in Mali and Guinea. Central and South American women had most of the HPV 39 and HPV 59 infections, and all 3 of the novel type W13B were found in specimens from the Philippines.

Conclusion.—Most cases of cervical cancer cases worldwide are associated with HPV infection. Therefore, HPV is the major risk factor for the development of invasive cervical lesions. The etiologic patterns for squamous cell tumors, adenocarcinomas, and adenosquamous carcinomas were consistent, even though HPV type-specific prevalences varied geographically. The existence of at least 20 HPV types associated with cancer presents complexities for diagnosis, management, and vaccine development.

▶ The association between infection with HPV and an increased risk for cervical cancer has long been known. This new report puts the problem in a global perspective. Of the 500,000 new cases of invasive cervical cancer worldwide, more than 90% are associated with HPV infection. The HPV 16– and HPV 18–related groups of virus accounted for the vast majority of virus-associated cancers; however, more than 20 different HPV types were found to be associated with cervical cancer. This finding has major implications in the search for a cervical cancer vaccine for this common sexually transmitted agent. That cervical cancer is the most common cancer in the developing world further complicates the global effort to decrease mortality, because health care resources in these countries are severely limited.

R.F. Ozols, M.D., Ph.D.

A Prospective Study of Family History and the Risk of Colorectal Cancer

Fuchs CS, Giovannucci EL, Colditz GA, Hunter DJ, Speizer FE, Willett WC (Brigham and Women's Hosp, Boston; Dana-Farber Cancer Inst, Boston; Harvard School of Public Health, Boston)
N Engl J Med 331:1669–1674, 1994   1–8

Purpose.—Several retrospective studies have found that a family history of colorectal cancer is an important risk factor for the disease. However, the strength of this association is unclear, particularly as influenced by the characteristics of the individual at risk and of the affected family members. These issues were addressed using data from two large prospective cohorts.

Methods.—The analysis used data from 2 continuing studies: the Nurses' Health Study and the Health Professionals Follow-Up Study. The subjects were 32,085 men and 87,031 women with no previous colonoscopic or sigmoidoscopic examination. All provided information on first-degree relatives with colorectal cancer, as well as on diet and other risk factors. A diagnosis of colorectal cancer was made during follow-up in 315 women and 148 men.

Results.—Overall, 9.4% of the men and 10% of the women reported a history of colorectal cancer in a first-degree relative. The subjects with and without a positive family history did not differ significantly in patterns of dietary intake, body mass index, physical activity level, or smoking history (Table 1). For subjects with a family history vs. those without a family history, the age-adjusted relative risk of the disease was 1.72 (Fig 1). For subjects with two or more affected first-degree relatives, the relative risk rose to 2.75. The relative risk for subjects younger than 45 years of age who had a positive family history was 5.37; this risk decreased with increasing age.

TABLE 1.—Characteristics of the Study Participants According to the Presence or Absence of a Family History of Colorectal Cancer

Characteristic	Men (N = 32,085)		Women (N = 87,031)	
	No Family History (n = 29,078)	Family History (n = 3,007)	No Family History (n = 78,304)	Family History (n = 8,727)
Age (yr)	51.3	53.7	48.9	51.3
Body-mass index†	25.5	25.5	23.7	23.7
Total energy intake				
(kcal/day)	1967	1981	1638	1660
Alcohol intake (g/day)	12.4	12.1	6.9	7.0
Dietary intake				
Folate (µg/day)‡	457	463	364	365
Methionine (g/day)	2.1	2.1	1.9	1.9
Animal fat (g/day)	39.9	39.1	52.4	52.0
Dietary fiber (g/day)	21.9	22.5	16.8	16.9
Red meat (g/day)	75.5	75.3	209	210
Calcium (mg/day)‡	939	939	731	731
Vitamin D (IU/day)‡	392	393	290	291
Regular aspirin use				
(% of participants)§	28.3	25.6	23.5	25.4
Screening endoscopy				
(% of participants)	20.2	34.1	4.5	12.8
Physical activity (met/day)¶	19.7	19.7	24.8	25.0
History of smoking	48.0	47.5	56.2	55.3
(% of participants)				

Note: Values for men and women are means directly standardized according to the age distribution of the respective cohort in its entirety. Dietary values represent the mean energy-adjusted intake for men and women.

† The weight in kilograms divided by the square of the height in meters.

‡ Includes the use of supplements.

§ Two or more days per week.

¶ Measured in metabolic equivalents (met).

(Reprinted by permission of *The New England Journal of Medicine*, Fuchs CS, Giovannucci EL, Colditz GA, et al: A prospective study of family history and the risk of colorectal cancer. 331:1669–1674, Copyright 1994, Massachusetts Medical Society.)

Conclusions.—Individuals with a family history of colorectal cancer are at increased risk of the disease. The increased risk is greatest in younger people and decreases with age. The findings support the American Cancer Society recommendation that younger people with a family history of colorectal cancer should receive earlier screening.

▶ Factors that may predict a higher frequency or an earlier onset of a common malignancy, such as colorectal cancer, are crucial because treatment for advanced and metastatic disease is poor and does not result in cure. Furthermore, earlier detection of disease may reduce the stage at which disease is found, thereby improving the results of surgery and adjuvant chemotherapy, if indicated. This study by Fuchs et al. was a prospective study of more than 32,000 men and 87,000 women who had not previously been examined by colonoscopy or sigmoidoscopy. Each had provided information regarding a family history of colorectal cancer. The preponderance of women in this study is the result of an analysis of data from the ongoing Nurses' Health Study, which began in 1976 and includes more than 121,000 women who were registered nurses between the ages of 30 and 55 years

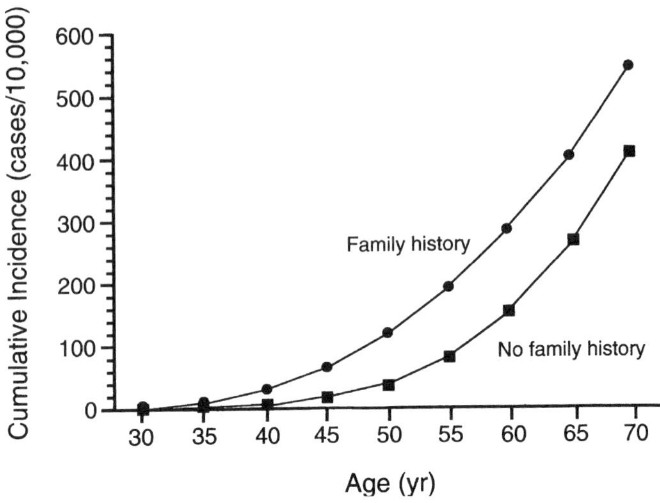

FIGURE 1.—Cumulative incidence of colorectal cancer according to age and the presence or absence of a family history of the disease. (Reprinted by permission of *The New England Journal of Medicine*, Fuchs CS, Giovannucci EL, Colditz GA, et al: A prospective study of family history and the risk of colorectal cancer. 331:1669–1674, Copyright 1994, Massachusetts Medical Society.)

and who completed a questionnaire regarding known or suspected risk factors for cancer.

Age, body mass index, total energy, alcohol and dietary intake, regular aspirin use, screening endoscopy, physical activity, and smoking history were analyzed according to the presence or absence of family history (see Table 1). Approximately 10% of the cohort reported a history of colorectal cancer in a first-degree relative. A family history of colorectal cancer was associated with a higher risk of colorectal cancer in a first-degree relative (see Fig 1). The age-adjusted relative risk was 1.72, with 95% confidence limits of 1.35 and 2.19. With two or more affected first-degree relatives, the relative risk was 2.75; for participants under the age of 45 who had one or more affected first-degree relatives, the relative risk was 5.37 (see Table 4 in the original article). Therefore, a family history of colorectal cancer in a first-degree relative was associated with a higher risk of colorectal cancer in all age groups, but especially among those of younger age.

G.J. Bosl, M.D.

Family History of Cancer, Body Weight, and p53 Nuclear Overexpression in Duke's C Colorectal Cancer

Zhang Z-F, Zeng Z-S, Sarkis AS, Klimstra DS, Charytonowicz E, Pollack D, Vena J, Guillem J, Marshall JR, Cordon-Cardo C, Cohen AM, Begg CB (Mem Sloan-Kettering Cancer Ctr, New York; State Univ of New York, Buffalo)
Br J Cancer 71:888–893, 1995   1–9

Background.—Colorectal cancer is the second most common malignancy of both sexes in developed countries, with an estimated 394,000 deaths occurring annually as a result of this disease. Because colorectal carcinomas with and without *TP53* mutations may be characterized by etiologic heterogeneity, a group of patients with primary Dukes' C colorectal cancers was studied. Specifically, associations between *p53* nuclear overexpression and risk factors including family history of cancer, body weight, occupational physical activity, smoking, drinking, and parity were investigated.

Patients and Methods.—The medical records of 107 consecutive patients seen at the Memorial Sloan-Kettering Cancer Center between 1986 and 1990 were evaluated. Thirty-four percent of the patients were less than 60 years of age, 35% were between 60 and 69 years, and 31% were aged 70 years or older. There were 48 females and 59 males. The overexpression of *p53* was assessed using the monoclonal antibody PAb 1801.

Results.—A *p53*-positive phenotype, defined as equal to or greater than 25% positive cells, was observed in 42 patients. Fifty-four of 107 patients had 1 or more relatives with cancer, 49 had 1 or more first-degree family members with cancer, and 21 had at least 2 first-degree relatives with cancer. An odds ratio of 2.9 for *p53* overexpression was noted in those patients with 2 or more first-degree relatives with cancer, compared with patients without a family history of cancer. A potential correlation between body weight and *p53* overexpression was observed, with an odds ratio of 3.4 for *p53* overexpression noted in patients at the highest quartile, compared with those at the lowest quartile. No significant association between height and *p53* overexpression was found. Additionally, associations between *p53* overexpression and smoking, drinking, occupational physical activity, and parity were not observed.

Conclusion.—The overexpression of *p53* may be related to a genetic predisposition of colorectal cancer, with possibly different etiologic pathways controlling *p53*-positive and *p53*-negative colorectal cancers.

▶ The literature is becoming filled with studies of the association of *p53* mutations and the occurrence or aggressiveness of a particular cancer. These types of studies are likely to grow as more tumor suppressor genes are discovered. The gist of this particular study is that patients with a strong family history of cancer were more likely to overexpress *p53* than were those without a family history of cancer.

Because the reader is likely to see many more studies of this type, I include with this article a cautionary note that is emphasized by the authors in their discussion. This warning has to do with the technique used for identifying *p53* overaccumulation, usually an immunohistochemical method. The specificity of the technique is open to some question. Furthermore, an arbitrary cutoff point must be used, as in many tests, to establish the line between a positive reading and a negative reading. In this study, the cutoff was equal to there being greater than 25% positive cells. These are the kind of data, therefore, that one may hold in abeyance until stronger and more definitive technology and associations are developed. Nonetheless, the prospect of an emerging genetic profile of each cancer is exciting for those who are interested in prevention, early detection, or novel treatment approaches.

J.V. Simone, M.D.

Aspirin and the Risk of Colorectal Cancer in Women
Giovannucci E, Egan KM, Hunter DJ, Stampfer MJ, Colditz GA, Willett WC, Speizer FE (Harvard Med School, Boston; Harvard School of Public Health, Boston)
N Engl J Med 333:609–614, 1995   1–10

Introduction.—Research on the effect of aspirin use on the risk of colorectal cancer has been inconsistent. The purpose of this study was to establish a correlation between colon and rectal cancers and aspirin use.

Methods.—Almost 90,000 women in the Nurses' Health Study, who had no diagnosis or family history of colorectal cancer, completed a baseline questionnaire on use of medication and diet. This was followed up every 2 years with another questionnaire on use of aspirin and other nonsteroidal anti-inflammatory drugs. Cases of adenomatous polyps of both participants, and their next of kin, were documented. The association between aspirin use and occurrence of a new colon or rectal cancer over 12 years was then analyzed.

Results.—During the 8 years of this study, 331 cases of not previously reported colorectal cancer were documented among women in the Nurses' Health Study. Individuals who in the initial questionnaire reported themselves as being regular aspirin users (those who took at least 2 aspirins per week) for a 4-year period had a lower risk of cancer developing than did nonusers. A reduction in risk was observed for women who had used aspirin regularly for at least 10 years, and this decrease became significant at 20 years of regular aspirin use. After controlling for other risk factors, women who, on 3 consecutive questionnaires (which were filled out every 2 years), reported regular aspirin use, were 38% less likely to have colorectal cancer develop. A significant inverse relationship was shown between the intake of 4–6 aspirins per week and the risk of development of colorectal cancer (Fig 1). These results are even more impressive because, over the course of the study, women who did take aspirin had a higher rate of endoscopy.

Discussion.—The results show that long-term use of aspirin (10 years or more) at a rate of 4–6 tablets per week results in decreases in the risk of colorectal cancer in women. Endoscopy, which could lead to a possibly earlier detection of tumors, actually showed a decrease in the actual number of colorectal tumors among aspirin users. The possible mechanisms for the action of aspirin in this instance include the inhibition of cyclooxygenase and subsequent inhibition of prostaglandin action, or the inhibition of phospholipase activity. It has also been documented that aspirin can modulate prostaglandin levels in the rectal epithelium. This

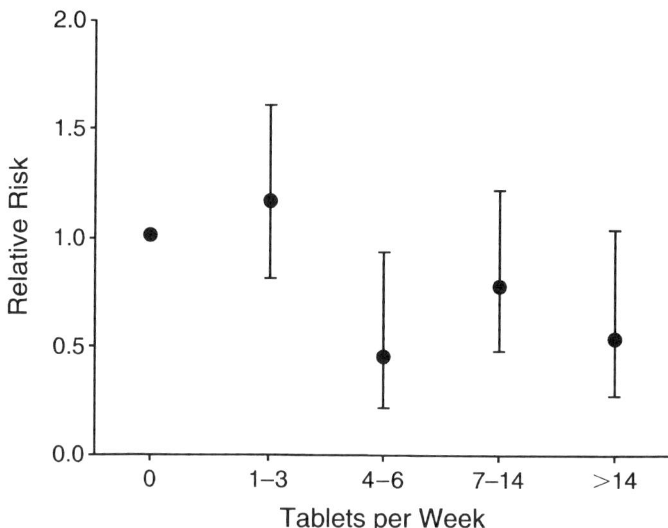

FIGURE 1.—Multivariate relative risks of colorectal cancer and 95% confidence intervals according to the level of aspirin use among women who used aspirin from 1980 through 1984 compared with nonusers. Relative risks were adjusted for age, family history of colorectal cancer, pack-years of smoking more than 35 years in the past, body mass index, physical activity index, physical activity level, and dietary intake of animal fat, dietary fiber, folate, methionine, alcohol, red meat, vitamin D, and calcium in 1980. (Reprinted by permission of *The New England Journal of Medicine*, Giovannucci E, Egan KM, Hunter DJ, et al: Aspirin and the risk of colorectal cancer in women. 333:609–614, 1995. Copyright 1995, Massachusetts Medical Society.)

work requires further research, especially because low-dose aspirin has been shown to decrease the incidence of cardiovascular disease.

Aspirin and Reduced Risk of Esophageal Carcinoma

Funkhouser EM, Sharp GB (Univ of Alabama, Birmingham; St Jude Children's Research Hosp, Memphis, Tenn)
Cancer 76:1116–1119, 1995
1–11

Introduction.—Aspirin and other nonsteroidal anti-inflammatory agents have been shown to suppress synthesis of prostaglandin and inhibit the growth of various tumors, including chemically induced esophageal cancers. A study of more than 600,000 American adults, followed for 6 years, indicated that aspirin use relates to a lower risk of dying of esophageal cancer.

Objective.—The association, if any, between aspirin use and esophageal cancer was examined by reviewing data from the National Health and Nutrition Examination Survey and the National Epidemiologic Follow-Up Studies. Of 14,407 individuals 25–74 years of age in the initial cohort, 13,300 with no history of cancer at baseline were followed for 12–16 years.

Findings.—Esophageal cancer developed in 15 persons. The occasional use of aspirin was associated with a 90% reduction in the risk of esophageal cancer developing. None of the patients was a regular aspirin user. The negative association between aspirin use and esophageal cancer persisted after adjusting for cigarette smoking ever vs. never and alcohol use (at least monthly vs. none).

Conclusion.—The regular, and even occasional, use of aspirin correlates with a substantial reduction in the risk of esophageal cancer. If confirmed, it might be feasible to use aspirin to prevent this cancer in high-risk groups such as individuals who have Barrett's syndrome.

▶ These are important epidemiologic studies in the assessment of the potential impact of regular aspirin use as a preventive agent in gastrointestinal cancer. Prior studies have not been conclusive. The benefits in the colorectal study (Abstract 1–10) required 20 years of regular aspirin use to reach statistical significance at a risk reduction of 44%. There was a risk reduction of 35% after 10 years. This did not reach statistical significance.

The esophageal study (Abstract 1–11) suggests a 90% decreased risk, which, so far, is the greatest effect seen at any site. The authors evaluated cigarette smoking and alcohol use in their analysis. These data provide additional information as to the value of nonsteroidal anti-inflammatory agents (NSAIDs) as preventative agents and demonstrate the need for further studies of the molecular basis of such growth inhibition. The very large cohort study in women (Abstract 1–10) provides additional data with regard to the role of NSAIDs as a chemopreventive agent, and it also provides additional encouragement for laboratory studies to better define the mechanism and to develop more specific chemopreventive agents that are involved in the prostaglandin pathway.

A.M. Cohen, M.D.

Adenocarcinoma of the Esophagus: Role of Obesity and Diet
Brown LM, Swanson CA, Gridley G, Swanson GM, Schoenberg JB, Greenberg RS, Silverman DT, Pottern LM, Hayes RB, Schwartz AG, Liff JM, Fraumeni JF Jr, Hoover RN (Natl Cancer Inst, Bethesda, Md; Michigan State Univ, East Lansing; New Jersey State Dept of Health, Trenton; et al)
J Natl Cancer Inst 87:104–109, 1995   1–12

Introduction.—The past two decades have seen a rapidly increasing incidence of esophageal adenocarcinoma, including that of the esophagogastric junction, in the United States. Aside from their association with Barrett's esophagus, there is little information on the causes of these tumors. The dietary and nutritional risk factors for adenocarcinoma of the esophagus were examined in a population-based, case-control study.

Methods.—The case patients were 174 white men (median age, 63 years) with adenocarcinoma of the esophagus, and there were 750 control subjects (median age, 61 years) living in 3 areas of the United States.

TABLE 1.—Odds Ratios (ORs) for Adenocarcinomas of the Esophagus and Esophagogastric Junction in White Men, According to Dietary Factors

Factor	No. of case patients	No. of control subjects	OR*	95% CI
BMI, kg/m²†				
<23.1	24	172	1.0	—
23.1–25.0	31	170	1.1	0.6–2.1
25.1–26.6	27	169	1.2	0.6–2.3
>26.6	79	171	3.1¶	1.8–5.3
Unknown	1	3		
Total calories from food‡				
<1397	28	171	1.0	—
1397–1769	39	171	1.3	0.7–2.3
1770–2136	34	172	1.0	0.6–1.8
≥2137	61	171	1.5	0.8–2.6
No. of meals/day§				
≥3	109	451	1.0	—
<3	53	234	0.9	0.6–1.4

* All estimates were adjusted for age, area, smoking, liquor use, and income.
† Estimates were adjusted for calories from food.
‡ Excludes calories from alcohol; estimates were adjusted for body mass index.
§ Estimates were adjusted for calories from food and body mass index.
¶ $P < .001$.
(Courtesy of Brown LM, Swanson CA, Gridley G, et al: Adenocarcinoma of the esophagus: Role of obesity and diet. *J Natl Cancer Inst* 87:104–109, 1995.)

In-person interviews, conducted from 1986 through 1989, were held to gather detailed data on medical and dental history, alcohol and tobacco use, usual occupation, sociodemographic factors, and usual adult diet.

Results.—Subjects in the heaviest quartile of body mass index were at significantly increased risk compared with those in the lightest quartile, for an odds ratio of 3.1 (Table 1). Total calories from food, the number of meals per day, the fat intake level, and coffee or tea consumption were not significantly associated with esophageal adenocarcinoma. Subjects who ate the least amount of vegetables were at greatest risk, and there was evidence of a dose response for cruciferous vegetables and raw vegetables. Subjects eating the least amount of raw fruit were also at significantly increased risk. Increasing dietary fiber intake had a significant protective effect. There were no apparent associations for intake of particular micronutrients, either overall or in supplements.

Conclusions.—Risk of adenocarcinoma of the esophagus appears to be influenced by obesity and diet. Risk increases with obesity and decreases with intake of raw fruits and vegetables and dietary fiber. The noted associations will be useful in directing further studies of this form of cancer. The link with obesity may help to explain the recent epidemic increases in the incidence of esophageal adenocarcinoma.

▶ Adenocarcinoma of the esophagus and the esophagogastric junction has been increasing in the United States during the past several years. Barrett's esophagus is a recognized precursor of adenocarcinoma of the esophagus, but it is the only known predisposing factor to the disease. Tobacco use predisposes to squamous cell carcinoma of the esophagus and was recently identified as a risk factor for adenocarcinoma as well. In this article, the authors report the results of a study of the impact of diet and weight on the incidence of esophageal adenocarcinoma. This case-controlled, population-based study examined 4 geographical areas and considered only male cases; the number of female cases would have been too few to analyze as a result of the higher incidence of adenocarcinoma of the esophagus in men compared with women. The observed odds ratio for the highest quartile of body weight showed a significantly increased risk of adenocarcinoma of the esophagus when compared with lower quartiles (see Table 1). There was no consistent pattern of increased risk among different food groups. Risk appeared to be reduced in subjects with the highest fiber, fruit, and vegetable intake when compared with those with lower intake.

The recent increase in the incidence of adenocarcinoma of the esophagus may be partly related to dietary habits leading to obesity. Vitamin supplements did not appear to alter the risk of this fatal disease developing. Thus, adenocarcinoma of the esophagus is another malignancy that is influenced by tobacco and diet.

G.J. Bosl, M.D.

Incidence of Human Immunodeficiency Virus–Related and Nonrelated Malignancies in a Large Cohort of Homosexual Men

Lyter DW, Bryant J, Thackeray R, Rinaldo CR, Kingsley LA (Univ of Pittsburgh, Pa; Pittsburgh Cancer Inst, Pa; the Multicenter AIDS Cohort Study)
J Clin Oncol 13:2540–2546, 1995   1–13

Objective.—The frequency of malignant conditions other than Kaposi's sarcoma (KS) and non-Hodgkin's lymphoma (NHL) was examined in 1,199 homosexual men living in Pittsburgh who were part of the Multicenter AIDS Cohort Study of the natural course of HIV infection.

Study Population.—There were 769 HIV-seronegative (SN) and 430 seropositive (SP) individuals in the study group. Person-years of follow-up totalled 5,708 for the SN group and 2,344 for the SP group. The overall average patient age at entry was 32.5 years. More than 90% of the study group were white men.

Findings.—There were 59 AIDS-defining malignancies (e.g., KS, NHL, and CNS lymphoma) in the SP group. The incidence of nonmelanoma skin cancer was not higher than expected in the SP group. All other malignancies combined were 3.4 times more frequent than predicted in the SP men. The increase was significant compared with both the SN cohort and the general population. Two SP men had testicular cancer, 1 had an extragonadal seminoma, and 2 had Hodgkin's disease.

Conclusion.—Both Hodgkin's disease and seminoma, tumors that are common in young men in general, are especially likely to be found in HIV-infected men.

▶ The association of HIV and malignancy is well known. Kaposi's sarcoma, NHL, and CNS lymphoma are well-recognized entities. Scattered reports have suggested that other malignancies are of higher incidence. This study addresses this issue in a large cohort of patients at risk for HIV-related cancers. Hodgkin's disease, germ cell tumors, anal squamous cell carcinoma, and cutaneous basal cell carcinoma were observed, but their frequency compared with that in the general population was not statistically increased; the confidence limits, however, were quite wide. When all malignancies except KS, lymphoma, and nonmelanoma skin malignancies were added together, there was a statistically significant increase in the rate of incidence. Which of these malignancies might be specifically associated with HIV is not clear.

Malignancies other than NHL may be seen in immunocompromised patients with HIV. Although further study is needed, the wide impact of HIV on health continues to evolve, and the appearance of malignancies other than KS and lymphoma should be considered in the management of these patients.

G.J. Bosl, M.D.

Association of Epstein–Barr Virus With Leiomyosarcomas in Young People With AIDS

McClain KL, Leach CT, Jenson HB, Joshi VV, Pollock BH, Parmley RT, DiCarlo FJ, Chadwick EG, Murphy SB (Baylor College of Medicine, Houston; Univ of Texas, San Antonio; East Carolina Univ, Greenville, NC; et al)
N Engl J Med 332:12–18, 1995   1–14

Introduction.—Children with AIDS have a high incidence of leiomyomas and leiomyosarcomas, tumors that otherwise are rarely seen in children. It has been suggested that the Epstein-Barr virus (EBV) may be involved in the development of spindle-cell sarcomas in liver transplant recipients, and it has been hypothesized that EBV may also be involved in the development of soft-tissue tumors in AIDS patients.

Methods.—Tumor samples were obtained from 6 patients with AIDS and leiomyoma and/or leiomyosarcoma, and from 7 HIV-negative children with either leiomyoma or leiomyosarcoma (Table 1). Tumor cells were analyzed with in situ hybridization and polymerase chain reaction (PCR) to test for the presence of HIV and EBV. The clonality of EBV was determined with Southern blot analysis. Immunostaining determined the presence of EBV receptors. Serologic testing was done to detect anti-EBV antibodies.

Results.—Light microscopy and immunostaining confirmed findings consistent with the smooth muscle origin of the tumor cells. All 4 of the plasma samples (from 1 HIV-negative and 3 HIV-positive patients) confirmed past EBV infection. In situ hybridization evidenced no intracellular HIV infection. Whereas EBV infection was present in all tumor cells in patients with AIDS. No normal smooth muscle cells or tumor cells in

TABLE 1.—Clinical Data on the Patients With Smooth-Muscle Tumors

Patient No.	Race or Ethnic Group	Age (yr) at Tumor Diagnosis/Sex	Tumor Site	Tumor Type	Age (yr) at Diagnosis of AIDS	Route of HIV Transmission	CD4 + Count (cells/mm^3) at Tumor Diagnosis
HIV-positive							
1	Hispanic	8/F	Lung	Leiomyosarcoma	4	Perinatal transfusion	3
			Colon	Leiomyoma			
2	Hispanic	4/F	Stomach	Leiomyosarcoma	2	Perinatal	43
3	Black	7/F	Intestine	Leiomyosarcoma	2	Perinatal	9
4	Hispanic	24/M	Liver	Leiomyosarcoma	18	Transfusion	20
5	White	5/F	Colon	Leiomyosarcoma	1	Perinatal	330
6	Black	4/M	Lung	Leiomyoma	4	Perinatal transfusion	6
HIV-negative							
7	Black	7/M	Rectum	Leiomyosarcoma	—	—	—
8	White	14/F	Stomach	Leiomyosarcoma	—	—	—
9	White	8/F	Labia majora	Leiomyosarcoma	—	—	—
10	White	12/F	Stomach	Leiomyoma	—	—	—
11	Hispanic	5/M	Ear	Leiomyoma	—	—	—
12	White	3/F	Ileocecum	Leiomyoma	—	—	—
13	White	3/M	Finger	Leiomyoma	—	—	—

(Reprinted by permission of *The New England Journal of Medicine,* McClain KL, Leach CT, Jenson HB, et al: Association of Epstein-Barr virus with leiomyosarcomas in young people with AIDS. *N Engl J Med* 332:12–18, Copyright 1995, Massachusetts Medical Society.)

HIV-negative patients showed the presence of EBV. Quantitative PCR found extremely high levels of EBV in the tumor samples of patients with AIDS. Clonality EBV could only be assessed in 2 patients, and the results were consistent with separate EBV infection or mixed monoclonal infections. The tissue sections from all of the patients demonstrated strong immunostaining for the EBV receptor.

Discussion.—These findings support the hypothesized causal association between EBV and the development of soft-tissue tumors in patients with AIDS. This suggests that EBV may play an etiologic role in the development of other smooth muscle tumors in patients with immunosuppression from other causes.

▶ This is an extremely important paper from a variety of vantage points. By demonstrating the strong association of EBV with leiomyosarcomas that develop in young people with AIDS, it leads one to the unavoidable conclusion that the virus has a role in causing the tumor. The Epstein-Barr virus has long been associated with a variety of tumors, most especially Burkitt's lymphoma and nasopharyngeal carcinoma.

It is instructive to review the sequence of events in these 6 patients, because it gives an indication of the time frame for the development of cancer of this type. Five of the 6 patients were exposed to HIV in the perinatal period, and all 6 received a diagnosis of AIDS within a few years following exposure. The tumor appeared 2–6 years after the diagnosis of AIDS in 5 of the patients and in the same year in 1 patient. One assumes that the immunosuppression created a favorable environment for EBV to participate in the carcinogenesis; it would appear that the latent period for these types of tumors in young people is relatively short.

Many of us have always believed that the investigation of carcinogenesis in children was a more favorable scientific approach because one expected a relatively short latency period since conception is the irreducible starting point. Although scientifically this observation is most interesting, it presents another worry in the already troubled and uncertain management of children with AIDS.

J.V. Simone, M.D.

The Association of Epstein–Barr Virus With Smooth-Muscle Tumors Occurring After Organ Transplantation
Lee ES, Locker J, Nalesnik M, Reyes J, Jaffe R, Alashari M, Nour B, Tzakis A, Dickman PS (Univ of Pittsburgh Med Ctr, Pa; Children's Hosp of Pittsburgh, Pa)
N Engl J Med 332:19–25, 1995   1–15

Introduction.—Immunodeficient patients, regardless of the cause of immunodeficiency, have an increased incidence of neoplastic disorders, including smooth muscle tumors. The clonal Epstein-Barr virus (EBV) genome has been isolated from lymphoproliferative tumors in many immunodeficient patients. The possibility of a causal role for EBV was explored in 3 pediatric organ transplant recipients who had smooth muscle tumors develop while receiving immunosuppressive drugs.

Methods.—Tissue was examined with light and electron microscopy from the lesions in 3 liver transplant recipients, aged 2.75 to 6.75 years at discovery of tumors. The masses were found in the left lobe of the liver in one patient who survived, in the lung, liver, retroperitoneum, stomach, and colon in one child who died, and in the anterior mediastinal and paravertebral lymph nodes, lung, and stomach of one child who died. Tissue sections were also analyzed immunohistochemically, with in situ hybridization for EBV *EBER,* a region of the EBV genome transcribed in latently infected cells, and with molecular genetic analysis.

Results.—Light microscopy revealed spindle cells with eosinophilic cytoplasm and long, blunt-ended nuclei in all of the tumors. Electron microscopy showed smooth muscle cell features. Cytoplasmic immunostaining was positive for vimentin, muscle-specific actin, and focal desmin, and was negative for EBV latent membrane protein and CD21. However, half of the tumor cells, but none of the parenchymal and stromal cells, stained for EBV nuclear antigen 2 (EBNA-2). In situ hybridization revealed that the nuclei of most tumor cells, but not of adjacent parenchymal and stromal cells, were strongly positive for *EBER.* All tumor tissue contained clonal EBV DNA.

Discussion.—The single form of EBV DNA with unique episomal bands that were found in each tumor suggests that the neoplasia developed from a single preexistent clone of cells. The expression of EBNA-2 is typically found only in lymphoproliferative tumors that occur after transplantation, suggesting that these tumors arise in response to immunosuppression. Expression of both EBNA-2 and *EBER* is associated with latent EBV infection. These findings strongly suggest a causal association between EBV and the post-transplant development of smooth muscle tumors.

▶ This paper, which followed the one by McClain et al. (Abstract 1–14) in *The New England Journal of Medicine,* provides another strong line of evidence that EBV either causes or participates in the causation of smooth muscle tumors in patients with immunosuppression. All 3 patients were young children, as were all but 1 of the subjects in Abstract 1–14. One wonders whether young children are particularly susceptible to oncogenesis by EBV and, if they are, why?

Many pediatric oncologists strongly believe that viruses play a far more important role in causing childhood cancers than we have been able to prove scientifically. I suspect that this is not the last we will hear of viruses associated with pediatric cancers.

J.V. Simone, M.D.

Childhood Cancer and Paternal Exposure to Ionizing Radiation: A Second Report From the Oxford Survey of Childhood Cancers
Sorahan T, Lancashire RJ, Temperton DH, Heighway WP (Univ of Birmingham, England; Queen Elizabeth Med Ctr, Birmingham, England)
Am J Ind Med 28:71–78, 1995   1–16

Background.—Several studies have been done on the association between paternal occupational exposure to ionizing radiation and cancer in their offspring. However, the results are difficult to interpret. It was hypothesized that if paternal preconception irradiation is an important risk factor for childhood cancers, then the risks associated with preconception work in certain occupations would be increased, whereas those associated with postconception work would not.

Methods.—Data on paternal occupation collected in the Oxford Survey of Childhood Cancers in England, Wales, and Scotland were analyzed. Job information was available both for the fathers of 14,869 children dying of cancer between 1953 and 1981 and for matched control subjects. The preconception occupations that were assessed were clinical radiology, surgery and anesthesiology, veterinary surgery, dental surgery, work in the nuclear industry, and industrial radiography.

Findings.—When compared with postconception employment, preconception employment in any of the occupations studied did not appear to be associated with greater risks of any childhood cancers and any childhood leukemias. Neither paternal preconception exposure to external ionizing radiation nor exposure to unsealed radionuclide sources was an important risk factor for these diseases.

Conclusion.—Men employed in occupations associated with external ionizing radiation exposure before conception did not have offspring with greater childhood risks of cancer than did men employed in these occupations after conception.

▶ Over the past several years, we have reviewed several papers on the role of preconceptual paternal exposure to ionizing radiation in the etiology of childhood cancer. Most of these studies have been from England and Scandinavia and have resulted from a study done in 1990 that reported an increased risk of leukemia among children born to fathers exposed to high recorded doses of external ionizing radiation before conception. Many other studies have followed, and most, including this one, have come to the conclusion that there is no relationship between paternal exposure to ionizing radiation and childhood cancer.

As is true of many epidemiology studies, the best they can do is to provide inferential evidence, which is seldom absolutely convincing by itself. This is because of the difficulty in accounting for all potential factors, particularly in the causation of diseases for which the etiology is unknown. I must say that I have become satisfied that no current evidence convinces me that paternal exposure to external ionizing radiation before conception raises the incidence of childhood cancer in subsequent offspring.

J.V. Simone, M.D.

Influence of Tobacco Marketing and Exposure to Smokers on Adolescent Susceptibility to Smoking

Evans N, Farkas A, Gilpin E, Berry C, Pierce JP (Indiana Univ, Bloomington; Univ of California, San Diego, La Jolla)
J Natl Cancer Inst 87:1538–1545, 1995

Rationale.—Adolescents continue to take up smoking despite 3 decades of sustained educational efforts to discourage this habit. More than one fourth of those 17 and 18 years of age in the United States are presently smokers. The tobacco industry insists that they do not overtly encourage adolescents to try smoking. Instead, they argue that exposure to other smokers is what prompts adolescents to begin smoking.

Study Plan.—The comparative influence of advertising and promotional efforts on the one hand, and exposure to smokers on the other, was studied in a series of 3,536 adolescents 12–17 years of age who had never so much as taken a puff of a cigarette. Data were taken from the 1993 California Tobacco Survey. Those who stated that they would not rule out trying smoking soon or smoking a cigarette if offered one by a friend were considered to be susceptible. Receptivity to tobacco advertising was rated on a 5-point scale and exposure to family and peer smoking on a 4-level scale.

Findings.—One fourth of the adolescents were considered to be susceptible to smoking (Fig 1). More than 80% of those aged 12–13 years believed that tobacco ads promote at least 1 benefit of smoking (Fig 2). About 40% of adolescents of all ages could name a brand of cigarettes that

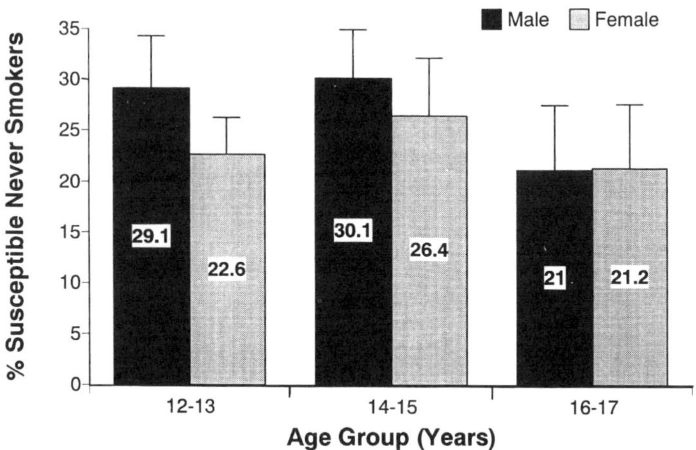

FIGURE 1.—Percentage of male and female adolescent never-smokers in California who were susceptible to beginning smoking, stratified by age group: 12–13 years (*n* = 1,500), 14–15 years (*n* = 1,167), and 16–17 years (*n* = 819). *Numbers in the bars* give weighted percents, and the upper limits of the 95% confidence intervals are shown. *Abbreviation:* CTS, California Tobacco Survey. (Courtesy of Evans N, Farkas A, Gilpin E, et al: Influence of tobacco marketing and exposure to smokers on adolescent susceptibility to smoking. *J Natl Cancer Inst* 87:1538–1545, 1995.)

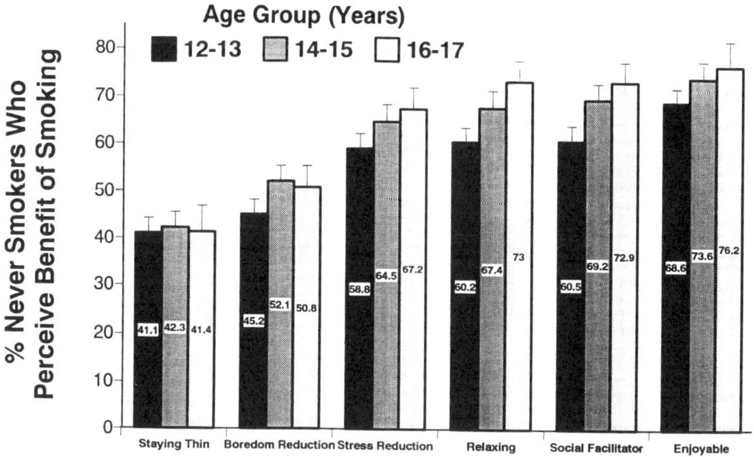

FIGURE 2.—Percentage of California adolescent never-smokers aged 12–13 years ($n = 1,550$), 14–15 years ($n = 1,167$), and 16–17 years ($n = 819$) who perceived a benefit of smoking as being promoted by cigarette advertisements by the 6 messages most frequently identified: staying thin, boredom reduction, stress reduction, relaxation, social facilitation, and enjoyment. *Numbers in the bars* are weighted percents, and the upper limits of the 95% confidence intervals are shown. *Abbreviation: CTS,* California Tobacco Survey. (Courtesy of Evans N, Farkas A, Gilpin E, et al: Influence of tobacco marketing and exposure to smokers on adolescent susceptibility to smoking. *J Natl Cancer Inst* 87:1538–1545, 1995.)

they would prefer purchasing. Both exposure to smokers and, more obviously, receptivity to tobacco advertising (Fig 4) were independently associated with susceptibility to smoking. Hispanic adolescents were relatively more likely to be susceptible, as were those who performed no better than average at school.

Implication.—The advertising and marketing of tobacco products strongly influence adolescents to try smoking.

▶ This is a fascinating and frightening study of a large number of California adolescents. It appears to me that more adolescents are smoking today than were 5 years ago. Although national statistics demonstrated a decrease in adolescent smoking from the mid-1970s to the mid-1980s and a leveling off thereafter, it is my view that data from the 1990s will ultimately show that smoking among adolescents has increased.

This study attempts to measure the effect of tobacco advertising on the likelihood that an adolescent will begin smoking. Because most smokers begin smoking during adolescence, this is an extremely important issue. Studies have consistently documented high awareness and recall of tobacco advertising among adolescents and even among young children. Also, adolescents are known to be highly adept at decoding cigarette advertisements, and an awareness of brand imagery and covert messages is already present in the preteen years. There are also data showing a high correlation between

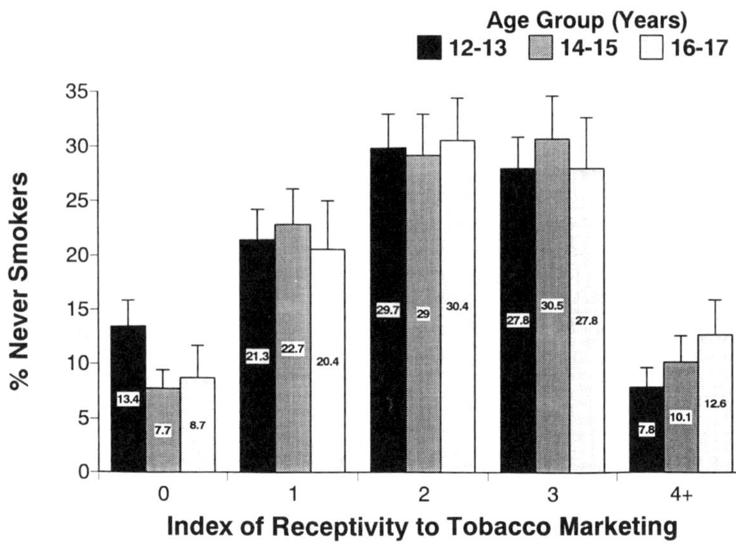

FIGURE 4.—Percentage of California adolescent never-smokers aged 12–13 years ($n = 1,550$), 14–15 years ($n = 1,167$), and 16–17 years ($n = 819$) according to their score of 0–4+ on the Index of Receptivity to Tobacco Marketing. *Numbers in the bars* are weighted percents, and the upper limits of the 95% confidence intervals are shown. *Abbreviation: CTS,* California Tobacco Survey. (Courtesy of Evans N, Farkas A, Gilpin E, et al: Influence of tobacco marketing and exposure to smokers on adolescent susceptibility to smoking. *J Natl Cancer Inst* 87:1538–1545, 1995.)

the timing of particular tobacco advertising campaigns and increases in the rates at which adolescents take up smoking.

This study provides substantial evidence that tobacco marketing may be a stronger influence in encouraging smoking among adolescents than exposure to either peer or family members who smoke. The cynical advertising campaigns of tobacco companies are a national disgrace. Not much better are the congressmen from tobacco states who protect tobacco companies for political gain, thereby retaining their jobs by standing on the graves of large numbers of fellow Americans.

J.V. Simone, M.D.

Residential Radon Exposure and Lung Cancer Among Nonsmoking Women

Alavanja MCR, Brownson RC, Lubin JH, Berger E, Chang J, Boice JD, Jr (Natl Cancer Inst, Bethesda, Md; Missouri Dept of Health, Columbia; Information Management Services, Rockville, Md)
J Natl Cancer Inst 86:1829–1837, 1994   1–18

Introduction.—Animal studies and epidemiologic studies of underground miners have established an association between high levels of radon exposure and an increase in lung cancer risk. However, the association between lung cancer and lower level residential radon exposure is more controversial. In a population-based case-control study, the radon-related risks in nonsmoking women were investigated.

Methods.—The subjects were 538 white women, aged 30–84 years, who were given a diagnosis of primary lung cancer over a 5-year period. The controls were age-matched white women who were randomly selected from the population files. All participants either had never smoked or had quit smoking at least 15 years earlier. All participants were interviewed by telephone to obtain information on demographic factors, occupational history, lifetime passive smoking, previous active smoking, previous nonmalignant lung disease, and diet. Measurements of year-long radon exposure were taken in current and past residences with alpha-track detectors. Tissue slides from 409 case patients were examined.

Results.—The two groups did not have significant demographic differences, but the case group had a higher proportion of former smokers and more previous nonmalignant lung disease, and ate more saturated fat than did the control group. The 2 groups had the same time-weighted average radon concentration exposures (Fig 1). Women exposed to the highest quintile of radon concentration had a 1.20 relative risk of lung cancer compared with women who were exposed to the lowest quintile of radon concentration (Table 3). However, there was no evidence of an exposure-response pattern, even when adjusting for other lung cancer risk factors, including age and smoking (Table 4, Fig 2). There was significant evidence

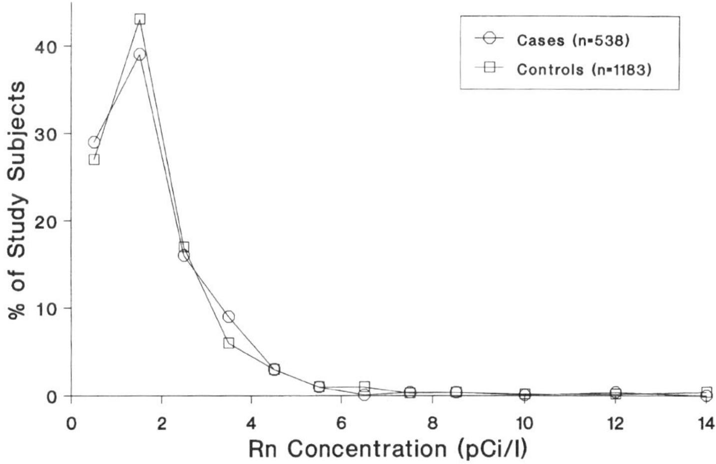

FIGURE 1.—Distribution of study subjects (and percent distribution) by time-weighted average residential radon concentrations for the 5- and 30-year period before study enrollment. Radon measurements were obtained for 78.4% of the relevant residential period. Missing radon concentrations were not imputed. (Courtesy of Alavanja MCR, Brownson RC, Lubin JH, et al: Residential radon exposure and lung cancer among nonsmoking women. *J Natl Cancer Inst* 86:1829–1837, 1994.)

TABLE 3.—Odds Ratio for Lung Cancer by Quintiles of Time-Weighted Average Residential Radon Concentration

| | TWA radon levels* | | | | | | P† | |
	I	II	III	IV	V	Total	Continuous	Categorical
Case patients	112	112	93	99	122	538		
Control subjects	233	242	233	252	223	1183		
Total	345	354	326	351	345	1721		
Mean pCi/L^{-1}	0.6	1.0	1.4	2.0	4.0			
OR‡	1.00	1.01	0.84	0.90	1.20		.99	.19
95% CI		0.7–1.4	0.6–1.2	0.6–1.3	0.9–1.7			
			ORs with additional adjustment					*Adjusted for age and*
	1.00	1.01	0.89	0.88	1.21		.98	.38 Previous smoker
	1.00	0.95	0.83	0.74	1.11		(−).70	.38 Pack-years
	1.00	0.95	0.84	0.77	1.11		(−).72	.38 Pack-years and years since smoking cessation
	1.00	1.03	0.89	0.91	1.21		(−).95	.19 Previous lung disease
	1.00	1.01	0.90	0.90	1.24		.95	.17 Passive smoking
	1.00	0.97	0.96	0.96	1.43		.30	.03 Amount saturated fat
	1.00	1.01	0.90	0.90	1.24		.92	.14 Education

* The quintile intervals are (I) .1–.79 pCi/L^{-1}, (II) .80–1.19 pCi/L^{-1}, (III) 1.20–1.69 pCi/L^{-1}, (IV) 1.70–2.45 pCi/L^{-1}, and (V) 2.46–15.3 pCi/L^{-1} and are based on the control distribution.

† *P* value for two-sided test of trend. *Columns Continuous* and *Categorical* denote *P* values based on trend test using the actual TWA radon concentrations for individuals (continuous variable) or the mean TWA value of each quintile as the quantitative variable. *Negative sign* denotes a decreasing trend with increasing level of exposure.

‡ Odds ratio adjusted for six categories of age at diagnosis of lung cancer for case patients and age at interview for control subjects.

Abbreviations: TWA, time-weighted average; *OR,* odds ratio.

(Courtesy of Alavanja MCR, Brownson RC, Lubin JH, et al: Residential radon exposure and lung cancer among nonsmoking women. *J Natl Cancer Inst* 86:1829–1837, 1994.)

TABLE 4.—Odds Ratio for All Lung Cancer by Quintiles of Time-Weighted Average (TWA) Residential Radon Concentration Within Categories of Age and Smoking Status

	TWA radon levels*					P†		No. of case patients/
	I	II	III	IV	V	Continuous	Categorical	control subjects
Age group, y								
<65	1.00	0.67	1.33	0.78	1.88	.24	.12	123/297
65–74	1.00	0.81	1.00	0.92	1.10	.95	.48	166/384
≥75	1.00	1.29	0.70	0.93	1.17	(−).56	.61	249/502
Smoking status								
Never smoked	1.00	1.13	0.90	0.91	1.20	(−).99	.38	377/983
Former smoker	1.00	0.80	0.88	0.90	1.32	.95	.24	161/200

* The quintile intervals are defined in Table 3 footnote. Odds ratios were adjusted for 6 categories of age at interview for control subjects or cancer diagnosis for case patients.

† *P* value for two-sided test of trend. *Columns Continuous* and *Categorical* are defined as in Table 3 footnote (†). *Negative sign* denotes a decreasing trend with increasing exposure level.

(Courtesy of Alavanja MCR, Brownson RC, Lubin JH, et al: Residential radon exposure and lung cancer among nonsmoking women. *J Natl Cancer Inst* 86:1829–1837, 1994.)

of a dose-response association between radon exposure and the risk of adenocarcinoma, but with no other histologic types.

Discussion.—These findings do not support an association between residential radon exposure and the risk of lung cancer.

▶ The subject of radon exposure in the home is a complicated one. The Environmental Protection Agency (EPA) has made a simple declaration of its dangers and classifies radon as the second leading cause of lung cancer. I do not agree with that, because I see little evidence of radon causing cancer in patients who do not smoke. The literature is very clear about the interaction of smoking and radon, but most of the data on which the radon risk depends rests on a population of uranium miners, most of whom smoked.

This particular study is the first one I have seen that pays close attention to the smoking habits of the population involved. The data presented in this

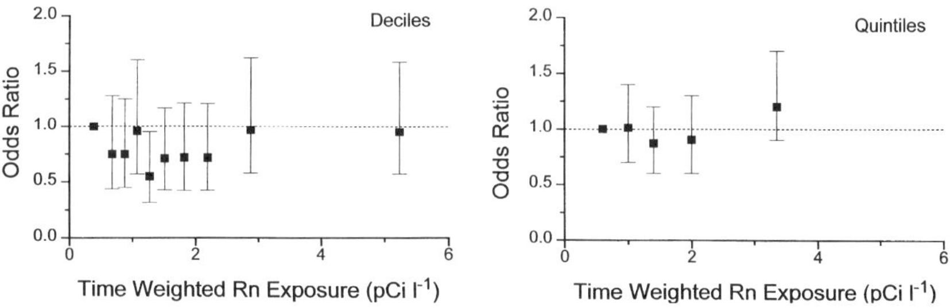

FIGURE 2.—Age-adjusted odds ratios for lung cancer by categories of time-weighted average (TWA) radon concentrations (pCi/L⁻¹). **Left panel** depicts the distribution of lung cancer risk according to deciles of TWA radon concentrations. **Right panel** depicts the distribution of lung cancer risk by quintiles of TWA radon concentrations. *Error bars* depict 95% confidence intervals on the point estimate of lung cancer risk. (Courtesy of Alavanja MCR, Brownson RC, Lubin JH, et al: Residential radon exposure and lung cancer among nonsmoking women. *J Natl Cancer Inst* 86:1829–1837, 1994.)

paper show very little in the way of a significant risk resulting from indoor radon. The quality of this particular study is the highest, I think, of any that have ever been done, and I think it should cause the EPA to look carefully at their own data and perhaps tone down the propaganda on radon. To the best of my knowledge, no one has ever identified a cancer in an individual patient as being radon-induced. In my own opinion, the people who are at real risk of radon exposure are those in the medical community who get exposed to significant amounts of radon, cumulatively over time, by inhalation. Technicians and young physicians-in-training who do a lot of research on radon are potentially at risk. What that true risk might be is still unclear.

In sum, I personally believe that radon is a risk, but not at the level that occurs in homes. The mammalian cell has a tremendous capacity for repair of radiation injury, and the cumulative exposure has to be able to saturate that capacity. This excellent paper calls into question a great deal of our presumptive thinking.

E. Glatstein, M.D.

Cancer Mortality in a Residential Cohort Exposed to Environmental Selenium Through Drinking Water

Vinceti M, Rovesti S, Gabrielli C, Marchesi C, Bergomi M, Martini M, Vivoli G (Univ of Modena, Italy; Local Health Unit of Reggio Emilia, Italy)
J Clin Epidemiol 48:1091–1097, 1995   1–19

Background.—Epidemiologic studies of the association between dietary intake of selenium and cancer in humans have yielded conflicting results. The findings of animal studies have also been inconsistent, with some suggesting a carcinogenic effect and some an anticarcinogenic effect. The cancer mortality rate was investigated in a cohort of residents exposed to environmental selenium through drinking water.

Methods.—A total of 4,419 residents of Reggio Emilia in northern Italy were studied. In this area, tap water with an unusually high selenium content was supplied by accident. Deaths from cancer between 1986 and 1992 were noted.

Findings.—Death rates from all cancers in male and female residents did not significantly differ from death rates in the rest of the population in that area. In males, there was no significant difference in mortality for site-specific cancers. Females had a greater mortality from malignancies of the lymphatic-hematopoietic tissue overall and from non-Hodgkin's lymphoma.

Conclusions.—These findings do not support the hypothesis that a selenium supplement greatly benefits cancer mortality in humans. A longer follow-up is needed to determine whether natural selenium supplementation has a slight beneficial effect on cancer death rates.

▶ Fad therapies are often the bane of an oncologist's practice. Shark cartilage is a recent fad, whereas Laetrile was debunked many years ago. Selenium supplements have been touted as an antineoplastic and antimetastatic agent. By chance, selenium levels were absent from all but 2 sources of drinking water in a specific municipality in Italy. The regions with selenium supplementation from the water supply showed no significant difference from the expected mortality for site-specific cancers or mortality from all cancers. If anything, women with hematopoietic malignancies and non-Hodgkin's lymphomas had a slightly higher death rate, not a lower death rate. This study provides evidence that selenium supplements are not useful, and it should be used by the treating physician as a reference when patients inquire about the value of selenium supplements.

G.J. Bosl, M.D.

Childhood Leukaemia and Non-Hodgkin's Lymphoma Near Large Rural Construction Sites, With a Comparison With Sellafield Nuclear Site

Kinlen LJ, Dickson M, Stiller CA (Univ of Oxford, England)
BMJ 310:763–768, 1995   1–20

Introduction.—An increased incidence of childhood leukemia and non-Hodgkin's lymphoma has been seen when large-scale mixing of rural and urban populations occurs (as in large rural construction projects), suggesting an infective cause. The incidence of childhood leukemia and non-Hodgkin's lymphoma in rural British areas near nonnuclear construction projects was studied.

Methods.—The nonnuclear construction projects selected for study were built after 1945, were located in a rural district more than 20 km from a large town, involved more than 1,000 workers, and took at least 3 years to build. National registry data were used to calculate the incidence of childhood leukemia and non-Hodgkin's lymphoma in the study areas during 3 periods: during and for 1 year after the construction period, the periods of overlap of construction and operation of the plants, and the 5 years preceding and following construction. The observed incidence was compared with the expected national incidence rate. Incidence rates were analyzed separately by social class.

Results.—Overall, there was at least a 35% excess incidence of childhood leukemia and non-Hodgkin's lymphoma in the study areas. The excesses were highest during the periods when construction and operation overlapped and, also, in areas of higher social class.

Discussion.—These findings support the hypothesized infective cause of increased incidence of childhood leukemia and non-Hodgkin's lymphoma. The highest excess incidence occurred during overlap periods of site contact between outside construction workers and local operating workers, which suggests that population mixing increases transmission of the underlying infective agent from infected to susceptible individuals.

▶ The apparent increase in the frequency of childhood leukemia among populations living near the Sellafield nuclear plant in England has been a source of many papers and much controversy. The assumption, of course, is that somehow either the children or their parents were exposed to excessive radiation from the nuclear plant and, therefore, were more likely to acquire leukemia. The authors explore the alternative theory that if leukemia were caused by an infectious agent, then any large-scale construction that causes an increase in airborne microbes might be a more likely target for study. In fact, they have demonstrated that the frequency of leukemia and non-Hodgkin's lymphoma was higher in children who lived near a nonnuclear construction site than among the population at large, and that it was similar to that seen among the children living around the Sellafield plant.

Sellafield also has a large workforce with many construction workers. In both cases, the frequency of leukemia was greater among residents in "social class I," i.e., a relatively high social class. The authors postulate that (1) large rural construction projects expose the population to more infectious agents, and (2) the influx of urban professionals and technicians not previously exposed to those agents increases the likelihood of an infection occurring in a nonimmune host at a critical time in lymphoid development, thereby causing an unusual reaction that leads to leukemia and lymphoma. This is a persuasive and prevailing theory in Britain today, and it may be true. All we need is some proof.

J.V. Simone, M.D.

Outcome of Treatment for Childhood Cancer in Black as Compared With White Children: The St Jude Children's Research Hospital Experience, 1962 Through 1992
Pui C-H, Boyett JM, Hancock ML, Pratt CB, Meyer WH, Crist WM (St Jude Children's Research Hosp, Memphis, Tenn)
JAMA 273:633–637, 1995   1–21

Background.—Cancer is the second leading cause of death among both black and white adults in the United States. Poorer survival has been associated with most of the common adulthood cancers in black Americans. However, it is unknown whether there are racial differences in cancer survival in children.

Methods.—A 30-year survival analysis (by race) was done. It was followed by separate studies done for early and recent treatment eras, which were defined by time points at which significantly improved outcome was shown for specific tumor types. The subjects were 798 black and 4,507 white children given a diagnosis of malignancies between 1962 and 1992.

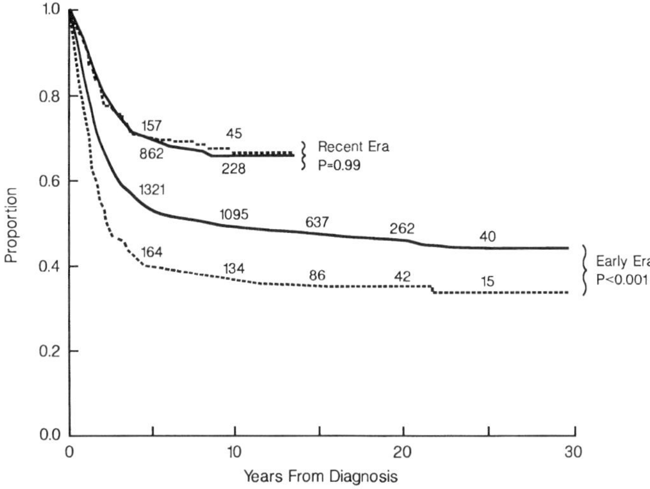

FIGURE.—Kaplan-Meier estimates of survival for black compared with white children with all forms of cancer treated in the early and recent treatment eras. *Dotted lines* represent black patients. *Numbers on the curves* represent patients at risk at specific time points. Survival was worse for black children during the early era but not the recent era ($P < .001$ and $P = .99$, respectively, by log-rank test). (Courtesy of Pui C-H, Boyett JM, Hancock ML, et al: *JAMA* 273:633–637, Copyright 1995, American Medical Association.)

These children were accepted for treatment regardless of their financial status. All were enrolled in disease-specific protocols.

Findings.—During the 30-year period, survival was significantly poorer among black children than among white children. In the early treatment era, there was a significant difference for all forms of cancer combined. The 10-year Kaplan-Meier estimates were 37% for black children and 50% for white children (Fig). This difference was primarily a reflection of the poorer prognosis of black children with acute lymphoblastic leukemia, the most common childhood cancer. No significant differences in treatment outcome by race were found for specific disease categories or for all forms of cancer combined. Black and white children had 10-year survival rates of 67% and 66%, respectively.

Conclusions.—The survival rates are comparable in black children and white children treated for malignancy with contemporary multimodality therapy. Therefore, with equal access to effective treatment, black children with cancer fare just as well as white children.

▶ This is an important and gratifying study of a large number of children with cancer treated at a single institution over 30 years. The figure tells the story of the improvement in survival seen when comparing the earlier era of treatment with the more recent era. The authors have wisely used different breakpoints for the two eras, depending on the disease-specific advances in treatment. The authors also explain the results as being caused by the improvement in therapeutic modalities and the equal access of patients, regardless of race, to such improved treatments. In a sense, the more effective treatments erased race as a prognostic factor, and equal access allowed the application. The improvement in therapies also includes the parallel improvement in supportive care, which has allowed the use of more intensive therapy and reduced the deaths from complications.

The biggest change among black children was the improvement in the outcome for acute lymphoblastic leukemia. From a 48% ten-year survival rate in the early era, the projected outcome is a 67% ten-year survival rate for black children compared with a rate of 66% for white children. This is both an astonishing improvement and a vivid reminder that, over time, prognostic factors change and evolve under the pressure of the single most important prognostic factor in any form of cancer: treatment.

J.V. Simone, M.D.

Incidence of Cancer in Children in the United States: Sex-, Race-, and 1-Year Age-Specific Rates by Histologic Type
Gurney JG, Severson RK, Davis S, Robison LL (Wayne State Univ, Detroit; Fred Hutchinson Cancer Research Ctr, Seattle; Univ of Washington, Seattle; et al)
Cancer 75:2186–2195, 1995   1–22

Introduction.—Estimates of the incidence rate of neoplasms among adults are usually presented in 5-year age categories stratified by topographic sites. This system is not ideal for understanding cancer among children, in whom there may be extensive variation in the rates of specific cancers across individual years of age. In addition, most childhood tumors are classified by histologic type rather than anatomical site. Histology-specific incidence rates of cancer among children in the United States within single-year age groups, stratified by sex and race, were calculated.

Methods.—The incidence rates of cancer among children younger than 15 years of age at diagnosis were calculated using data from the National Cancer Institute's Surveillance, Epidemiology, and End Results (SEER) Program. The analysis included 10,555 primary malignant neoplasms recorded from 1974 through 1989. Single-year age rates were calculated by modification of the SEER population denominator file.

Results.—For all histologic types of cancer in children combined, the annual incidence rate was 133.3 per 1 million children (Fig 1). Although the rate was higher among children younger than 5 years of age, many histologic types showed wide variation in rates within 5-year age groups. For retinoblastoma and Wilms' tumor, up to eightfold differences were noted within the 1- to 5-year and 5- to 9-year age groups, respectively. Other histologic types showing substantial differences included non-Hodgkin's lymphoma, acute lymphoid leukemia, acute myeloid leukemia, and osteosarcoma (Figs 2 to 4). The incidence rates were generally higher for boys than for girls, although young girls often had higher rates than young boys. Particularly in the first 5 years of life, the incidence rates were generally higher in white children than in black children; the difference in

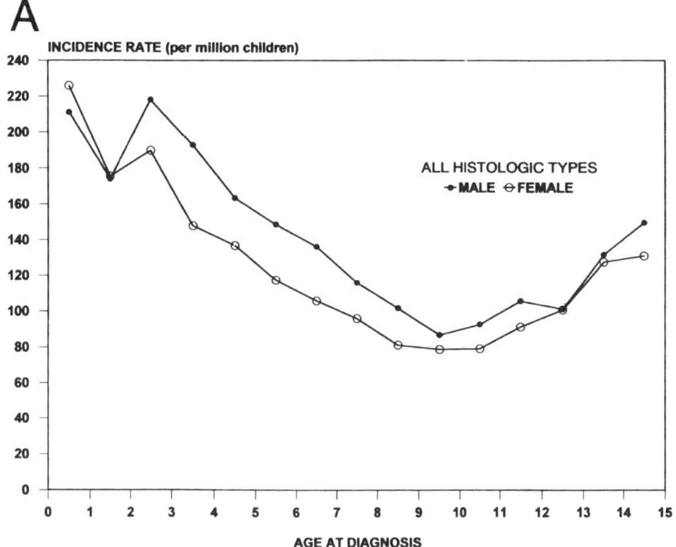

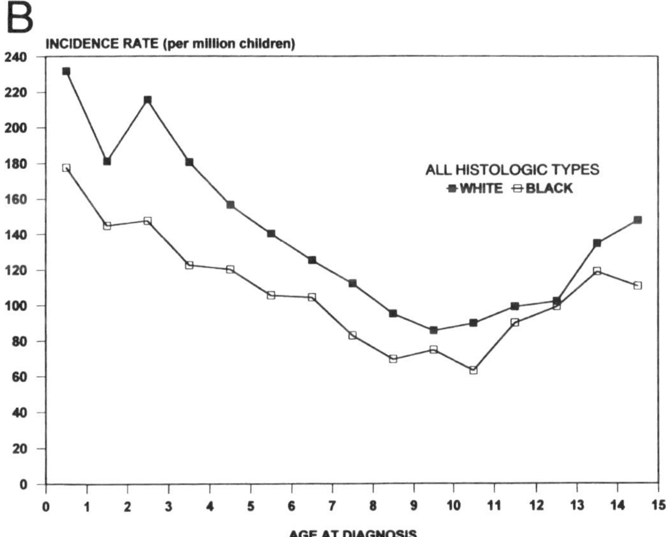

FIGURE 1.—**A,** age- and sex-specific incidence rates of all histologic types combined among children in the United States younger than 15 years of age. **B,** age-specific incidence rates of all histologic types combined among white and black children in the United States who are younger than 15 years of age. (Courtesy of Gurney JG, Severson RK, Davis S, et al: Incidence of cancer in children in the United States: Sex-, race-, and 1-year age-specific rates by histologic type. *Cancer* 75:2186–2195, copyright © 1995. Reprinted by permission of Wiley-Liss, Inc., a division of John Wiley & Sons, Inc.)

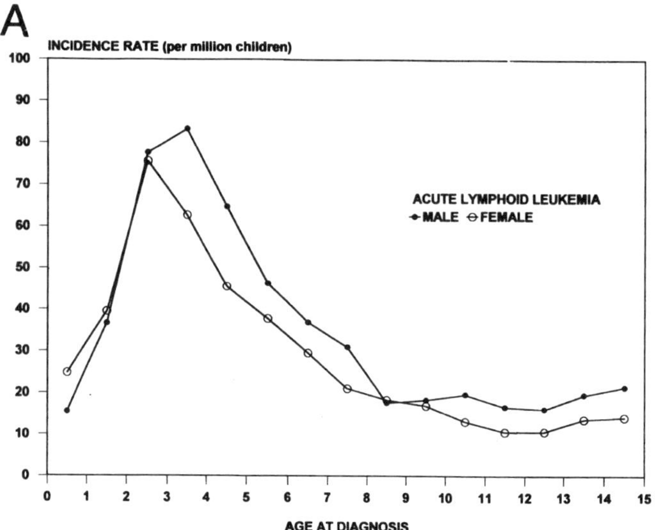

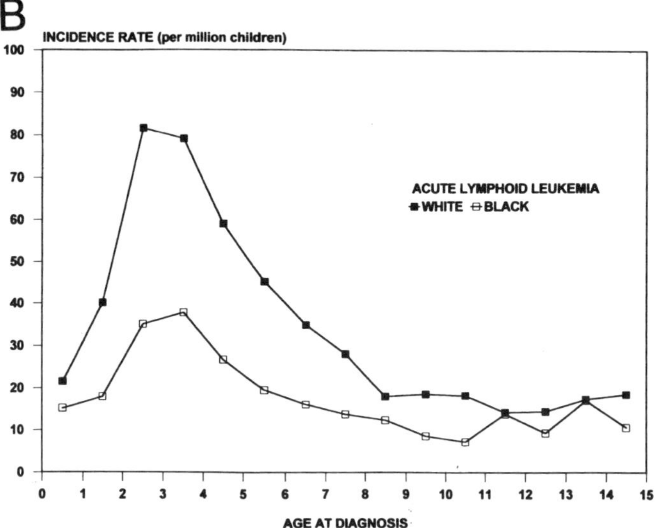

FIGURE 2.—**A,** age- and sex-specific incidence rates of acute lymphoid leukemia among children in the United States younger than 15 years of age. **B,** age-specific rates of acute lymphoid leukemia among white and black children in the United States who are younger than 15 years of age. (Courtesy of Gurney JG, Severson RK, Davis S, et al: Incidence of cancer in children in the United States: Sex-, race-, and 1-year age-specific rates by histologic type. *Cancer* 75:2186–2195, copyright © 1995. Reprinted by permission of Wiley-Liss, Inc., a division of John Wiley & Sons, Inc.)

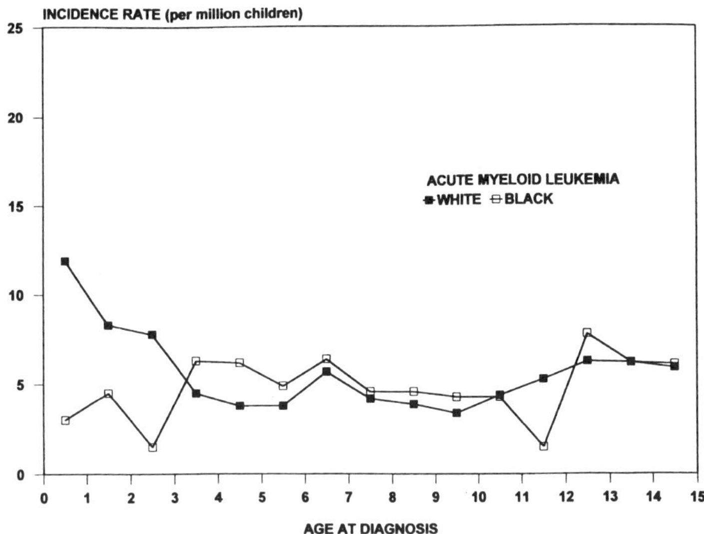

FIGURE 3.—Age-specific incidence rate of acute myeloid leukemia among white and black children in the United States who are younger than 15 years of age. (Courtesy of Gurney JG, Severson RK, Davis S, et al: Incidence of cancer in children in the United States: Sex-, race-, and 1-year age-specific rates by histologic type. *Cancer* 75:2186-2195, copyright © 1995. Reprinted by permission of Wiley-Liss, Inc., a division of John Wiley & Sons, Inc.)

acute lymphoid leukemia was particularly striking. Most neoplasms occurring in the first 2 years of life were embryonal tumors.

Conclusion.—The practice of summarizing the incidence rates of childhood cancers into 5-year age groups obscures some important demographic patterns. Whenever possible, these rates should be calculated and reported in single-year age groups. Cancer trends in children may be better explained if they are characterized in finer age groups.

▶ This paper is included for several reasons. The SEER data include more than 10,500 primary malignant neoplasms in children younger than age 15 years. Some of the more interesting findings are illustrated in the figures. Figure 1 demonstrates the higher frequency of all histologic types of cancer at virtually every age among males compared with females and among whites compared with blacks. Figure 2 shows a somewhat higher frequency of acute lymphoid leukemia among boys compared with girls but a strikingly greater incidence among whites compared with blacks. The higher frequency in whites is most striking in the first 6 years of life. This difference has been recognized for many years, but the reason has been unclear. Compare that with the data in Figure 3 which show very little difference in the frequency of acute myeloid leukemia between white and black children, with the exception of the first year of life. With regard to non-Hodgkin's lymphoma, as shown in Figure 4, males have a far greater frequency than females and whites have a far greater frequency than blacks.

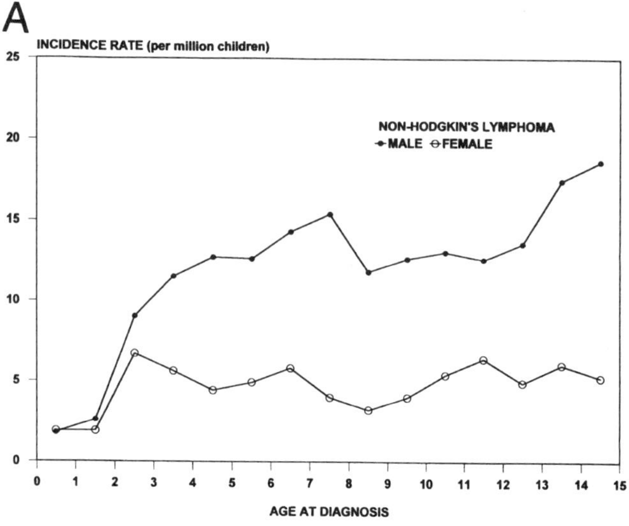

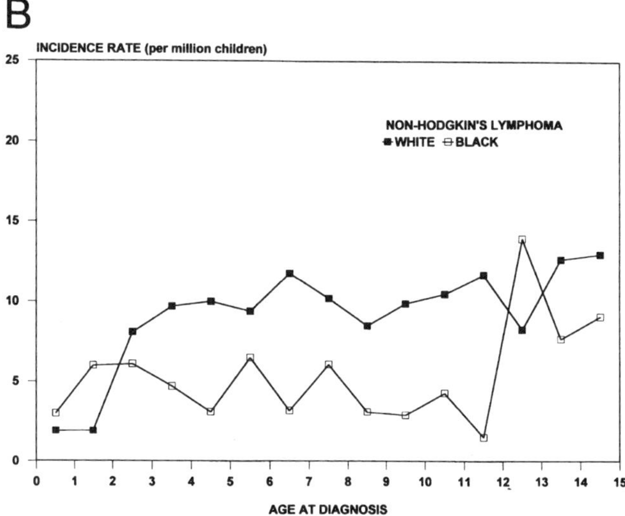

FIGURE 4.—A, age- and sex-specific incidence rates of non-Hodgkin's lymphoma among children in the United States younger than 15 years of age. **B,** age-specific rates of acute non-Hodgkin's lymphoma among white and black children in the United States who are younger than 15 years of age. (Courtesy of Gurney JG, Severson RK, Davis S, et al: Incidence of cancer in children in the United States: Sex-, race-, and 1-year age-specific rates by histologic type. *Cancer* 75:2186–2195, copyright © 1995. Reprinted by permission of Wiley-Liss, Inc., a division of John Wiley & Sons, Inc.)

These observations are not new and have been tantalizing epidemiologists and pediatric oncologists for many years. There are important clues to the etiology of these cancers hidden within these data. A variety of etiologic theories have been proposed, the most prominent being the differences in exposure to viral infections—or even the specific age or timing of exposure to viral infections—in childhood and the subsequent lymphoid reaction. As yet, no predisposing genetic factor has been identified to explain these differences; for the time being, they shall continue to intrigue and baffle us.

J.V. Simone, M.D.

Preliminary Evidence of an Association Between HLA-DPB1*0201 and Childhood Common Acute Lymphoblastic Leukaemia Supports an Infectious Aetiology
Taylor GM, Robinson MD, Binchy A, Birch JM, Stevens RF, Jones PM, Carr T, Dearden S, Gokhale DA (St Mary's Hosp, Manchester, England; Christie Hosp, Manchester, England; Royal Manchester Children's Hosp, England)
Leukemia 9:440–443, 1995   1–23

Objective.—There is a renewed emphasis on the possible etiologic role of infection in childhood common acute lymphoblastic leukemia (c-ALL). Several lines of evidence suggest that c-ALL may be a rare outcome of a common infection in genetically nonimmune individuals. In a previous study, it was found that there is an increased frequency of certain HLA-DP alleles in ALL. In a preliminary study, it was determined whether these DP alleles affect susceptibility to c-ALL.

Methods.—The prospective series included 63 children with the diagnosis of c-ALL, as confirmed by cytology and immunophenotyping. Blood samples for DNA analysis were obtained from these patients, from adult blood donors, and from normal full-term infants. Genomic DNA was extracted, polymerase chain reaction amplifications were performed, and HLA-DPB1 molecular typing was done using various sequence-specific oligonucleotide probes.

Results.—The children with c-ALL carried the HLA-DPB1 locus allele*0201 twice as frequently as infant controls and 3 times as frequently as adult controls. The children with c-ALL were also 3–4 times more likely to be heterozygous for DPB1*0201/*0301, /*0401, and /*0402. Single-strand conformation polymorphism analysis suggested that exon 2 of DPB1*0201 was probably not mutated in c-ALL.

Conclusion.—The HLA-DPB1*0201 allele—on its own or with other DPB1 alleles—may contribute to the risk of childhood c-ALL. This etiologic influence may occur via increased susceptibility to some infectious agent. For a child who types for DPB1*0201, the risk of c-ALL is increased from about 1 in 25,000 if there is no association between this allele and c-ALL to 1 in 13,800 if such an association does exist.

▶ There has been increasing interest in pursuing the possibility of an infectious etiology for childhood c-ALL. This is not a new idea by any means. The peak age of incidence (3–6 years of age) coincides with the greatest exposure to viral diseases and with the rapid proliferation of lymphoid tissue. This has long been a seductive combination for those who suspect an infectious cause of this disease, and this paper adds a bit more evidence to support that theory.

One line of thought has been that c-ALL results from the infection of nonimmune individuals with a common etiologic agent. Because the peak incidence occurs more commonly in communities with a high socioeconomic status, there is an implication that protection from the common infections at an earlier age exposes the patients to these agents at a critical time during the rapid growth of lymphoid tissue.

Another view is that genetic susceptibility plays a role in this process. The authors have provided some evidence to support the latter by demonstrating a higher-than-normal frequency of a specific HLA allele in childhood c-ALL. Therefore, the sequence might be as follows: Infection in a genetically susceptible and nonimmune host at a critical time during lymphoid development increases the likelihood of malignant transformation among B lymphocytes resulting in childhood c-ALL. If confirmed, this could be an extremely important finding.

J.V. Simone, M.D.

2 Cancer Biology, Markers, and Diagnosis

Small Renal Parenchymal Neoplasms: Further Observations on Growth
Bosniak MA, Birnbaum BA, Krinsky GA, Waisman J (New York Univ)
Radiology 197:589–597, 1995   2–1

Background.—It is unclear whether all small, incidentally detected renal parenchymal neoplasms will progress to the point where they are life-threatening or whether some will not grow or will grow so slowly that the patient's longevity is unaffected. The growth rate and behavior of renal parenchymal tumors 3.5 cm in diameter or smaller were investigated.

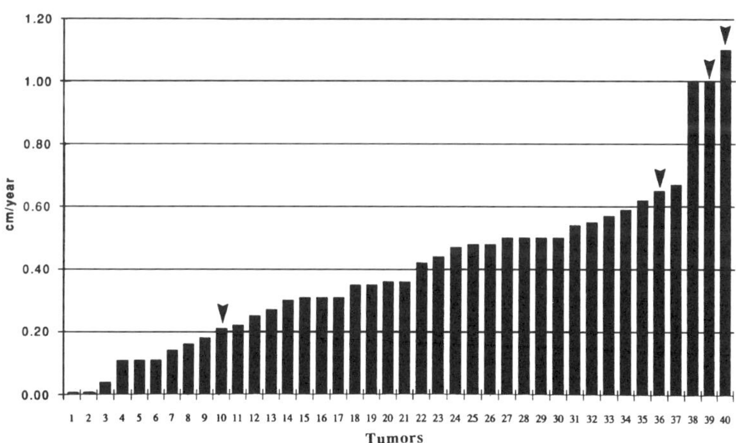

FIGURE 2.—Growth rate based on diameter (centimeters per year) in tumors in series. *Arrowheads* indicate grade 2 tumors proved at pathologic examination. Tumor numbers are shown at bottom of graph. (Courtesy of Bosniak MA, Birnbaum BA, Krinsky GA, et al: Small renal parenchymal neoplasms: Further observations on growth. *Radiology* 197:589–597, 1995. Radiological Society of North America.)

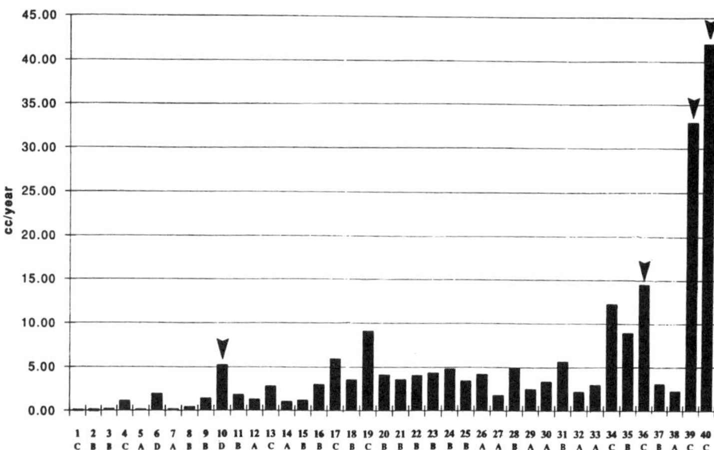

FIGURE 3.—Growth rate based on volume (cubic centimeters) per year. *Arrowheads* indicate grade 2 tumors proved at pathologic examination; these are among the fastest growing neoplasms. *Letters under tumor numbers* indicate the initial diameter and volume, respectively, of the neoplasm: A = 0–1 cm, 0–0.52 cm^3; B = 1.1–2 cm, 0.68–419 cm^3; C = 2.1–3 cm, 4.85–14.14 cm^3; D = > 3.0 cm, > 14.14 c^3. (Courtesy of Bosniak MA, Birnbaum BA, Krinsky GA, et al: Small renal parenchymal neoplasms: Further observations on growth. *Radiology* 197:589–597, 1995. Radiological Society of North America.)

Methods.—Thirty-seven adults with 40 renal parenchymal tumors were followed with CT and ultrasonography for 1.8–8.5 years. The patients were 26 men and 11 women with a mean age of 65.5 years. Twenty-six tumors were removed surgically. These tumors were proved and graded pathologically. Fourteen tumors meeting CT criteria for neoplasms underwent observation.

Findings.—Overall, the tumors grew at a rate of 0–1.1 cm per year. Thirty tumors grew at a rate of 0.5 cm or less per year. Nineteen grew very slowly—at a rate of 0.35 cm or less per year. Metastases did not develop in any of the patients. Twenty-four percent of the patients had multiple neoplasms (Figs 2 and 3).

Conclusion.—Most small, incidentally detected, well-marginated renal parenchymal neoplasms grow slowly and do not pose an immediate threat to the patient's life. Careful observation may be more appropriate than surgical removal, particularly in elderly patients or in those who may not survive the operation.

▶ This provocative paper looks at the growth rates of relatively small (3.5 cm or smaller) renal parenchymal neoplasms. A number of assumptions are made, including one that the growth rate of these tumors is constant. This assumption is not borne out by any specific data; in fact, based on what we know about carcinogenesis, these tumors represent a cascade of mutations, and it is reasonable to assume that the growth rate is not constant but, rather, changes over time as some of these mutations occur. There is an enormous heterogeneity in terms of the growth rates that are expressed within any 1 tumor mass, and it is hard for me to look at data from a paper like this without making the point that it is almost certainly fallacious to assume that the rate of growth is a constant either for or within any 1 tumor. The authors point out that most of the renal cell carcinomas that they describe represent the largest—and probably the only—series with careful prospective measurements to appear in the literature over time.

This paper is very provocative in terms of its advocacy for watchful waiting rather than surgical intervention. Although there are times when such an approach is reasonable—especially in elderly patients who are fragile—what is not clear about the "watch-and-wait" option is the type of change in parameters that will justify intervention at some point down the road. How large does one let the mass become? What kinds of enzymatic abnormalities will be tolerated without intervention? Does the development of visible adenopathy mean that the chance for cure with intervention has been compromised by delay? What are the medicolegal implications?

These kinds of questions do not have answers at this time, and before one routinely advocates the conservative approach, I think one has to address the issue of what is wrong with intervening as soon as the diagnosis is made, at least when patients have a reasonably good performance status. I have trouble with the watch-and-wait approach, except in the most elderly and fragile of patients.

E. Glatstein, M.D.

Telomeres, Telomerase, and Immortality
Rhyu MS (Natl Cancer Inst, Bethesda, Md)
J Natl Cancer Inst 87:884–894, 1995   2–2

Introduction.—There is increasing evidence that activation of the enzyme telomerase may play an important role in malignant tumor cells. Therefore, there is increasing interest in targeting telomerase for anticancer therapy. The current knowledge of telomeres and telomerase and the current evidence supporting the telomerase activation theory were reviewed.

Telomeres.—The telomeres, or chromosome ends, are essential for maintaining chromosomal integrity, which, in turn, allows normal cell division. Telomeric repeats typically have 5–8 base-pairs with numerous G bases. They appear to maintain chromosomal integrity in 2 ways. Telomeric binding with proteins in the nuclear membrane may shield chromosomal ends from degrading enzymes. Because an RNA primer sequence that is annealed to the end of each strand of DNA is required to begin cell division, the telomeric repeats provide expendable noncoding sequences that delay the shortening of chromosomal DNA with replication.

Telomerase.—Telomerase has been found to consist of a ribonucleoprotein complex that contains a region within the RNA component that serves as a template for repeat synthesis of the telomeric repeat. Telomerase activity has been observed specifically in germ cells but not in most somatic cells, which, therefore, have gradual depletion of their telomeric sequences, reflecting mitotic age, eventually leading to cell mortality by senescence (Fig 4). Telomerase activity prolongs the cellular life span and has been observed in immortal human cell lines and in tumor cells.

Therapeutic Implications.—Studies are under way to investigate the clinical usefulness of inhibiting telomerase to combat cancer. There are, however, cautionary notes. Although there is a correlation between telomerase and cancer, the relationship may not be causal. If the relationship is causal, there may also be other mechanisms involved in prolonging telomeric DNA, which may not be controlled with antitelomerase therapy. Because the lengths and patterns of telomeres vary considerably, development of antitelomerase drugs may be limited by the need for specificity. Nevertheless, studies of telomerase activation, both as a prognostic indicator and as a target for therapeutic intervention, hold great promise. Either the RNA or the protein components of telomerase may provide reasonable targets for inhibition.

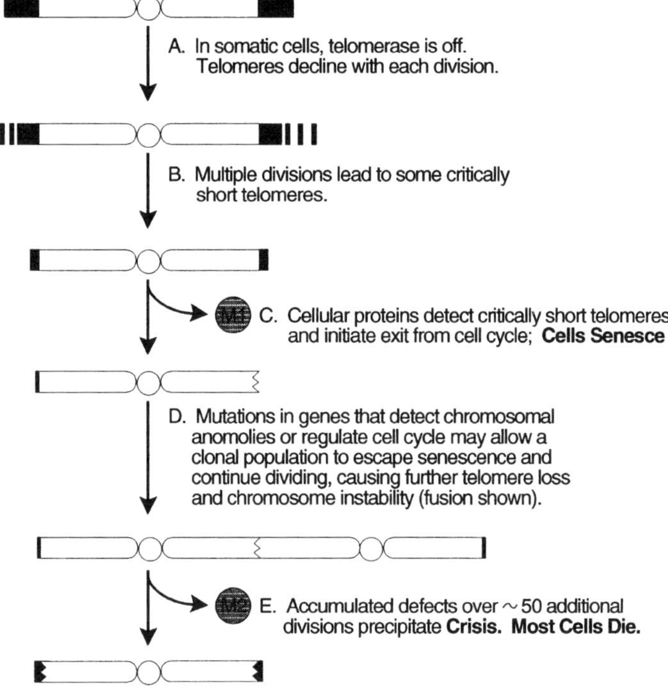

FIGURE 4.—Model for telomere role in aging and immortality. (Courtesy of Rhyu MS: Telomeres, telomerase, and immortality. *J Natl Cancer Inst* 87:884–894, 1995.)

Conclusion.—Inhibition of telomerase has potential as a cancer therapy. However, its usefulness is dependent upon (1) the establishment of a causal relationship between telomerase and cancer, and (2) an understanding of how and when telomerase is activated in tumor cells.

▶ What are telomeres, what is telomerase, and why is everybody talking about them? Telomeres are chromosomal ends that are responsible for the stabilization of chromosomes and are essential for maintaining the length of chromosomal DNA required for multiple cell division to occur. Telomerase is a ribonucleoprotein complex that overcomes the "end replication problem" associated with cell division by synthesizing the G-rich tandem repeats of telomeres needed for cellular immortality. The telomeres of normal somatic cells shorten with repeat cell division (in the absence of telomerase), leading to cellular senescence. Tumor cells with activated telomerase will divide indefinitely.

This difference in telomerase activity between normal and tumor cells has led to an intensive research effort to inhibit this enzyme in tumor cells and, thereby, make tumor cells "mortal." Of particular interest is the observation that telomerase activity is essentially absent in normal cells, thereby providing guarded optimism that a high degree of selectivity is possible by targeting telomerase. This timely review describes the potential strategies for inhibiting telomerase, and their clinical evaluation is eagerly anticipated.

R.F. Ozols, M.D., Ph.D.

Catalytic Specificity of Protein-Tyrosine Kinases Is Critical for Selective Signalling
Songyang Z, Carraway KL III, Eck MJ, Harrison SC, Feldman RA, Mohammadi M, Schlessinger J, Hubbard SR, Smith DP, Eng C, Lorenzo MJ, Ponder BAJ, Mayer BJ, Cantley LC (Harvard Med School, Boston; Tufts Univ, Boston; Howard Hughes Med Inst, Boston; et al)
Nature 373:536–539, 1995   2–3

Background.—The manner in which protein-tyrosine kinases (PTKs) are able to activate specific downstream events is presumed to involve the recognition of phosphotyrosine in a specific sequence context, either by Src-homology-2 (SH2) domains on tyrosine kinases or by targets of these kinases. The role of the catalytic site of tyrosine kinases in determining the specificity of potential targets remains uncertain.

Objective.—A new method of determining the substrate preference of protein kinases is based on the use of an oriented library of degenerate peptides. This method was used to identify the optimal peptide substrates for PTKs.

Findings.—Each of the 9 PTKs studied was found to have its own optimal substrate. Most of them selected peptides with Glu or Asp residues at specific sites in the N-terminal of the Tyr. Selectivity most often was dominated by a preference for specific hydrophobic amino acids at key positions. The cytosolic tyrosine kinases preferentially phosphorylated peptides recognized by their own SH2 domains or closely related domains. Receptor tyrosine kinases preferentially phosphorylated peptides recognized by subsets of group III SH2 domains.

Implications.—Protein-tyrosine kinases are specific for distinct substrates. Along with SH2 domains, they provide a "double" selectivity that maintains the fidelity of particular signaling events. In some instances, the ability of the SH2 domain of a given PTK to bind a site phosphorylated by the catalytic domain of the same enzyme may permit the phosphorylation of key substrates.

▶ Abnormal signal transduction is an important component of malignant transformation. Many "oncogenes" are normal transmembrane tyrosine kinase growth factor receptors that are important in normal growth regulation. Overexpression of these receptors and/or their ligands can result in a persistent state of growth stimulation leading to malignant transformation. The mechanisms by which these tyrosine kinases regulate subsequent ("downstream") events that ultimately result in growth regulation are unknown. One possible explanation is reported by Songyang and colleagues.

Several different families of growth factor receptors are known, and each has some substrate specificity at their respective catalytic binding sites. Songyang and colleagues found that each tyrosine kinase has its own optimal peptide substrate. The optimal peptides were synthesized and shown to have a very high affinity for its specific tyrosine kinase receptor. The authors also present evidence that this specificity is critical to the proper downstream signaling for that specific tyrosine kinase. Multiple endocrine neoplasia type-2B (MEN2B) is the result of a germline mutation affecting the RET tyrosine kinase transmembrane receptor. The nonmutated RET protein normally phosphorylates the peptide substrate for the epidermal growth factor receptor. However, the mutant RET protein is shown to phosphorylate the substrates usually optimal for two other tyrosine kinases. Therefore, alternative pathways, rather than the expected pathway, are stimulated.

Understanding the mechanism by which abnormal signaling results in malignant transformation and tumor growth is critical to learning how to inhibit these abnormal signals. As monoclonal antibodies to growth factor receptors and other forms of "targeted therapy" develop, better knowledge of the mechanisms of growth regulation may permit the synthesis or discovery of specific therapeutic agents directed against the dysregulated growth message signal. Such specificity would theoretically lead to either restoration of normal signaling or transformed cell death resulting from the interruption of a critical dysregulated growth regulatory pathway.

G.J. Bosl, M.D.

Spatial Heterogeneity in Tumor Perfusion Measured with Functional Computed Tomography at 0.05 µl Resolution
Hamberg LM, Kristjansen PEG, Hunter GJ, Wolf GL, Jain RK (Massachusetts General Hospital, Boston; Harvard Medical School, Boston)
Cancer Res 54:6032–6036, 1994   2–4

Background.—Tumor growth, metastasis, detection and treatment are affected by tumor blood flow and vascular morphology. Current methods for obtaining information on vascular tumor physiology include counting the vascular density of biopsied tissue, or noninvasive perfusion imaging with MRI, positron emission tomography, or conventional CT. The former method is invasive and restricted to biopsied tumor regions, whereas the latter techniques are limited by poor spatial and temporal resolution. Recently developed CT scanners using slip-ring technology currently permit very high spatial resolution to be obtained at rapid intervals. The combined high spatial and temporal resolutions make this tool, known as functional CT (fCT), an ideal method for the investigation of tissue vascular physiology. To verify the value of fCT, small-cell lung cancer lines from the same tumor with different physiologic and pharmacokinetic characteristics were studied, and the ability for fCT to detect the differences was examined.

Methods.—High-speed (200 ms of temporal resolution) fCT was used to investigate tumor vascular heterogeneity with 0.05 µl of spatial resolution. Vascular topologies were studied in 2 different human small-cell lung cancer lines originally derived from the same tumor. The tumor lines were implanted either subcutaneously or as a tissue-isolated tumor in immunodeficient nude mice.

Findings.—Peripheral vascular topology was detected in the subcutaneous preparations, whereas central vascular topology was noted in the tissue-isolated tumors. Pharmacokinetic analysis showed that tumor physiology was influenced by cell line, rather than by location.

Conclusions.—In patients with minimal tumor invasiveness, fCT may play a potential role in individual tumor characterization. Accordingly, this new technique may facilitate more detailed prognoses and help define optimal management strategies for unique tumor/patient combinations.

► It is my honest belief that our knowledge of tumor physiology is pathetically limited. We give a lot of lip service to a variety of issues, such as tumor vascularity, etc., without having a lot of specific information to which we can refer. This research team from Massachusetts General Hospital is generating what I think is very valuable information in the area of tumor physiology. These authors looked at functional high-speed CT, which they are using to demonstrate heterogeneity within the tumor's vascular system. They are appropriately investigating human cancer cells lines, which are grown either subcutaneously or as an isolated tissue preparation in immunocompromised mice.

The findings that these investigators generated are of interest, but more importantly, they are setting the pace in terms of new techniques for studying tumor physiology. This is something from which every oncologist (radiation, surgical, and medical) can benefit in the long haul.

E. Glatstein, M.D.

Inhibition of Human Tumor Xenograft Growth by Treatment With the Farnesyl Transferase Inhibitor B956
Nagasu T, Yoshimatsu K, Rowell C, Lewis MD, Garcia AM (Eisai Ltd, Tsukuba, Japan; Eisai Research Inst, Andover, Mass)
Cancer Res 55:5310–5314, 1995   2–5

Introduction.—The presence of oncogenic forms of *ras* has been seen in up to 50% of colon cancers, 30% of all types of human cancers, and 80% of pancreatic carcinomas. As a means of developing therapies for these types of cancer, *ras* is being targeted for drug development. In several types of tumors, the *ras* protein switches between inactive and active states and remains permanently activated to cause uncontrolled cell proliferation and differentiation. After posttranslational farnesylation, *ras* is localized at the plasma membrane. Inhibition of farnesylation has been a major target for the potential inhibition of tumor growth in those tumors in which *ras* is continually activated. A new peptidomimetic inhibitor of farnesyl was described.

Methods.—In vivo data were obtained with the potent new inhibitor, B956. The growth of tumors was induced in nude mice by *ras*-transformed cells, and they were treated with B956. Three human xenografts expressing different types of oncogenic *ras* were also treated with B956. A panel of 19 human tumor cell lines representing a variety of tissues, as well as *ras* mutations, and 2 model cell lines, zH1 and DK1, were used to test the effect of B956.

Results.—Inhibition of tumor growth is correlated with inhibition of *ras* post-translational processing in the tumor. The peptidomimetic inhibitor of farnesylation, B956, inhibited the growth of tumors induced in nude mice by *ras*-transformed cells. The formation of colonies in the soft agar of 14 human tumor cell lines expressing different *ras* oncogenes at concentrations between 0.2 and 60 µM were inhibited by B956 and its methyl ester B1086. To inhibit colony formation by 5 tumor cell lines with *ras* mutations, higher concentrations of B956, at 10–80 µM, were required. At 100 mg/kg, B956/B1086 inhibited tumor growth by HT1080 human fibrosarcoma, EJ-1 human bladder carcinoma and, to a lesser extent, HCT116 human colon carcinoma in nude mice.

Conclusion.—Inhibition of *ras* farnesylation as antitumor drug therapy appears promising, although differences in sensitivity to the inhibitor were observed in different cell lines. Other synthetic inhibitors of farnesyl transferase are being developed, and this strategy must still be evaluated clinically.

▶ In several types of tumors, the *ras* protein has switched between inactive and active states and remains permanently activated, leading to uncontrolled cell proliferation and differentiation. The *ras* protein is localized at the plasma membrane after posttranslational farnesylation. This process is critical for membrane localization and function of the *ras* protein. Consequently, inhibition of farnesylation has been a major target for the potential inhibition of tumor growth in those tumors in which *ras* is continually activated. This study demonstrates that a peptidomimetic inhibitor of farnesylation, B956, inhibits the growth of tumors induced in nude mice by *ras*-transformed cells. Furthermore, 3 human xenografts expressing different types of oncogenic *ras* were also inhibited by B956. There are other synthetic inhibitors of farnesyl transferase being developed, and early clinical evaluation of this novel strategy is eagerly awaited.

R.F. Ozols, M.D., Ph.D.

Glutathione *S*-Transferase Activity and Glutathione *S*-Transferase μ Expression in Subjects With Risk for Colorectal Cancer
Szarka CE, Pfeiffer GR, Hum ST, Everley LC, Balshem AM, Moore DF, Litwin S, Goosenberg EB, Frucht H, Engstrom PF, Clapper ML (Fox Chase Cancer Ctr, Philadelphia; Temple Univ, Philadelphia)
Cancer Res 55:2789–2793, 1995   2–6

Background.—Developing strategies and treatments for the prevention of colorectal cancer will require methods of identifying asymptomatic individuals who are at high risk. The glutathione *S*-transferases (GSTs), a family of phase II detoxication enzymes, protect the colon mucosa by catalyzing the conjugation of electrophilic compounds with glutathione, creating less cytotoxic soluble complexes. Studies have found correlations between deficiencies in GST-μ and an increased risk of lung, bladder, and larynx cancer. Both the total GST activity in blood lymphocytes and colon mucosa and the expression of GST-μ were investigated in individuals at increased risk for colorectal cancer and compared with those in normal controls.

Methods.—Blood samples and multiple sigmoid colon tissue biopsy samples were obtained from 60 individuals at increased risk for colorectal cancer and from 67 healthy individuals. Patients were considered at increased risk if they had a family or personal history of colorectal cancer (at least 2 years after definitive therapy) or a personal history of colon polyps. Expression of GST-μ in whole blood was determined with an enzyme-linked immunosorbent assay. Total GST activity in tissue samples and in isolated blood lymphocytes was determined spectrophotometrically.

Results.—Although GST activity in blood lymphocytes varied between subjects by more than eightfold, it was consistent over time within individuals. Total GST activity was significantly reduced in high-risk individuals compared with control individuals. The data suggest that the GST activity in blood lymphocytes decreased further with greater numbers of risk factors. The GST-μ null phenotype was found in 41% of the controls and 37% of the high-risk patients. Expression of GST-μ was significant for predicting risk only for males. Activity of GST in the blood lymphocytes and in the colon mucosa was strongly correlated.

Conclusion.—Decreased GST activity was associated with increased risk for colorectal cancer. The usefulness of GST activity as a biomarker of cancer susceptibility should be evaluated further. This biomarker may identify individuals who are likely to benefit from chemopreventive regimens that modify phase II detoxication enzymes.

▶ Although theoretically appealing, there are numerous practical concerns regarding the potential of agents for cancer prevention. If an effective agent is found, individuals may be required to take medication for a lifetime. The identification of high-risk individuals and the validation both of biomarkers of risk assessment and the efficacy of intervention will be needed to advance the field of cancer prevention. This interesting study from a pioneering clinical-laboratory group of investigators in the field of cancer prevention has identified GST to be a potentially critical biomarker in prevention of colorectal cancer. The observation that GST activity was lower in high-risk individuals will facilitate the evaluation of the potential efficacy of chemopreventive agents, because they would be expected to modify the activity of phase II detoxifying enzymes, such as GST, if they are to decrease the incidence of colorectal cancers.

R.F. Ozols, M.D., Ph.D.

Genetic Alterations at 5p15: A Potential Marker for Progression of Precancerous Lesions of the Uterine Cervix
Mitra AB, Murty VVVS, Singh V, Li R-G, Pratap M, Sodhani P, Luthra UK, Chaganti RSK (Mem Sloan-Kettering Cancer Ctr, New York; Inst of Cytology and Preventive Oncology, New Delhi, India)
J Natl Cancer Inst 87:742–745, 1995   2–7

Background.—Although distinct preneoplastic epithelial changes precede most cervical carcinomas, the course of progression from dysplasia to invasive carcinoma varies, suggesting that specific etiologic agents or genetic alterations may mediate this progression. In a recent study, it was discovered that loss of heterozygosity (LOH) in the short arm of chromosome 5 (5p) occurred in the majority of cervical tumor DNAs, suggesting that this region may contain a tumor suppressor gene. To investigate this possibility further, 5 loci mapped to 5p14-ter were analyzed in precancerous and cancerous cervical lesions.

Methods.—Archival paraffin-embedded tumor biopsy specimens and peripheral blood samples were obtained from 46 patients with untreated primary invasive carcinomas, 5 patients with carcinoma in situ (CIS), and 14 patients with precancerous lesions. Deoxyribonucleic acid was isolated from the peripheral blood mononuclear cells and from microdissected tissue sections, and it was analyzed by polymerase chain reaction, using 5 sets of primer pairs for polymorphic microsatellite loci mapped to 5p14-ter (D5S392, D5S117, D5S208, D5S406, and D5S432) to identify LOH or instability.

Results.—All lesions except for 1 invasive carcinoma showed LOH or instability in at least 1 of the markers tested. The LOH occurred in 55.6% of the invasive carcinomas, 20% of the CIS lesions, and 21% of the precancerous lesions, most frequently at D5S208 and D5S406 in carcinomas and at D5S406 in precancerous lesions. In all but 1 lesion with LOH, the losses were simple deletions with complete, terminal, or interstitial losses; 1 tumor had complex deletions. Microsatellite in stability at D5S406, D5S432, and D5S117 was observed in 13% of the invasive carcinomas, 40% of the CIS lesions, and 21% of the precancerous lesions. Ten of the 11 patients had instability at just 1 locus; the other patient (with moderate dysplasia) had microsatellite instability at 2 loci. Microsatellite instability was observed most frequently (8 of 12 instances) at D5S406. Five of the 11 patients with microsatellite instability also had LOH.

Conclusion.—A high frequency of LOH and microsatellite instability at 5p15.1-15.2, which includes the D5S406 locus, in precancerous and cancerous cervical lesions shows that this is a novel site for a candidate tumor suppressor gene. Alterations at this site may function as a marker of risk for progression of dysplasias to invasive cervical carcinoma. This possibility should be evaluated prospectively.

▶ The progression from preneoplastic proliferative changes in the cervical epithelium (intraepithelial neoplasia) to dysplasia to frank invasive carcinoma can be histologically documented in the development of cervical cancer. However, the genetic mechanisms controlling both the development and progression of such preneoplastic lesions have not been elucidated. Previous studies have demonstrated a high frequency of LOH in chromosome 5p in cervical carcinoma, which has suggested the possible existence of a candidate suppressor gene on this chromosomal arm. This study revealed frequent replication error (microsatellite instability) in precancerous lesions as well as in carcinomas, which suggests that the genetic instability in 5p is an early change in cervical carcinogenesis.

The investigators have also identified a novel site for a candidate suppressor gene. Identification of these changes in precancerous lesions may serve as a potential marker of risk for identifying patients at a high risk for progression to invasive carcinoma. The relationship between infection with human papillomavirus and alterations in a putative suppressor gene remains to be determined, but this is an area of obvious interest.

R.F. Ozols, M.D., Ph.D.

Microsatellite Instability in Gynecological Sarcomas and in *hMSH2* Mutant Uterine Sarcoma Cell Lines Defective in Mismatch Repair Activity

Risinger JI, Umar A, Boyer JC, Evans AC, Berchuck A, Kunkel TA, Barrett JC (Natl Inst of Environmental Health Sciences, Research Triangle Park, NC; Univ of North Carolina, Chapel Hill; Duke Univ, Durham, NC)
Cancer Res 55:5664–5669, 1995

2–8

Introduction.—Tumors from hereditary nonpolyposis colorectal cancer kindreds are associated with somatic instability of simple repetitive sequences, otherwise known as microsatellites. Compared with normal DNA, in tumor DNA this defect is apparent as an expansion or contraction of microsatellites. Recently, it has been shown that this defect is common in many sporadic tumors, including endometrial, colon, gastric, and pancreatic cancer. A panel of gynecologic sarcomas were examined for microsatellite instability.

Methods.—A panel of 44 primary genital tract sarcomas and their matched normal tissues and 3 cell lines were examined for microsatellite instability. Two unstable cell lines were found, which were examined for the nature of the underlying genetic defect and mismatch repair activity.

Results.—Of the 44 sarcomas, 11 had altered mobility of alleles for at least 1 marker, 6 of which showed altered mobility at 2 or more loci. Of the 44 patients whose tissues were examined, 8 remain free of disease, and 3 of these had microsatellite instability. No statistical correlation was seen between alterations in microsatellites and clinical outcome between tumors with microsatellite alterations at a single locus, tumors showing multiple cases of alterations, and tumors without an indication of alterations. In 2 cell lines derived from a uterine mixed mesodermal tumor, ditetranucleotide, tritetranucleotide, and tetranucleotide microsatellites were found to be highly unstable in single cell clones. An examination of the mismatch repair activity showed that both extracts were repair deficient, whereas the other cell line that did not have microsatellite instability was proficient in repair. A colon tumor cell extract complemented the repair deficiency, which was defective in the hMLH1 protein but not by an extract defective in hMSH2 protein. This means that in the uterine sarcoma line, the defect could be hMSH2.

Conclusion.—The mutator phenotype has been shown to be associated with mutations in mismatch repair genes. The defective mismatch repair capacity leads to microsatellite instability. Sarcomas are added to the growing list of solid tumors in which a microsatellite instability phenotype has been identified.

▶ Instability of simple or repetitive sequences, termed microsatellites, was initially shown to be associated with tumors from hereditary nonpolyposis colorectal cancer. This defect has proven common in sporadic tumors such as endometrial, colon, gastric, and pancreatic cancer. The mutator phenotype has been shown to be associated with mutations in mismatched repair genes. The defective mismatch repair capacity leads to microsatellite instability. Sarcomas are among the solid tumors in which a microsatellite instability phenotype has been identified.

R.F. Ozols, M.D., Ph.D.

A Collaborative Survey of 80 Mutations in the *BRCA* 1 Breast and Ovarian Cancer Susceptibility Gene: Implications for Presymptomatic Testing and Screening
Shattuck-Eidens D, McClure M, Simard J, Labrie F, Narod S, Couch F, Hoskins K, Weber B, Castilla L, Erdos M, Brody L, Friedman L, Ostermeyer E, Szabo C, King M-C, Jhanwar S, Offit K, Norton L, Gilewski T, Lubin M Osborne M, Black D, Boyd M, Steel M, Ingles S, Haile R, Lindblom A, Olsson H, Borg A, Bishop DT, Solomon E, Radice P, Spatti G, Gayther S, Ponder B, Warren W, Stratton M, Liu Q, Fugimura F, Lewis C, Skolnick MH, Goldgar DE (Myriad Genetics, Salt Lake City, Utah; HUL Research Ctr and Laval Univ, Quebec City, Quebec; McGill Univ, Montreal; et al)
JAMA 273:535–541, 1995   2–9

Background.—The discovery of a particular gene, *BRCA1*, which confers markedly increased vulnerability to both breast and ovarian cancers, has aroused much interest among oncologists. The implications for women who have a personal or family history of breast cancer are obvious.

Objective.—A review was done of the preliminary experience gained by an international group of investigators in North America and the United Kingdom in identifying mutations of *BRCA1*.

Study Population.—Nine laboratories analyzed DNA samples from 372 unrelated women having breast or ovarian cancer. Most of the women were from high-risk families. In addition, 3 of the laboratories analyzed 714 further samples from women with breast or ovarian cancer, 557 of whom were unselected for family history, to identify 2 particular mutations seen to recur in the familial samples.

Findings.—Mutations in *BRCA1* were found in 80 patient samples. Among 38 distinct mutations, 3 appeared to be relatively prevalent, occurring 8, 7, and 5 times, respectively. Specific testing for the 2 most common mutations demonstrated their presence in 17 additional patients. Eighty-six percent of all mutations were predicted to result in a truncated protein.

Implications.—That a relatively simple test could be developed for detecting mutations of *BRCA1* is conceivable. At present, the failure to discover such a mutation in an individual who is at risk is clinically meaningful only if a *BRCA1* mutation is present in a first-degree relative who has cancer. All risk calculations should include nongenetic risk factors, especially those that may interact with the genetic risk conferred by *BRCA1*.

► This very important collaborative study followed on the heels of the identification of the *BRCA1* breast and ovarian cancer susceptibility gene. I include this article because it underscores some of the difficulties that will be faced in applying information obtained by the search for specific genes associated with a higher incidence of cancer. The first important point is that the *BRCA1* gene was identified in 80 patient samples, but 38 distinct mutations were found. This finding means that it would be possible to use a simple, highly specific test for identifying a focal mutation in the gene. This also means that unless the probe is broad enough, a mutation might be missed because of the wide variety of possible mutants in such a large gene. Nonetheless, the authors found that it was possible to group some of the mutations into classes that might, in the long run, make it possible to develop a useful test for most of the mutations. Mutations usually remain true within a family tree. Therefore, failure to identify a mutant gene allows no definitive conclusion as to its absence, unless the gene—in one of its forms—has already been identified in another family member.

Another caution to keep in mind as the story of *BRCA1* continues to evolve is that neither its actual frequency in the general population nor its frequency among all women with breast cancer is known. The samples reported in this study were primarily gathered from patients in high-risk families so that there would be a sufficient number with which to begin to determine the range of genetic mutations. We will not know the impact of the discovery of this particular gene until general population studies of women with breast cancer can be completed. Also, the search for BRCA2 has now begun, and undoubtedly there will be a third and fourth gene and so on. We have merely crossed the threshold of a major new era in cancer control—one that will be arduous but extremely promising in helping us to reduce the fatalities resulting from breast and ovarian cancer.

J.V. Simone, M.D.

▶ The recent isolation of a specific gene, *BRCA1,* which confers increased susceptibility to breast and ovarian cancer, has generated a great deal of interest not only among oncologists, but, also, among thousands of women with a personal family history of either of these diseases. The strongest risk factor for breast cancer is a positive family history, and genetic screening holds promise for identifying those women who are carriers of a mutated gene. This abstracted study demonstrates that screening for *BRCA1* mutations may only be useful when the mutation has already been identified in an affected first-degree relative. Women who have not inherited the mutant *BRCA1* allele that is present in their effected relative will still have risks for breast and ovarian cancer that are equal to those in the general population. The *BRCA1* mutations have not been identified in the sporadic ovarian and breast tumors. In ovarian cancer, screening for *BRCA1* mutations is likely to identify very few women who are carriers, because hereditary ovarian cancer (defined as more than two affected first-degree relatives) is extraordinarily uncommon. Multiple laboratories are searching for additional loci that may be associated with the predisposition to early-onset breast cancer and ovarian cancer. The *BRCA1* gene remains the first of what promises to be multiple genes that can increase susceptibility to breast cancer and ovarian cancer.

R.F. Ozols, M.D., Ph.D.

Expression of Vascular Endothelial Growth Factor and Its Receptors flt and KDR in Ovarian Carcinoma
Boocock CA, Charnock-Jones DS, Sharkey AM, McLaren J, Barker PJ, Wright KA, Twentyman PR, Smith SK (Univ of Cambridge, England; Babraham Inst, Cambridge, England; Med Research Council Ctr, Cambridge, England)
J Natl Cancer Inst 87:506–516, 1995   2–10

Background.—Two thirds of patients with ovarian carcinoma have advanced disease at diagnosis. Their prognosis is poor because highly invasive carcinoma cells and rapidly accumulating ascitic fluid are present. Ovarian carcinomas, together with other tumors, produce increased amounts of vascular endothelial growth factor (VEGF), a potent mitogen of endothelial cells. Acting through the known human receptors for VEGF, flt and KDR, VEGF may stimulate angiogenesis and promote tumor progression. The function of VEGF in tumor development was further clarified by identifying the cells in ovarian carcinoma tissue that express VEGF and its receptors.

Methods.—Samples of primary tumors were obtained from 5 patients with ovarian carcinoma and from the metastases of ovarian carcinoma from another 3 patients. Using in situ hybridization and immunohistochemistry in frozen sections, VEGF, flt, and KDR expression was localized. Reverse transcription followed by polymerase chain reaction (RT-PCR) and an enzyme-linked immunosorbent assay were used to assess the expression of VEGF, flt, and KDR in 6 epithelial cell lines derived from ovarian carcinoma ascites from another 5 patients.

Findings.—Primary ascitic cells and 3 of the 4 ovarian carcinoma cell lines assessed by RT-PCR showed messenger RNAs (mRNAs) encoding VEGF, flt, and KDR. Culture media conditioned by the cell lines showed VEGF levels of 20–120 p*M*. Increased VEGF mRNA expression occurred in all primary tumors and metastases, especially at the margins of tumor acini. Vascular endothelial growth factor immunoreactivity was concentrated in tumor cell clusters and stromal matrix patches, and flt immunoreactivity was confined to tumor blood vessels. However, in situ hybridization did not detect flt mRNA. By contrast, KDR mRNA was present in vascular endothelial cells and in tumor cells at primary malignant sites.

Conclusion.—Tumor cells in primary and metastatic ovarian carcinoma express VEGF, which accumulates in the stromal matrix. Some tumor blood vessels express flt and KDR. In addition, KDR is expressed by some tumor cells that co-express VEGF. Such co-expression raises the possibilities of autocrine stimulation and treatment strategies that target this receptor-ligand interaction.

▶ The morbidity and mortality of ovarian cancer primarily relate to intraperitoneal carcinomatosis. Malignant cells from the ovary can spread throughout peritoneal surfaces, producing innumerable metastatic deposits that ultimately lead to obstruction of critical organs. Vascular endothelial growth factor plays a critical role in the pathogenesis of ovarian cancer by stimulating angiogenesis and promoting tumor progression. This study demonstrates that VEGF is expressed by tumor cells both in primary and metastatic ovarian carcinomas and that its receptors, flt and KDR, are also expressed by some tumor blood vessels, with the latter receptor also being expressed in tumor cells that co-express VEGF.

This receptor-ligand interaction is an attractive target for new therapeutic strategies in ovarian cancer. It may be possible to inhibit VEGF activity by anti-VEGF monoclonal antibodies. Such antibodies have already been shown to suppress tumor vascularization and decrease the growth of some human tumors in nude mouse xenografts. The intraperitoneal administration of such monoclonal antibodies may be a particularly effective way to inhibit angiogenesis of small tumors on peritoneal surfaces.

R.F. Ozols, M.D. Ph.D.

Characterization of Human Ovarian Epithelial Tumors (*ex vivo*) by Proton Magnetic Resonance Spectroscopy

Mackinnon WB, Russell P, May GL, Mountford CE (Univ of Sydney, Australia; Royal Prince Alfred Hosp, Camperdown, Australia)
Int J Gynecol Cancer 5:211–221, 1995   2–11

Purpose.—It has been suggested that ovarian cancer should be considered as an adenoma-to-carcinoma sequence, but this concept remains ill defined. It would be clinically useful to establish the precise position of proliferating tumors along a neoplastic scale ranging from benign epithelial tumors at one end to frankly invasive malignancies at the other end. The alternative investigational modality, proton MR spectroscopy (^{1}H MRS), has the potential for assisting current pathologic techniques in the detection and staging of ovarian cancer. The ability of altered cellular chemistry, as determined by ^{1}H MRS, to provide a reliable indicator of ovarian epithelial tumor development and progression was assessed.

Methods.—Ex vivo ^{1}H MRS studies were performed on human ovarian tissue specimens ranging from normal to frankly malignant. The study included 12 histologically normal specimens; 3 benign ovarian fibromas; and 18 benign, 9 proliferating, and 30 frankly malignant surface epithelial-stromal tumors. One-dimensional ^{1}H MR spectra were used to distinguish between carcinomatous and benign or normal tissue, based on differences in the resonance intensities of cellular lipid, creatine/phosphocreatine, and lysine.

Results.—The ^{1}H MRS technique had a sensitivity of 87% and a specificity of 91%. Multiple crosspeaks attributable to cell-surface fucosylation were noted on 2-dimensional MRS of the carcinomatous biopsy specimens. Those crosspeaks, which correlated with tumor grade and loss of cellular differentiation, were absent in spectra from normal ovary and benign tumors. The finding of MR-visible fucosylation distinguished between carcinomatous and normal or benign tissue with a sensitivity of 88% and a specificity of 97%. The specimens of proliferating tumors showed a range of cell-surface fucosylation patterns indicating their malignant potential.

Conclusion.—In ^{1}H MRS studies of ovarian epithelial tumor specimens, the progression from normal tissue and benign tumors to proliferating and carcinomatous tissue is characterized by increasing cell-surface fucosylation, lipid signals, and altered cellular metabolism. This investigational modality may be helpful in the pathologic diagnosis of human ovarian epithelial-stromal neoplasms. These findings provide strong support for the concept of an adenoma–carcinoma sequence in ovarian cancer.

▶ The existence of a premalignant lesion for invasive epithelial ovarian tumors remains to be established. Some investigators believe that, similar to the pathogenesis of colon carcinomas, there is a stepwise progression from an adenoma of the ovary to a borderline tumor to a frankly invasive malignant carcinoma. Careful histologic examination of tumors and molecular typing have failed to unequivocally establish such a sequence. The identification of a precursor lesion may facilitate earlier diagnosis and screening and permit intervention at a more curable stage. Proton MR spectroscopy provides supportive evidence for a sequential progression from adenomas to carcinomas.

This study shows that the progression from normal and benign tissues to invasive carcinomas of the ovary is characterized by increasing cell-surface fucosylation, lipid signals, and altered cellular metabolism, which can be measured by ^{1}H MRS. In addition to providing support for the concept of an adenoma–carcinoma sequence in ovarian cancer, the data suggest that ^{1}H MRS may be a useful modality for assisting in the diagnosis and evaluation of the invasive characteristics of epithelial neoplasms.

R.F. Ozols, M.D., Ph.D.

Mutation Analysis of the *BRCA1* Gene in Ovarian Cancers

Takahashi H, Behbakht K, McGovern PE, Chiu H-C, Couch FJ, Weber BL, Friedman LS, King M-C, Furusato M, LiVolsi VA, Menzin AW, Liu PC, Benjamin I, Morgan MA, King SA, Rebane BA, Cardonick A, Mikuta JJ, Rubin SC, Boyd J (Univ of Pennsylvania, Philadelphia; Univ of California, Berkeley; Jikei Univ, Tokyo)
Cancer Res 55:2998–3002, 1995

Background.—Ovarian carcinoma has been associated with allelic deletion on chromosome 17, with loss of heterozygosity on 17q demonstrated in up to 75% of ovarian tumors. Germline mutations at the *BRCA1* locus on chromosome 17q21 have been linked to both breast and ovarian cancer. However, subsequent studies have suggested that *BRCA1* is a tumor suppressor gene that is important in hereditary, but not sporadic, ovarian tumors. A large number of both sporadic and familial forms of ovarian carcinomas were examined to determine *BRCA1* involvement.

Methods.—Genomic DNA was extracted from epithelial ovarian carcinomas from 115 patients with ovarian carcinoma that had not been treated with chemotherapy or radiation and from lymphocytes or uninvolved reproductive tract tissue. Twenty-two exons, including exon 7, were amplified by polymerase chain reaction and analyzed for mutations with single-strand conformation polymorphism, sequencing, and allelotyping.

Results.—Ten sequencing variants, which represented 2-allele polymorphisms in exons 11, 13, and 16 and introns 8, 11, and 18, were found in multiple tissue samples. Eight other sequencing variants, representing mutations of the *BRCA1* gene, were found in one specimen each. Of these 8 variants, 5 were frameshift mutations that created a premature stop codon, which would truncate the production of the BRCA1 protein. One was a missense mutation, which would probably alter the function of the protein's "zinc-finger" motif. The functional impact of the intronic mutation could not be definitively determined, but it may prevent the correct splicing of exons 20 and 21. Only patients with medical and/or family histories of breast and/or ovarian cancer had these 8 *BRCA1* germline sequence variants.

Conclusion.—Inherited mutations of the *BRCA1* allele are important in a significant number of patients with dual primary breast and ovarian cancer and hereditary ovarian cancer alone. However, somatic mutations of *BRCA1* are rare in patients with sporadic ovarian carcinomas. The frequent loss of heterozygosity noted on chromosome 17q in these patients suggests that mutations of other tumor suppressor genes may be involved. These findings will require confirmation with mutational analysis of a larger number of ovarian cancers.

▶ Conventional methods (determination of CA 125 levels and transvaginal ultrasound) of screening for ovarian cancer have not been established to be effective and are not recommended for the general population. Even in women who have a family history of ovarian cancer, there remains controversy as to how these patients should be followed. It is clear that *BRCA1* plays an important role in hereditary ovarian cancer, which accounts for approximately 5% of epithelial ovarian cancers. In the vastly more common sporadic ovarian cancers, *BRCA1* mutations in tumors have been infrequently reported. The potential for genetic screening is obvious. However, multiple different *BRCA1* mutations have been noted, and only some are associated with a markedly increased predisposition to ovarian cancer.

Currently, the best evidence that *BRCA1* is involved in a specific pedigree is to establish that a mutation is present in an affected individual with ovarian cancer and, consequently, any family member having the identical germline *BRCA1* mutation would be at risk. A great deal more information is needed to define risks associated with *BRCA1* mutations. It is certain that other genes will also be involved in some hereditary ovarian cancers.

Caution must be exercised when the results of these genetic tests are made available to individual women. It seems prudent that highly skilled genetic counselors discuss with women the implications of genetic "screening" before and after their tissues are analyzed for *BRCA1* mutations. The development of standards for screening, quality assurance, and guidelines for counseling and confidentiality are urgently needed.

R.F. Ozols, M.D., Ph.D.

Phase Ia/Ib Trial of Bispecific Antibody MDX-210 in Patients With Advanced Breast or Ovarian Cancer That Overexpresses the Proto-Oncogene HER-2/*neu*
Valone FH, Kaufman PA, Guyre PM, Lewis LD, Memoli V, Deo Y, Graziano R, Fisher JL, Meyer L, Mrozek-Orlowski M, Wardwell K, Guyre V, Morley TL, Arvizu C, Fanger MW (Dartmouth-Hitchcock Med Ctr, Lebanon, NH; Norris Cotton Cancer Ctr, Lebanon, NH; Medarex Inc, Annandale, NJ)
J Clin Oncol 13:2281–2292, 1995   2–13

Objective.—Although specific monoclonal antibodies have been developed, none has been shown to be immunologically effective. On the other hand, bispecific antibodies (BsAbs), 1 specific for the tumor target cell and the other for the immune-effector cells, lead to tumor destruction. The results of a phase Ia/Ib study of a single IV infusion of MDX-210, a bispecific antibody that binds to type I Fc receptors for immunoglobulin G (IgG) (FcγRI) and to the HER-2/*neu* oncogene protein, were evaluated to define the tolerability and safety, and maximum and therapeutic dosages for patients with advanced breast or ovarian cancers.

Methods.—The MDX-210 antibody was given IV to 15 patients (age, 39–69 years) with breast cancer (9 patients) and ovarian cancer (6 patients) in doses of 0.35, 1.0, 3.5, 7.0, and 10.0 mg/m², until the maximum-tolerated dose (MTD) or optimal biological dose (OBD) was delivered. The MTD was defined as the dose resulting in a toxicity of grade 3 or greater in fewer than half the patients. The OBD was defined as the dose yielding maximal saturation of monocyte FcγRI and optimized cytokine release and human leukocyte antigen expression.

Results.—The treatment was generally well tolerated, with low-grade fever, mild hypotension, and nausea as the main adverse effects at higher doses. Peripheral blood monocytes decreased significantly, and lymphocytes decreased slightly after infusion but returned to normal by 24 hours. At doses of 3.5 mg/m^2 or more, MDX-210 bound to more than 80% of FcγRI on monocytes reaching plasma concentrations of 1 µg/mL or more. Increased plasma levels of tumor necrosis factor-α, interleukin-6, granulocyte colony-stimulating factor, and neopterin were detected at MDX-210 concentrations of 7.0 mg/m^2 or more. In 2 patients, there was MDX-210 localization in tumors at 10 mg/m^2. Antibodies to MDX-210 were detected in 6 patients and appeared to be dose-related. Two patients had reduction of more than 50% or almost complete resolution of tumors but experienced spread of other tumors.

Conclusion.—The side effects of treatment were unremarkable and expected. The OBD of a single IV infusion of MDX-210 is 7–10 mg/m^2. The MTD is 7.0 mg/m^2. The BsAb MDX-210 antibody can deliver cytotoxins to tumor sites overexpressing the HER-2/*neu* protein.

▶ Bispecific monoclonal antibodies are hybrids constructed from 2 parent antibodies, with one having specificity for the tumor target cell and the other having specificity for immune-effector cells. Such bispecific monoclonal antibodies have been shown to be able to effectively eradicate tumor cells in vitro and in vivo by the cytotoxic activation of monocytes, monocyte-derived macrophages, T cells, and natural-killer cells.

This study reports a clinical trial of a bispecific antibody that binds to the HER-2/*neu* oncogene protein expressed on the tumors of some patients with breast cancer and ovarian cancer, as well as to type I Fc receptors for immunoglobulin G (IgG) (FcγRI). The biological activity of the bispecific antibody was established by increased plasma levels of monocyte products such as tumor necrosis factor and interleukin-6. Furthermore, the antibody was localized in tumor tissue in 2 patients. The efficacy of this approach depends on the identification of patients whose tumors express a high proportion of HER-2/*neu*–positive cells.

In this trial, 15 patients were treated, but it would be of interest to know how many patients were screened for eligibility to determine whether their tumor cells were high expressors of HER-2/*neu*. Nevertheless, the data demonstrate that bispecific antibodies can be safely administered, resulting in doses required for optimal monocyte-macrophage activation in vitro and that they produce the corresponding biological effect in patients. Clinical trials of efficacy are warranted.

R.F. Ozols, M.D., Ph.D.

Gene Transfer of Wild-Type p53 Results in Restoration of Tumor-Suppressor Function in a Medulloblastoma Cell Line

Rosenfeld MR, Meneses P, Dalmau J, Drobnjak M, Cordon-Cardo C, Kaplitt MG (Mem Sloan Kettering Cancer Ctr, New York; Rockefeller Univ, New York)
Neurology 45:1533–1539, 1995   2–14

Background.—Multiple genetic defects appear to be involved in tumorigenesis. However, the replacement of critical genes in cancer cells may suppress cell growth or induce cell death. There is a high frequency of mutations of the *p53* tumor-suppressor gene in human cancers, including primary brain tumors. This high frequency suggests that *p53* may play a critical role in carcinogenesis and tumor progression.

Methods and Findings.—In a set of experiments, wild-type *p53* was introduced into a human medulloblastoma cell line—DAOY cells—expressing mutant p53 using a defective herpes simplex viral (HSV) vector. After gene transfer, a novel expression of wild-type p53 protein was observed in the cells. The p53 protein was functionally active. Gene transfer resulted in elevated levels of mdm2 proteins and induced cell cycle arrest in most of the transduced cells.

Conclusions.—A defective HSV vector was used in to replace wild-type *p53* in DAOY cells expressing mutant *p53*. Examination of changes in the expression of mdm2 protein and effects on cell cycle progression showed that wild-type *p53* gene transfer results in the production of functionally active wild-type p53 protein.

▶ I include this report of an in vitro experiment because it is emblematic of what gene therapists hope to achieve in patients. As the reader probably knows, some forms of cancer are caused by a mutation of the *p53* gene, which, in its normal state, suppresses the development of cancer. The mutated gene does not have that capacity, thus allowing the cancer to develop. The wild-type *p53,* which is normal, was injected into a medulloblastoma cell line, and the authors demonstrated that they could restore the tumor suppressor function that was absent in the cancer. They used a herpes simplex viral vector, a common means of transferring genes in the laboratory. Most important, the p53 protein produced by the injected gene was functionally active. Once again, an exciting demonstration of changing the nature of a cancer cell has been demonstrated in the laboratory.

Making this process work in patients, however, faces major obstacles. From what we know of cancer, one must reverse the malignant potential of virtually all cancer cells to prevent a recurrence of the tumor. The efficiency of this type of gene transfer is not 100% even in vitro; it is likely to be far less efficient in vivo because one cannot ensure the approximation of the vector and all the cancer cells and because one also cannot ensure the entry of that vector with a functional gene in each of those cells. It is possible that the efficiency of this transfer will improve with time, but an informed and healthy skepticism should be the attitude of the day. Clinical oncologists have enormous respect for the ability of cancer cells to adapt to adverse circumstances such as exposure to radiation or chemotherapy. Nonetheless, the elegance and novelty of injecting functional genes into cancer and reversing its malignant potential are so attractive that this research must be encouraged and supported.

J.V. Simone, M.D.

3 Breast Cancer

Patient Preferences for Treatment of Metastatic Breast Cancer: A Study of Women With Early-Stage Breast Cancer
McQuellon RP, Muss HB, Hoffman SL, Russell G, Craven B, Yellen SB (Wake Forest Univ, Winston-Salem, NC; Rush Presbyterian/St Luke's Med Ctr, Chicago)
J Clin Oncol 13:858–868, 1995   3–1

Introduction.—For a number of reasons, there is renewed interest in the research of patient preferences for treatment. Such research may help patients and oncologists to select from among treatment alternatives with similar survival but differing toxicity. However, there are few data on patient preferences for cancer treatment. Preferences regarding treatment for metastatic breast cancer were studied among women with early-stage breast cancer.

Methods.—One hundred fifteen patients with stage I–IIIA breast cancer were interviewed. All had received primary treatment with mastectomy or lumpectomy plus radiotherapy. Fifty-eight percent had received adjuvant chemotherapy. The patients were presented with 4 hypothetical treatment scenarios describing a woman with metastatic breast cancer and a life expectancy of 18 months. As in common clinical situations, the side effects of treatment varied from low (with hormonal therapy) to life-threatening (with high-dose experimental therapy). The women were asked to indicate which of the 4 treatments they would accept and prefer for a 50% chance of increased life expectancy in increments ranging from 1 week to 5 years.

Results.—Contrary to the investigators' expectations, patient preferences were unaffected by quality of life at the time of the interview, previous chemotherapy, and difficulty of previous treatments. As the potential toxicity of the treatment increased, patients became less likely to accept it. Still, about 15% of patients said they would prefer high-risk treatment to gain as little as 1 month of additional life expectancy. Most patients would accept experimental treatment for a 5-year increase in survival; 34% to 82% of patients preferred different therapies for a 6-month increase (Table 3).

Younger patients were more likely to accept the risks of treatment for a small increase in survival. Fifty-four percent to 78% of the patients would choose to start treatment even if they had no symptoms of metastatic disease. Seventy-six percent would choose standard treatment or an ex-

TABLE 3.—Treatment Preferences vs. Additional Time Added to Survival

Clinical Scenario	1 Week		1 Month		6 Months		1 Year		18 Months		5 Years	
	No.	%	No.	%	No.	%	No.	%	No.	%	No.	%
Standard chemotherapy*	14	12	21	18	51	44	73	63	83	72	105	91
Experimental chemotherapy†	15	13	19	17	38	33	66	57	74	64	100	87
Standard chemotherapy‡§	8	16	14	24	36	62	46	79	50	86	57	98
vs. hormonal therapy	30	54	34	61	46	82	52	93	55	98	56	100
Standard chemotherapy‡‖	10	20	13	26	26	52	36	72	38	76	47	94
vs. high-dose experimental chemotherapy	4	8	5	9	18	34	34	64	39	74	53	100

* Ten subjects (9%) preferred no treatment.

† Fifteen subjects (13%) preferred no treatment.

‡ Subjects were asked to choose 1 of 2 treatment alternatives in these scenarios. After treatment selection, as in scenario 1 and 2, they were asked if they would take the treatment if it gave them a 50% chance of living an additional 5 years, 18 months, 1 year, etc., until they no longer would accept treatment.

§ One subject (1%) preferred no treatment. Fifty-eight subjects (50%) chose standard chemotherapy; 56 subjects (49%) chose hormonal therapy.

‖ Twelve subjects (10%) preferred no treatment. Fifty subjects (44%) chose standard therapy; 53 subjects (46%) chose high-dose experimental chemotherapy.

(Courtesy of McQuellon RP, Muss HB, Hoffman SL, et al: Patient preferences for treatment of metastatic breast cancer: A study of women with early-stage breast cancer. *J Clin Oncol* 13:858–868, 1995.)

perimental treatment to reduce symptoms or pain, even if there was no increase in life expectancy. Just 10% of patients would accept randomization to a clinical trial of high-dose vs. standard chemotherapy. Most patients reported no distress associated with participating in the study.

Conclusion.—When presented with hypothetical treatment scenarios, patients with early breast cancer report clear preferences for specific treatments. Patient preferences vary widely according to the risks and benefits of treatment. However, a significant proportion of patients would assume the risk of major toxicity if it yielded a minimal increase in overall survival.

▶ This interesting study sought to identify patient treatment preferences for metastatic breast cancer. Patients with early-stage breast cancer, but not those with metastatic disease, were studied. Four scenarios were developed—standard chemotherapy, experimental chemotherapy (designed to simulate a phase II trial), a choice of standard chemotherapy or hormonal therapy, and a randomized trial comparing standard chemotherapy to high-dose chemotherapy. Not surprisingly, patients with higher physical function scores on a self-report questionnaire measuring health-related quality of life were more likely to choose standard chemotherapy in the absence of symptoms, as were patients who had previously received adjuvant chemotherapy. A minority would accept experimental or standard chemotherapy (17% to 18%) for a prolongation of survival of even 1 month, and 33% to 44% would accept therapy for prolongation of 6 months or more. In considering a choice of standard chemotherapy or hormonal therapy, 24% of patients would select standard chemotherapy for a 1-month increase in survival, whereas 61% would accept hormonal therapies (see Table 3).

The fourth scenario, however, shows why it will be very difficult to prove that high-dose chemotherapy improves survival in patients with breast cancer (or, for that matter, in individuals with any other malignancy). This scenario was designed to simulate a randomized trial comparing standard chemotherapy with high-dose chemotherapy. Fewer than 10% of the patients would accept high-dose experimental chemotherapy for a 1-month improvement in survival, and only 34% would accept it for a 6-month improvement in survival. Sadly, but not surprisingly, 90% of patients would not permit randomization to decide on a treatment, although 64% would receive high-dose therapy for a 1-year improvement in survival.

This study has flaws. First, more than 90% of patients were white, and more than 50% had some college education. In addition, the patients studied were not those actually about to undergo treatment. In any case, this study provides some insight into the factors that influence a patient's choice regarding treatment of metastatic breast cancer and should be taken into consideration when offering them their treatment options. It also provides an impetus to find an acceptable strategy for incorporating these patients into clinical trials, particularly those requiring randomization. Otherwise, we may never know the answers to critical questions regarding the ultimate value of a new therapy, particularly high-dose chemotherapy, in this or other diseases.

G.J. Bosl, M.D.

Mammography in the Follow-Up After Breast-Conserving Treatment in Cancer of the Breast: Suitability for Mammographic Interpretation, Validity and Interobserver Variation
Jager JJ, Langendijk JA, Dohmen JP, Schreutelkamp IL, Volovics L, Van Engelshoven JM, De Jong JM, Schouten LJ, Hupperets PS, Blijham GH (Radiotherapeutisch Instituut Limburg, Heerlen, The Netherlands; St Jans Gasthuis, Weert, The Netherlands; Univ of Limburg, Maastricht, The Netherlands; et al)
Br J Radiol 68:754–760, 1995   3–2

Background.—The prognosis of patients with local relapse after breast-conserving surgery and radiotherapy for early-stage breast cancer relies on the extent of the relapse. Therefore, early detection is extremely important. However, little is known about the reliability and accuracy of mammography in detecting tumor in operated, irradiated breasts.

Methods.—Two radiologists reviewed mammographs, from 100 consecutive patients obtained before and after treatment. Minimum follow-up was 5 years. A total of 86 initial and 534 posttreatment mammograms from 92 patients were included in the final analysis.

Findings.—Mammogram suitability for interpretation did not differ from pretreatment mammograms. Suitability was significantly correlated with patient age and was greater in patients older than 50 years. Suitability for interpretation was not associated with treatment-related factors, even when irradiation was combined with concurrent chemotherapy. Interobserver agreement on classification was moderate. Receiver operating characteristic (ROC) analysis indicated that the optimal decision threshold lay between the categories of "uncertain" and "suspect" malignancy, with a sensitivity of 86% and a specificity of 98%. The most important malignant feature predicting local relapse seemed to be the appearance of new abnormal microcalcifications with or without tumor mass.

Conclusions.—Breast-conserving therapy did not appear to change the suitability of mammograms for interpretation, even when radiation treatment was combined with concurrent chemotherapy. Although mammography may be slightly less sensitive after breast-conserving treatment, it is just as specific as when used for screening.

▶ Breast conservation treatment strategies are now used for a significant proportion of women with early-stage breast cancer. Monitoring for recurrent mammary disease is a critical part of follow-up. The reliability of mammography in this setting has been challenged because of potential artifacts caused by soft-tissue alterations resulting from operations or radiation therapy. This study supports the use and value of follow-up mammography after breast conservation management. In my opinion, there should be no reluctance in the routine use of mammography to screen for recurrent disease in the previously treated breast. Careful follow-up for "uncertain" findings and immediate workup for "suspicious" or "malignant" findings are required.

G.J. Bosl, M.D.

Women's Attitudes About Receiving Mammographic Results Directly From Radiologists
Liu S, Bassett LW, Sayre J (Univ of California, Los Angeles)
Radiology 193:783–786, 1994   3–3

Background.—For medicolegal reasons, some radiologists are communicating mammographic findings and recommendations directly to patients. The attitudes of women toward this practice were investigated.

Methods and Findings.—At the time of mammographic assessment, 307 women completed a survey eliciting their opinions on the direct communication of mammographic findings by the radiologist. Most agreed that the radiologist should directly report normal and abnormal findings on site. The women also agreed that the radiologist should send to them a report written in lay language. The women also wanted the radiologist to inform them of recommendations for short-term follow-up examinations and to monitor their compliance.

Conclusions.—Most women agreed that radiologists should report mammographic results directly to their patients on site, regardless of whether these findings are normal or abnormal. Further research is needed to determine what women in diverse socioeconomic backgrounds and geographic locations think about this issue.

▶ Failure to diagnose cancer is the most common cause of malpractice against physicians who care for patients with cancer. This is particularly true for breast cancer, a disease in which a reduction in mortality resulting from early diagnosis based on mammographic screening is well established. Current practice dictates that abnormal results are provided directly to the referring health care provider. However, many patients undergoing screening may not have a primary health care provider. This study evaluated the reaction of patients who received their mammography results directly from the radiologist, rather than from their primary health care provider. A questionnaire was answered by 307 women. Between 87% and 94% of the patients either agreed or agreed strongly that mammography results should be directly communicated to them by the radiologist. An occasional patient disagreed, usually preferring the primary health care provider to provide the results and an explanation.

Involving the patient in her care is important. The stress of waiting for a report, as well as the increasing proportion of patients without primary physicians who undergo screening, suggests that results communicated by the radiologist may be preferable to sending a report to another provider. Such a report is still required, but direct communication eliminates one delay in communicating a diagnosis. However, this study does not address the follow-up of these patients to ascertain that those with abnormal results proceeded with appropriate diagnostic medical care.

G.J. Bosl, M.D.

Cured of Breast Cancer?
Joensuu H, Toikkanen S (Univ Central Hosp of Turku, Finland; Univ of Helsinki, Finland)
J Clin Oncol 13:62–69, 1995   3–4

Background.—Late deaths caused by breast cancer have been observed up to several decades after initial diagnosis. Therefore, the ultimate curability of this disease remains controversial. Late mortality caused by breast cancer was investigated.

Patients and Methods.—All patients with histologically confirmed breast cancer were identified from the files of hospitals located within a defined urban area of Finland, and the Finnish Cancer Registry. The clinical data and histologic and autopsy slides of 563 patients were reviewed. Sixty-six of these women had been followed for a median of 29 years (range, 22–44 years). The remaining 497 patients were monitored until death.

Findings.—Mortality from breast cancer was observed even during the fourth decade of follow-up. When excluding the 30 patients with diagnosed contralateral breast cancer, however, no disease-related deaths were identified after the 27th year of follow-up (Fig 2). In patients with axillary pN0 (node-negative) cancer, the 30-year survival rate was 62%. Compa-

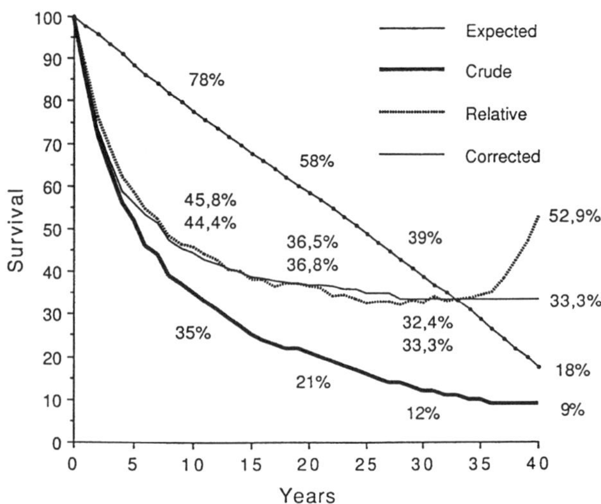

FIGURE 2.—Crude survival, expected survival, relative survival, and survival corrected for intercurrent deaths among 533 women with unilateral invasive breast cancer. Survival figures at 10, 20, and 30 years of follow-up are shown. (Courtesy of Joensuu H, Toikkanen S: Cured of breast cancer? *J Clin Oncol* 13:62–69, 1995.)

rable rates of 25% and 0% were observed in women with pN1 and pN2 (node-positive) cancers (Fig 3). The high 30-year survival rates in women with small (pT1N0M0) unilateral cancer was 80%; 45% for those with lobular cancer and 81% for those with special histologic types (Table 2).

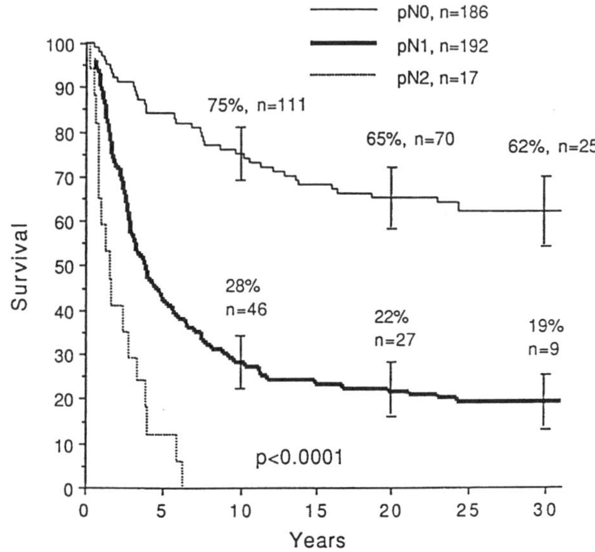

FIGURE 3.—Survival corrected for intercurrent deaths by postsurgical axillary nodal status (pN). Women with bilateral cancer, those with distant metastases at the time of diagnosis, and those treated with palliative surgery only have been excluded. The 95% confidence interval is shown by *bars*. (Courtesy of Joensuu H, Toikkanen S: Cured of breast cancer? *J Clin Oncol* 13:62–69, 1995.)

TABLE 2.—Long-Term Survival in Some Subgroups of Breast Cancer

Subgroup	No. of Patients	Survival Corrected for Intercurrent Deaths, Years (%)				χ^2	$P*$
		10	20	30	40		
Axillary nodal status†							
pN0	186	75	65	62	62	120.2	<.0001
pN1	192	28	22	19	19		
pN2	17	0	0	0	0		
Histologic grade							
grade 1	123	74	62	58	58	97.3	<.0001
grade 2	192	53	43	39	39		
grade 3	155	29	23	20	20		
Postsurgical stage							
stage I (pT1N0)	51	96	85	80	80	94.8	<.0001
stage II	242	51	43	41	41		
stage III	96	19	13	11	—		
Primary tumor size‡							
pT1	68	89	75	65	65	80.6	<.0001
pT2	273	52	44	41	41		
pT3–4	123	26	18	16	—		
Histologic type							
Special	49	93	87	81	81	43.1	<.0001
Lobular	66	57	45	45	45		
Ductal	355	43	35	30	30		

Women with bilateral cancer ($n = 30$), those who had distant metastases at the time of the diagnosis (M1, $n = 37$), and those treated with palliative surgery only ($n = 26$) have been excluded.
 * Log-rank test.
 † Postsurgical axillary nodal status was not available in 75 cases.
 ‡ Postsurgical tumor/node/metastasis (TNM) classification was not available in 6 cases.
 (Courtesy of Joensuu H, Toikkanen S: Cured of breast cancer? *J Clin Oncol* 13:62–69, 1995.)

These rates were achieved after adjusting for known intercurrent deaths or for mortality in the age- and sex-matched general population.

Conclusions.—Node-negative and node-positive breast cancer may be permanently cured even if managed with locoregional treatment only. The reported survival determinations may be considered as minimum values, because patients with breast cancer diagnosed between 1970 and 1984 showed significantly improved short-term survival rates (less than 20 years) compared with women with breast cancer diagnosed from 1945 to 1969 (Fig 4).

▶ Although most of us in the field of oncology strongly believe in the curability of breast cancer, there have always been a few people, mostly in other fields of medicine, who believe that breast cancer cannot be cured. To crystallize this controversy, one has to decide how much time is required before one can be confident of a "cure". Is 20 years long enough? It is surprising how little literature one can find on this point, and there are virtually no data beyond 30 years. In the real scheme of the natural history of breast cancer, 5 years—and even 10 years—is a woefully inadequate period.

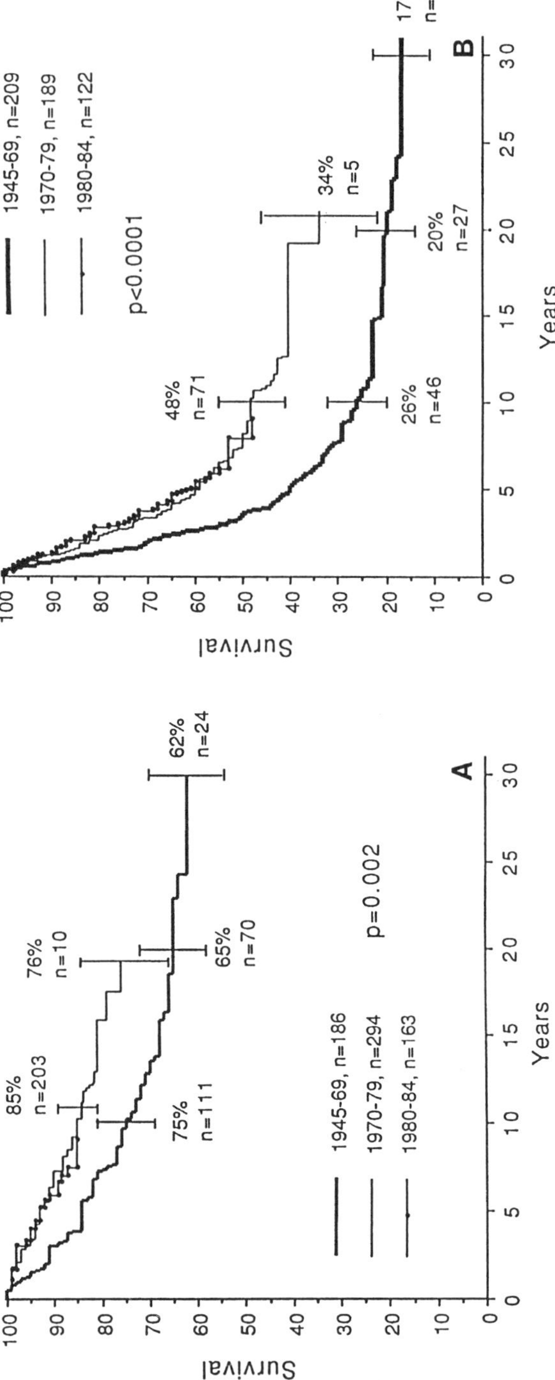

FIGURE 4.—Survival corrected for intercurrent deaths by decade of diagnosis. A, women with invasive pNO breast cancer; B, women with invasive pN+ cancer. The 95% confidence intervals are shown by *bars*. (Courtesy of Joensuu H, Toikkanen S: Cured of breast cancer? *J Clin Oncol* 13:62–69, 1994.)

This provocative series from Finland represents a very defined population that does not move around a great deal. I doubt this kind of information can ever really be generated in this country, where the population is so mobile. The median follow-up in this series was 29 years, a truly remarkable figure.

The problem of interpreting the available data revolves around competing causes of death over multiple decades. This argument is similar to that regarding prostate cancer, largely because of the very slow natural history associated with these 2 cancers in particular, as compared with most neoplasms. A special problem in breast cancer interpretation has to do with a second breast cancer in the contralateral breast. It is unclear whether this contralateral lesion represents a metastasis or a new primary caused by the enigmatic etiology associated with this cancer. In this series, the authors show that if one interprets this as a new cancer and excludes those patients, there appears to be a plateau after approximately 25 years. It should be emphasized that if one includes those patients who have a second contralateral breast cancer, the plateau still does not hold up.

I think this paper is essential reading for students of breast cancer because it may to look at their data carefully and to take a long-range approach of 30–40 years, where possible. For those who are interested in the natural history of untreated breast cancer, I would also like to mention what I think is probably the most important paper on the history of breast cancer ever written, that by Bloom, Richardson, and Harries.[1] This paper, taken from the bowels of the Middlesex Hospital in London, looks at patients from the 19th century and early 20th century for whom *no specific* treatment was given. It is important to realize that some patients lived 20 years or more *without any specific* treatment. Obviously they were subject to lots of problems, and the proportion of patients living 20 years was very modest; however, the point is that it was not necessarily an immediate death sentence. I think these two papers are important reading in today's climate in which sweeping conclusions are made on the basis of a 5-year actuarial projection, sometimes with only 1 patient out at the 5-year mark.

E. Glatstein, M.D.

Reference

1. Bloom HJ, Richardson WW, Harries EJ: Natural history of untreated breast cancer (1805–1933). Comparison of untreated and treated cases according to histological grade of malignancy. *BMJ* 5299:213, 1962.

Medical Outcomes of Care for Breast Cancer Among Health Maintenance Organization and Fee-for-Service Patients
Vernon SW, Heckel V, Jackson GL (Univ of Texas, Houston; The Kelsey-Seybold Found for Med Research and Education, Houston)
Clin Cancer Res 1:179–184, 1995   3–5

Objective.—Until recently, there have been few studies of the effects of various types of health insurance coverage on the quality of medical care, particularly among patients with cancer. A good topic for such studies is breast cancer, as it is relatively easy to diagnose and to treat effectively if detected early. The outcomes of breast cancer care were compared for patients with HMO vs. fee-for-service (FFS) health insurance.

Methods.—The historical cohort study used tumor registry data to compare treatment type, stage at diagnosis, and survival for 425 women with newly diagnosed breast cancer over an 8-year period. All patients were covered by FFS with third-party coverage or HMO plans offered by the same medical practice. Fifty-four percent of the patients were HMO members, and 46% were covered by various FFS plans. Survival status was known for all but 16 patients.

Results.—The median survival was 4.3 years for the HMO patients and 4.8 years for the FFS patients. Neither were there any significant differences in type of treatment or stage at diagnosis; about 40% of both groups had their cancer diagnosed at an early stage. The FFS patients were used as the reference group for Cox regression analysis. The unadjusted mortality rate ratio for survival was 0.66; after adjustment for age, race, and tumor stage, the rate ratio was 0.80.

Conclusions.—Among women with breast cancer treated by the same medical care provider, there are no systematic differences in outcomes for HMO members versus FFS patients. This result is in line with the findings of previous studies indicating similar disease-related outcomes for HMO members and persons with other types of health insurance coverage.

▶ The ability of different health care organizations to provide quality medical care is being critically evaluated. Attempts will be made to compare cost effectiveness and outcomes in health care systems ranging from HMOs to FFS physicians, to cancer research centers. Although survival remains the most obvious outcome by which to compare different medical health care systems, numerous other factors will need to be evaluated to develop a true comparison. Parameters such as patient satisfaction and morbidity of treatment, in addition to survival, are important factors in cancer care.

R.F. Ozols, M.D., Ph.D.

Potential for Cost Economies in Guiding Therapy in Patients With Metastatic Breast Cancer
Robertson JFR, Whynes DK, Dixon A, Blamey RW (City Hosp, Nottingham; Univ of Nottingham, England)
Br J Cancer 72:174–177, 1995   3–6

Background.—Treatment response in patients with advanced breast cancer has traditionally been evaluated using the International Union Against Cancer, or UICC, criteria. However, it may be possible to attain comparably effective assessment at a lower cost by using serum markers. Potential cost savings from the use of serum markers instead of conventional assessment were estimated.

Methods.—Cost savings estimates were based on data from 2 sources: broad retrospective clinical parameters established from the accumulated research done at 1 breast cancer unit in Nottingham, England, and the unit costs of monitoring, hormone treatment, and chemotherapy incurred at the City Hospital in Nottingham. To avoid overstating the cost savings, it was assumed that serum marker assessment at diagnosis would include a chest radiograph, bone scan, and liver ultrasound study. Both assessment methods require full blood counts and biochemistry before each cycle of chemotherapy.

Findings.—The UICC assessment was shown to be about 50% more expensive than serum marker assessment. The use of serum marker assessment would cost £189.07 per patient. After the first year, the annual cost of UICC assessment would be £304.62, and that of serum marker assessment would be £123.50. Nationally, the average savings would be estimated at £10.83 to £13.74 million per year. Assuming that only about half the patients with metastatic breast cancer receive any chemotherapy, this estimate would be £8.16 to £10.35 million.

Conclusions.—The estimates based on this model suggest that the use of serum marker assessment instead of UICC criteria for determining treatment response in patients with advanced breast cancer may be more cost-effective. A randomized, controlled trial is now needed to provide further support for this possibility.

▶ What is the appropriate policy by which women receiving treatment for metastatic breast cancer should be followed for progressive disease? Re-evaluation of established metastatic sites is generally needed to establish therapeutic response. Periodic biochemical and radiographic assessment is expensive, however, and relatively little is known about whether such follow-up care improves survival. Robertson and colleagues suggest a biochemical index of response that incorporates markers such as CA 15-3, carcinoembryonic antigen (CEA), and sedimentation rate. Compared with a recommended UICC assessment recommendation, the biochemical index is reportedly less expensive.

The trouble with this study is that it presents a hypothetical scenario. Real patients are not followed. I do not perform the tests recommended in the UICC assessment (skeletal survey and chest radiograph every 3 months in all patients). Moreover, I do not necessarily change therapy based solely on an increasing CA 15-3 or CEA level if the patient is completely asymptomatic. However, this study points out a significant problem: There are few data that address the "efficacy" of the follow-up programs that we use. Assessment of known metastatic sites at regular intervals appears logical, but how frequently should it be done in the patient who has improved or who is asymptomatic? How often should tests be done in the absence of known disease at that site (a chest radiograph in the absence of known pulmonary metastases)? We must spend more time addressing these end points while continuing to perform therapeutic studies. For now, I would recommend periodic reevaluation of known visceral metastatic sites, bone scans when clinically indicated, blood studies to measure the known effects of chemotherapy or hormonal therapy on end organ function, and clinical judgment in the frequency of test ordering. Both too many and too few tests will have a negative impact on patient care.

G.J. Bosl, M.D.

Breast Implants and Breast Cancer: Reanalysis of a Linkage Study
Bryant H, Brasher P (Alberta Cancer Board, Calgary, Canada)
N Engl J Med 332:1535–1539, 1995   3–7

Background.—In 1992, a study by Berkel et al. concluded that women who had breast augmentation had a significantly lower risk of breast cancer development than did the general population. However, several problems with the analysis were noted. The rounding of dates, failure to adjust for women who moved out of the study area, failure to identify patients after changes in marital status, and the use of a limited number of variables conferred the potential for underlinkage. Hence, the data were reanalyzed.

Methods.—Eligible women with bilateral breast augmentation were identified, using a data set from the Alberta Health Care insurance plan. To identify breast cancers developing during the study, these data were linked to the Alberta Cancer registry, using a combination of deterministic and probabilistic methods. Differing study eligibility rates, induction periods (the time after augmentation during which a developing malignancy is presumed to have a presurgical origin) and types of breast cancer were considered in the calculation of standardized incidence ratios. The study was also updated with the addition of 9 cases of breast cancer occurring in 1991.

Results.—The original study reported an overall standardized incidence ratio for breast cancer of 0.48 in women who had undergone breast augmentation; with consideration of a 10-year induction period, the ratio was 0.16. Using 1973 as the starting point, the revised analysis showed a standardized incidence ratio of 0.68 with a 10-year induction period. The ratios for 0- and 5-year induction periods were 0.76 and 0.85, respectively. None of these ratios differed significantly from 1. The higher standardized incidence ratios of the reanalysis were the result of substantial differences in the numbers of person-years at risk. At reanalysis, the cohort size was reduced by 7%, primarily because of the exclusion of women with unilateral implants and revision of the starting and ending dates.

Discussion.—The reanalysis derived a lesser number of person-years at risk, not only because of reduced cohort size but also because of the failure of the original protocol to account for out-migration and because of its consistent overestimation of follow-up time (caused by the rounding of dates). Underlinkage may exist, even in the reanalysis, partly because of the difficulties in tracing women whose registry identification numbers changed because of marital status. Regardless, the reanalysis does not support the original conclusion of the study. The apparent risk of breast cancer occurring among the women studied during the determined period cannot be deemed to be either significantly higher or lower than that seen in the general population.

▶ In 1992, Berkel and colleagues[1] reported the results of a large study analyzing the potential relationship between breast implantation and the subsequent development of breast cancer. Their analysis linked 2 large databases: a provincially funded health insurance plan (Alberta Health Care) and the Alberta Cancer Registry. The analysis suggested that the likelihood of breast cancer developing was markedly reduced in women undergoing implantation for a (standardized incidence ratio of 0.16, assuming a 10-year induction period).

In 1994, Bryant et al.[2] suggested that there were significant flaws in the original analysis of the data. Among the potential problems, there was a consistent over calculation of half a year for every woman in the cohort, because dates were rounded in the original study. Second, women who moved out of the province were lost to follow-up in the Alberta Cancer Registry. Third, the Alberta Health Care number, which identified patients within the health plan, was not unique over a patient's lifetime, and if events such as marriage, divorce, or other changes occurred, another patient number could have been assigned. Fourth, the manner in which patients were identified included procedures with a specific fee code, which may have introduced patients undergoing surgical procedures other than implantation or breast surgery.

The new analysis of these original databases takes into consideration the problems with the original study. With reanalysis, the cohort size was reduced by approximately 7%. In addition, there is a significant discrepancy between the 2 analyses in terms of the number of person-years at risk used to calculate the risk of breast cancer. The original study estimated in excess of 120,000 person-years at risk, whereas the maximal estimate in the present analysis was 89,000. The reduced number of person-years at risk is attributed to the following: (1) a large proportion of women removed from the cohort were excluded early, taking with them a disproportionally high number of years of follow-up; (2) migration was not accounted for in the original study but was considered in this study; and (3) an overestimation of approximately one half year per woman in the original study accounted for additional reduction in the number of person-years at risk.

Despite the flaws identified in the original study, the number of postimplantation cancers identified in this study is 45 compared with 41 cancers identified in the original study. Because the number of person-years at risk for the 10-year induction period was significantly overestimated in the original work, there is a marked discrepancy between the standardized incidence ratios calculated between the original study and the reanalysis. The standardized incidence ratio calculated for the 10-year induction period in the reanalysis is 0.68 compared with 0.16 in the original study.

The reanalysis indicates that over the period considered, the risk of breast cancer was not higher or significantly lower than that of the general population. The analysis did not consider the type of implant used and its potential relationship to the development of breast cancer. The use of polyurethane-covered implants is considered low in Alberta. Longer follow-up of this cohort will be necessary to determine whether a longer induction period is needed to induce breast cancer in patients undergoing implantation.

W.J. Gradishar, M.D.

References

1. Berkel H, Birdsell DC, Jenkins H: Breast augmentation: A risk factor for breast cancer? *N Engl J Med* 326:1649–1653, 1992.
2. Bryant H, Brasher PMA, van de Sande JH, et al: Review of methods in "Breast augmentation: A risk factor for breast cancer?"*N Engl J Med* 330:293, 1994.

Discovery Method and Stage of Breast Cancer in Two Different Patient Populations

Tigges S, Monticciolo DL, Kessler L (Emory Univ, Atlanta, Ga)
South Med J 88:1114–1117, 1995   3–8

Background.—Previous research has found that a very low percentage of breast malignancies in a given series is detected by mammography. This is almost undoubtedly because of underuse. The stage and method of discovery of newly diagnosed breast cancers in 2 separate patient populations were reported.

Methods.—Medical records at an urban and a suburban teaching hospital were reviewed retrospectively. Three hundred four patients with breast cancer were seen at the suburban center in 1992, and 155 such patients were seen at the urban hospital during 1991 and 1992. Patients who were younger than 40 years, male, or who were being seen for recurrent disease were excluded, leaving 100 and 112 patients at the 2 centers, respectively.

Findings.—Cancers were discovered mammographically in only 26% of the patients at the urban hospital and in 38% of those at the surburban hospital. At both centers, cancers identified on mammography were of a lower stage than were those discovered by clinical assessment. Eighty-three percent of mammographically detected cancers at the urban hospital and 79% at the suburban hospital were stage I or 0 compared with 20.5% and 35.5% detected clinically at the respective centers.

Conclusion.—Mammography was almost certainly underused in these 2 patient populations. Further efforts are needed to educate the public as well as clinicians regarding the benefits of mammographic screening for breast cancer.

▶ This study from Emory University suggests that the use of mammography still is not satisfactory. Fewer lesions were detected by mammography at the urban hospital than at the suburban hospital. Mammographically discovered cancers appear to be lower stage than those that were detected clinically and, thus, had a better prognosis. The numbers in this particular study are too small to make any sweeping conclusion, but the data give a provocative implication that urban centers need to exploit mammography to a far greater degree than has been done until now.

E. Glatstein, M.D.

Prediction of Axillary Lymph Node Status in Breast Cancer Patients by Use of Prognostic Indicators
Ravdin PM, De Laurentiis M, Vendely T, Clark GM (Univ of Texas Health Science Ctr, San Antonio; Nichols Inst, San Juan Capistrano, Calif)
J Natl Cancer Inst 86:1771–1775, 1994   3–9

Objective.—Many women with breast cancer could be spared the morbidity and expense of axillary lymph node dissection if it were possible to accurately predict their nodal status from basic clinical information and primary tumor characteristics. A very low or very high risk of axillary node positivity cannot be predicted by tumor size alone. The ability of prognostic indicators to predict axillary node status in patients with primary breast cancer was assessed.

Methods.—The analysis used data from 26,683 patients from the National Breast Cancer Tissue Resource. The patients were randomized into 2 groups: a training set, in which patient information was used to construct predictive models, and a validation set, in which the prospective models were evaluated prospectively. Complete prognostic factors were available for 11,964 patients: 5,963 in the training set and 6,001 in the validation set. All had tumors measuring no more than 5 cm and had undergone evaluation of at least 15 axillary lymph nodes. The factors considered in the construction of prognostic models included tumor size, number of positive nodes, age, measured levels of estrogen receptors and progesterone receptors (PgR), ploidy as determined from DNA flow cytometry, and S-phase fraction. Nodal status was predicted using logistic regression models.

Results.—The multivariate predictive models constructed included tumor size, age, S phase, and PgR as independent predictors (Table 2). Using these models, the investigators were able to identify patient risks of node positivity ranging from 6% to 79%. Identified risks of having 10 or more

TABLE 2.—Logistic Regression β-Coefficients

Variable	≥1 positive node	β coefficients (SE) ≥4 positive nodes	≥10 positive nodes
Log (tumor size + 1)	4.342 (0.216)	4.522(0.270)	4.555(0.383)
Log (S phase + 1)	0.3992 (0.0918)	0.4241(0.112)	0.8471(0.161)
Age	−0.01343 (0.0021)	−0.00843(0.0026)	—
Log (PgR + 1)	0.06919 (0.0259)	—	—
Constant	−2.201 (0.193)	−3.720(0.239)	−5.625(0.247)

Abbreviation: SE, standard error.
(Courtesy of Ravdin PM, De Laurentis M, Vendely T, et al: *J Natl Cancer Inst* 86:1771–1775, 1994.)

TABLE 5.—Practical Application of Equation Projections for a 60-Year-Old Woman

Tumor size, cm	% node positive (95% confidence interval)	
	Low S phase and low PgR	High S phase and high PgR
1.0	15.1 (13.2–16.8)	31.1 (17.9–34.1)
2.0	25.7 (22.8–28.4)	46.6 (43.9–49.2)
3.0	35.6 (32.9–38.3)	58.2 (55.2–61.2)
4.0	44.2 (41.0–47.5)	66.7 (63.8–69.8)
5.0	51.6 (48.2–55.4)	73.0 (70.3–75.8)

(Courtesy of Ravdin PM, De Laurentis M, Vendely T, et al: *J Natl Cancer Inst* 86:1771–1775, 1994.)

positive nodes ranged from less than 1% to about 30%. In no case, however, was it possible to identify patient subsets with more than a 95% likelihood of node negativity or positivity (Table 5).

Conclusions.—Prognostic indicators added to tumor size can improve estimates of axillary node status in breast cancer patients. However, the predictive models constructed cannot avoid the need for axillary node dissection in patients for whom information on node status would influence treatment decisions. There are some patient subsets with less than a 5% chance of having 10 or more positive nodes. Therefore, if the only goal of axillary dissection were to identify patients with this high-risk feature, the procedure could be avoided in some patients.

▶ As the therapy of patients with stage I, II, and III breast cancer evolves, there is a greater urgency to identify high-, intermediate-, and low-risk patient subgroups who might derive benefit from lesser (hormonal therapy alone) and dose-intensive (with stem-cell support) treatment. Unfortunately, the size of the primary tumor does not provide for clear stratification. Ravdin and colleagues examined data from 26,683 patients from the National Breast Cancer Tissue Resource. The patients in this resource were randomly assigned to a training set or validation set to prospectively evaluate predictive factors. Tumor size, S-phase fraction, age, estrogen and PgR status, ploidy, and the number of examined lymph nodes were all investigated.

A regression model that enabled prediction of involved node subgroups ranging between 6% involved and 79% involved was developed. Similar analyses could predict whether a patient was likely to have 4 or more involved lymph nodes or 10 or more involved lymph nodes. Tumor size, S-phase fraction, patient age, and PgR status were independent predictor variables with a decreasing impact on the likelihood of involved lymph nodes. Curiously, PgR status was found to be directly related to the likelihood of an involved lymph node, contrary to an expected inverse relationship. For predicting 10 or more involved lymph nodes, however, only tumor size and S-phase fraction appear to be predictor variables (see Table 2). A practical application would be to project the likelihood of involved lymph nodes for a patient of a specific age. The authors performed this analysis for a 60-year-old woman (see Table 5). Although the model improves the ability to predict whether lymph nodes will be involved, the degree of improvement is small. Therefore, with current predictive factors, it seems unlikely that good models can be developed that would eliminate the need for axillary lymph node dissection in the staging of patients with breast cancer.

G.J. Bosl, M.D.

Expression of the bcl-2 Gene Family in Normal and Malignant Breast Tissue: Low *bax*-α Expression in Tumor Cells Correlates With Resistance Towards Apoptosis
Bargou RC, Daniel PT, Mapara MY, Bommert K, Wagener C, Kallinich B, Royer HD, Dörken B (Max Delbrück Ctr for Molecular Medicine, Berlin-Buch, Germany)
Int J Cancer 60:854–859, 1995   3–10

Introduction.—Because apoptosis (programmed cell death) has been shown to be an important regulator of tissue development, differentiation, and homeostasis, it was hypothesized that dysregulation of apoptosis may play a role in the pathogenesis of cancer. The hypothesis was investigated by analyzing, in both normal and malignant cells, the expression of genes known to regulate apoptosis: *bcl-2, bcl-x,* and *bax.*

Methods.—Using Northern blotting of messenger RNA preparations and polymerase chain reaction analysis, the expression of the apoptosis-regulating genes was evaluated and compared in human breast cancer cell lines and normal breast epithelial cell lines, and in breast cancer tissue samples and normal breast tissue obtained at mastectomy. To investigate the sensitivity of *bas* expression to apoptosis, apoptosis was induced with either serum (growth-factor) depletion or with monoclonal immunoglobulin 3 antibody (anti-APO-1 antibody), and the dead cells were excluded with propidium iodide staining.

Results.—Both normal and cancer cell lines and normal and cancer tissue cells expressed comparable levels of *bcl-x* and *bcl-2*, with nearly all expressing the long splice variant of *bcl-x_s*. The normal tissue and epithelial cell lines expressed relatively high levels of the *bax*-α variant compared with cancer tissue and cell lines, which expressed little or none of this 1-kb splice variant. One of the cancer cell lines had no detectable *bax* expression. Normal cell lines, with high expression of *bax*-α, demonstrated nearly 100% cell death within 7 days after serum depletion, whereas cancer cell lines, with low levels of *bax*-α expression, demonstrated prolonged survival, even after serum depletion. Similar results were obtained in the normal and cancer tissue cells and with anti-APO-1–induced apoptosis.

Conclusion.—These findings suggest that an imbalance between the anti-apoptosis genes and apoptosis-promoting genes could result in dysregulation of apoptosis in breast cancer. Other studies have found that *p53*, the tumor suppressor gene involved in the pathogenesis of breast cancer, may be involved in regulating *bcl-2* and *bax* inversely lends further support for the hypothesized role for dysregulation of apoptosis in the pathogenesis of breast cancer.

▶ Apoptosis (programmed cell death) is a critical cell process involved in the regulation of tissue development and organism homeostasis. It is under the control of several genes and requires intact *p53* function. In the breast and prostate, hormone ablation results in cell death and organ involution. Therefore, disruption of the genetic events that regulate apoptosis might be expected to result in deregulated cell growth and the formation of neoplasms.

The *bcl-2* gene was first recognized as involved in the t(14; 18) chromosomal translocation characteristic of many B-cell lymphomas. This translocation results in the increased expression of *bcl-2* and deregulated lymphoid cell growth. In normal cell systems, what balances normal *bcl-2* expression, thereby permitting apoptosis and regulation of cell proliferation? A counteracting protein product must be present. Recently, the *bax* gene family was discovered to have significant homology to *bcl-2,* and its protein product was shown to promote apoptosis. Its protein product forms a complex (heterodimer) with the *bcl-2* protein product, thereby regulating the antiapoptotic effect of *bcl-2.* Therefore, under normal circumstances, overexpression of *bcl-2* or low expression or failure to express *bax* would result in a fundamentally similar physiologic state: relatively high *bcl-2* levels. Either situation could theoretically support neoplastic growth.

In this study, Bargou and colleagues examined several human breast cancer cell lines, 2 cell lines derived from nonmalignant breast epithelium and 10 tumor samples for *bcl-2* and *bax* family genes. The *bcl-2* gene and *bcl-x$_L$* (a closely related gene with a similar antiapoptotic effect) were found to be expressed at similar levels in normal breast cell lines, breast cancer–derived cell lines, and breast tumors. However, the *bax*-α message (one form of *bax* gene expression) was similar to that of *bcl-2* in the 2 normal cell lines and in nonmalignant tissue but was low-to-absent in tumor cell lines and tumor samples. Therefore, although *bcl-2* expression is not increased, its relative expression compared with *bax* is high.

This study indicates that in normal and malignant breast tissue, resistance to apoptosis may be mediated through aberrant expression of *bax* and not overexpression of *bcl-2.* In a more general sense, this study shows that identifying the reasons for neoplastic transformation and drug resistance will be difficult and that multiple gene families are involved in the control of apoptosis. Further study will be necessary in other tumor systems to determine the degree to which different malignancies are resistant to apoptosis and the mechanisms by which this resistance is induced. As a tumor marker, high *bcl-2* or low *bax* expression have similar physiologic effects, and the relative ratio of one to the other will need to be evaluated.

G.J. Bosl, M.D.

_p53_ in Node-Negative Breast Carcinoma: An Immunohistochemical Study of Epidemiologic Risk Factors, Histologic Features, and Prognosis

Rosen PP, Lesser ML, Arroyo CD, Cranor M, Borgen P, Norton L (Mem Sloan-Kettering Cancer Ctr, New York; North Shore Univ Hosp, Manhasset, NY)

J Clin Oncol 13:821–830, 1995   3–11

Background.—The oncogene *p53* has been widely studied for its role in the origin and prognosis of breast cancer. Immunohistochemical techniques can detect protein changes resulting from alterations or overexpression of *p53*. The relationships between *p53* expression and various aspects of node-negative breast carcinoma—epidemiologic risk factors, tumor histopathologic findings, prognosis, and *HER2/neu* (HER) expression—were examined.

Methods.—Immunohistochemical staining was performed for *p53* in formaldehyde-fixed, paraffin-embedded primary invasive carcinomas from 440 node-negative patients with breast carcinoma. The patients were prospectively followed for a median of 119 months.

Results.—Expression of *p53*, on its own or in combination with HER, was not a significant prognostic factor, nor was *p53* consistently associated with any of the epidemiologic risk factors for breast cancer. Sixty-eight percent of medullary carcinomas expressed *p53* compared with 9% of the lobular and 23% of the ductal carcinomas. No low-grade tubular or papillary carcinomas and few mucinous carcinomas expressed *p53*. Expression of the oncogene was significantly more frequent in high-grade or poorly differentiated nuclear grade tumors than in low- or intermediate-grade tumors. A significant inverse relationship was noted between estrogen receptor positivity and *p53* expression. When the tumor immunophenotype was *p53* (+)/HER(−), the tumors were more likely to be medullary or ductal carcinomas with a marked lymphoplasmacytic reaction. Infiltrating lobular carcinomas tended to be *p53* (−)/HER(−). The prognosis was best for *p53* (+)/HER(+) carcinomas and worst for *p53* (−)/HER(+) tumors. For patients with T1N0M0 infiltrating duct carcinoma, this trend was significant for recurrence-free and overall survival.

Conclusion.—In patients with node-negative breast carcinoma, *p53* expression is not a reliable prognostic indicator and is not associated with epidemiologic risk factors for the disease. However, the combined immunophenotypic expression of *p53* and HER is significantly associated with some histologic types of breast cancer and with prognosis in patients with T1N0M0 disease. Combined oncogene immunophenotypes may be associated with seemingly paradoxical relationships to prognosis; these relationships may offer clues to the mechanisms of oncogene interaction in the biology of breast cancer.

▶ In a paper recently published in *Cancer* by the same authors,[1] overexpression of *HER* was not found to be a prognostic factor in patients with T1 or

T2, node-negative breast cancer. In this study, *p53* expression determined by immunohistochemistry was evaluated. *TP53*, the gene encoding *p53*, is known to be mutated in about 50% of breast cancers. The oncogene *p53* has tumor-suppressor functions. Mutant *p53* has a prolonged half-life, permitting detection by immunohistochemistry. However, the antibody recognizes both wild-type and mutant *p53*, and it relies on the prolonged half-life of mutant *p53* for its association with mutations in *TP53*. There are other reasons for detection of *p53* that is not mutated, and false positives implicating *TP53* mutations do exist.

In this study, immunohistochemical detection of *p53* was expressed in about two thirds of medullary carcinomas and much less frequently in lobular and ductal carcinomas. There was no significant difference in the frequency of a positive reaction between T1 and T2 primary tumors; *p53* immunoreactivity could not be shown to be significantly related to survival or time to recurrence. Associations between the expression of *p53* and HER was observed. The expression of *p53* was associated with an absence of estrogen receptor expression. The most favorable outcome in the combined series of T1 and T2 tumors was noted for tumors that were both *p53* (+) and HER (+); recurrence patterns paralleled those of survival and were noted to be highest in tumors that were *p53* (+)/HER(−). However, none of these differences were statistically significant.

This study shows the importance of the evaluation of multiple prognostic factors. Mutations in *TP53* and both overexpression and the importance of HER implicate multiple pathways of cell growth deregulation in tumors and imply the need to evaluate them together when drawing clinical associations. Based on the data in this study, neither *p53* nor HER should be part of the routine evaluation of node-negative T1 and T2 breast cancers and the decisions that need to be made regarding adjuvant chemotherapy.

G.J. Bosl, M.D.

Reference

1. Rosen PP, Lesser ML, Arroyo CD, et al: Immunohistochemical detection of HER2/neu in patients with axillary lymph node negative breast carcinoma. A study of epidemiologic risk factors, histologic features, and prognosis. *Cancer* 75:1320–1326, 1995.

Immunohistochemical Detection of *HER2/neu* in Patients With Axillary Lymph Node Negative Breast Carcinoma: A Study of Epidemiologic Risk Factors, Histologic Features, and Prognosis

Rosen PP, Lesser ML, Arroyo CD, Cranor M, Borgen P, Norton L (Mem Sloan-Kettering Cancer Ctr, New York; North Shore Univ Hosp, Manhasset, NY)

Cancer 75:1320–1326, 1995   3–12

Introduction.—Several recent studies have evaluated the prognostic importance of the *HER2/neu* (HER) oncogene in axillary lymph node–

negative breast carcinoma. Some of these studies have suggested that altered expression of HER is an unfavorable prognostic factor, but this conclusion is controversial. Relationships of HER expression, as detected by immunohistochemistry, with epidemiologic risk factors, tumor histopathologic findings, and prognosis were examined.

Methods.—The analysis included 440 patients with primary breast cancer and pathologically negative axillary lymph nodes. The median follow-up was 119 months. Immunohistochemical staining was performed for HER on 10% formalin-fixed, paraffin-embedded tumor specimens.

Findings.—Forty-four percent of the tumors showed positive membrane immunoreactivity for HER. The patients' HER status was not a significant prognostic factor (Fig 2), nor was it consistently associated with epide-

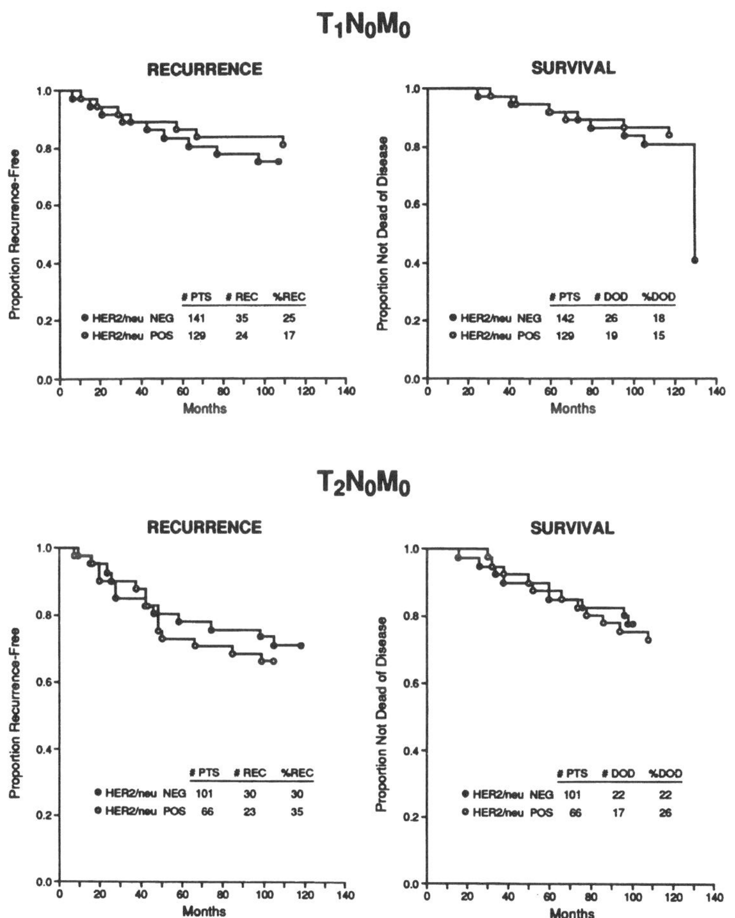

FIGURE 2.—Effect of *HER2/neu* on recurrence-free and disease-related survival in axillary lymph node-negative breast carcinoma stratified by tumor/node/metastasis stage. (Courtesy of Rosen PP, Lesser ML, Arroyo CD, et al: *Cancer* 75:1320–1326, copyright © 1995. Reprinted by permission of Wiley-Liss, Inc., a division of John Wiley & Sons, Inc.)

miologic risk factors. Only 10% of medullary carcinomas were HER-positive compared with 49% of other ductal carcinomas and 43% of lobular carcinomas. Therefore, there was a significant correlation between HER and the histopathologic features of the carcinomas.

Conclusion.—In patients with axillary lymph node–negative breast carcinoma, immunohistochemical demonstration of HER does not appear to be a significant prognostic factor. It is not associated with major epidemiologic risk factors for breast cancer, although it is significantly correlated with the phenotypic features. The latter associations may be useful in individual diagnosis, but they probably are not strong enough for use in refining the classification of breast carcinoma. The immunohistochemical changes in HER identified in this study most likely do not occur in the earliest stages of carcinogenesis.

▶ The use of prognostic factors to direct treatment decisions is well established. In breast cancer management, primary tumor size and axillary lymph node status are the most powerful independent predictors of outcome. Recently, overexpression of the *HER2/neu* (HER) oncogene has been touted as an additional independent prognostic factor. In a recent study,[1] HER overexpression (also called c-*erb*B-2) was found to be an independent prognostic factor in patients receiving adjuvant chemotherapy with a combination of cyclophosphamide, doxorubicin, and 5-fluorouracil in women with node-positive breast cancer. The question arises: Is HER overexpression a prognostic factor in women with axillary node–negative breast cancer?

Rosen and colleagues evaluated 440 primary tumors from women with negative axillary lymph nodes. For patients with both T1 and T2 primary tumors, survival was not influenced by HER overexpression in the primary tumor (see Fig 2). The authors did not find that a very low proportion of medullary breast cancers overexpressed HER (10%) when compared with other cell types. Based on these data, an immunohistochemical evaluation for HER overexpression is not justified as a routine test in tumors without axillary lymph node involvement.

G.J. Bosl, M.D.

Reference

1. Muss HB, Thor AD, Berry DA, et al: c-*erb*B-2 Expression and response to adjuvant therapy in women with node-positive early breast cancer. *N Engl J Med* 330:1260–1266, 1994.

Chromosome Abnormalities in Bilateral Breast Carcinomas: Cytogenetic Evaluation of the Clonal Origin of Multiple Primary Tumors

Pandis N, Teixeira MR, Gerdes A-M, Limon J, Bardi G, Andersen JA, Idvall I, Mandahl N, Mitelman F, Heim S (Odense Univ, Denmark; Univ Hosp, Lund, Sweden; Norwegian Radium Hosp, Oslo, Norway)
Cancer 76:250–258, 1995   3–13

Background.—Presumably, acquired somatic mutations are crucial in carcinogenesis. However, nothing is known about the chromosome aberrations of bilateral breast carcinomas. The first characterization of the karyotypic profile of bilateral breast carcinomas was recently presented.

Methods.—Sixteen breast carcinomas from 8 patients with bilateral disease were obtained for analysis. Cytogenetic examination was performed on 18 specimens. Fluorescence in situ hybridization with painting probes was used to supplement the banding analysis.

Findings.—The same clonal abnormalities were found in samples from both breasts in 2 cases, indicating that the bilaterality was the product of a metastatic process. The absence of such similarities in the rest of the specimens indicated that the 2 carcinomas had an independent origin. Examples of both karyotypically related and unrelated clones were found in multifocal lesions in the same breast. A total of 9 specimens showed multiple clones without similarities, sometimes together with other karyotypically related clones. Bilateral carcinomas did not appear to be cytogenetically different from unilateral ones. Recurrent chromosomal abnormalities included der(1;16)(q10;p10), del(1)(q11-n12), del(1)(q42), and del(3)(p12-n13p14-n21).

Conclusions.—Bilateral and unilateral breast carcinomas have the same cytogenetic aberrations, including evidence of polyclonality. Most bilateral breast cancers appear to occur independently, although some result from metastasis from one breast to the other. Bilateral breast carcinomas are similar to multifocal breast cancers in this sense. Bilateral tumors may be a special case of multifocal disease.

Identification of Multiple Breast Cancers of Multicentric Origin by Histological Observations and Distribution of Allele Loss on Chromosome 16q

Tsuda H, Hirohashi S (Natl Cancer Ctr Research Inst, Tokyo, Japan)
Cancer Res 55:3395–3398, 1995   3–14

Background.—Frequently, breast cancer is clinically and/or histopathologically detected as multiple lesions. It is not known whether the origin of such lesions can be objectively identified by comparing their loss of heterozygosity (LOH) patterns.

Methods and Findings.—Loss of heterozygosity on chromosome 16q was investigated in 60 cases of multiple breast cancer. Southern blot analysis was used. Thirty unilateral multiple cancers were morphologically classified into 3 groups on the basis of continuity among tumors and satellite nodule features: group A included 11 cases of multicentric origin; group B, 15 cases of multifocal invasion of 1 intraductal carcinoma; and group C, 4 cases of intramammary metastases. Two groups of cancers were studied for comparison: 11 in group D were synchronously bilateral and 19 in group E were sets of a primary tumor and a lymph node metastasis. Assuming that LOH on chromosome 16q occurred randomly in half the breast cancers at an early stage, the number of cases showing a concordant LOH pattern on chromosome 16q among tumors was compared, and the value was estimated from a normal distribution model in each group. The allele pattern on chromosome 16q among tumors in groups A and D was concordant in 5 of 11 cases each, supporting their independent occurrence and multicentric origin. The LOH pattern among tumors was identical in all cancers in groups B, C, and E, indicating their monocentric origin.

Conclusions.—The findings of this comparison of the LOH pattern in multiple breast cancer were consistent with those of the morphological classification. Loss of heterozygosity on chromosome 16q appears to occur at the preinvasive stage and usually does not change during the process of stromal tumor invasion. Comparisons of LOH patterns may be of diagnostic value.

▶ Multifocal and bilateral breast cancers are well-known phenomena. In general, management is dictated by the presumption that these cancers are separate and distinct from the initial primary tumor and do not represent metastases. Clinically this makes sense, but the biological basis for this clinical management has been lacking. These 2 papers (Abstracts 3–13 and 3–14) show that multifocal breast cancer and bilateral breast cancers are polyclonal in origin. The patterns of loss of heterozygosity on the long arm of chromosome 16q were similar among tumors arising from a single intraductal carcinoma and in primary tumors with lymph node metastases, whereas they were discordant in multicentric tumors. Macroscopic karyotypic abnormalities similar to those in breast cancers were found in bilateral breast tumors.

These data provide the biological evidence for management of multicentric and bilateral breast cancers as independent entities from the first tumor. They also provide the underpinning of future studies that will also allow us to test tumor material directly to determine whether histologically similar tumors from the same or different sites are from the same or different primary tumors.

G.J. Bosl, M.D.

Absence of Breast Cancer Cells in a Single-Day Peripheral Blood Progenitor Cell Collection After Priming With Cyclophosphamide and Granulocyte-Macrophage Colony-Stimulatinig Factor

Passos-Coelho JL, Ross AA, Moss TJ, Davis JM, Huelskamp A-M, Noga SJ, Davidson NE, Kennedy MJ (Johns Hopkins Oncology Ctr, Baltimore, Md; Immunologic Sciences Labs, Reseda, Calif; Cedars-Sinai Med Ctr, Los Angeles)

Blood 85:1138–1143, 1995

3–15

Background.—Peripheral blood progenitor cells (PBPCs) are increasingly being used for hematopoietic rescue in recipients of high-dose chemotherapy. They are preferable to bone marrow grafts in patients who have overt tumor involvement of the marrow or harvest sites that have previously been irradiated, but the low concentration of hematopoietic progenitor cells in the peripheral blood has been a problem. Sensitive methods have shown that some patients have occult contamination of the bone marrow by tumor cells.

Objective.—The effects of PBPC priming on tumor-cell contamination were examined by analyzing hematopoietic specimens for both PBPC and occult tumor cells in 28 patients with stage IIIB or stage IV breast cancer sensitive to chemotherapy.

Methods.—Tumor cells were detected by immunocytochemical techniques and tumor clonogenic assays specific for epithelium-derived tumor cells. Cyclophosphamide and granulocyte-macrophage colony-stimulating factor were administered for 15 days, starting the day after marrow was harvested. A single leukapheresis was then performed and, 1 week later, ablative chemotherapy was given with cyclophosphamide and thiotepa, followed by the infusion of PBPCs and purged bone marrow.

Results.—Initially, tumor cells were identified in the peripheral blood in 1 of 23 patients (4%), and in bone marrow harvests from 4 of 27 patients (15%). After priming, 2 of 28 patients (7%) had tumor cells in their PBPC samples. The PBPC fraction had been amplified by a median of 19-fold.

Conclusion.—Patients with advanced breast cancer and histologically negative bone marrow specimens may rarely have tumor cells in their marrow and peripheral blood after cytoreduction treatment. These patients may benefit from the reinfusion of primed PBPCs without an increased risk of relapse.

▶ Patients with metastatic breast cancer have an incurable disease. Given the chemosensitivity of breast cancer cells, the strategy of using high-dose chemotherapy followed by bone marrow transplantation in patients with both metastatic and early-stage breast cancer has been explored. Initially, bone marrow was used as a source of progenitor cells for hematopoietic reconstitution. However, technological advances are such that for patients with overt tumor involvement in the marrow, fibrosis of the marrow, or previous irradiation, PBPCs may be easily procured from the circulation. To decrease the number of leukaphereses required and to improve the rapidity of engraftment, cytokine or chemotherapy mobilization of PBPCs has been the focus of intense research.

Passos-Coelho and colleagues address their concern that mobilization of PBPCs may increase the level of occult tumor-cell contamination of the product. Fortunately, they report a low percentage of occult tumor-cell contamination in both steady-state collections and those primed with cyclophosphamide and granulocyte macrophage–colony-stimulating factor. Sensitive immunocytochemical and tumor clonogenic assays specific for epithelial-derived tumor cells were used. It is possible that prior cytoreductive systemic chemotherapy may contribute to the low frequency of occult tumor-cell contamination. Therefore, the results reported in this study cannot necessarily be extrapolated to patients with untreated disease. Furthermore, the patients in this study had no evidence of disease involving the bone marrow, a setting in which the issue of PBPC collection of contaminated progenitor cell collections is particularly important. The precise role of high-dose chemotherapy with stem-cell transplantation in the setting of metastatic breast cancer has not been clearly defined, primarily because of a high relapse rate. Results with translation in this setting have been encouraging enough to prompt tests of this strategy in patients with early-stage breast cancer. The progress made in our ability to deliver high-dose chemotherapy safely and the use of mobilized PBPCs have contributed to early engraftment (often less than 10 days in the setting of breast cancer). However, relapse among patients who have undergone transplantation for metastatic disease remains a formidable challenge. Although we certainly need more effective chemotherapy or immune modulation post transplant, the authors of this manuscript have contributed to our progress in improving treatment for patients with breast cancer. These results reassure us that we should continue to improve our ability to collect purified stem cells in the setting of metastatic breast cancer, for use in hematopoietic reconstitution, because they appear to be relatively free of significant tumor contamination.

M.S. Tallman, M.D.

Ten-Year Results of a Comparison of Conservation With Mastectomy in the Treatment of Stage I and II Breast Cancer
Jacobson JA, Danforth DN, Cowan KH, D'Angelo T, Steinberg SM, Pierce L, Lippman ME, Lichter AS, Glatstein E, Okunieff P (Natl Cancer Inst, Bethesda, Md; Univ of Michigan, Ann Arbor; Lombardt Cancer Ctr, Washington, DC; et al)
N Engl J Med 332:907–911, 1995   3–16

Objective.—Because it remains uncertain whether breast conservation treatment is as effective as mastectomy in women with early-stage breast cancer, the National Cancer Institute conducted a randomized trial in the years 1979–1987 to compare these two approaches in 247 women having clinical stage I and II breast cancers.

TABLE 2.—Comparison of Randomized Trials of Breast Conservation Therapy

Trial	Follow-up	Eligibility Criteria	No. of Patients	Recurrence DFS	Local or Regional OS		Recurrence Within the Breast
	yr				percent		
NSABP B-06*	8	Stage I or II: T <4 cm; N0–1					
Mastectomy			590	58	71	8	NA
Breast conservation			629	59	71	8	10
Gustave-Roussy	10	Stage I; T <2 cm; N0–1					
Mastectomy			91	58	80	10	NA
Breast conservation			88	66	79	5†	—
Milan	13	Stage I; T <2 cm; N0–1					
Mastectomy			349		69	2	NA
Breast conservation			352		71	3†	—
EORTC	8	Stage I or II					
Mastectomy			426		63‡	9	NA
Breast conservation			456		58‡	13†	—
Danish Breast Cancer Group	6	Stage I or II					
Mastectomy			429	66	82	6	NA
Breast conservation			430	70	79	5	3
Present study	10	Stage I or II					
Mastectomy			116	69	75	10	NA
Breast conservation			121	72	77	5	18

* There was an episode of misconduct in the National Surgical Adjuvant Breast Project (NSABP) B-06 trial. The reanalysis of the study, after completion of an audit, has yet to be published.
† The rate of recurrence within the breast is included in the value.
‡ The value was obtained from the survival curve.
Abbreviations: DFS, disease-free survival; *OS*, overall survival; *NA*, not applicable; *EORTC*, European Organization for Research and Treatment of Cancer.
(Reprinted by permission of *The New England Journal of Medicine,* Jacobson JA, Danforth DN, Cowan KH, et al: Ten-year results of a comparison of conservation with mastectomy in the treatment of stage I and II breast cancer. *N Engl J Med* 332:907–911, Copyright 1995, Massachusetts Medical Society.)

Study Plan.—A total of 237 patients were randomized and have been followed up for a median of 10.1 years. Conservation treatment included lumpectomy, axillary dissection, and irradiation. Women randomized to undergo mastectomy also underwent axillary dissection. Radiotherapy consisted of 4,500–5,040 cGy to the whole breast, delivered in 180-cGy fractions 5 days a week. Patients with node involvement received cyclophosphamide and doxorubicin.

Results.—Disease-free survival and overall survival were comparable in the 2 treatment groups. Disease-free survival at 10 years was 69% in the mastectomy group and 72% for those assigned to conservation treatment. Locoregional recurrence, as an isolated first event, developed in 4% of the patients in each group, but it was more frequent in the mastectomy group when patients with concomitant distant disease were included. The risk of recurrence limited to the ipsilateral breast after lumpectomy was 18% at 10 years. The only factors significantly predicting disease-free survival were tumor stage and axillary node involvement.

Conclusion.—These results affirm those obtained in 5 similar randomized trials (Table 2). Lumpectomy combined with axillary node dissection and radiotherapy eliminates stage I/II breast cancer as effectively as mastectomy.

▶ Treatment with lumpectomy and axillary lymph node dissection has become part of the standard management of women with early-stage breast cancer. Provided that radiation therapy is administered after lumpectomy, randomized trials have shown that local recurrence rates are low and comparable with those seen in mastectomy. Because breast cancer often has a natural history that exceeds 10 years, some physicians have expressed the fear that late relapses will occur.

The trial reported by Jacobson and colleagues was a randomized trial from the Radiation Oncology Branch of the National Cancer Institute. Two hundred and forty-seven patients were randomized, and the results have a median follow-up of 10.1 years. Disease-free and overall survival were essentially identical ($P = 0.93$ and 0.89, respectively) at 10 years, and the local recurrence rate was 10% after mastectomy and 5% after lumpectomy plus radiation therapy ($P = 0.17$).

The authors summarize the results of 6 randomized trials of breast conservation therapy (see Table 2). Three of these trials now have follow-up of more than 10 years and, in each trial, the disease-free and overall survival rates have been similar. In the breast conservation and mastectomy groups, the risk of a recurrence confined to the residual breast tissue ranged from 3% to 18%, indicating the need for careful, long-term follow-up. However, "salvage" mastectomy done at the time of such recurrence is effective therapy. In the abstracted study, 15 of the 18 patients with recurrence in the breast had no further local or regional disease after "salvage" mastectomy, with follow-up ranging from 3 months to 9.9 years.

Lumpectomy with radiation therapy is an appropriate alternative to mastectomy in appropriately selected patients. Early detection of disease by mammography may increase the proportion of women who are eligible for breast conservation therapy. It is both good and responsible practice to offer patients both options during the process of informed consent.

G.J. Bosl, M.D.

Sequential or Alternating Doxorubicin and CMF Regimens in Breast Cancer With More Than Three Positive Nodes: Ten-Year Results

Bonadonna G, Zambetti M, Valagussa P (Istituto Nazionale Tumori, Milan, Italy)

JAMA 273:542–547, 1995

3–17

Introduction.—Clinical results have supported the biological concept of adjuvant systemic therapy in the treatment of high-risk resectable breast cancer. The prototype chemotherapy combination of cyclophosphamide (600 mg/m²), methotrexate (40 mg/m²), and fluorouracil (600 mg/m²) has significantly improved long-term survival and stood the test of validation studies. Doxorubicin (DOX) is a drug with very high efficacy and has been shown to be effective in treating patients with breast disease involving more than 3 lymph nodes. The combination of the drugs is effective, and the order of delivery appears to be of importance. The 10-year results comparing sequential or alternating chemotherapy were reported.

Methods.—A total of 403 women younger than 70 years of age participated in the study. All had unilateral disease and underwent surgery with

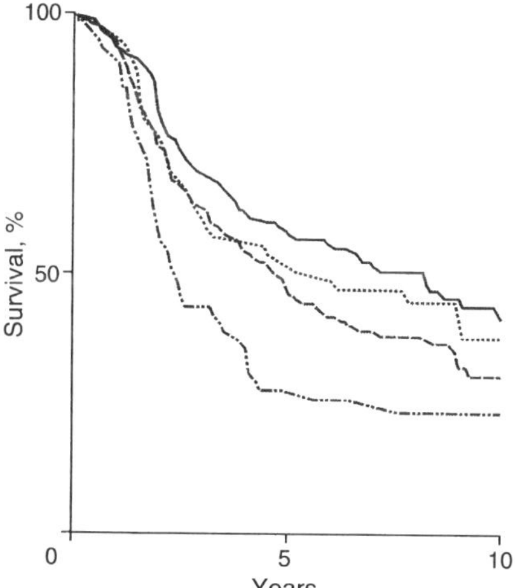

FIGURE 3.—Comparative 10-year relapse-free survival in breast cancer with more than 3 positive nodes relative to menopausal status. *Solid line* indicates DOX → CMF, premenopause; *dotted line* indicates DOX → CMF, postmenopause. *Dashed line* indicates CMF/DOX, premenopause; and *dashed and dotted line* indicates CMF/DOX, postmenopause. *Abbreviations: DOX → CMF,* sequential administration of doxorubicin and a combination of cyclophosphamide, methotrexate, and fluorouracil; *CMF/DOX,* alternating administration of a combination of cyclophosphamide, methotrexate, and fluorouracil, and doxorubicin. (Courtesy of Bonadonna G, Zambetti M, Valagussa P: *JAMA* 273:542–547, Copyright 1995, American Medical Association.)

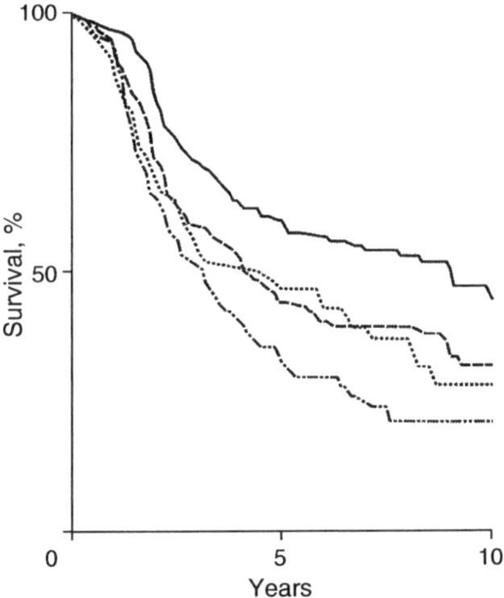

FIGURE 4.—Comparative 10-year relapse-free survival in breast cancer with more than 3 positive nodes relative to extent of nodal involvement. *Solid line* indicates DOX → CMF, 4–10 positive nodes; *dotted line* indicates DOX → CMF, more than 10 positive nodes. *Dashed line* indicates CMF/DOX, 4–10 positive nodes; and *dashed and dotted line* indicates CMF/DOX, more than 10 positive nodes. See legend to **Figure 2** for an explanation of abbreviations. (Courtesy of Bonadonna G, Zambetti M, Valagussa P: *JAMA* 273:542–547, Copyright 1995, American Medical Association.)

full nodal dissection. Involvement of at least 3 lymph nodes was necessary for inclusion in the study. Patients were randomly assigned to 1 or 2 groups. One group, the sequential group, received 4 courses of IV doxorubicin (75 mg/m²) followed by 8 courses of IV CMF (DOX→CMF). The other group, the alternating group, received 2 IV courses of CMF alternated with 1 course of doxorubicin (CMF/DOX), for a total of 12 courses. Chemotherapy was started between 2 and 4 weeks after surgery. After randomization, the only difference between the 2 groups was that the sequential group had fewer women with more than 10 lymph nodes involved. Relapse-free survival and death from all causes was the end point for total survival.

Results.—In the sequential group, 107 woman had new disease develop; in the alternating group, 134 women had new disease. The relapse-free survival rate was 42% and 28%, whereas the total survival probability was 58% and 44%, respectively, in the sequential and alternating group. The superiority of the sequential treatment was evident in all subsets of patients. For example, survival curves varied according to menopausal status (Fig 3) and extent of nodal involvement (Fig 4). Overall, the treatment was well tolerated by the patient; however, there were 4 cases of congestive heart failure, 2 of which were fatal.

Conclusion.—The mechanism for the differences between the 2 treatment protocols is unknown. These results are of sufficient maturity to warrant suggesting that the classical routine of CMF be replaced with a sequential method (DOX→CMF) in patients with extensive nodal involvement.

▶ In 1982, Bonadonna and colleagues initiated a randomized trial of DOX and CMF administered in either a sequential or alternating fashion (1). Available data on Hodgkin's disease at that time suggested that the alternating treatment with MOPP (mechlorethame, Oncovin [vincristine sulfate], procarbazine, and prednisone) and ABVD (Adriamycin [doxorubicin], bleomycin, vinblastine, and dacarbazine) was superior to MOPP alone. The concept of using an alternating non–cross-resistant regimen to enhance outcome had to be considered in the context of dose-intensity therapy, which suggested that such alternation of regimens would result in a lower dose intensity of all drugs administered and could be detrimental.

The randomized trial described in this abstract attempted to answer that question in the context of patients with breast cancer who had more than 3 positive axillary lymph nodes. At 10 years, the probability of patients remaining disease-free was 42% in the sequential treatment arm and 28% in the alternating arm ($P = 0.002$). This observation was true in patients with 4–10 positive lymph nodes and in those with more than 10 positive lymph nodes (see Figure 4). Similar results were obtained in both premenopausal and postmenopausal patients (see Figure 3). The results of the alternating treatment arm were similar to those seen with the use of CMF alone in this patient population. Sequential Adriamycin followed by CMF appears to be the treatment of choice for patients with breast cancer who have multiple positive lymph nodes.

G.J. Bosl, M.D.

Reference

1. Bonnadonna G, Zambetti M, Valagussa P: Sequential or alternating doxorubicin and CMF regimens in breast cancer with more than three positive nodes: Ten-year results. *JAMA* 273:542–547, 1995.

Reduced Expression of Proapoptotic Gene *BAX* Is Associated With Poor Response Rates to Combination Chemotherapy and Shorter Survival in Women With Metastatic Breast Adenocarcinoma
Krajewski S, Blomqvist C, Franssila K, Krajewska M, Wasenius V-M, Niskanen E, Nordling S, Reed JC (La Jolla Cancer Research Found, Calif; Univ of Helsinki)
Cancer Res 55:4471–4478, 1995

3–18

Background.—There is good evidence that the protein encoded by the gene *bcl-2* is a key regulator of apoptosis, which in turn has a critical role in normal tissue homeostasis. The gene *bax* is 1 of a family of genes whose encoded proteins share amino acid sequence homology with *bcl-2*. The *bax* protein itself promotes cell death, and the ratio of these 2 genes may determine the relative sensitivity of cells to apoptotic stimuli.

Objective.—Levels of *bax* protein were estimated immunohistochemically in 121 women having metastatic adenocarcinoma of the breast. All participants had a performance index of 2 or less. None had received anthracyclines previously.

Findings.—In contrast to the findings in normal breast epithelium or in situ carcinoma, immunostaining for *bax* was markedly reduced in 34% of the 119 evaluable tumors. Reduced expression of *bax* correlated with shorter survival (8 vs. 16 months), a shorter time to tumor progression, and failure to respond to chemotherapy. On multivariate analysis, reduced immunostaining for *bax* correlated closely with both shorter survival and more rapid progression of disease.

Therapeutic Implication.—Women with metastatic breast cancer whose tumors fail to express *bax* protein may benefit from more aggressive treatment.

▶ An article by Bargou et al. (Abstract 3–10) suggests that low *bax* expression in tumor cells correlated with resistance to apoptosis. By way of review, *bax* and *bcl-2* act in a coordinated way to promote or inhibit apoptosis. A relatively "high" ratio of *bcl-2* to *bax* expression, caused either by overexpression of *bcl-2* or low expression of *bax,* might have a negative impact on response and survival. Bargou et al. studied breast cancer cell lines and 10 tumor samples.

This abstracted paper by Krajewski et. al. reports on the next step. Antibodies to the *bax* protein were developed, and tissue sections from paraffin-embedded breast tumors were evaluated for the relative expression of the *bax* protein. The clinical courses of 119 patients were evaluated in relation to *bax* expression. Importantly, other potential prognostic factors were also evaluated in multivariate analysis. It was hypothesized that low *bax* protein expression would be associated with an inferior survival. In this study, both the progression-free survival (not shown) and the overall survival were longer in patients with tumors expressing *bax* protein compared with those whose tumor did not express *bax* protein. Curiously, the effect was most pronounced in patients receiving weekly adjuvant treatment regimens compared with those receiving monthly regimens. By multivariate analysis, *bax* protein expression, tumor grade, and treatment group (monthly *or* weekly) were significantly associated with progression and shorter survival.

This preliminary study indicates that *bax* protein expression—and the ability of treatment to induce apoptosis in breast cancer cells—may be an important prognostic factor. The data also imply that different treatment regimens may have different effects in patients with various tumor subgroups. This is a story that will bear watching, and future analyses of prognostic factors in patients with breast cancer will probably need to include *bax* protein immunostaining to properly evaluate the many potential prognostic factors in this disease.

G.J. Bosl, M.D.

Adjuvant Cyclophosphamide, Methotrexate, and Fluorouracil in Node-Positive Breast Cancer: The Results of 20 Years of Follow-Up

Bonadonna G, Valagussa P, Moliterni A, Zambetti M, Brambilla C (Istituto Nazionale Tumori, Milan, Italy)
N Engl J Med 332:901–906, 1995

3–19

Introduction.—Earlier studies reported the short-term survival benefits associated with adjuvant treatment with cyclophosphamide, methotrexate, and fluorouracil (CMF) in patients with node-positive breast cancer. The CMF therapy has become the most common treatment combination in patients with cancers. The results of long-term follow-up of a randomized trial of CMF chemotherapy in women with breast cancer were evaluated.

Methods.—Between 1973 and 1975, 391 patients with node-positive breast carcinoma were stratified by age, number of involved axillary nodes, and the type of radical mastectomy performed and were then randomly assigned to receive either 12 monthly cycles of CMF or no adjuvant treatment. The patients were followed for a median of 19.4 years with physical examination, biochemical tests, chest roentgenography, bone roentgenography or scanning, and mammography. Relapse-free and event-free survival were calculated for the 2 groups.

Results.—Both relapse-free and overall survival were significantly longer in the patients treated with surgery and adjuvant chemotherapy than in patients treated with surgery alone (Fig 1). The median time to relapse was 40 months in the control group and 83 months in the CMF group. The median overall survival was 104 months in the control group and 137 months in the CMF group. Adjuvant CMF therapy improved overall survival in all subgroups of patients except postmenopausal women and those with 4–10 postive nodes. There were no significant

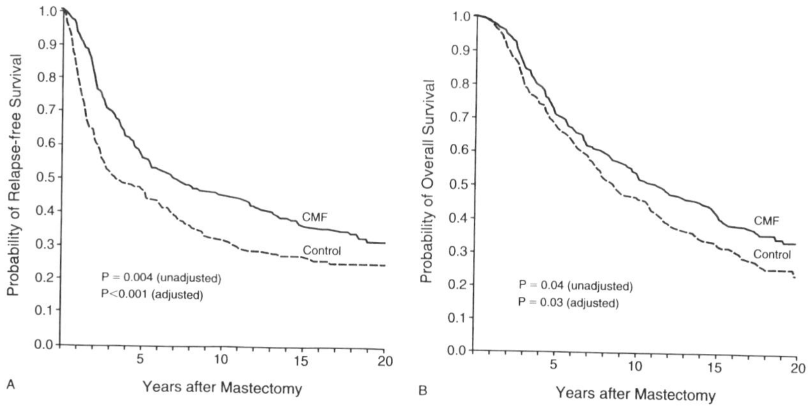

FIGURE 1.—Relapse-free survival (**A**) and overall survival (**B**) according to treatment group. With respect to relapse-free survival, 48 of 179 controls were disease-free at 20 years, as compared with 74 of 207 patients in the cyclophosphamide-methotrexate/fluorouracil (CMF)-treated group. With respect to overall survival, 44 of 179 controls were alive at 20 years, as compared with 70 of 207 CMF-treated patients. (Reprinted by permission of *The New England Journal of Medicine*, Bonadonna G, Valagussa P, Moliterni A, et al: Adjuvant cyclophosphamide, methotrexate, and fluorouracil in node-positive breast cancer: The results of 20 years of follow-up. 332:901–906, Copyright 1995, Massachusetts Medical Society.)

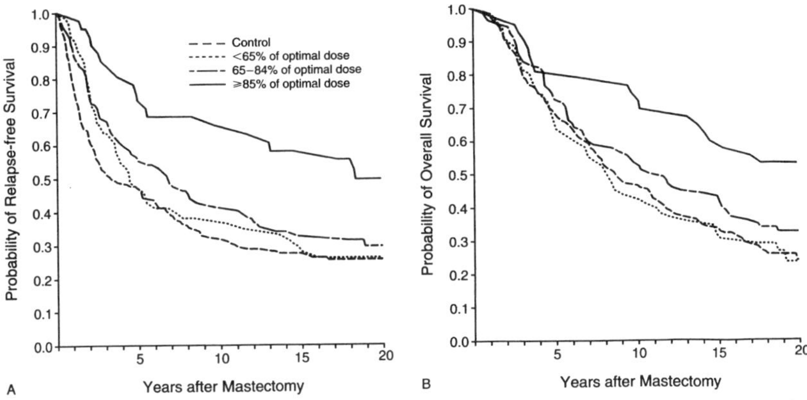

FIGURE 2.—Relapse-free survival (**A**) and overall survival (**B**) according to percentage of optimal dose administered. With respect to relapse-free survival, 48 of 179 controls were disease-free at 20 years, as compared with 21 of 71 patients given < 65% of the optimal dose of cyclophosphamide/methotrexate/fluorouracil (CMF), 31 of 94 patients given 65% to 84% of the optimal dose, and 22 of 42 patients given ≥ 85% of the optimal dose. With respect to overall survival, 44 of 179 controls were alive at 20 years, compared with 18 of 71 patients given < 65% of the optimal dose of CMF, 30 of 94 patients given 65% to 84% of the optimal dose, and 22 of 42 patients given ≥ 85% of the optimal dose. (Reprinted by permission of *The New England Journal of Medicine,* Bonadonna G, Valagussa P, Moliterni A, et al: Adjuvant cyclophosphamide, methotrexate, and fluorouracil in node-positive breast cancer: The results of 20 years of follow-up. 332:901–906, Copyright 1995, Massachusetts Medical Society.)

differences in survival between perimenopausal women and women with or without drug-induced amenorrhea. The 2 treatment groups did not have significant differences in the incidence of locoregional and contralateral breast relapse, but the CMF group had a significantly reduced incidence of distant metastases.

Discussion.—These data indicate that combination chemotherapy with CMF confers a significant overall and relapse-free survival advantage lasting at least 20 years after surgery. Overall, the relative risk of relapse was reduced by 34% and the relative risk of death was reduced by 26% in patients treated with adjuvant CMF. The lack of improved outcome seen in postmenopausal women may have been attributable to the low dose of chemotherapy often given to these patients, suggesting that maximal benefit is dependent on using optimal doses (Fig 2).

▶ Almost 20 years ago, Bonadonna and colleagues first reported the improved outcome of patients receiving CMF as adjuvant treatment for node-positive breast cancer. Multiple updates of this study, which have been provided over the years, show sustained improvement in the patients receiving adjuvant therapy. In this most recent report, with a median follow-up of 19.4 years, the patients who received adjuvant chemotherapy continued to have significantly improved relapse-free and total survival (see Fig 1). Locoregional recurrence rates remain < 15% at 20 years. It is important that the association of improved survival with optimal dose administration (see Fig 2) was again observed, emphasizing the importance of avoiding dose reduction. These data attest to the increment of patients *cured* after appropriately administered adjuvant chemotherapy. Although this may not be surprising, it is reassuring to know that the therapy eradicates, rather than merely delays, the disease in some proportion of patients.

G.J. Bosl, M.D.

Adjuvant CMFVP Versus Tamoxifen Versus Concurrent CMFVP and Tamoxifen for Postmenopausal, Node-Positive, and Estrogen Receptor–Positive Breast Cancer Patients: A Southwest Oncology Group Study
Rivkin SE, Green S, Metch B, Cruz AB, Abeloff MD, Jewell WR, Costanzi JJ, Farrar WB, Minton JP, Osborne CK (Puget Sound Oncology Consortium, Seattle; Southwest Oncology Group Statistical Ctr, Seattle; Univ of Texas Health Science Ctr, San Antonio; et al)
J Clin Oncol 12:2078–2085, 1994   3–20

Introduction.—Previous studies have shown that the estrogen receptor (ER) status of the primary breast tumor can predict the response to endocrine therapy. In addition, it has been suggested that chemotherapy may be less effective in postmenopausal patients than in premenopausal patients. The relative efficacy of chemotherapy or hormonal therapy, either alone or in combination, was determined in postmenopausal patients with ER-positive breast cancer.

Methods.—Women with breast cancer and at least 1 involved axillary node, no distant metastases, and an ER-positive tumor were stratified by the number of positive nodes and by the type of primary surgery. They were then assigned to receive 1 year of treatment with either tamoxifen (295 patients), chemotherapy (300 patients), or both (303 patients). The chemotherapy regimen included cyclophosphamide, methotrexate, fluorouracil, vincristine, and prednisone (CMFVP). Disease-free and overall survival were compared.

Results.—With a median follow-up of 6.5 years, neither disease-free nor overall survival differed significantly in either the entire population or in the subsets defined by the number of positive nodes. There was a 5-year survival rate of 77% in the tamoxifen group, 78% in the CMFVP group, and 75% in the combination group. The 5-year disease-free rates were 61% in the tomoxifen group, 55% in the CMFVP group, and 49% in the combination group. Tamoxifen alone was better tolerated than either of the other treatment regimens; 5% of the tamoxifen-treated patients, 56% of the CMFVP-treated patients, and 61% of the patients treated with both experienced severe or life-threatening toxicity.

Conclusion.—These findings suggest that tamoxifen alone provides comparable benefits and control of disease recurrence to chemotherapy with CMFVP and also causes significantly less toxicity in postmenopausal women with ER-positive, node-positive breast cancer. The combination of tamoxifen and CMFVP increases toxicity but not survival.

▶ This randomized trial performed by the Southwest Oncology Group tested the efficacy of tamoxifen as monotherapy for postmenopausal node-positive and ER-positive patients with breast cancer, comparing it to a 5-drug combination alone and the 5-drug combination plus tamoxifen. The 5-drug combination was one that was popular in the late 1970s and was administered for one year. Tamoxifen was administered for only one year. With a median follow-up of 6.5 years, no difference in survival was noted in any of the node-positive subgroups. Approximately 60% of the patients receiving the 5-drug regimen experienced "severe" or "life-threatening" toxicity. Ten patients experienced thromboembolic phenomena in the combined chemohormonal arm. Four cases were noted on the chemotherapy arm alone, and no cases were observed on the tamoxifen arm.

At face value, the results of this trial do not support the use of chemotherapy in postmenopausal, node-positive women with breast cancer. However, the chemotherapy regimen used was not among the most widely applied variations of CMF, and the duration of therapy with tamoxifen was shorter than what we now believe to be ideal (3–5 years or more). In addition, about 25% of the patients assigned to each of the chemotherapy arms did not complete the planned treatment. Therefore, the results of this trial should be viewed with some caution. At least one large study (NSABP B-16) suggests that this same group of patients (node- and receptor-positive, postmenopausal) benefits dramatically from the combination of chemotherapy plus tamoxifen as compared with tamoxifen alone, and the Early Breast Cancer Trialists' Collaborative Group[1] concludes similarly.

The conclusion of this article, which indicates that tamoxifen is the preferred treatment for node-positive receptor-positive women with breast cancers, stands in contrast to the convincing evidence of there being an additive benefit for chemotherapy plus tamoxifen, as described above. Hence, clinicians should not rely on the results of this single trial but, rather, should base their treatment on the Oxford data, which incorporate numerous trials and thousands of patients. Although it remains true that patients in this subgroup can be treated with tamoxifen alone, it is also clear that adding chemotherapy adds benefit. The decision to use either tamoxifen or tamoxifen plus 4–6 months of chemotherapy for patients outside of clinical trials should be made on an individualized basis. This requires a discussion with the patient of the modest, but real, additive impact of chemotherapy, as well as the toxicities of treatment. Patients and their physicians can then arrive at appropriate individualized decisions.

G.J. Bosl, M.D.

Reference

1. Early Breast Cancer Trialists' Collaborative Group: Systemic treatment of early breast cancer by hormonal, cytotoxic, or immune therapy: 133 randomised trials involving 31,000 recurrences and 24,000 deaths among 75,000 women. *Lancet* 339:1–15, 71–84, 1992.

The Importance of the Lumpectomy Surgical Margin Status in Long Term Results of Breast Conservation

Smitt MC, Nowels KW, Zdeblick MJ, Jeffrey S, Carlson RW, Stockdale FE, Goffinet DR (Stanford Univ, Calif; Redwood Microsystems, Menlo Park, Calif)
Cancer 76:259–267, 1995   3–21

Introduction.—For selected patients with early breast cancer, lumpectomy followed by radiation therapy offers freedom from relapse and overall survival similar to that of mastectomy. However, reported long-term local failure rates have varied considerably. Although leaving gross residual disease in the breast clearly increases local recurrence rates, there is controversy regarding the need to achieve microscopically negative resection margins. Patients with breast cancer undergoing lumpectomy and radiation therapy were studied to determine the effects of surgical margin status on long-term local control rates.

Methods.—The retrospective study included 289 women treated with lumpectomy and radiation therapy for 303 invasive breast cancers. The initial biopsy findings and any re-excision specimens were examined to classify the surgical margins as positive, close (i.e., within 2 mm), negative, or indeterminate. Margin status was analyzed as a potential prognostic factor for local recurrence, along with other factors such as tumor and node classification, age, histologic features, and use of adjuvant therapy. The patients were followed for a mean of 6.25 years.

Results.—The overall actuarial probability of freedom from local recurrence was 94% at 5 years and 87% at 10 years. The 10-year actuarial probability of local control was 98% for patients with negative surgical

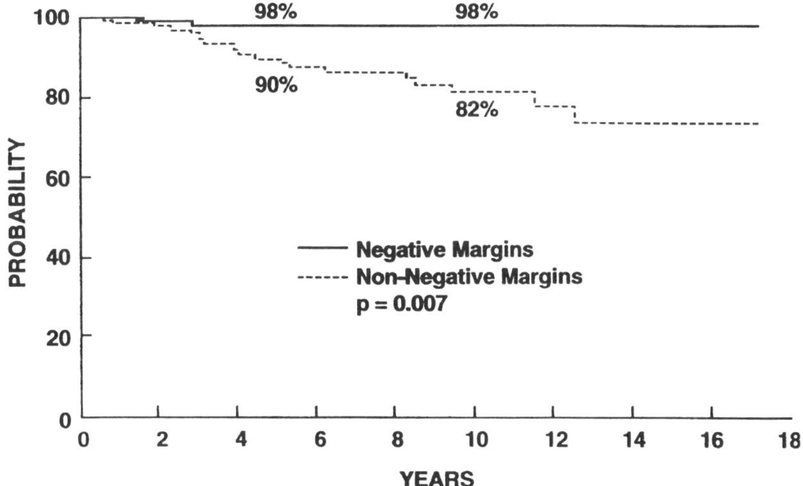

FIGURE 2.—Freedom from local recurrence by margin status: negative (*solid line*); all others (*broken line*). (Courtesy of Smitt MC, Nowels KW, Zdeblick MJ, et al: The importance of the lumpectomy surgical margin status in long term results of breast conservation. *Cancer* 76:259–267, copyright © 1995. Reprinted by permission of Wiley-Liss, Inc., a division of John Wiley & Sons, Inc.)

margins vs. 82% for all other patients (Fig 2). Patients who underwent re-excision had a 10-year local control rate compared with 84% for those who did not have re-excision. On univariate analysis, final margin status was the most significant prognostic factor in local recurrence. Multivariate analysis showed that final marginal status and adjuvant chemotherapy were the significant prognostic factors.

Conclusions.—For patients with early-stage breast cancer who were undergoing lumpectomy and radiation therapy, negative surgical margins are the strongest predictor of local control. For patients with close, indeterminate, or positive margins after their initial resection, re-excision appears to yield a local control benefit, as long as negative final margins are obtained.

▶ The use of the term "lumpectomy" rather than "wide local excision" in the surgical treatment of breast cancer suggests a rather imprecise operative procedure that involves removal of only all macroscopic or gross tumor. It has been accepted that postoperative radiation therapy, including a boost radiation dose to the tumor site, will then reduce the risk of local recurrence. In this experience with almost 300 women with a median follow-up of 6 years, the issue of surgical margins as well as other potential prognostic factors for local recurrence was explored. Their results, as demonstrated in Figure 2, indicate the importance of obtaining negative margins, assuming this can be done with adequate cosmesis. The extent of the local operation is frequently determined by cosmetic considerations, because breast conservation without adequate cosmesis defeats the major goal of this alternative to mastectomy. Of importance, 42% of patients who underwent a reexcision of the prior biopsy site had residual carcinoma, which included 25% residual carcinoma in patients with negative margins on the initial excisional biopsy specimen. If extensive intraductal cancer was present, 82% of patients had residual carcinoma. All of these data demonstrate the importance of careful communication between the initial surgeon obtaining the pathology for review before definitive treatment and then performing careful re-excision in most patients within the limits of an acceptable cosmetic result.

A.M. Cohen, M.D.

Local Recurrences and Distant Metastases After Conservative Breast Cancer Treatments: Partly Independent Events
Veronesi U, Marubini E, Del Vecchio M, Manzari A, Andreola S, Greco M, Luini A, Merson M, Saccozzi R, Rilke F, Salvadori B (Istituto Nazionale Tumori, Milan, Italy; Istituto di Statistica Medica e Biometria, Milan, Italy)
J Natl Cancer Inst 87:19–27, 1995   3–22

Background.—Local recurrence is a major concern in conservative breast cancer therapy. The incidences of local and distant recurrences according to demographic, biological, and pathologic variables were determined in a large group of women undergoing conservative treatment. The objective was to identify women in whom local failure predicts distant metastases and who are therefore candidates for aggressive systemic therapy.

Methods.—The medical records of 2,233 women treated at one center from 1970 to 1987 were analyzed. All underwent quadrantectomy and axillary lymph node dissection followed by breast radiotherapy.

Findings.—One hundred nineteen local recurrences were documented. There were also 32 new ipsilateral carcinomas and 414 distant metastases as first events. The annual probability of local failures was approximately 1% up to the 10th year, whereas that of distant metastases was 5% in the second year, declining progressively until year 8. An important risk factor was young age. Peritumoral lymphatic invasion also predicted local and distant recurrences. Tumor size and axillary lymph node involvement were unassociated with local recurrence but were important predictors of distant metastases. An extensive intraductal component was a risk factor only for local recurrence. Compared with later failure, early local failure predicted distant metastases. Patients with local failure had a 5-year survival rate of 69%.

Conclusions.—Local recurrences and distant metastases are partially independent events occurring at different times. Several predictors also differ. However, the risk of distant metastases in women with local recurrences was significant. Those women who are 35 years of age or younger at first diagnosis and had initial peritumoral lymphatic invasion and local recurrence within 2 years have a high risk for distant spread. A lower risk of recurrence is associated with an extensive intraductal component and, possibly, inadequate surgery.

▶ For some time there has been a discussion of the meaning of a local recurrence in the breast after conservative breast cancer surgery. One of the real problems and paradoxes in the field of breast cancer is that when a tumor is detected either in the breast or in the axillary nodes, after so-called definitive treatment to the breast itself, there is no good evidence that such locoregional recurrences have a negative impact on the survival. This is a real problem in terms of developing our logic of how to approach this disease.

This paper from Milan is a jewel in terms of its data. It represents a study of more than 2,200 women with at least 7 years of follow-up. The data are most impressive, with 119 local recurrences, 32 new primary ipsilateral carcinomas, and 110 contralateral breast carcinomas. A total of 414 women had distant metastases develop. It is interesting to see that the *rates* of local failure and of distant metastases were somewhat different; local failures were manifested at approximately 1% per year for the first decade of follow-up. The rate of distant metastases appeared to hit a peak of approximately about 5% at approximately 2 years and experienced a steady decline thereafter. Age was an important factor, although tumor size and axillary node involvement were important only as predictors for distant metastases.

In all honesty, the take-home message of this paper it is not clear to me, but this is largely because an enormous amount of data is included. One is left with the basic idea that there may well be more than one disease that comes under the heading of breast cancer with variable degrees of expression of some of these prognostic indicators. For patients who have small-volume primaries, this reference will probably serve as the standard for the next decade or so.

E. Glatstein, M.D.

Irradiation of Bone Metastases in Breast Cancer Patients: A Randomized Study With 1 Year Follow-Up
Rasmusson B, Vejborg I, Jensen AB, Andersson M, Banning A-M, Hoffmann T, Pfeiffer P, Nielsen HK, Sjøfgren P (Rigshospitalet, Copenhagen; Odense Univ, Denmark)
Radiother Oncol 34:179–184, 1995   3–23

Objective.—A simplified irradiation schedule was compared with the standard regimen for bone metastases of breast cancer. Two hundred patients who had painful osteolytic and/or osteosclerotic metastases in the spine, sternum, pelvis, or extremities were included in the trial. Those with bone fracture in their metastases were not included.

Management.—Patients received either a tumor dose of 30 Gy in 10 fractions over 12–14 days (regimen A), or 15 Gy in 3 fractions in an overall time of 8–9 days (regimen B). Photon energies were 1.2, 4, or 6 MV.

Results.—The median survival from the start of radiotherapy was 1 year for group A patients and 11 months for those in group B. Bone pain was significantly relieved in both groups after 1 month, and it remained reduced through the first year of follow-up. Approximately two thirds of the patients had a good response at 3 months. Activity levels significantly improved in both groups, and there was no difference in analgesic consumption (Table 4). The radiographic response rates were also comparable (Table 5). There were no substantial side effects from radiotherapy, and there were no differences between the 2 regimens.

Conclusion.—A radiotherapy regimen of 15 Gy, given in 3 fractions at 2 fractions per week, appears to be as effective as conventional treatment for women with symptomatic bone metastases of breast cancer.

▶ When we get to palliative issues, the bean counters in managed care organizations will undoubtedly require us to look carefully at ways of hypofractionation that do not compromise the patient's outcome. This study from Denmark randomized patients with breast cancer and metastatic disease to the bone to receive a conventional regimen of 3,000 rad given in 10 fractions in 2 weeks vs. 1,500 rad given in 3 fractions over 8–9 days. No differences were seen in pain assessment, radiologic response, or side effects. I must say I would be reluctant to give less than 3 fractions, but it is quite correct

TABLE 4.—Consumption of Analgesic

	Months since randomization									
	0		1		3		6		12	
	A	B	A	B	A	B	A	B	A	B
Morphine 5	3 (3)	5 (6)	3 (5)	3 (5)	3 (6)	2 (5)	2 (6)	2 (7)	1 (7)	1 (8)
Morphine 4	10 (12)	7 (9)	7 (11)	3 (5)	6 (12)	3 (7)	5 (16)	1 (4)	3 (21)	1 (8)
Morphine 3	14 (16)	8 (10)	12 (18)	7 (11)	8 (16)	6 (14)	5 (16)	2 (7)	2 (14)	1 (8)
Peripheral 2	36 (42)	44 (54)	20 (30)	31 (51)	18 (37)	20 (45)	9 (29)	15 (54)	6 (43)	5 (38)
P.n. 1	20 (23)	16 (20)	12 (18)	9 (15)	4 (8)	7 (16)	4 (13)	2 (7)	0 (0)	2 (15)
None	3 (3)	1 (1)	10 (15)	7 (11)	10 (20)	6 (14)	6 (19)	6 (21)	2 (14)	3 (23)
No data	0 (0)	0 (0)	2 (3)	1 (2)	0 (0)	0 (0)	0 (0)	0 (0)	0 (0)	0 (0)
All	86 (100)	81 (100)	66 (100)	61 (100)	49 (100)	44 (100)	31 (100)	28 (100)	14 (100)	13 (100)

Analgesics: Morphine 5, oral morphine (or equianalgesic doses of other opioids), > 100–400 mg/day; *Morphine 4*, oral morphine (or equianalgesic doses of other opioids), 40–100 mg/day; *Morphine 3*, oral morphine (or equianalgesic doses of other opioids), < 40 mg/day; *Peripheral 2*, peripheral analgesics fixed daily doses; *P.n. 1*, peripheral analgesics p.n.

(Reprinted from *Radiother Oncol,* Vol. 34, Rasmusson B, Vejborg I, Jensen AB, et al: Irradiation of bone metastases in breast cancer patients: A randomized study with 1 year follow-up, pp 179–184, 1995, with kind permission of Elsevier Science–NL, Sara Burgerhartstraat 25, 1055 KV Amsterdam, The Netherlands.)

TABLE 5.—Radiologic Response According to Time After Irradiation

	Time after irradiation (months)							
	1		3		6		12	
	A	B	A	B	A	B	A	B
Complete or partial response	13 (24)	15 (30)	32 (60)	41 (79)	31 (70)	28 (76)	18 (72)	21 (81)
No change	34 (63)	29 (58)	16 (30)	9 (17)	10 (23)	4 (11)	6 (24)	2 (8)
Progression or mixed response	7 (13)	6 (12)	5 (10)	2 (4)	3 (7)	5 (13)	1 (4)	3 (11)
N	54	50	53	52	44	37	25	26

Note: Percentage of the total number of evaluable patients in *parentheses.*
(Reprinted from *Radiother Oncol,* vol. 34, Rasmusson B, Vejborg I, Jensen AB, et al: Irradiation of bone metastases in breast cancer patients: A randomized study with 1 year follow-up, pp 179–184, 1995, with kind permission of Elsevier Science–NL, Sara Burgerhartstraat 25, 1055 KV Amsterdam, The Netherlands.)

that these 3 fractions should be much more convenient to the patient and less costly to society as a whole. Have no doubts: You will see more studies like this in the future.

E. Glatstein, M.D.

Tumor Biology of Infiltrating Lobular Carcinoma: Implications for Management

Yeatman TJ, Cantor AB, Smith TJ, Smith SK, Reintgen DS, Miller MS, Ku NNK, Baekey PA, Cox CE (Univ of South Florida, Tampa)
Ann Surg 222:549–561, 1995   3–24

Background.—Invasive lobular (IL) carcinoma can have a subtle presentation that is difficult to detect mammographically and that may be multicentric and more invasive than suspected. However, several reports have supported conservative surgical treatment of IL tumors. It was hypothesized that IL tumors had biological characteristics that distinguished them from infiltrating ductal (ID) tumors. This hypothesis was tested in a retrospective analysis of patients with breast cancer of 3 different histologic subtypes who were treated and followed.

Methods.—Of 1,548 patients seen with breast cancer, there were treatment and follow-up data available for 917 patients. Of these patients, complete data, including pathologic and mammographic findings, were available for 777 patients in 3 histologic categories: ID (661 patients), IL (74 patients), and mixed ID and IL (42 patients). The clinical, treatment, survival, and follow-up variables were compared in the 3 groups.

Results.—The 3 groups had similar age distributions, except the IL tumor group had fewer patients who were younger than 39 years (Fig 2). Tumor size was significantly larger in the IL tumor group than in the ID

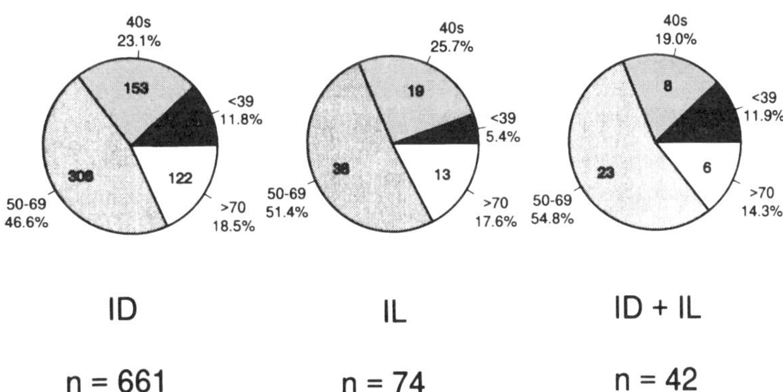

FIGURE 2.—Age distribution of all patients entered in the breast cancer database. All distributions were similar, with the exception of the invasive lobular (IL) carcinoma group, in which only 5.4% of patients were younger than 39 years of age at presentation. (Courtesy of Yeatman TJ, Cantor AB, Smith TJ, et al: Tumor biology of infiltrating lobular carcinoma: Implications for management. *Ann Surg* 222:549–561, 1995.)

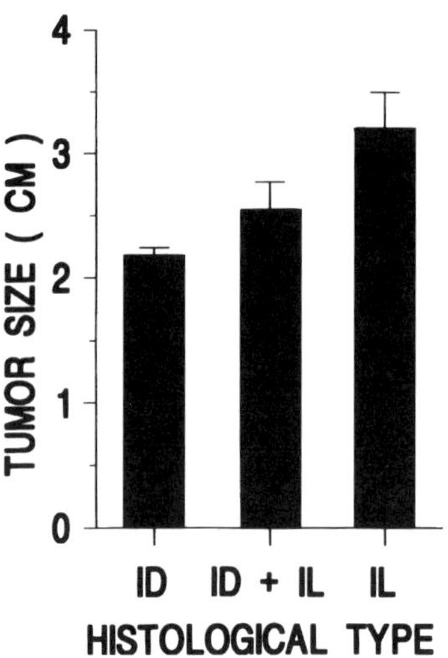

FIGURE 3.—Mean tumor size derived from final pathologic reports was plotted for each tumor subgroup. Infiltrating lobular (*IL*) tumor sizes were found to be significantly larger than infiltrating ductal (*ID*) tumor sizes. (Courtesy of Yeatman TJ, Cantor AB, Smith TJ, et al: Tumor biology of infiltrating lobular carcinoma: Implications for management. *Ann Surg* 222:549–561, 1995.)

tumor group, with the mixed group having tumor sizes in between those of the other 2 groups (Fig 3). Although mammography significantly undersized tumors in all 3 groups, the mean difference between pathologic and mammographic tumor size was larger in the IL tumor group (Table 4). There was a higher incidence of nodal positivity, although the number of positive nodes correlated less with tumor size in the IL tumor group compared with the other 2 groups (Table 5, Fig 4). Patients with IL tumors tended to have more advanced tumors at diagnosis. The incidence of estrogen receptor positivity was highest in the IL tumor group, but there were no significant differences in the 3 groups regarding progesterone receptor positivity. Mastectomy was a significantly more common treat-

TABLE 4.—Comparison of Means for Differences Between Pathologic and Mammographic Tumor Sizes

Tumor Histology	n*	Mean Tumor Size [Δ(pathologic— mammographic)(mm)]	p Value†
ID	297	5.2	< 0.0001
ID + IL	21	6.9	0.0216
IL	38	10.6	0.0016

* Mammographic data were not available on all patients in the study population.
† P values derived using paired *t*-test. P = 0.08 for a comparison of ID differences vs. IL differences, pooled *t*-test.
Abbreviations: ID, infiltrating ductal tumor; *IL*, infiltrating lobular tumor.
(Courtesy of Yeatman TJ, Cantor AB, Smith TJ, et al: Tumor biology of infiltrating lobular carcinoma: Implications for management. *Ann Surg* 222:549–561, 1995.)

TABLE 5.—Incidence of Positive Lymph Nodes

Tumor Histology	Incidence	% Positive	Positive LN/Patient (mean ± SD)*
ID	237/661	36	5.1 ± 6.6
ID + IL	18/42	43	3.1 ± 3.3
IL	38/74	51	6.6 ± 9.0
p value		0.025†	NS‡

* Only patients with at least 1 positive node were included in this analysis.
† Chi square.
‡ ANOVA.
Abbreviations: ID, infiltrating ductal tumor; *IL*, infiltrating lobular tumor; *LN*, lymph node; *NS*, not significant.
(Courtesy of Yeatman TJ, Cantor AB, Smith TJ, et al: Tumor biology of infiltrating lobular carcinoma: Implications for management. *Ann Surg* 222:549–561, 1995.)

ment in the IL tumor group than in the ID tumor group; patients with IL tumors had a 2.5-fold greater incidence of conversion from lumpectomy to mastectomy than did patients with ID tumors. Analysis of the intraoperative touch-preparation margins showed a greater tendency for false nega-

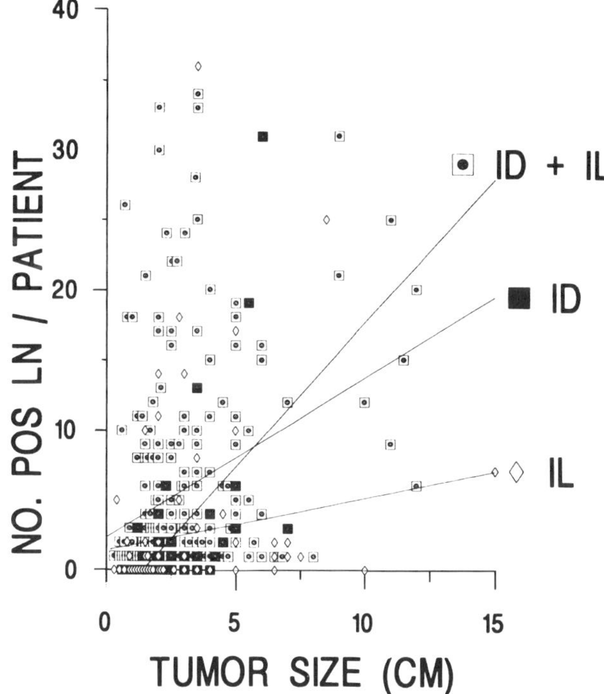

FIGURE 4.—Linear regression analysis of pathologic tumor size vs. the number of positive lymph nodes per patient for 3 tumor histologic types. Infiltrating lobular (*IL*) tumors were significantly different from infiltrating ductal (*ID*)-plus-IL tumors (*P* = 0.02) and marginally different from ID tumors (*P* = 0.09) (Fisher's z-test). These data suggest that IL tumors, unlike ID and ID-plus-IL tumors, are less likely to produce more positive nodes as they grow. (Courtesy of Yeatman TJ, Cantor AB, Smith TJ, et al: Tumor biology of infiltrating lobular carcinoma: Implications for management. *Ann Surg* 222:549–561, 1995.)

tive results with IL tumors than with ID tumors. The overall and disease-free survival rates were similar in the 3 groups.

Conclusion.—Infiltrating lobular cancer is an insidious variant of breast cancer with biological characteristics that distinguish it from infiltrating ductal cancer. Lumpectomy can be a safe and effective treatment for certain patients with infiltrating lobular cancer, but these patients must be selected judiciously.

▶ This paper presents a very good comparison of ID cancer of the breast and IL cancer of the breast. The latter represents only 10% to 15% of patients, but there seems to be some confusion in the minds of many individuals concerning the differences between IL and the "common garden-variety" type of IL lesions. The authors also include an analysis of a mixed-tumor population.

The conclusions the authors reach are probably correct, although I do not think they sufficiently emphasize that there is a major overlap in the biological characteristics of these groups of patients. Even so, the generalizations put forth are certainly reasonable and represent biological characteristics of which the physician should be aware.

E. Glatstein, M.D.

4 Gynecologic Malignancies

Ovarian Cancer Screening
Mackey SE, Creasman WT (Med Univ of South Carolina, Charleston)
J Clin Oncol 13:783–793, 1995   4–1

General Principles.—The goal of a screening program is to test an asymptomatic population in a way that is relatively simple and inexpensive so as to classify individuals according to whether they are likely or unlikely to have a given form of cancer. Ultimately, the purpose of screening is to decrease complications and deaths. Conditions that have potentially serious consequences, such as ovarian cancer, are suitable for screening efforts. There should be a preclinical phase that is long enough to permit convenient screening intervals. Treatment that is most effective when used early should be available. The validity of a given test is reflected by its sensitivity, specificity, and positive and negative predictive values.

Specific Screening Measures.—Of the many serum tumor markers evaluated for use in screening asymptomatic women for ovarian cancer, the most widely used is the glycoprotein CA 125. The specificity of the CA 125 assay is much improved by adding pelvic examination or follow-up ultrasonography. Ultrasound studies have been done by both the transabdominal and transvaginal routes. The latter method precludes the need for a full bladder and is effective in assessing obese patients. In addition, clearer images are obtained than with abdominal examination. Color Doppler imaging appears to be a useful adjunct to transvaginal ultrasound examination. The transvaginal study is acceptable to patients and is highly sensitive and specific. It remains uncertain, however, whether any current screening method will prevent deaths from ovarian cancer.

▶ Frequently, the patient—not the physician—brings up the issue of whether she should be screened for ovarian cancer. It often is easier to order the screening tests than to explain to the patient why routine screening for ovarian cancer is not recommended. As pointed out by the authors of this timely review, the major problem with screening tests that are currently used for ovarian cancer is that they have an unacceptably high positive predictive value. This is perhaps the most important predictive value in assessing the potential benefit of a screening program because it reflects the number of false positive procedures that will be performed on patients who do not have the disease. For example, in patients with ovarian cancer, if a test has a 10% positive predictive value, then for every patient identified as actually having ovarian cancer, 10 laparotomies would be performed on patients who were positive on this screen.

Because the laparotomy is not a benign procedure and has a defined morbidity and mortality rate, particularly in elderly patients in whom the incidence of ovarian cancer is highest, screening may actually do more harm than good. Consequently, it is the obligation of the caregiver to discuss with the patient the fact that she may be harmed by undergoing screening for ovarian cancer. Furthermore, in some prior screening studies, the majority of patients who had been found to have ovarian cancer actually had advanced-stage disease. This suggests that screening, with the currently available clinical tests will not be of benefit.

R.F. Ozols, M.D., Ph.D.

Preliminary Analysis of the Behavior of Stage I Ovarian Serous Tumors of Low Malignant Potential: A Gynecologic Oncology Group Study
Barnhill DR, Kurman RJ, Brady MF, Omura GA, Yordan E, Given FT, Kucera PR, Roman LD (Walter Reed Army Med Ctr, Washington, DC; Johns Hopkins Med Insts, Baltimore, Md; Roswell Park Cancer Inst, Buffalo, NY; et al)
J Clin Oncol 13:2752–2756, 1995   4–2

Objectives.—Consensus on the management of ovarian epithelial tumors of low malignant potential (LMP) has yet to be reached. To investigate further, the Gynecologic Oncology Group conducted a long-term prospective study to evaluate the biological behavior of ovarian LMP tumors, the effectiveness of melphalan chemotherapy both in patients with clinically detectable residual disease after surgical staging and in those whose tumors progress or recur after surgical therapy, and the response rate to cisplastin in those who failed to respond to melphalan therapy.

Management.—Between 1983 and 1992, 146 patients with stage I serous LMP tumors underwent removal of the affected ovary (or ovaries) and a complete staging operation. None of the patients had endosalpingiosis. The median patient age was 43.7 years. Twenty-one patients had a unilateral salpingo-oophorectomy with retention of the uterus and a normal-appearing contralateral ovary; 123 had total bilateral abdominal hysterectomy and bilateral salpingo-oophorectomy. The tumor was ruptured in 10% of patients, the peritoneal cytology was positive in 12%, and external surface excrescences were present in 15%. In 7 patients who initially had an ovarian cystectomy and were then surgically explored, none had residual tumor in the ovary in which the cystectomy had been performed or in the contralateral normal-appearing ovary. None of the patients received adjuvant chemotherapy or radiation therapy.

Outcome.—All patients survived without recurrence during a median follow-up of 42.4 months (range, 1.6–108 months).

Conclusion.—Ovarian serous LMP tumors limited to the ovaries rarely, if ever, recur. These findings support a conservative surgical approach for the treatment of ovarian LMP tumors. After careful surgical exploration and thorough pathologic sampling with negative findings, unilateral salpingo-oophorectomy or, possibly, ovarian cystectomy is adequate therapy for women of reproductive age.

▶ This study defines the biology of serous tumors of LMP, which, in turn, has important clinical implications. Survival for patients with invasive malignant epithelial tumors of the ovary is markedly worse than for patients with LMP tumors. Virtually all patients with invasive epithelial tumors are treated with aggressive surgery followed by intensive chemotherapy. In the past, a similar approach had been used for patients with LMP tumors. However, it is clear from this study that stage I serous LMP tumors are curable in the vast majority of patients, and even recurrences are extremely unusual. Consequently, because these tumors frequently occur in women of reproductive age, conservative treatment—including a unilateral salpingo-oophorectomy or, possibly, even an ovarian cystectomy—is adequate therapy. There is no need for any form of postoperative adjuvant therapy in this group of patients.

R.F. Ozols, M.D., Ph.D.

Genetic Disparity Between Morphologically Benign Cysts Contiguous to Ovarian Carcinomas and Solitary Cystadenomas

Zheng J, Benedict WF, Xu H-J, Hu S-X, Kim TM, Velicescu M, Wan M, Cofer KF, Dubeau L (Univ of Southern California, Los Angeles; Baylor College of Medicine, The Woodlands, Tex)
J Natl Cancer Inst 87:1146–1153, 1995   4–3

Introduction.—It is uncertain whether the benign cysts found contiguous to clearly malignant areas in certain ovarian carcinomas (known as cystadenocarcinomas) represent the remnants of preexisting benign cystadenomas or integral components of the carcinomas themselves. The answer to this question has important implications for our understanding of ovarian carcinogenesis and tumor heterogeneity and for the clinical management of ovarian cystadenomas. An attempt was made to confirm whether mutations of the *p53* tumor suppressor gene are markers of malignancy in ovarian tumors, and the distribution of these mutations in cystadenocarcinomas was assessed.

Methods.—The presence of *p53* mutations was evaluated by immunohistochemistry and DNA sequencing in 46 ovarian carcinomas, 21 ovarian tumors of low malignant potential, and 16 solitary cystadenomas. The distribution of *p53* mutations in various parts of cystadenocarcinomas was then evaluated using similar techniques.

Results.—Fifty-two percent of the carcinomas studied showed *p53* mutations compared with none of the tumors of low malignant potential or solitary cystadenomas. Of 6 cystadenocarcinomas that had *p53* mutations, the same mutation was seen in adjacent, histologically benign cysts. The mutations occurred throughout the morphologically benign cysts, not just in areas immediately adjacent to the carcinomas. Of 24 tumors showing mutation of 1 *p53* allele, 20 also showed loss of genetic heterozygosity; this finding suggested deletion of the other *p53* allele. When allelic loss was found in the morphologically malignant parts of cystadenocarcinomas, it was also present in the contiguous cysts.

Conclusion.—Analysis of *p53* mutations can differentiate ovarian carcinomas from ovarian cystadenomas and tumors of low malignant potential. Mutations of this tumor suppressor gene are found in histologically benign cysts that are contiguous with ovarian carcinomas. Therefore, these cysts do not appear to be typical cystadenomas, and they may carry a genetic predisposition to carcinogenesis not found in ordinary cystadenomas.

▶ There has been a long search to identify the precursors to epithelial ovarian carcinomas. It has been postulated that benign cysts may lead to cystadenomas, which, in turn, may be the precursors to borderline tumors of the ovary, which then become invasive carcinomas. In this study, mutations of the *p53* gene were seen both in the cells immediately adjacent to the carcinomas and throughout morphologically benign cysts contiguous to ovarian carcinomas. This suggests that such cysts may carry a genetic predisposition to carcinogenesis that is not present in ordinary cysts and cystadenomas.

Liu and Nuzum,[1] in an intriguing editorial accompanying this paper, provide 2 explanations for the observations reported by Zheng et al. It is possible that some of the benign ovarian cysts or tumors of low malignant potential that harbor *p53* mutations identify those tissues predestined to become ovarian carcinomas. Alternatively, it is possible that benign cysts are differentiated cells derived from the adjacent carcinoma. Because one half of ovarian adenocarcinomas have discernible mutations in the *p53* gene, these mutations may be useful in the detection of residual disease or for molecular staging.

R.F. Ozols, M.D., Ph.D.

Reference

1. Liu E, Nuzum C: Molecular sleuthing: Tracking ovarian cancer progression. *J Natl Cancer Inst* 87:1099–1101, 1995.

Value of P-Glycoprotein, Glutathione S-Transferase pi, c-*erb*B-2, and p53 as Prognostic Factors in Ovarian Carcinomas

van der Zee AGJ, Hollema H, Suurmeijer AJH, Krans M, Sluiter WJ, Willemse PHB, Aalders JG, de Vries EGE (Univ Hosp Groningen, The Netherlands; Martini Hosp, Groningen, The Netherlands)
J Clin Oncol 13:70–78, 1995   4–4

Background.—In combination, available prognostic factors can predict the long-term survival of patients with ovarian carcinoma. However, there is no current way of predicting the response to chemotherapy in an individual patient. Expression of tumor-suppressor genes and/or oncogenes, in addition to their implications for tumor aggressiveness, may also influence the drug sensitivity of tumors. The prognostic value of immunostaining for various tumor-suppressor genes and oncogenes—P-glycoprotein (P-gp), glutathione S-transferase (GST) pi, c-*erb*B-2, and p53—was examined in patients with advanced-stage ovarian carcinoma.

Methods.—Immunostaining was performed for P-gp, GST pi, c-*erb*B-2, and p53 on 89 primary tumors in patients with advanced ovarian carcinoma. They also analyzed P-gp and GST pi in 38 residual tumors after treatment with platinum- and doxorubicin-containing chemotherapy. The immunostaining results were read independently and correlated with the clinicopathologic prognostic factors, chemotherapy response, progression-free survival (PFS), and overall survival.

Results.—Sixty-five percent of patients had progressive disease after chemotherapy. Immunoreactivity was noted for P-gp in 15% of cases and for GST pi in 89%. These findings were unrelated to any other prognostic factor or to overall survival. Twenty percent of cases showed c-*erb*B-2 immunoreactivity, which was associated with an undifferentiated histiotype but not with PFS or overall survival. Thirty-five percent of cases showed immunoreactivity in the nuclei and 10% in the cytoplasm. The factors associated with nuclear p53 staining were grade III tumor, presence of more than 1-L ascites, and more than 2 cm of residual tumor after initial laparotomy. Progression-free survival was shorter in patients with nuclear p53 staining (relative risk, 3.3). However, nuclear p53 staining lost its independent prognostic significance in stage III/IV tumors after adjustment for the presence of more than 1-L ascites or age over 50 years.

Forty-seven percent of residual tumors studied after chemotherapy showed P-gp staining compared with 15% of untreated tumors. The response to chemotherapy could not be adequately predicted by any combination of prognostic factors.

Conclusions.—In patients with advanced ovarian carcinoma, nuclear immunoreactivity of p53 is associated with a shorter PFS and overall survival and with determinants of increased tumor aggressiveness. Residual tumors in patients treated with chemotherapy show an increased frequency of P-gp immunoreactivity; therefore, doxorubicin-containing chemotherapy may induce P-gp in ovarian carcinomas. Response to chemotherapy is not improved by immunostaining of P-gp, GST pi, c-*erb*B-2, and p53.

▶ The list of clinically useful and proposed prognostic factors in epithelial ovarian carcinomas continues to grow. Stage, histology, tumor grade, age, performance status, and volume of residual disease have been accepted as clinically useful prognostic factors. More recently, ovarian cancers and other solid tumors have been examined for the presence of specific oncogenes, tumor-suppressor genes, and biochemical factors identified to be associated with drug resistance in experimental models of cancer.

This study demonstrates that there is a negative prognostic impact of immunostaining for the tumor suppressor gene p53, which appears to be correlated with more aggressive tumor growth. However, it failed to confirm the results of earlier studies, which indicated a negative prognostic impact of immunostaining for the oncogene c-*erb*B-2. Furthermore, determination of factors associated with drug resistance were not predictive for a response to chemotherapy. The selection of chemotherapy for ovarian cancer should be on the basis of prospective randomized trials comparing different regimens and *not* on the basis of molecular and biochemical parameters assayed in tumor biopsy specimens.

R.F. Ozols, M.D., Ph.D.

The Differential Expression of Cytokeratin 18 in Cisplatin-Sensitive and -Resistant Human Ovarian Adenocarcinoma Cells and Its Association With Drug Sensitivity
Parekh HK, Simpkins H (Temple Univ, Philadelphia; Fels Inst of Molecular Biology and Cancer Research, Philadelphia)
Cancer Res 55:5203–5206, 1995   4–5

Introduction.—Treatment of various cancers involves cisplatin, which interacts with the cellular cytoskeleton composed of microtubules and intermediate filaments. DNA is the primary target of cisplatin, which binds to the N7 position of guanosine and forms intrastrand and interstrand cross-links. A major problem in the use of cisplatin is the development of resistance to this anticancer drug. Cytokeratins are intermediate filament proteins that play a key role in the maintenance of cell shape, spatial organization of cellular organelles, and modulation of membrane transport. Intermediate filaments may be involved with DNA function and structure. The role of intermediate filaments in the development of cisplatin resistance in human ovarian carcinoma cells and their cisplatin-resistant variants was studied.

Methods.—The sensitivity of human ovarian carcinoma cells (2008 and 2780) and their cisplatin-resistant variants (2008/C13 and C70) to the cytotoxic effect of cisplatin was evaluated. The protein content of the cytoskeletal fractions was determined. The intracellular levels of the cytoskeletal proteins cytokeratin and vimentin were determined. Deoxyribonucleic acid was extracted from the 2 cell lines and was analyzed and digested with *Hpa*II and its methylation-sensitive isoschizomer.

Results.—When compared with the cisplatin-sensitive 2008 cell line, the cisplatin-resistant 2008/C13 cell line contained a sixfold lower level of cytokeratin 18. In the resistant cell line, there was a markedly decreased level of cytokeratin 18 messenger RNA. No detectable differences were seen in the methylation status of the cytokeratin gene. The expression of cytokeratin 18 could not be enhanced in the resistant cell line using 5 azacytodime (5 µM) or retinoic acid (1 µM). However, clones with increased levels of cytokeratin 18 were created from transfection of full-length cytokeratin 18 cDNA into the cisplatin-resistant 2008/C13 cells. These clones had a marked increase in their sensitivity to cisplatin.

Conclusion.—Sensitization of a drug-resistant human ovarian cell line to cisplatin results from modulating the expression of an intermediate filament protein. It is possible that the formation of cytokeratin-DNA cross-links is associated with cisplatin toxicity and that the reduced expression of cytokeratin 18 in platinum-resistant cells may lead to a reduced formation of protein-DNA cross-links, thereby mitigating the cytotoxic effects of cisplatin.

▶ Cytokeratins are intermediate filament proteins and play a key role in maintenance of cell shape, spatial organization of cellular organelles, and modulation of membrane transport. Furthermore, intermediate filaments may also be involved with DNA function and structure. It is possible that the formation of cytokeratin-DNA cross-links is associated with cisplatin toxicity and that the reduced expression of cytokeratin 18 in platinum-resistant cells may lead to a reduced formation of protein-DNA cross-links, thereby mitigating the cytotoxic effects of cisplatin.

R.F. Ozols, M.D., Ph.D.

Dose Escalation of Paclitaxel With High-Dose Cyclophosphamide, With Analysis of Progenitor-Cell Mobilization and Hematologic Support of Advanced Ovarian Cancer Patients Receiving Rapidly Sequenced High-Dose Carboplatin/Cyclophosphamide Courses
Fennelly D, Schneider J, Spriggs D, Bengala C, Hakes T, Reich L, Barakat R, Curtin J, Moore MAS, Hoskins W, Norton L, Crown J (Mem Sloan-Kettering Cancer Ctr, New York)
J Clin Oncol 13:1160–1166, 1995   4–6

Introduction.—The use of hematopoietic growth factors and peripheral-blood progenitors (PBPs) has facilitated the use of multiple courses of higher-dose chemotherapy. Several investigations have reported that Taxol may not be excessively toxic to hematopoietic stem cells. It is possible that its inclusion with cyclophosphamide in the PBP-mobilizing phase of the regimen may augment antitumor activity without compromising PBP collection. A phase I inquiry was commenced with escalating doses of Taxol to assess its impact on antitumor efficacy and mobilization of PBP cells in patients with stage IIC to IV ovarian cancer.

Methods.—Sixteen patients (age, 22–63 years) underwent infusion of cyclophosphamide, 3 g/m², and escalating-dose Taxol in cohorts of 3 (dose levels I to IV were 150, 200, 250, and 300 mg/², respectively). Filgrastim granulocyte colony-stimulating factor (G-CSF) and leukapheresis to harvest PBP were followed by 4 courses of rapidly cycled carboplatin and cyclophosphamide.

Results.—All 16 patients completed all planned cycles (32 courses) of Taxol/cyclophosphamide therapy. The median interval for treatment courses was 14 days. Twelve patients completed 54 cycles of carboplatin/cyclophosphamide that were administered and rescued with PBP. The median interval for treatment courses was 17 days. There were medians of 8 and 11 days to recovery of an absolute neutrophil count greater than .5 and a self-sustaining platelet count greater than 20×10^9/L, respectively. One patient died of sepsis. Thirteen patients were assessable for response. Five patients (38.5%) had pathologic complete responses, 6 patients (46%) had microscopic residual disease, and 2 patients (15%) had pathologic partial responses, for an overall response rate of 100%.

Conclusion.—The PBP mobilization was not compromised with the addition of escalating-dose Taxol to high-dose cyclophosphamide. Although antitumor activity was not the primary end point, the overall response rate of 100% deserves further investigation.

▶ The importance of dose intensity in ovarian cancer has long been an area of clinical investigation. Restrospective studies have suggested that survival is correlated with the administered dose intensity of platinum compounds. However, most prospective studies have failed to demonstrate any benefit from platinum regimens that were twofold greater in dose intensity than standard therapies. In addition, high-dose therapy that has required peripheral stem cell support and/or bone marrow transplantation has also been studied in patients with ovarian cancer. Although the response rates are high in patients with recurrent disease, the duration of remission is short, and survival does not appear to be influenced. If high-dose therapy that requires hematologic support is going to have a role in ovarian cancer, it will be in patients who have drug-sensitive disease and who have small-volume tumors. The ideal patient population to study would be optimal stage III patients, either at the time of initiation of chemotherapy or after several cycles of standard induction therapy.

This important study by Fennelly et al. shows that high-dose chemotherapy with paclitaxel and carboplatin can be administered for multiple courses if hematologic support is used. This study lays the groundwork for a pilot study within the Gynecologic Oncology Group to determine the feasibility of such an approach in previously untreated patients. If successful, the pilot study should then lead to a definitive study of high-dose chemotherapy with hematologic support, compared with standard paclitaxel plus platinum-based chemotherapy. It should be noted that in this study the pathologic complete remission rate was 38.5% in a patient population in which 62.5% were suboptimally debulked at initial surgery. Although encouraging, these results demonstrate the potential limitations of high-dose therapy in patients with suboptimal disease.

R.F. Ozols, M.D., Ph.D.

European-Canadian Randomized Trial of Paclitaxel in Relapsed Ovarian Cancer: High-Dose Versus Low-Dose and Long Versus Short Infusion
Eisenhauer EA, ten Bokkel Huinink WW, Swenerton KD, Gianni L, Myles J, van der Burg MEL, Kerr I, Vermorken JB, Buser K, Colombo N, Bacon M, Santabárbara P, Onetto N, Winograd B, Canetta R (Natl Cancer Inst of Canada Clinical Trials Group, Kingston; British Columbia Cancer Agency, Vancouver; Toronto Bayview Regional Cancer Centre; et al)
J Clin Oncol 12:2654–2666, 1994   4–7

Introduction.—The new anticancer agent paclitaxel (Taxol) has demonstrated activity against epithelial ovarian cancer, in addition to a number of other human tumors. Doses of paclitaxel studied in nonrandomized trials have ranged from 135 to 250 mg/m² given over 24 hours, along with premedication to prevent hypersensitivity reactions (HSRs). The dose-response relationship of paclitaxel in patients with relapsed ovarian cancer was assessed, and the safety of a short infusion administered along with premedication was evaluated in a randomized trial.

Methods.—Four hundred seven women with platinum-pretreated epithelial ovarian cancer and measurable recurrent disease were studied. The patients were randomized in a bifactorial design to receive paclitaxel in a dose of 175 or 135 mg /m² over 24 or 3 hours. Premedication consisted of 20 mg of oral dexamethasone given 12 and 6 hours before paclitaxel infusion, plus 50 mg of IV diphenhydramine and 50 mg of IV ranitidine given 30 minutes before infusion. If toxic effects were not prohibitive and there was no evidence of tumor progression, treatment cycles were repeated every 3 weeks. The main end points were frequency of significant HSRs and objective response rate; secondary end points were progression-free and overall survival.

Results.—Three hundred ninety-one of the 407 patients randomized were eligible, and 382 were evaluable for response. Severe HSRs occurred in only 1.5% of patients and were unaffected by the paclitaxel dose or administration schedule. Response rates were 20% at the 175 mg/m² dose and 15% at the 135 mg/m² dose; the difference was not significant. There was a significant difference in progression-free survival, 19 weeks in the high-dose group vs. 14 weeks in the low-dose group. The 24-hour paclitaxel infusion schedule was associated with significantly more neutropenia. Response rates were not significantly different between the 2 schedules: 19% in the 24-hour group and 16% in the 3-hour group. Survival was similar in the 2 treatment schedules.

Conclusions.—When given with premedication, 3-hour paclitaxel infusion is safe and is associated with less neutropenia. A longer time to progression is noted at a dose of 175 mg/m², reflecting a modest dose effect. Longer paclitaxel infusion leads to more myelosuppression without increasing response rates; therefore, future studies should focus on determining the optimal dose and schedule of this novel anticancer agent.

▶ Determination of the optimal dose and administration schedule of paclitaxel remains an area of active clinical investigation. Acute hypersensitivity reactions observed in the early phase I trials were essentially eliminated by a 24-hour infusion of paclitaxel together with premedication. This study establishes that premedication is effective in eliminating such hypersensitive reactions, even in a 3-hour infusion. Of particular interest in this study was the significantly lower incidence of neutropenia associated with the 3-hour infusion compared with the 24-hour infusion. There also did not seem to be a deleterious effect on survival in previously treated patients receiving the short infusion compared with the 24-hour schedule. Furthermore, there also appeared to be a modest dose effect with a longer time to progression at higher doses. Consequently, a 3-hour infusion of 175 mg/m² has become the accepted dose and administration schedule for relapsed ovarian cancer patients. The same schedule facilitated the development of paclitaxel combinations together with platinum compounds, particularly carboplatin. Finally, 1-hour infusion schedules have been studied, as have prolonged 96-hour infusions. Clinical trials comparing short and long infusions are in progress. Until results are available from these trials, a 3-hour infusion at 175 mg/m² can be considered "standard" schedule, particularly for patients with relapsed ovarian cancer.

R.F. Ozols, M.D., Ph.D.

Ovarian Malignant Mixed Müllerian Tumors Treated With Platinum-Based Chemotherapy

Bicher A, Levenback C, Silva EG, Burke TW, Morris M, Gershenson DM (MD Anderson Cancer Ctr, Houston)
Obstet Gynecol 85:735–739, 1995   4–8

Background.—Malignant mixed müllerian tumors of the ovary are rare tumors that have malignant epithelial and mesenchymal components and are associated with a poor prognosis. These tumors are generally initially treated surgically, with a variety of postoperative therapies. The efficacy of platinum-based chemotherapy was evaluated retrospectively.

Methods.—The records and histologic material, if available, were reviewed for 36 patients receiving a diagnosis of ovarian malignant mixed müllerian tumors and treated with platinum-based chemotherapy. The treatment regimens included combination cisplatin, doxorubicin, and cyclophosphamide in 16 patients; cisplatin and ifosfamide in 5; cisplatin and cyclophosphamide in 4; cisplatinum and doxorubicin in 3; carboplatinum in 3; and other platinum-based combination regimens in 2.

Results.—The patients had a mean age of 59 years; 83% were postmenopausal. There was 1 patient with stage IA disease; 2 had stage IIIB disease, 21 had stage IIIC, and 2 had stage IV; 10 were unstaged. Of the 16 patients evaluated for clinical response to chemotherapy, 7 (44%) had a complete response, 4 (25%) had a partial response, and 5 (31%) had no response. Of the 9 patients who underwent a second-look laparotomy, 5 (56%) had a complete surgical response, 1 (11%) had a partial surgical response, and 3 (33%) had no response. All 5 patients with a complete surgical response had less than 2 cm of residual tumor after primary excision. The median progression-free survival from diagnosis was 15.4 months in the 25 patients evaluated. Overall, the survival rates were 82% at 1 year, 47% at 2 years, and 30% at 5 years, with a median survival of 18 months.

Conclusion.—Ovarian malignant mixed müllerian tumors have response rates to platinum-based chemotherapy and survival rates similar to those seen in patients with advanced-stage epithelial ovarian cancer. As with epithelial ovarian cancer, an aggressive, combined modality treatment approach is recommended.

▶ The malignant mixed müllerian tumors of the ovary are composed of malignant epithelial and mesenchymal components. These aggressive tumors have often been treated with combination chemotherapy regimens designed to treat both histologic components. Doxorubicin and dacarbazine, which have been shown to have activity in sarcomas, have been coupled with drugs with demonstrable activity in epithelial ovarian cancer, such as cisplatin and cyclophosphamide.

This study confirms the efficacy of platinum-based chemotherapy with a complete response rate of 44% and an overall response rate of 69%. However, the survival rate for this group of patients remains poor, and improvements in chemotherapy are needed. Based on the marked activity of paclitaxel in epithelial ovarian cancer, this agent should be tested in combination with other drugs in the treatment of mixed müllerian tumors. A potentially interesting combination would be paclitaxel plus doxorubicin, because this combination is already shown to have an extremely high response rate (> 90%) in patients with metastatic breast cancer.

R.F. Ozols, M.D., Ph.D.

Impact of Doxorubicin on Survival in Advanced Ovarian Cancer
A'Hern RP, Gore ME (Royal Marsden Hosp, London)
J Clin Oncol 13:726–732, 1995   4–9

Introduction.—Previous research examining the use of various chemotherapy regimens for the management of patients with ovarian cancer has found a survival advantage associated with platinum treatment. However, none of these overview studies have examined the role of doxorubicin in the treatment of advanced epithelial ovarian cancer. The data from 2 overview studies were reexamined to determine the effect of doxorubicin on survival and to compare its impact with that of platinum.

Methods.—The data from the Advanced Ovarian Cancer Trialists Group (AOCTG) and the Ovarian Cancer Meta-Analysis Project (OCMP) were analyzed to determine the effect of the addition of doxorubicin or platinum to a treatment regimen. Data were analyzed with and without controlling for the confounding effects of other agents and the relative effects of combination or single-agent therapy with either doxorubicin or platinum.

Results.—The data suggested that adding doxorubicin to a chemotherapy regimen significantly reduced the relative risk of death and had a beneficial impact similar to that associated with the addition of platinum.

Discussion.—Meta-analysis revealed that including doxorubicin in the chemotherapy regimen significantly improves survival in patients with advanced epithelial ovarian cancer. In addition, the data suggest that treatment with a doxorubicin-containing therapy would be more effective than a nondoxorubicin, nonplatinum therapy. Therefore, it is recommended that both doxorubicin and platinum be used in the standard treatment regimen for patients with advanced epithelial ovarian cancer. This drug combination should be used as the standard against which other experimental treatments, such as a paclitaxel/platinum combination, are compared in clinical trials.

▶ The importance of doxorubicin's effect on survival in patients with advanced ovarian cancer, when used in combination with platinum compounds, has been an area of considerable debate. Prospective randomized trials have failed to demonstrate individually any significant impact of doxorubicin when it is combined with platinum. However, the meta-analysis described by A'Hern and Gore suggests that doxorubicin improves the overall survival rates by approximately 5%. How does this information relate to the standard therapy regimen for ovarian cancer? In the United States, standard therapy should include paclitaxel plus a platinum compound. Previous "standard" therapy regimens involving the use of platinum compound plus cyclophosphamide are inferior. At this time, it would not be possible to perform a randomized trial of paclitaxel combined with a platinum compound vs. a nonpaclitaxel combination, even if it did include doxorubicin.

Although paclitaxel is easily combined with platinum compounds, the situation with doxorubicin is not as simple. The combination of paclitaxel and doxorubicin has been studied most extensively in breast cancer, and toxicity has been formidable. Whether a platinum compound can be added to such a combination is problematic. The "best" treatment for patients with advanced ovarian cancer currently consists of using paclitaxel plus a platinum compound.

R.F. Ozols, M.D., Ph.D.

Laparoscopic Surgical Staging of Ovarian Cancer

Childers JM, Lang J, Surwit EA, Hatch KD (Univ of Arizona, Tucson)
Gynecol Oncol 59:25–33, 1995   4–10

Objective.—Although laparoscopy has been used to identify extraovarian metastases, its value in the surgical staging of ovarian cancer has yet to be determined. The accuracy, advantages, and disadvantages of laparoscopic staging of ovarian cancers were studied retrospectively.

Methods.—In the first group of women, aged 27–80 years, 40 had 44 second-look laparoscopic staging procedures for advanced disease after surgical debulking and chemotherapy. In the second group, there were 14 women, aged 17–75 years, with presumed early ovarian cancer, 5 of whom were unstaged when their tumors were surgically removed.

Results.—In the second-look group, 24 patients (56%) had persistent cancer. At surgery, 5 patients had microscopic disease located in the omentum, in para-aortic nodes (2 patients), pelvic peritoneum, and peritoneal washings. All of those patients had recurrences. In 20 of the patients who had restaging procedures, no metastatic disease was found, but 8 of those patients had recurrences. Six patients with second-look procedures had serious complications, and 3 required laparotomy. Eight of the 14 patients undergoing staging for the first time had metastatic disease including 2 with adenocarcinoma, 3 with pelvic disease, 1 with carcinoma of the fallopian tubes, 2 with carcinoma of the pelvic peritoneum, and 3 with metastatic adenocarcinoma of the para-aortic lymph nodes. Two patients had significant complications. Hospital stays ranged from 0 to 3 days.

Conclusion.—Laparoscopic surgical staging of ovarian cancer is effective and accurate. Additional validation studies are recommended.

▶ Ovarian cancer is characterized by widespread dissemination throughout the peritoneal cavity, frequently involving multiple peritoneal surfaces, the mesentery, and lymph nodes. Accurate assessment of histopathologic features has been critical in the selection of postoperative chemotherapy. Consequently, a formal staging laparotomy has traditionally been an essential part of the overall management of patients with ovarian cancer. Because of recent improvements in techniques, a laparoscopy may actually have some advantages over a traditional laparotomy in selected patients with ovarian cancer. Certainly, in the evaluation of patients following systemic chemotherapy who are in a clinical complete remission, a laparoscopy can frequently identify patients with residual disease and consequently obviate the need for a laparotomy. In patients with presumed early-stage disease, the situation is more difficult. Patients with isolated adnexal masses frequently will have very small metastases to diaphragmatic and other peritoneal surfaces. Laparoscopic visualization, because of illumination and enhanced magnification, can actually provide a better view of these areas of high risk and lead to identification of occult areas of metastases.

In the past, laparoscopy was limited because of the inability to evaluate lymph nodes, but modern laparoscopy does permit evaluation of peritoneal lymph nodes. The authors correctly emphasize that this is a technically demanding procedure and that expert laparoscopists should be performing staging procedures if critical decisions will be made on the basis of an accurate assessment of stage. It is apparent from this study that expert laparoscopy can decrease the number of laparotomies that are required in the management of patients with ovarian cancer.

R.F. Ozols, M.D., Ph.D.

Abdomino Pelvic Irradiation After Second-Look Laparotomy for Stage III Ovarian Carcinoma

Chapet S, Berger C, Fignon A, Calais G, Fetissof F, Reynaud-Bougnoux A, Descamps P, Body G, Lansac J, le Floch O (Centre Hospitalier et Universitaire, Tours, France)
Eur J Obstet Gynecol Reprod Biol 62:43–48, 1995   4–11

Introduction.—Optimal debulking surgery and systemic chemotherapy are the treatments of choice for patients with advanced ovarian carcinoma. Patients with minimal residual disease after chemotherapy should then receive further chemotherapy or radiotherapy. Several adjuvant treatment regimens have been proposed, including whole abdominal irradiation. The results and toxicity of whole abdominal irradiation given after surgery and chemotherapy in stage III patients without macroscopic residual disease were studied retrospectively.

Methods.—Over 9 years, 34 patients with invasive stage III ovarian carcinoma were initially treated with surgery and chemotherapy and achieved complete clinical and radiologic remission. At second-look lap-

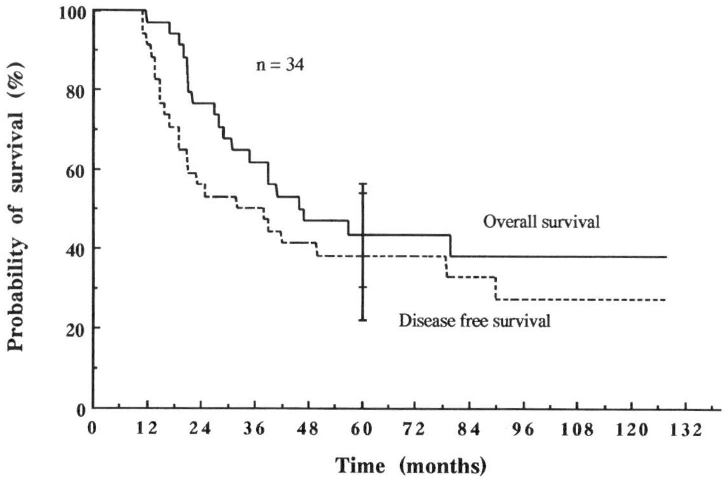

FIGURE 1.—Five-year overall and disease-free survival of the population (*n* = 34). (Reprinted from Chapet S, Berger C, Fignon A, et al: Abdominal pelvic irradiation after second-look laparotomy for stage III ovarian carcinoma. *Eur J Obstet Gynecol Reprod Biol* 62:43–48, 1995, with kind permission from Elsevier Science Ireland Ltd, Bay 15K, Shannon Industrial Estate, Co. Clare, Ireland.)

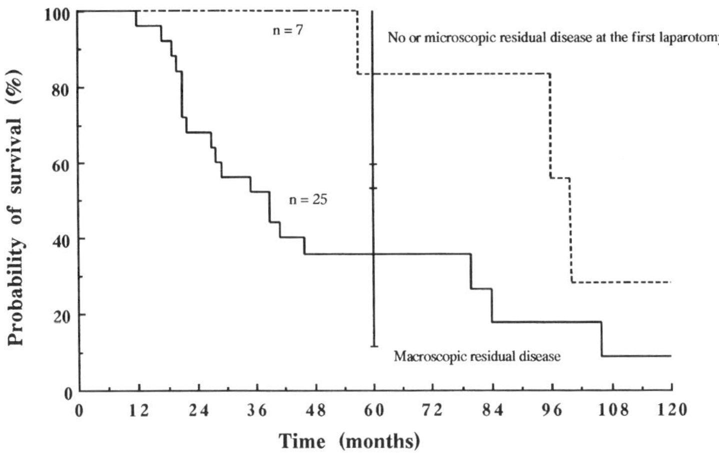

FIGURE 2.—Five-year overall survival according to the size of the residual disease at the first laparotomy. Patients with minimal residual disease or no residual disease had a better survival. The 2 patients who had no hysterectomy were excluded from the analysis. (Reprinted from Chapet S, Berger C, Fignon A, et al: Abdominal pelvic irradiation after second-look laparotomy for stage III ovarian carcinoma. *Eur J Obstet Gynecol Reprod Biol* 62:43–48, 1995, with kind permission from Elsevier Science Ireland Ltd, Bay 15K, Shannon Industrial Estate, Co. Clare, Ireland.)

arotomy, they had either no or minimal (< 2 cm) residual disease. Whole abdominal irradiation was administered in a midplane total dose of 22.5 Gy with a 22.5-Gy pelvic boost. The median follow-up was 94 months and ranged from 45 to 166 months. The survival rates were calculated, and prognostic factors were analyzed.

Results.—Of the 34 patients, 7 (21%) had no macroscopic residual disease after the first laparotomy; 7 had no macroscopic residual disease and 19 had completely resected macroscopic residuum after the second laparotomy. The overall survival rates were 62% at 3 years and 43% at 5 years. Disease-free survival rates were 53% at 3 years and 38% at 5 years (Fig 1). There was a 100% recurrence rate among patients with nonresectable macroscopic residual disease compared with 61% among patients with no macroscopic residual disease after the second laparoscopy. At 5 years, the survival rate was 35% in patients with unresected residual disease and 83% in patients with resected or microscopic residual disease (Fig 2). Treatment morbidity included grade 3 myelosuppression in 35%, grade 2 intestinal acute toxicity in 61%, grade 3 gastrointestinal toxicity in 4 patients, and fatal radiation enteritis in 1.

Conclusion.—Whole abdominal irradiation may be useful in the management of stage III ovarian carcinoma with minimal residual disease after surgery and chemotherapy. Further study with prospective randomized trials is required to establish the value of whole abdominal irradiation in this setting.

▶ The authors of this paper looked at 34 patients with stage III ovarian carcinoma who were thought to have achieved a complete clinical remission after initial surgery and chemotherapy. Patients then had a second-look laparotomy and underwent whole abdominal irradiation. Most patients had small residual disease at the time of treatment. The whole abdomen received 2,250 rad, and the pelvis was boosted for an additional 2,250 rad. The authors reported a 5-year overall survival rate of 43%, which is surprisingly good. Thirty-eight percent of the patients were disease free at 5 years. Even so, 68% had local relapse or local disease progression. There was 1 treatment-related death caused by radiation enteritis.

I think the authors have arrived at the correct conclusion that although there is curative potential with radiation administered after chemotherapy, when a patient has had a complete clinical response, the long-term benefits have not yet been established for the role of whole abdominal radiation in the treatment of ovarian cancer. Frankly, it is hard for me to see whether whole abdominal radiation has a great future because of the significant morbidities patients experience with this kind of treatment. On the other hand, I would be delighted if someone would prove me wrong.

E. Glatstein, M.D.

The Effect of Debulking Surgery After Induction Chemotherapy on the Prognosis in Advanced Epithelial Ovarian Cancer
Van Der Burg MEL for the Gynecological Cancer Cooperative Group of the European Organization for Research and Treatment of Cancer (Rotterdam Cancer Inst, The Netherlands)
N Engl J Med 332:629–634, 1995   4–12

Introduction.—The value of cytoreductive surgery for epithelial ovarian cancer is well established. Large, poorly perfused tumors with slow growth rates are relatively resistant to cytotoxic drugs, whereas smaller, perfused tumors with more rapid growth rates respond to chemotherapy. Removal of large tumors reduces the chance that drug-resistant clones will develop, whereas removal of small tumors means less chemotherapy will be needed, thereby decreasing the possibility of drug resistance. The use of debulking surgery after induction is less well defined. Survival has been reported to be similar in patients who undergo cytoreduction after induction chemotherapy and patients who had cytoreduction at their primary surgery.

Methods.—To be eligible, patients had to have a lesion greater than 1 cm after primary surgery. After 3 cycles of cyclophosphamide and cisplatin, the patients were randomly assigned to either the debulking group or the no surgery group. Each group had 3 further cycles of the medication. Progression-free and overall survival rates were calculated.

Results.—A total of 319 patients underwent the randomization procedure, with 278 eventually being evaluated; 140 patients had surgery and 138 did not. A total of 65% of the patients had a tumor larger than 1 cm. In this group, 45% of the lesions were reduced, surgically, to less than 1 cm. The surgery was not associated with death or any severe morbidity. The 2-year survival rate was 56% in the surgery group and 46% in the nonsurgery group. Surgery significantly increased both the overall and progression-free survival from 20 to 26 months. After adjusting for prognostic factors (e.g., number of tumors, ascites, tumor grade, International Federation of Gynecology and Obstetrics [FIGO] stage, World Health Organization [WHO] status, and chemotherapy response), surgery resulted in a 33% reduction in fatalities.

Conclusion.—The use of debulking surgery significantly increased progression-free and overall survival in patients with ovarian cancer. There was a 33% reduction in the risk of death, after adjusting for a variety of prognostic factors.

▶ Even though this is the largest randomized trial examining the role of debulking surgery in ovarian cancer, unfortunately it does not provide a definitive answer as to the impact of such a procedure on survival. Patients who were randomized to undergo debulking surgery had modest prolongation of progression-free survival and overall survival. A careful analysis of the results of debulking surgery after 3 cycles of chemotherapy raises some interesting questions. Of the 127 patients who underwent debulking surgery, 46 (36%) still had residual disease greater than 1 cm, consequently, optimal debulking was not achieved, and these patients did not benefit from this interval debulking procedure. In an additional 22 (17%) patients who underwent debulking surgery, no microscopic disease was found at the time of this interval laparotomy; therefore, these patients also did not benefit from the procedure. An additional 22 patients were found to have less than 1 cm disease at the time of interval debulking surgery, and 15 patients (12%) were still left with the same volume of disease after the attempt at interval debulking. Thus, in this study, 65% of the patients who underwent interval debulking surgery did not undergo a clinically meaningful alteration in disease volume on the basis of the surgical procedure. It appears that, theoretically, internal debulking surgery could only have benefited one third of the patients.

With so many investigators participating in this study it is probable that there were meaningful differences in the aggressiveness of the initial surgery. Until better chemotherapeutic regimens are developed, debulking surgery should be a major component of the overall treatment of patients with advanced ovarian cancer. It is probable that there is little difference in the end results seen when the debulking surgery is effectively performed at the time of diagnosis rather than subsequent to a few cycles of chemotherapy. This issue is being reevaluated in the United States by the Gynecologic Oncology Group (GOG), which is using a nationwide trial of similar design. More importantly, in the GOG study, a superior regimen of paclitaxel plus cisplatin is being used instead of the cyclophosphamide plus cisplatin regimen used in the European Organization for Research and Treatment of Cancer (EORTC) study.

R.F. Ozols, M.D., Ph.D.

Assessment of Dose-Intensive Therapy in Suboptimally Debulked Ovarian Cancer: A Gynecologic Oncology Group Study

McGuire WP, Hoskins WJ, Brady MF, Homesley HD, Creasman WT, Berman ML, Ball H, Berek JS, Woodward J (Emory Univ, Atlanta, Ga; Univ of the Health Sciences, Bethesda, Md; Mem Sloan-Kettering Cancer Ctr, New York; et al)
J Clin Oncol 13:1589–1599, 1995   4–13

Background.—A prospective trial of dose intensity and its effect in ovarian cancer using the current standard 2-drug therapy has not been reported. In a multi-institutional, prospective, randomized trial in women with advanced ovarian cancer, the effect of chemotherapy dose intensity on survival and progression-free survival was evaluated.

Methods.—Four hundred eighty-five patients with epithelial ovarian cancer and residual masses greater than 1 cm after surgery (stage III presentation) or with stage IV presentation were randomly assigned to receive either standard therapy or intense therapy. Standard therapy consisted of cyclophosphamide, 500 mg/m^2, and cisplatin, 50 mg/m^2, IV every 3 weeks for 8 courses. Intense therapy consisted of cyclophosphamide, 1,000 mg/m^2, and cisplatin, 100 mg/m^2, given every 3 weeks for 4 courses. Patients were not allowed to have any deviations in doses, but deviations were allowed in timing of subsequent doses. Before the next course could be administered, patients were required to have a white blood cell count greater than or equal to 3 × 10^9/L and a platelet count greater than or equal to 100 × 10^9/L.

Results.—Of the 485 patients, 458 met all eligibility criteria and were assessed for survival and progression-free survival. The intense-therapy group received the same total dose of the 2 drugs as the standard-therapy group, but the dose intensity was 1.97 times greater. Both groups of patients had similar clinical and pathologic response rates, response duration, and survival. The intense-therapy group had significantly more frequent and more severe hematologic, gastrointestinal, and renal toxicities, and more febrile episodes and septic events than did the standard therapy group. Seventeen percent of the patients in the intense-therapy group and 7% of patients in the standard-therapy group were removed from the study because of toxicity.

Summary.—In patients with bulky ovarian epithelial cancers, modest increases in chemotherapy dose intensity (without increasing the total dose) did not improve survival or progression-free survival. The increased-intensity treatment did, however, cause more severe toxicity.

▶ This study is the final blow for "high-dose cisplatin." Although retrospective studies have suggested there is a strong correlation between cisplatin dose intensity and outcome, this trial and others have failed to prospectively demonstrate that doses of cisplatin, 100 mg/m^2, add anything but toxicity to the treatment of ovarian cancer. It is possible that doubling the dose of cisplatin was insufficient to produce a clinical benefit and that a fivefold to tenfold increase in dose intensity is essential. This tenuous hypothesis is frequently used to justify high-dose chemotherapy that requires hematologic support (i.e., a bone marrow transplant or peripheral blood stem cell transfusions) in patients with ovarian cancer. However, outside of a clinical trial setting, there is no accepted role for high-dose therapy with hematologic support in ovarian cancer.

R.F. Ozols, M.D., Ph.D.

Can Fenretinide Protect Women Against Ovarian Cancer?

De Palo G, Veronesi U, Camerini T, Formelli F, Mascotti G, Boni C, Fosser V, Del Vecchio M, Campa T, Costa A, Marubini E (Istituto Nazionale Tumori, Milan, Italy)
J Natl Cancer Inst 87:146–147, 1995   4–14

Introduction.—In animal studies, the synthetic retinoid, fenretinide, has been shown to inhibit chemically induced mammary carcinomas and to enhance the effectiveness of tamoxifen. Its potential as a chemopreventive agent in patients with breast cancer who are at risk for another primary tumor developing in the contralateral breast was investigated in a randomized clinical trial.

Methods.—Patients who had undergone surgical treatment for T1–T2 breast cancer and had no evidence of axillary node involvement, local recurrence, or distant metastases were randomly assigned to receive either 200 mg of fenretinide daily for 5 years or no treatment.

Results.—With a median follow-up of 51.9 months, 21 patients in the treatment group and 22 patients in the control group had a new primary tumor develop in sites other than the breast. The sites were not significantly different in the 2 groups, with 1 exception. Six patients in the control group and none in the treatment group had ovarian cancer develop. The difference was statistically significant. After 5 years of fenretinide treatment, 2 patients had ovarian cancer, 1 at 10 months and the other at 30 months after the completion of treatment. The posttreatment incidence of ovarian cancer was not significantly different between the 2 groups.

Discussion.—These findings suggest that fenretinide may have a chemopreventive effect against the development of ovarian cancer during intervention, which does not continue after treatment is discontinued. These data support results seen in animal studies and suggest that fenretinide may prevent both breast and ovarian cancer, which could have profound benefits for women who are found to have the breast-ovarian cancer susceptibility gene.

▶ Chemoprevention is an exciting new approach to the cancer problem. It has long been known that a history of oral contraceptive use decreases the risk of ovarian cancer. Similarly, a correlation between either nulliparity or a family history and a subsequent increased risk of ovarian cancer has also been established. Recently, epidemiologic evidence demonstrated that a history of prolonged use of oral contraceptive pills (5 years or more) decreases the risk of ovarian cancer in women who have either a positive family history or who are nulliparous to almost the same level as that which exists for the general parous population. Preliminary data, as reported in this study, coupled with the epidemiologic data on oral contraceptive use provide optimism that prevention will be a real possibility, particularly when coupled with genetic studies to identify high-risk individuals.

R.F. Ozols, M.D., Ph.D.

Predicting Endometrial Cancer Among Older Women Who Present With Abnormal Vaginal Bleeding

Feldman S, Cook EF, Harlow BL, Berkowitz RS (Brigham and Women's Hosp, Boston; Harvard Med School, Boston; Harvard School of Public Health, Boston)
Gynecol Oncol 56:376–381, 1995

4–15

Background.—Generally, all older women with abnormal vaginal bleeding undergo endometrial sampling, either by office biopsy or dilation and curettage. However, fewer than 10% of women with abnormal perimenopausal or postmenopausal bleeding actually have endometrial cancer, which means that there is much unnecessary morbidity and expense.

Objective.—The clinical history was reviewed in 203 women, age 49 years and older, who were seen with abnormal vaginal bleeding and underwent either endometrial biopsy or dilation and curettage. Thirty-six of them were found to have endometrial cancer, and 16 had complex endometrial hyperplasia.

Observations.—On univariate analysis, cases were more likely to be nulliparous than were control women with neither index condition. They

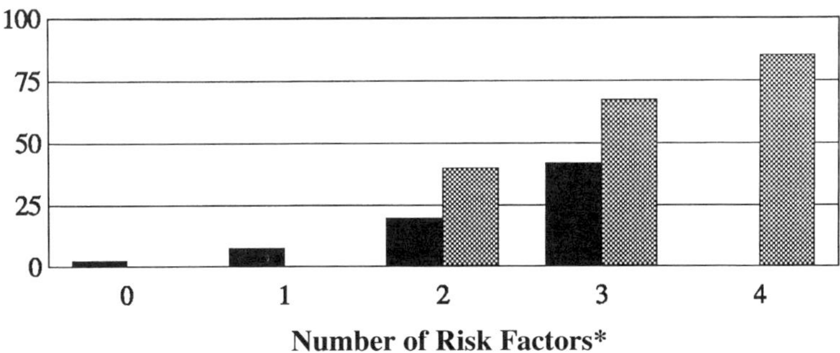

FIGURE 1.—Average estimated risk (percentage) of endometrial cancer/complex endometrial hyperplasia, according to the number of risk factors. *Filled bar* represents patients younger than 70 years; *hatched bar*, patients 70 years or older; all of whom are menopausal. *Asterisk* indicates risk factors evaluated: age of 70 years or greater, diabetes, nulliparity, and menopause. (Courtesy of Feldman S, Cook EF, Harlow BL, et al: Predicting endometrial cancer among older women who present with abnormal vaginal bleeding. *Gynecol Oncol* 56:376–381, 1995.)

also were more likely to have a history of unopposed estrogen use and to have had cancer other than breast cancer, diabetes, and hypertension. Multivariate analysis yielded 3 factors that were significant predictors of disease: age 70 years or older, diabetes, and nulliparity. When a model was constructed based on these factors and on a history of menopause, the risk ranged from 2.6% for individuals lacking all risk factors to 87% for those possessing all 4 risk factors (Fig 1).

Conclusion.—This model provides a convenient and inexpensive means of estimating the risk of endometrial cancer or complex endometrial hyperplasia in perimenopausal and postmenopausal women who have abnormal vaginal bleeding develop.

▶ Of all of the warning signs for cancer, postmenopausal bleeding has been among the most recognized because of its association with either endometrial cancer or an immediate precursor of endometrial cancer, such as complex endometrial hyperplasia. However, it should be noted that in several recent series, fewer than 10% of women who are seen with abnormal perimenopausal or postmenopausal bleeding actually have endometrial cancer (or its histologic precursor). Women with abnormal vaginal bleeding usually have undergone endometrial sampling, either by biopsy or by dilatation and curettage (D&C).

This important study identified the factors associated with endometrial cancer/complex hyperplasia. Age of 70 years or older, diabetes, and nulliparity were all associated with an increased risk of carcinoma in patients who were seen with abnormal vaginal bleeding (see Fig 1). In fact, if a woman possessed all 3 of these characteristics, her risk was 87%; her risk was less an 7% if she had none of the characteristics. This study may provide a useful model in which to identify those women who should undergo endometrial sampling, with its associated expense and morbidity, compared with those women for whom counseling and follow-up may be appropriate.

R.F. Ozols, M.D., Ph.D.

Endometrial Cancer: Stage at Diagnosis and Associated Factors in Black and White Patients
Barrett RJ II, Harlan LC, Wesley MN, Hill HA, Chen VW, Clayton LA, Kotz HL, Eley JW, Robboy SJ, Edwards BK (Wake Forest Univ, Winston-Salem, NC; Natl Cancer Inst, Bethesda, Md; Information Management Services Inc, Silver Spring, Md; et al)
Am J Obstet Gynecol 173:414–423, 1995   4–16

Objective.—There is a 30% difference in survival between black and white women with endometrial cancer, primarily because of the stage of the disease at the time of diagnosis. A comprehensive population-based matched case study was conducted to determine the clinicopathologic, health status, medical system, and socioeconomic factors responsible for this difference.

Methods.—Between January 1, 1985 and December 31, 1987, medical records, demographic data, and personal interviews were reviewed and analyzed for 130 black and 329 white patients with invasive endometrial cancer.

Results.—Of the patients with stage I or II disease, 75% were black and 91% were white; of those with stage IV disease, 11% were black and 3% were white. Black patients were less likely to have been interviewed, had less education and a lower poverty index, were less likely to have private insurance, and were more likely to use outpatient clinics, emergency departments, and public clinics. Body mass was a factor, with 72% of blacks being overweight or very overweight compared with 36.5% of whites. Blacks were much more likely to have hypertension and diabetes and were much less likely to be taking estrogen. Whereas adenocarcinomas were the most common cancer, adenoacanthoma occurred 4 times more often in white patients, and clear-cell and serous carcinoma were more common in blacks.

At diagnosis, 40.8% of women with stage I disease had at least some college education, whereas only 7.7% of women with stage IV disease had some college education. Early diagnosis was related to higher income and use of estrogen. Poorly differentiated tumors were found in 54% of the women with stage IV disease and 14.2% of those with stage I disease.

Conclusion.—Black women have higher stage and more aggressive and poorly differentiated endometrial cancers at diagnosis. The reasons for these more aggressive lesions are not known.

▶ This large study helps define the reasons that may exist for the observed difference in survival rates between black and white patients with endometrial cancer. Higher grade lesions and more aggressive histologic subtypes occur more frequently in black patients with endometrial cancer. It has been suggested that there may be 2 pathogenetic types of endometrial carcinoma. The more common type—the one that is most prevalent in the white population—is associated with endometrial hyperplasia, signs of hyperestrogenism, and better overall survival. The second type does not appear to be associated with increased estrogen and is characterized by a predominance of poorly differentiated carcinomas that have a more aggressive biological behavior. Why blacks have a higher predisposition for the more aggressive endometrial cancer remains to be determined.

R.F. Ozols, M.D., Ph.D.

The Effect of Diagnosis and Treatment Delay on Prognostic Factors and Survival in Endometrial Carcinoma
Menczer J, Krissi H, Chetrit A, Gaylor J, Lerner L, Ben-Baruch G, Modan B
(Chaim Sheba Med Ctr, Tel Hashomer, Israel)
Am J Obstet Gynecol 173:774–778, 1995   4–17

Objective.—Whether treatment delay (the time elapsing from the first symptom of endometrial carcinoma to the diagnosis) influences outcome was studied in 181 consecutive women given a diagnosis of endometrial carcinoma in the years 1970–1986.

Observations.—The study population was primarily postmenopausal and older than 50 years of age. More than two thirds of the patients were seen with postmenopausal bleeding. Approximately three fourths of the patients had stage I disease. The diagnosis was delayed longer than 3 months in half the patients and for more than 6 months in about one fourth of the group. On multivariate analysis, older patients, those with higher-grade tumors, and those of higher clinical state all did relatively poorly. The duration of diagnostic delay did not correlate with either the significant prognostic factors or survival.

Conclusion.—Endometrial carcinoma tends to progress slowly. Prompt diagnosis is always desirable, but a delay of less than 4 months is not likely to compromise the outcome in most patients.

▶ It is generally accepted as good medical practice not to delay treatment once the diagnosis of malignancy has been made. However, this well-established clinical principle is being tested, both by clinical trials and by economic realities. This study demonstrates that there is no adverse effect on survival in patients with endometrial cancer in whom the diagnosis of cancer was delayed for as long as a year and in whom treatment was delayed for less than 4 months from the time of diagnosis.

However, there is no benefit to be derived from not evaluating postmenopausal bleeding in a timely manner and from delaying a curative therapy once the diagnosis of endometrial cancer is made. This study's findings primarily reflect the natural history of endometrial cancer as a slowly progressing disease. The standard of care should remain a prompt evaluation of postmenopausal bleeding followed by definitive treatment for endometrial cancer.

R.F. Ozols, M.D., Ph.D.

Adenocarcinoma of the Endometrium: Survival Comparisons of Patients With and Without Pelvic Node Sampling

Kilgore LC, Partridge EE, Alvarez RD, Austin JM, Shingleton HM, Noojin F III, Conner W (Univ of Alabama, Birmingham)
Gynecol Oncol 56:29–33, 1995   4–18

Introduction.—Approximately 10% of patients with clinical stage I endometrial adenocarcinoma have pelvic node metastases. Patients with endometrial adenocarcinoma were reviewed retrospectively to evaluate survival traits of patients with and without pelvic node sampling.

Methods.—The mean patient age was 63.2 years. A total of 649 patients underwent total abdominal hysterectomy and bilateral salpingo-oophorectomy with peritoneal washings. The decision to sample nodes was surgeon-dependent and influenced by patient age, obesity, referral biopsy, and the desire to enroll patients in surgical staging protocols. Tumor grades were as follows: 165 grade 1, 351 grade 2, and 98 grade 3. Patients were categorized as low risk (disease confined to the uterine corpus) or high risk (disease outside the uterine corpus). A total of 212 patients had multiple-site pelvic node sampling (mean, 11 nodes), 205 patients had limited pelvic node sampling (mean, 4 nodes), and 208 had no node sampling.

Results.—The overall survival rate of patients undergoing multiple-site pelvic node sampling was significantly better than for those without node sampling, in both high- and low-risk groups. Patients in both categories had significantly better survival rates when treated with whole pelvic radiation with multiple-node sampling compared with no node sampling. Patients in both categories who did not receive radiation had statistically better survival rates if multiple-node sampling vs. no node sampling was done. The only patients benefiting from limited node sampling were those in the high-risk category who received whole pelvic radiation. The mean follow-up was 3 years.

Conclusion.—Multiple-site pelvic node sampling was associated with a significantly better survival rate than no node sampling. Multiple-site node sampling may be helpful in focusing treatment strategies.

▶ In many cancers, including endometrial cancer, there is a controversy regarding the prognostic vs. the therapeutic effect of lymphadenectomy or lymph node sampling. In this retrospective study, there was a surprisingly consistent survival advantage for patients with endometrial cancer who underwent multiple-site pelvic node sampling whether they were considered low or high risk. Although the use of radiation therapy and its influence on the recurrence risk and survival of patients with endometrial cancer remain controversial, in this study, the low-risk patients who received postoperative and whole pelvic radiation for grade 3 tumors, deep myometrial invasion, or disease outside the fundus had improved survival if the nodes were sampled from multiple sites (see Fig 1 in the original article), when compared with patients who did not undergo node sampling. Similar improvements were noted in high-risk patients as well. It is possible that improved survival is somehow related to node sampling. Unfortunately, the retrospective nature of this study cannot establish causality; prospective studies are needed.

R.F. Ozols, M.D., Ph.D.

Amplification and Overexpression of HER-2/*neu* (c-*erb*B2) in Endometrial Cancers: Correlation With Overall Survival
Saffari B, Jones LA, El-Naggar A, Felix JC, George J, Press MF (Univ of Southern California, Los Angeles; MD Anderson Cancer Ctr, Houston; Oncor Inc, Gaithersburg, Md)
Cancer Res 55:5693–5698, 1995   4–19

Introduction.—In the United States, the most common cancer of the female genital tract is endometrial cancer; about 33,000 new cases are diagnosed every year. Few studies have identified molecular genetic alterations in endometrial cancer to help predict poor clinical outcome. A poor prognosis has previously been associated with overexpression of HER-2/*neu*, transforming growth factor–α, and p53 proteins. The HER-2/*neu* gene was predictive in conjunction with the more established prognostic factors of extent of disease, nuclear grade, histopathology, DNA ploidy, and lymphovascular space invasion. The HER-2/*neu* gene amplification and overexpression were evaluated in a series of endometrial cancers. The results were compared with established prognostic markers and with overall survival. The response of patients with endometrial cancer to adjuvant therapies was also compared with the level of HER-2/*neu* expression.

Methods.—Ninety-two women with endometrial cancer had their level of HER-2-*neu* gene amplification and expression characterized. To characterize HER-2/*neu* gene copy number, fluorescence in situ hybridization was used. To characterize expression, immunohistochemistry was used. Women were followed for 3–123 months (mean, 67 months). Two women had chemotherapy, and 30 had radiation therapy.

Results.—Moderate or high immunostaining was seen in 47 of 90 endometrial cancers (52%). In 17 of 81 women (21%), HER-2/*neu* gene amplification was detected. Eighty women had both immunohistochemical staining and fluorescence in situ hybridization; among these 80, there were moderate or high immunostaining and gene amplification in 14. A shorter overall survival was seen for women in whom endometrial cancer exhibited HER-2/*neu* gene amplification by fluorescence in situ hybridization than for women whose endometrial cancer did not have amplification. Lower cumulative overall survival was seen with tumors with moderate or high HER-2/*neu* immunostaining than with tumor with low immunostaining. Overexpression of HER-2/*neu* was an independent predictor of overall survival. Adjuvant chemotherapy or radiation therapy was associated with an improved overall survival among those women with overexpression of HER-2/*neu*. However, overall survival was not improved by adjuvant therapy among women whose tumor lacked overexpression.

Conclusion.—Women whose endometrial cancers had overexpression of HER-2/*neu*—which, by itself, was associated with an inferior prognosis—had an improved overall survival if they received adjuvant chemotherapy or radiation therapy compared with those women who also expressed HER-2/*neu* but did not receive such therapies. It appears that HER-2/*neu* may be useful in helping select women who would benefit from postoperative treatment.

▶ The most useful prognostic factors are those that identify a subset of patients with an unfavorable prognosis who experience an improvement in outcome when they are treated on the basis of the identified prognostic factor. In endomentrial cancer, expression of HER-2/*neu* has previously been identified as a prognostic factor. In this regard, it was predictive in conjunction with the more established prognostic factors, such as extent of disease (stage), nuclear grade, histopathology, DNA ploidy, and lymphovascular space invasion.

What makes this study of particular interest is the observation that women whose endometrial cancers had overexpression of HER-2/*neu*—which, by itself, was associated with an inferior prognosis—had an improved overall survival if they received adjuvant chemotherapy or radiation therapy compared with those women who also expressed HER-2/*neu* but did not receive such therapies. In contrast to other prognostic factors, HER-2/*neu* may be useful as an aid in selecting women who would benefit from postoperative treatment.

R.F. Ozols, M.D., Ph.D.

Endometrioid Adenocarcinoma of the Ovary and Its Relationship to Endometriosis
McMeekin DS, Burger RA, Manetta A, DiSaia P, Berman ML (UCI Med Ctr, Orange, Calif; Long Beach Mem Med Ctr, Calif)
Gynecol Oncol 59:81–86, 1995   4–20

Background.—The clinical presentation of patients with endometriosis-related tumors has not been well documented. In addition, the biological behavior of these tumors is poorly understood. The study of a 13-year historical cohort determined whether endometriosis-associated tumors were different from typical endometrioid adenocarcinomas in clinico-pathologic variables and disease outcome.

Methods.—All women with endometrioid adenocarcinoma of the ovary (ECO) diagnosed between 1979 and 1991 were included in the review. Pathology reports were analyzed to determine whether coexisting endometriosis was present. Cancers adjacent to endometriosis on the same ovary or arising within endometriosis were classified as endometriosis-associated endometrioid adenocarcinoma (EAEA). All others were considered typical endometrioid adenocarcinoma (TEA).

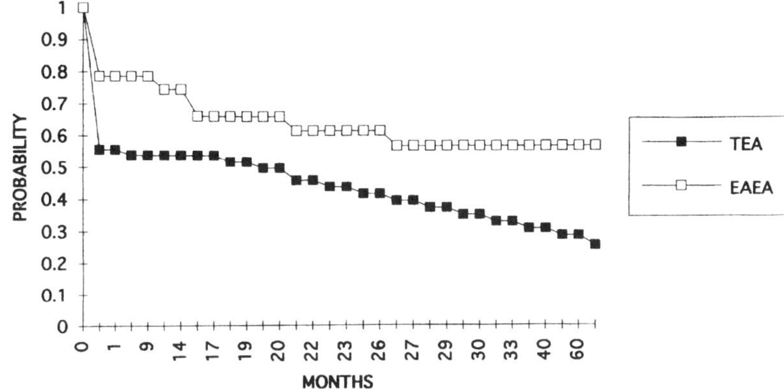

FIGURE 2.—Comparison of disease-free interval for typical endometrioid adenocarcinoma (*TEA*) and endometriosis-associated endometrioid adenocarcinoma (*EAEA*) cohorts. (Courtesy of McMeekin DS, Burger RA, Manetta A, et al: Endometrioid adenocarcinoma of the ovary and its relationship to endometriosis. *Gynecol Oncol* 59:81–86, 1995.)

Findings.—Sixty-nine percent of the 91 patients with ECO had TEA, and 31% had EAEA. Patients with TEA and those with EAEA differed significantly in age at diagnosis, with more patients with TEA being older than 55 years; nulliparity, with more patients with EAEA being nulliparous; stage, with I and II being more common among patients with EAEA; and disease status at the completion of primary surgery, with a greater proportion of patients with EAEA undergoing complete tumor resection. Eleven percent of patients with TEA and 25% of those with EAEA had synchronous atypical endometrial hyperplasia of uterine carcinoma. The estimated 5-year disease-free interval (DFI) was significantly longer in patients with EAEA than in those with TEA (Fig 2). However, the 5-year survival difference was nonsignificant. Disease stage was the only independent prognostic factor that predicted both DFI and survival.

Conclusions.—Endometrioid adenocarcinoma of the ovary associated with endometriosis may have a more favorable biological behavior than TEA. Women with EAEA are significantly younger, have an earlier disease stage on presentation, and have a longer disease-free survival than patients with TEA.

▶ There has been controversy regarding the relationship between endometriosis and the development of endometrioid adenocarcinoma of the ovary. Endometrioid adenocarcinoma of the ovary is a histologic subtype of epithelial ovarian cancer and is frequently diagnosed without any evidence of endometriosis. However, as noted by the authors, approximately 200 cases in which endometrioid adenocarcinoma appears to have developed from a malignant transformation of endometriosis have been reported in the literature.

This retrospective study has 2 important conclusions. First, it demonstrates that in approximately one third of patients with endometrioid adenocarcinoma of the ovary, the diagnosis is made in association with endometriosis. Second, women with endometrioid adenocarcinoma of the ovary who do have endometriosis are younger, are seen with earlier stage disease, and have a longer disease-free survival than do those with the more common typical endometrioid adenocarcinoma not associated with endometriosis. The mechanism involved in the transformation process, however, remains to be established.

R.F. Ozols, M.D., Ph.D.

Combinations of Multiple Serum Markers Are Superior to Individual Assays for Discriminating Malignant From Benign Pelvic Masses
Woolas RP, Conaway MR, Xu F, Jacobs IJ, Yu Y, Daly L, Davies AP, O'Briant K, Berchuck A, Soper JT, Clarke-Pearson DL, Rodriguez G, Oram DH, Bast RC Jr (Duke Univ, Durham, NC; Royal London Hosp)
Gynecol Oncol 59:111–116, 1995   4–21

Background.—Most studies of preoperative diagnosis in patients with pelvic masses include relatively few markers, and many have used simple thresholds for analysis. The use of larger panels of markers linked to novel analytic methods may increase sensitivity and specificity. Eight markers and 4 analytic methods were used to differentiate malignant from benign disease with greater sensitivity and specificity than can be achieved using CA 125 alone.

Methods.—Sera from 429 patients were assayed for CA 125, macrophage colony-stimulating factor, OVX1, lipid-associated sialic acid (LASA), CA15-3, CA72-4, CA19-9, and CA54/61. One hundred ninety-two patients had malignant histology.

Findings.—By itself, CA 125 had a sensitivity of 78.1% and a specificity of 76.8%. The sensitivity and specificity of a panel consisting of CA 125, OVX1, LASA, CA15-3, and CA72-4 were 83.3% and 84%, respectively, when 2 or more markers were increased. Logistic regression analysis, including the concentrations of these 5 markers, had a sensitivity of 85.4% and a specificity of 83.1%. When the values of markers were considered in different sequences, a classification and regression tree analysis increased sensitivity and specificity to 90.6% and 93.2%, respectively.

Conclusion.—Multiple serum markers are significantly more effective than the CA 125 assay for differentiating malignant from benign pelvic masses. Classification and regression tree analysis, applied in clinical practice, may improve the management of women with a pelvic mass. It may also be useful in screening for ovarian cancer.

► The diagnostic workup for a pelvic mass depends on a complexity of clinical factors, including symptoms, the size of the mass, and menopausal status. In a postmenopausal woman, a pelvic mass should lead to an ultrasonographic evaluation together with a serum CA 125 level to help differentiate a malignant tumor from a benign process. In this regard, CA 125 has been particularly useful.

This study demonstrates that there can be a further increase in sensitivity and specificity when combinations of serum markers are used. Furthermore, the use of multiple serum markers may also prove useful in screening for ovarian cancer.

However, although the results presented in this study are encouraging, they do not change the standard practice. Screening with serum markers and transvaginal ultrasonography has not been established to be useful in the asymptomatic population. In postmenopausal women with a pelvic mass, surgical exploration will likely be indicated in the majority of cases, with serum markers and ultrasonography only helping to establish the probability that ovarian cancer will be detected at surgery.

R.F. Ozols, M.D., Ph.D.

Improving Compliance Among Women With Abnormal Papanicolaou Smears
Paskett ED, Phillips KC, Miller ME (Wake Forest Univ, Winston-Salem, NC)
Obstet Gynecol 86:353–359, 1995   4–22

Purpose.—For various reasons, Papanicolaou smear screening has not been entirely successful in eliminating cervical cancer. A great deal is known about the reasons why women do and do not have Papanicolaou smears. However, there are few data on why women with abnormal smears do not receive appropriate treatment and surveillance. A clinic-based intervention to increase adherence to treatment recommendations by women with abnormal Papanicolaou smears was developed and tested.

Methods.—The intervention consisted of motivational brochures and a clinic-based tracking system. One brochure was aimed at women with a diagnosis of atypia, and it included key issues related to adherence. The other was for women with dysplasia, and it covered the definition, known causes, treatment, and curability of dysplasia. The tracking system consisted of a paper record with an accompanying tickler file.

Two family planning clinics, 2 family practice clinics, and 2 dysplasia clinics participated in the trial. One clinic of each type was randomly assigned to provide the clinic-based intervention for women with abnormal Papanicolaou smears, and the other was assigned to maintain its usual contact procedures. The clinics in the intervention group used the tracking system and sent the motivational brochures to women who were notified of abnormal cervical smear results. The comparison clinics used the tracking system but did not send the brochures. For each clinic, prospective data on adherence were available from about 100 consecutive women with abnormal smear results, including patients with inflammatory benign atypia or cervical intraepithelial neoplasia I, II, or III.

Results.—Baseline adherence rates, based on data from the year before the study, ranged from 33.3% to 69.3% for women with atypia and from 33.3% to 87.5% for those with dysplasia. Adherence by women with dysplasia significantly improved in the intervention clinics. However, there was no significant difference in adherence by women with atypia. More extensive analyses were performed using the data from the family planning clinics. Women at the intervention clinic were nearly 3 times more likely to obtain follow-up treatment for their abnormal cervical smear (odds ratio, 2.6). The intervention may have been more effective among black women (odds ratio, 15.7) than white women (odds ratio, 1.8). This difference was nonsignificant, however, because of the small number of black women enrolled. White women, women with dysplasia, and nonsmokers were most likely to adhere to treatment recommendations.

Conclusions.—The clinic-based intervention used in this study may improve adherence to recommended treatment among women whose Papanicolaou smears show atypia or dysplasia. Further efforts are needed to improve adherence among more resistant patients. The findings underscore the need for some user-friendly tracking system that is not unduly burdensome to clinic staff.

▶ The cure rate for cervical cancer is very high if the disease is detected in the preinvasive stages. The Papanicolaou smear has been established to decrease mortality from this disease by diagnosing it in preinvasive stages. One reason cervical cancer remains to be eliminated is the failure to treat precancerous lesions that are detected on the Papanicolaou smear properly. For undetermined reasons, a significant percentage of women, although making the effort to get the initial smear, do not undergo the appropriate follow-up treatments. This problem appears to be greater in black women than in white women, and it may account, in part, for the increased mortality from this disease in black Americans.

This study demonstrates that a motivational brochure can enhance adherence to treatment recommendations for women who do have abnormal Papanicolaou smears. However, white women with dysplasia on a Papanicolaou smear were still more likely to adhere to treatment recommendations than were black women. Clinics need to develop user-friendly tracking systems to ensure that women who do have an abnormal Papanicolaou smear return for further follow-up. It is the responsibility of both the individual and the medical care system to ensure that all women not only get screened for cervical cancer, but also that an abnormal Papanicolaou smear does result in the appropriate follow-up.

R.F. Ozols, M.D., Ph.D.

Correlation of High Lactate Levels in Human Cervical Cancer With Incidence of Metastasis
Schwickert G, Walenta S, Sundfør K, Rofstad EK, Mueller-Klieser W (Univ of Mainz, Germany; Norwegian Radium Hosp, Oslo, Norway)
Cancer Res 55:4757–4759, 1995   4–23

Introduction.—Several previous studies have documented early developments of abnormalities of tumor microcirculation and marked heterogeneities in the metabolic milieu within malignancies. Aspects of the metabolic milieu and their relationship with clinical parameters were studied in human cervical cancer to assess the importance of pathophysiologic prognostic parameters.

Methods.—Eleven tumor specimens from 10 patients were sectioned and stained with enzymes to measure the tissue concentrations of adenosine triphosphate (ATP), glucose, and lactate by averaging pixel values and then determining the differences in section values. Clinical data were also documented and analyzed for correlation with the metabolic parameters.

Results.—There was extreme heterogeneity in the metabolite distributions in all of the tumors, but the distribution patterns were clearly similar in serial sections. The concentrations of the 3 metabolites within specific locations were strongly correlated. The mean intratumoral concentrations of lactate were significantly higher in patients with metastases than in patients without metastases. There were no correlations with clinical parameters for mean intratumoral ATP or glucose concentrations.

Conclusion.—Generally, the pixel values of ATP, glucose, and lactate correlated well with each other. Although none of the 3 metabolites studied correlated with clinical staging or pathohistologic grading of the tumors, high lactate levels were significantly predictive of metastasis. Therefore, metabolic imaging may provide prognostic information in patients with cervical cancer, which can be useful in making treatment decisions.

▶ Classic prognostic factors such as tumor size, histologic grade, and depth of invasion will continue to be important in assessing gynecologic malignancies for the foreseeable future. However, several new prognostic factors have recently been developed from an increasing understanding of the microenvironment of human tumors. Cervical carcinoma is a prototype tumor in this regard because it is accessible for repeated biopsies. Furthermore, a technique of quantitative bioluminescence and single-photon imaging has been developed that permits biopsy specimens obtained in the clinic to be analyzed for a series of metabolic parameters.

Although this study is limited with regard to the number of patients examined, an interesting observation is made with regard to the high levels of lactate found in cervical cancer and the incidence of metastases. The reasons for such an association remain to be defined. It is possible that tumor lactate levels may facilitate neovascularization. In fact, tumor vascularity has already been identified to be a new prognostic factor in patients with advanced cervical carcinoma.[1] Neovascularization has also been shown to be an important prognostic factor in breast tumors. In addition, factors associated with angiogenesis have now become a potential target for therapeutic strategies. Antibodies and drugs that may disrupt angiogenesis are currently being evaluated in clinical trials.

R.F. Ozols, M.D., Ph.D.

Reference

1. Schlenger K, Hockel M, Mitze M, et al: Tumor vascularity: A novel prognostic factor in advanced cervical carcinoma. *Gynecol Oncol* 59:57–66, 1995.

Improved Control of Invasive Cervical Cancer in Sweden Over Six Decades by Earlier Clinical Detection and Better Treatment
Sparén P, Gustafsson L, Friberg L-G, Pontén J, Bergström R, Adami H-O
(Univ Hosp, Uppsala, Sweden; Univ of Uppsala, Sweden; Univ of Gothenburg, Sweden; et al)
J Clin Oncol 13:715–725, 1995   4–24

Introduction.—The most common type of cancer seen in developing countries is cervical cancer. Because this cancer affects young women, it is an important factor in reducing the life span. Cytologic screening is the most efficient method of disease control, but clinical detection and basic irradiation could be instituted with a minimum of resources. Data on the crude 5-year survival rate since 1914 show that mortality was reduced before advent of screenings. Using a large database on Swedish women, incidence and survival rates by stage, time, and age at diagnosis were analyzed. The database contains information dating back to the 1930s.

Methods.—Data on women from western Sweden from 1930 to 1990 were analyzed. The cohort included, 6,044 women. The patients were followed for at least 10 years after admission. A number of demographic and clinical variables were tabulated on all patients. The basic staging of cervical cancer has remained relatively intact since 1914. Actual and relative survival rates were determined. These were compared with the mortality tables for Swedish women in 5-year intervals from 1926 to 1990.

Findings.—Each higher stage of cancer at diagnosis increased the risk of death by 2.5 times. Prognosis improved over the years, with the 5- and 10-year survival probabilities being parallel during the review. Five-year survival probabilities were 4% to 5% higher. The 10-year survival rate increased from 33% in the 1930s to 55% in the 1950s and beyond. Clinical stage was a significant predictor of 10-year survival; 80% for stage I, 50% for stage II, 20% for stage III and 8% for stage IV.

Comments.—There has been little improvement in the survival rates of women with cervical cancer since the advent of more advanced treatment technologies. Improvement in survival are the result of public and professional awareness that has resulted in patients being given a diagnosis at earlier stages. These data are significant in that substantial reduction in mortality can be obtained without cytologic screening. This means that countries with limited resources can improve survivability with basic education and irradiation.

▶ It is well accepted dogma that in the West, the improved survival rates seen among patients with cervical cancer are primarily the results of screening. It is of interest that, in this study from Sweden, there was a marked improvement in survival from cervical cancer that developed before the widespread use of cytologic screening. The reason given for this improvement primarily relates to an increased clinical awareness leading to earlier clinical detection combined with effective therapy. The authors' interesting conclusion is that in developing countries where cervical cancer remains the leading cause of death from gynecologic cancer, public health efforts focus on increasing the awareness of cervical cancer instead of promoting a comprehensive screening program. Furthermore, the authors also suggest that the establishment of specialized centers that have diagnostic and therapeutic resources but do not require high-dose intracavitary therapy or external-beam radiation may lead to effective and inexpensive treatment for the majority of patients with cervical cancer.

R.F. Ozols, M.D., Ph.D.

Long-Term Results of Treatment of Cervical Carcinoma in the United States in 1973, 1978, and 1983: Patterns of Care Study (PCS)
Komaki R, Brickner TJ, Hanlon AL, Owen JB, Hanks GE (Univ of Texas MD Anderson Cancer Ctr, Houston; St Francis Hosp-NWBCC, Tulsa, Okla; Am College of Radiology, Philadelphia; et al)
Int J Radiat Oncol Biol Phys 31:973–982, 1995   4-25

Objective.—Data from the Patterns of Care Study (PCS) were analyzed to compare local control and survival rates in women treated for cervical carcinoma in 1973, 1978, and 1983, with respective follow-ups of at least 15, 10, and 5 years.

Database.—The PCS is a nationwide survey of practice patterns in patients with squamous carcinoma of the cervix who receive radiotherapy. A mail survey was conducted to update outcome data for each of the 3 follow-up cohorts. The numbers of patients surveyed totalled 937 in 1973; 565 in 1978; and 184 in 1983.

Findings.—Brachytherapy was increasingly used during the period under review. It was used in 60.5% of patients with stage III disease treated in 1973, 76.5% of those treated in 1978, and 88% of those treated in 1983. The use of higher energy external pelvic radiotherapy (instead of cobalt-60) also became more prevalent, increasing from 28% of patients in the 1973 cohort to 87% in the most recent cohort. Patients with stage III disease had improved local control in 1983 (Fig 2), as well as better overall and disease-free survival rates, but this was not the case for those patients

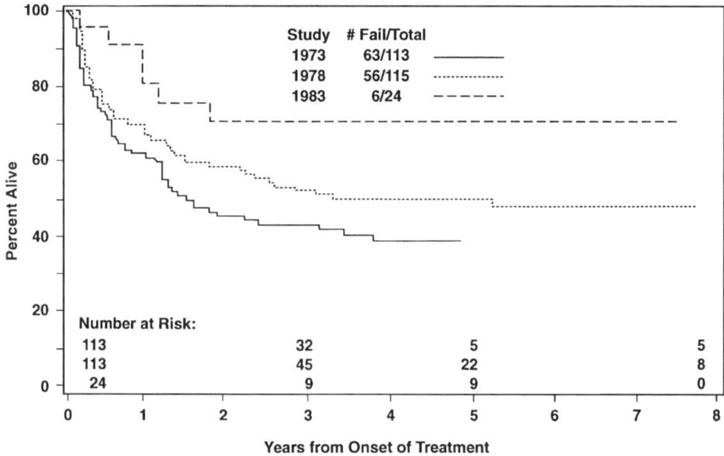

FIGURE 2.—The PCS (Patterns of Care Study) Cervix: 1973, 1978, 1983. Local control rates for patients with stage III cervical carcinoma. (Reprinted from *Int J Radiat Oncol Biol Phys*, Vol. 31, Komaki R, Brickner TJ, Hanlon AL, et al: Long-term results of treatment of cervical carcinoma in the United States in 1973, 1978, and 1983: Patterns of case study [PCS], pp 973–982, Copyright 1995, with kind permission from Elsevier Science Ltd, The Boulevard, Langford Lane, Kidlington 0X5 1GB, UK.)

with less advanced disease. Five-year survival for patients with stage III disease increased from 25% in the 1973 cohort to 47% in the 1983 cohort, a significant change.

Interpretation.—The improving prognosis for patients with stage III cervical carcinoma probably is a result of the wider use of brachytherapy as well as higher energy pelvic irradiation.

▶ Effective treatment for cervical cancer involves controlling the disease locally as well as distantly. The Patterns of Care Study (PCS) provides an important process by which to determine the impact of new treatments on the nationwide mortality of cervical cancer and other tumors as well. As shown in Figure 2, there has been a substantial improvement in local control rates for patients with stage III cervical carcinomas, probably as a result of the increase in the mean paracentral dose administered to such patients in the past decade. This has usually been accomplished by the combination of high-energy pelvic irradiation and increased use of brachytherapy. Not only has this led to improvement in local control, but it has also produced an improvement in 5-year survival, from 25% in 1973 to 47% in 1983. It is particularly encouraging that this marked improvement in end results has been accomplished without an increase in complications. Such improvement is possible because of superior dose distribution resulting from an increased use of linear accelerators/betatrons during the past decade. However, distant metastases remain a major problem for approximately one third of all patients with stage III disease. Whether new combined-modality approaches can decrease this rate of distant metastases remains to be determined.

R.F. Ozols, M.D., Ph.D.

Adenocarcinoma as an Independent Risk Factor for Disease Recurrence in Patients With Stage IB Cervical Carcinoma

Eifel PJ, Burke TW, Morris M, Smith TL (Univ of Texas MD Anderson Cancer Ctr, Houston)
Gynecol Oncol 59:38–44, 1995

4–26

Background.—The many studies of the effect of histologic type of tumor on prognosis among patients with International Federation of Gynecology and Obstetrics stage IB adenocarcinoma (AC) and with squamous cell carcinoma (SCC) of the cervix have yielded inconsistent results. Previous studies have been limited by methodological problems, such as small patient numbers. The influence of histologic type on outcome was investigated in 1,767 radiation-treated patients with stage IB AC and SCC of the cervix.

Methods and Findings.—The patients were treated between 1960 and 1989. Two hundred twenty-nine had AC, and 1,538 had SCC. The overall 5-year survival rate for patients with SCC was 81% and for those with AC, 72%. Maximum cervical diameter of less than 4 cm was more frequently documented in those with AC (53%) than in those with SCC (47%). Among the 903 patients with tumors measuring 4 cm or greater, 73% with SCC and 59% with AC survived for 5 years or longer (Fig 2). The rate of pelvic disease recurrence did not differ significantly between groups, but

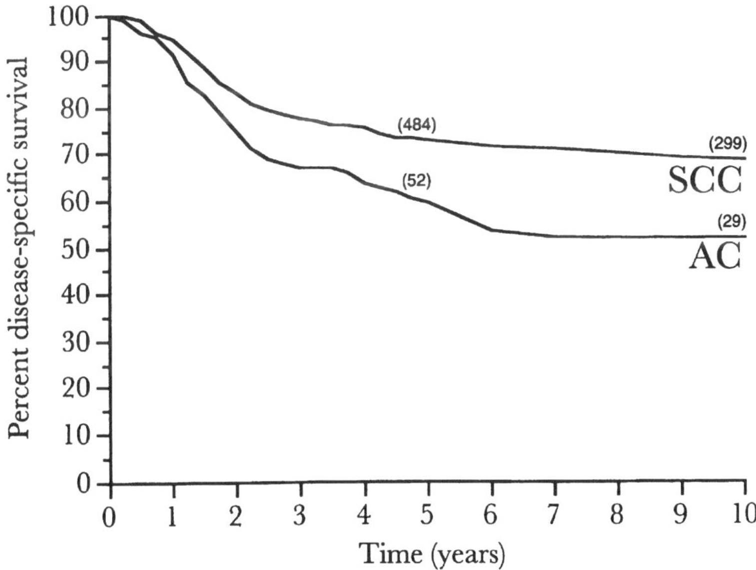

FIGURE 2.—Relationship between histologic type and disease-free survival rates of 903 patients with tumors 4 cm or greater in diameter. *Numbers in parentheses* indicate the number of patients at risk 5 or 10 years after treatment. *Abbreviations: AC,* adenocarcinoma; *SCC,* small-cell carcinoma. (Courtesy of Eifel PJ, Burke TW, Morris M, et al: Adenocarcinoma as an independent risk factor for disease recurrence in patients with stage IB cervical carcinoma. *Gynecol Oncol* 59:38–44, 1995.)

the rate of distant metastases was greater for patients with AC. Prognosis was strongly associated with tumor size and lymphangiogram findings but not with age or tumor morphologic type in patients with tumors of 4 cm or greater. There was a nonsignificant trend toward better survival in 165 patients undergoing adjuvant hysterectomy. In a multivariate analysis, the association between histologic type and survival was highly significant and independent. Patients with AC of 4 cm or greater in diameter had a 1.9 times higher estimated risk of death than patients with SCC.

Conclusions.—The prognosis of patients with AC of the cervix does appear to be worse than that of patients with similar stage and diameter SCC. This difference mainly reflects a greater rate of distant metasases in patients with AC.

▶ There has been a controversy regarding the influence of tumor histologic type on the prognosis of patients with early-stage cervix cancer. Some initial studies suggested that AC conferred an inferior prognosis compared with that of patients with SCC of the cervix. However, other studies did not report any such difference. This large retrospective review from the University of Texas M.D. Anderson Cancer Center establishes that AC is clearly an adverse prognosis factor in patients with stage IB cervical carcinoma. Although there is a slightly increased rate of central or pelvic recurrences in patients with stage IB ACs who are treated with radiation therapy compared with those with SCC, the major difference in prognosis relates to a higher degree of distant metastases for patients with AC of the cervix. These patients should be prime candidates for clinical trials evaluating the role of systemic therapy in preventing development of distant metastases.

R.F. Ozols, M.D., Ph.D.

Differential Expression of M_r 70,000 Heat Shock Protein in Normal, Premalignant, and Malignant Human Uterine Cervix

Ralhan R, Kaur J (All India Inst of Med Sciences, New Delhi)
Clin Cancer Res 1:1217–1222, 1995   4–27

Objective.—Heat shock proteins, or stress proteins, are produced by cells under normal conditions, but levels of HSPs are higher in cancer cells. Although not much is known about HSP expression in human normal and malignant cells, HSPs are suspected of being involved in the carcinogenesis of some cancers. The M_r 70,000 HSP (HSP70) expression in human uterine cervical cancer, cervical dysplasia, and normal uterine cervix was studied, as was the predictive value of HSP70 expression on disease outcome.

Methods.—Mouse antibody IgG_2 against HSP70 was used to measure HSP70 expression by an enzyme-linked immunosorbent assay method in 20 samples of human squamous carcinoma of the uterine cervix and in 11 dysplastic and 11 normal uterine cervical cell samples. Heat-shocked and non–heat-shocked HeLa cells were used as the standard.

Results.—There was significantly more HSP70 immunoreactivity detected in non–heat-shocked malignant cells than in non–heat-shocked normal or dysplastic cells. There was no significant difference between levels of HSP70 in heat-shocked normal and dysplastic cells. Whereas there was a significant increase in HSP70 levels in heat-shocked malignant cells, induction was less than in normal or dysplastic cells. Although no staining was detected in normal or dysplastic specimens, cytoplasmic and nuclear staining were seen in malignant specimens using mouse antibodies against HSP70, horseradish peroxidase-conjugated rabbit antimouse immunoglobulins, and diaminobenzidine tetrachloride.

Conclusion.—There is significantly more expression of HSP70 in cancer cells than in normal or dysplastic cells. The HSP70 levels are correlated with tumor size.

▶ Heat shock proteins (HSP) are stress proteins whose levels are frequently higher in cancer cells than in normal tissues. This study demonstrated an increased expression of HSPs in squamous cell carcinomas of the cervix compared with normal—or even with premalignant—lesions in the uterine cervix. It appears that HSPs are involved in the progression from cervical dysplasia to carcinoma in the cervix. Heat shock protein expression may also have a clinical prognostic significance, as there was a correlation between an increase in tumor size and the level of HSP70 expression.

R.F. Ozols, M.D., Ph.D.

Randomized Trial of Epirubicin and Cisplatin Chemotherapy Followed by Pelvic Radiation in Locally Advanced Cervical Cancer

Tattersall MHN, for the Cervical Cancer Study Group of the Asian Oceanian Clinical Oncology Association (Univ of Sydney, Australia; Chang Mai University, Mahidol University, et al)
J Clin Oncol 13:444–451, 1995   4–28

Introduction.—Although early detection of cervical cancer has improved with Papanicolaou smear screening, treatment choices have not changed and outcome has not improved recently. Patients with locally advanced disease are usually treated with radiotherapy, frequently with disappointing results. Studies of primary chemotherapy followed by radiotherapy have not conclusively proven to be beneficial. A large, randomized, multicenter trial of primary chemotherapy was conducted in several countries.

Methods.—Over 4 years, 260 patients with histologically confirmed cervical cancer (stage IIB to IVA) who had not received prior radiotherapy or chemotherapy were randomly assigned to receive pelvic radiotherapy beginning either immediately or within 3 weeks after chemotherapy. The chemotherapy regimen was 3 cycles of a combination of epirubicin and cisplatin administered at 3-week intervals. The radiotherapy regimen con-

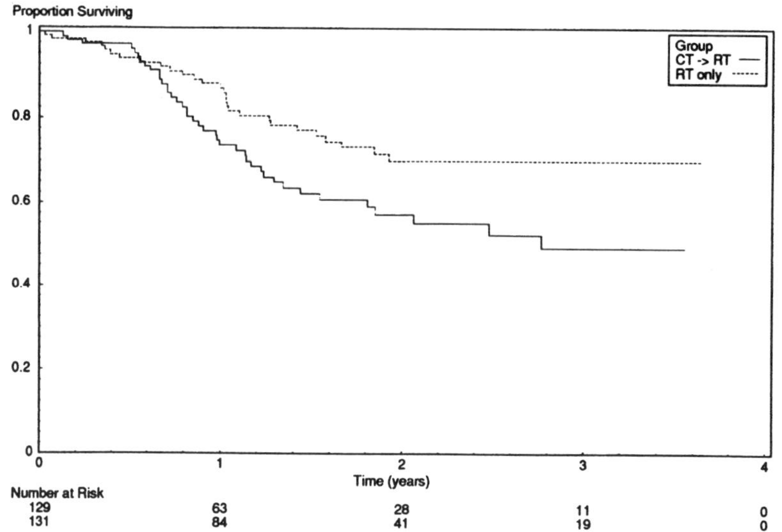

FIGURE 6.—Overall survival according to randomization group. (Courtesy of Tattersall MHN, for the Cervical Cancer Study Group of the Asian Oceanian Clinical Oncology Association: Randomized trial of epirubicin and cisplatin chemotherapy followed by pelvic radiation in locally advanced cervical cancer. *J Clin Oncol* 13:444–451, 1995.)

sisted of 40–55 Gy of external beam whole pelvis radiotherapy followed by 30–35 Gy of intracavitary radiotherapy. Tumor response was monitored, and survival was calculated.

Results.—The 2 treatment groups were comparable for prognostic factors. Before radiotherapy began, primary chemotherapy resulted in a 63% tumor response. In 62 of the 99 patients who had treatment failure, the relapse occurred in the pelvis. The pelvic failure rate was significantly higher and the survival rate was significantly lower (Fig 6) among patients treated with primary chemotherapy and radiotherapy than among patients treated with radiotherapy alone.

Discussion.—These data indicate that although a significant number of patients experience tumor regression with primary chemotherapy, these patients have reduced survival and control rate compared with patients treated with pelvic radiotherapy alone. Therefore, primary chemotherapy followed by radiotherapy is not recommended in the treatment of patients with locally advanced cervical cancer.

▶ Combined cancer treatment with chemotherapy and radiation has usually resulted in either improvement or no benefit compared with treatment with either modality. In this large randomized trial in patients with locally advanced cervical cancer, primary chemotherapy with epirubicin and cisplatin before pelvic radiation not only produced inferior local control, but also had a deleterious effect on overall survival compared with patients treated with standard pelvic radiation therapy. The mechanism(s) of why pretreatment with chemotherapy reduced the effectiveness of radiation therapy remain to be determined, particularly in view of the fact that chemotherapy was associated with a high objective response rate (63%). The adverse effect of chemotherapy was most apparent in the group of patients who did not have a good response to initial chemotherapy.

Among the mechanistic possibilities requiring further exploration are the impact of chemotherapy on cross resistance to radiation and drug-induced alterations in the cell kinetics of the residual tumor. Because chemotherapy was effective in reducing the size of the cervical tumors in most of these patients, it is possible that primary chemotherapy followed by surgery may be advantageous. Further trials of such a combined modality approach are needed.

R.F. Ozols, M.D., Ph.D.

5 Prostate Cancer

The Role of Increasing Detection in the Rising Incidence of Prostate Cancer
Potosky AL, Miller BA, Albertsen PC, Kramer BS (Natl Cancer Inst, Bethesda, Md; Univ of Connecticut, Farmington)
JAMA 273:548–552, 1995

5–1

Background.—The diagnosis of prostate cancer has increased so dramatically that prostate cancer has surpassed lung cancer as the most diagnosed nonskin cancer in men. This is likely the result of early detection methods or the finding of incidental cancer during transurethral resection procedures (TURP). If so, then age-adjusted death rates should begin to decrease.

Methods.—Data from the National Cancer Institute's Surveillance, Epidemiology, and End Results (SEER) program were analyzed from 1973 to 1991. The SEER program is considered the definitive source of data on cancer survival and incidence. Prostate cancer incidence was determined from surgical stage at diagnosis and match-adjusted per 100,000 Medicare enrollees.

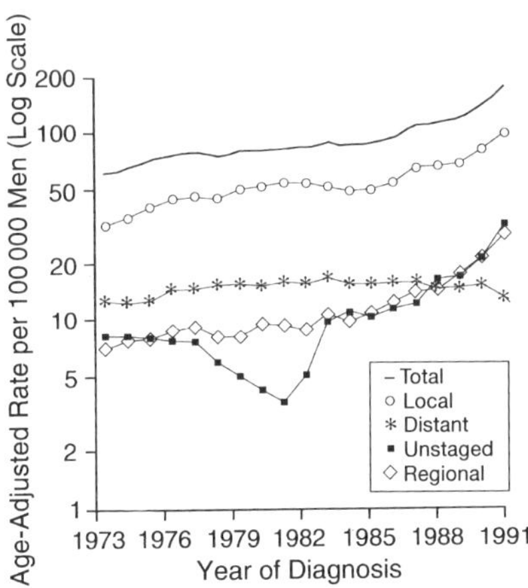

FIGURE 1.—Prostate cancer incidence by stage for all ages. Data are from 4 Surveillance, Epidemiology, and End Results areas. (Courtesy of Potosky AL, Miller BA, Albertsen PC, et al: *JAMA* 273:548–552, Copyright 1995, American Medical Association.)

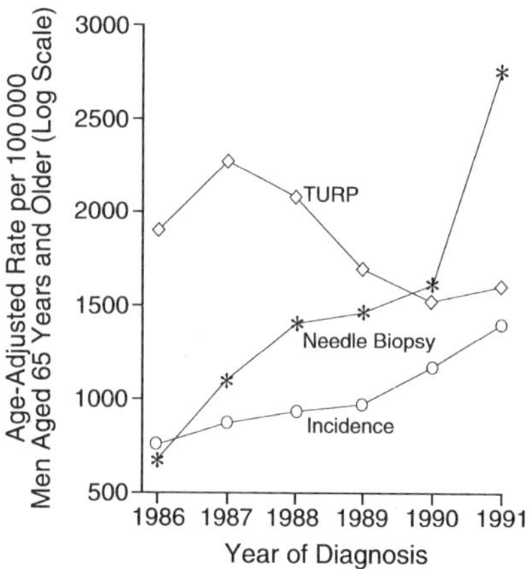

FIGURE 2.—Changes in the method of diagnosis of prostate cancer among men aged 65 years and older. Data are from Medicare enrollees in 4 Surveillance, Epidemiology, and End Results areas. *Abbreviation: TURP,* transurethral resection of the prostate. (Courtesy of Potosky AL, Miller BA, Albertsen PC, et al: *JAMA* 273:548–552, Copyright 1995, American Medical Association.)

Findings.—Over the 20-year period, the age-adjusted incidence of prostate cancer increased by 178% from 64 to 178 per 100,000 (Fig 1). Transurethral resection procedures and needle biopsies seem to be responsible for detecting prostate cancer as evidenced by the age-adjusted incidence rate compared with TURP and needle biopsies (Fig 2). From its peak, the rate of use of TURP has declined by 29% whereas the rate of needle biopsy has nearly tripled. The hypothesis was that the use of needle biopsies were driven by the use of transrectal ultrasound and prostate-specific antigen (Fig 3).

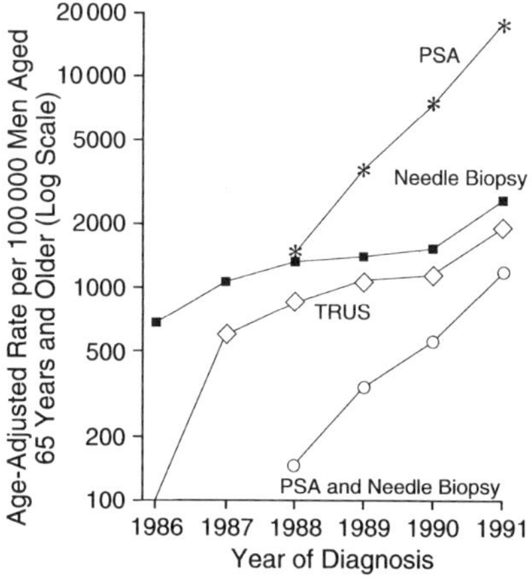

FIGURE 3.—Trends in the use of procedures to detect prostate cancer. Data are from Medicare enrollees in 4 Surveillance, Epidemiology, and End Results areas. The 1986 TRUS value was less than 100. *Abbreviations: PSA,* prostate-specific antigen; *TRUS,* transrectal ultrasound of the prostate. (Courtesy of Potosky AL, Miller BA, Albertsen PC, et al: *JAMA* 273:548–552, Copyright 1995, American Medical Association.)

Conclusion.—The apparent epidemic of prostate cancer is caused by an increase in the detection of tumors from prostate-specific antigen screening. The more intense attitude of the medical community toward surveillance explains the trend. There is wide geographic variability in the use of the screening procedure, which suggests that there is not widespread agreement on the value of the test in reducing mortality from prostate cancer.

▶ In the mid-1980s, data indicating that measurements of serum prostate-specific antigen (PSA) could result in the early detection of prostate cancer became available. Subsequent screening studies have confirmed this observation, and the use of PSA as a screening tool in men older than 50 years of age has been widely recommended. Between 1989 and 1991, the incidence of prostate cancer dramatically increased by more than 40% in this short interval. By 1994, approximately 200,000 new cases of prostate cancer were predicted, and approximately 38,000 men were predicted to die of the disease (see Fig 1). Is there evidence that early detection has resulted in an improvement in survival?

In this study, Medicare physician claims data were used to study the frequency of use of procedures to detect and diagnose prostate cancer. Data from 4 SEER (Surveillance, Epidemiology, and End Results) tumor registries were used. Between 1973 and 1986, the incidence of prostate cancer increased by 178%. The greatest increase occurred between 1986 and 1991. During this same 5-year period, the frequency of use of needle biopsy for diagnosing prostate cancer increased dramatically whereas that for TURP (transurethral resection of the prostate) decreased (see Fig 2). Between 1988 and 1991, the rate of PSA testing increased more than tenfold, and the combination of PSA followed by needle biopsy paralleled this growth between 1988 and 1991.

These data strongly suggest that the very rapid increase in the incidence of prostate cancer is the result of earlier diagnosis made possible by PSA testing and is associated with many more biopsy procedures to confirm disease. If the rapid rise in incidence is the result of screening procedures for detecting occult disease, then it might be expected that this increase will plateau at some point. The costs of PSA screening and subsequent diagnosis of prostate cancer are substantial, and they will be a worthy investment only if mortality decreases. However, this will be difficult to determine for many years. Because of the profound impact of lead time bias in a disease with a very long natural history, earlier diagnosis can in no way be used to predict reduced mortality. Better treatment for locally advanced and metastatic disease must be accomplished before a decrease in long-term mortality can be appreciated.

G.J. Bosl, M.D.

Are Pelvic Computed Tomography, Bone Scan and Pelvic Lymphadenectomy Necessary in the Staging of Prostatic Cancer?

Levran Z, Gonzalez JA, Diokno AC, Jafri SZH, Steinert BW (William Beaumont Hosp, Royal Oak, Mich)
Br J Urol 75:778–781, 1995

5–2

Background.—A significant risk of local recurrence is associated with prostate carcinoma with extracapsular involvement. The efficacy and cost-effectiveness of CT scanning, bone scanning, and pelvic lymphadenectomy as staging modalities in patients undergoing radical prostatectomy were investigated.

Methods.—Eight hundred sixty-one men with prostate cancer diagnosed between 1990 and 1993 were included in the study. Four hundred nine underwent surgery. Pelvic CT scans and prostate-specific antigen (PSA) analysis were performed in all patients. Those having surgery underwent preoperative bone scans and Gleason's scoring of pathologic tissue.

Findings.—Pelvic CT scans were positive in only 1.5% of the 861 patients. All those undergoing surgery had negative pelvic CT and bone scans. Forty-seven percent of those men had extracapsular disease at modified pelvic lymphadenectomy. Only 3.7% of the patients undergoing surgery had positive nodes.

Conclusions.—Pelvic CT and bone scans have a very low yield and are not cost-effective in the clinical staging of patients with PSA levels of 20 ng/mL or less. The role of a modified pelvic lymphadenectomy for the purposes of staging, whether by open or laparoscopic procedure, is also questionable, as the yield of positive diagnoses with this procedure is also very low.

▶ This retrospective study addresses an increasing concern: What staging tests are necessary in patients with organ-confined prostate cancer? This study evaluates the clinical tests (bone scan and CT) that were performed in 861 patients, and it compares the results of the tests to known pathologic outcomes. Only 13 of 861 patients with newly diagnosed prostate cancer (1.5%) had a positive pelvic CT scan. All of those patients had a serum PSA > 20 ng/mL. All 409 patients who elected to undergo radical prostatectomy had negative pelvic CT scans and bone scans. Only 15 of the 409 (3.7%) patients had involved lymph nodes. In addition, the pelvic CT scan was very poor at detecting extracapsular disease; 192 of 409 reported patients (47%) had extracapsular disease. These facts imply that abdominal and pelvic CT scan are not useful in the staging of patients with prostate cancer. Only 8 patients (0.9%) had a positive bone scan; all 8 patients had serum PSA values greater than 20 ng/mL. Clearly, pelvic CT scan and bone scan do not provide much information if the serum PSA is low.

G.J. Bosl, M.D.

Prostate-Specific Antigen Values at the Time of Prostate Cancer Diagnosis in African-American Men
Moul JW, Sesterhenn IA, Connelly RR, Douglas T, Srivastava S, Mostofi FK, McLeod DG (Walter Reed Army Med Ctr, Washington, DC; Armed Forces Inst of Pathology, Washington, DC; Uniformed Services Univ of the Health Sciences, Bethesda, Md)
JAMA 274:1277–1281, 1995   5–3

Background.—Black men have a 50% higher incidence of prostate cancer than do white men after adjusting for age; they have the highest incidence in the world. Hormonal, genetic, nutritional, and socioeconomic reasons have all been considered. Analyzing the levels of prostate-specific antigen (PSA) in military patients with prostate cancer should provide an opportunity to assess the importance of access to care and socioeconomic status.

Study Population.—Complete records were available for 541 patients treated for newly diagnosed prostatic adenocarcinoma at Walter Reed Army Medical Center in the years 1990–1994. Data on tumor volume were analyzed in 91 patients having radical prostatectomy in 1993 and 1994.

Observations.—Geometric mean levels of PSA were significantly higher in black than in white patients (14 vs. 8.3 ng/mL). Blacks had higher levels for all categories of age, stage, and tumor grade. They were also 2.2-fold more likely than whites to have a PSA level exceeding 10 ng/mL.

Radical Prostatectomy Cohort.—Comparable numbers of black and white patients underwent biopsy on the basis of PSA screening. Black patients had tumor volumes that were more than twice as large as those of whites, but differences in prostate weight were not significant. There was no radial difference in prostatitis. On linear regression analysis, tumor volume predicted the PSA levels, but race no longer was a significant factor.

Conclusion.—Even when given equal access to health care, black men with prostate cancer have higher levels of PSA at the time of diagnosis than do white patients of similar age who have comparably advanced disease.

▶ Epidemiologic studies have shown that black men with prostate cancer appear to be seen with more advanced disease and have a worse overall survival compared with white men. This study sheds some light on these racial differences. It encompassed 541 men in military service who had newly diagnosed prostate cancer. Not only were black men seen with significantly higher levels of PSA than were white men, but they were more likely to have larger tumor volume and a higher stage of disease. Even within a clinical stage, black men had a higher tumor volume. In multivariate analysis, race, grade, and age at presentation were not significant independent variables, whereas tumor volume and stage were significant.

This study would strongly suggest that important genetic differences exist in prostate cancer arising in black and white patients, particularly because all patients came from within an equal-access military health care system. The differences in tumor volume within stage suggest that the disease is perhaps inherently more aggressive in black men and that screening strategies need to be applied more urgently in this patient population.

G.J. Bosl, M.D.

Overexpression of bcl-2 Protects Prostate Cancer Cells From Apoptosis *In Vitro* and Confers Resistance to Androgen Depletion *In Vivo*
Raffo AJ, Perlman H, Chen M-W, Day ML, Streitman JS, Buttyan R (Columbia Univ, New York; Univ of Michigan, Ann Arbor)
Cancer Res 55:4438–4445, 1995   5–4

Background.—The oncoprotein encoded by the gene *bcl-2* appears to contribute to the development of human follicular B-cell lymphomas, and it may also have a role in breast and prostate cancers. The secretory epithelial cells of the normal human prostate do not express *bcl-2* protein, but some cells of primary untreated adenocarcinomas do express this protein, which suppresses apoptosis. Expression is consistently seen in tumors that are resistant to hormonal measures.

Objective.—Both in vitro and in vivo studies were undertaken to learn to what extent the overexpression of *bcl-2* protein can protect prostate cancer cells against factors promoting apoptosis. Human prostate cancer cells were transfected with a eukaryotic expression vector containing complementary DNA encoding human *bcl-2*. The tumorigenic potential of cells overexpressing *bcl-2* was determined by injecting them into male nude mice.

Results.—Transfected human prostate cancer cells that expressed *bcl-2* protein grew at the expected rate in medium containing 10% serum and expressed usual amounts of prostate-specific antigen and androgen receptor protein. When grown in charcoal-stripped serum lacking dihydrotestosterone, however, the cells grew more rapidly than expected and proved very resistant to such apoptotic stimuli as serum starvation and phorbol ester. Subcutaneous injections of transfected cells resulted in the earlier appearance of tumors and the formation of larger tumors. The cells gave rise to tumors when injected into castrated mice, whereas nontransfected cells had no such effect. In addition, castration did not inhibit tumor growth.

Implication.—The development of hormone-resistant prostate tumors is associated with the presence of *bcl-2* oncoprotein, which protects the cancer cells against apoptosis.

▶ In the past few months, we have seen articles describing interactions between the *bcl-2* and *bax* genes and their relative importance to the control of apoptosis in breast cancer.[1, 2] In prostate cancer, the situation may be reversed. Prostate adenocarcinoma cells were recently found to overexpress the *bcl-2* protein. This would theoretically shift the *bcl-2/bax* ratio toward the inhibition of apoptosis. In this study, a human prostate adenocarcinoma cell line was altered to overexpress *bcl-2* protein. These cells were resistant to stimuli that would lead to apoptosis. More important, the cells became resistant to the effects of castration in nude mouse xenografts. This suggests that overexpression of *bcl-2* protein is important in the evolution of hormone-refractory prostate cancer. The study of *bcl-2* and *bax* in prostate cancer will shed light on the importance of this pathway in the evolution of advanced and hormone-resistant prostatic adenocarcinoma.

G.J. Bosl, M.D.

References

1. Krajewski S, Blomquist C, Franssila K, et al: Reduced expression of proapoptic gene BAX is associated with poor response rates to combination chemotherapy and shorter survival in women with metastatic breast adenocarcinoma. *Cancer Res* 55:4471–4478, 1995.
2. Bargou RC, Daniel PT, Mapara MY, et al: Expression of the bcl-2 gene family in normal and malignant breast tissue: Low bax-expression in tumor cells correlates with resistance towards apoptosis. *Int J Cancer* 60:854–859, 1995.

Long-Term Survival Among Men With Conservatively Treated Localized Prostate Cancer
Albertsen PC, Fryback DG, Storer BE, Kolon TF, Fine J (Univ of Connecticut, Farmington; Univ of Wisconsin, Madison; Yale Univ, New Haven, Conn)
JAMA 274:626–631, 1995   5–5

Purpose.—More men with localized prostate cancer are being treated with either radiation therapy or radical surgery. However, there are insufficient data to document the therapeutic benefits of these treatments, compared with the more conservative alternative of deferred therapy, for patients aged 65–75 years. The debate over the use of widespread screening and treatment for men in this age group depends on inferences about the natural history of conservatively managed localized prostate cancer. A population-based study was performed to analyze mortality and life expectancy for 65- to 75-year-old men with newly diagnosed, clinically localized prostate cancer who were treated only with immediate or delayed hormonal therapy.

Methods.—The retrospective analysis used identified cases from the Connecticut Tumor Registry. It included all men with clinically localized prostate cancer diagnosed in 1971–1976, who were 65–75 years old at the time of diagnosis, and were either untreated or treated with immediate or delayed hormonal therapy. The final cohort included 451 men with a mean age of 70.9 years at the time of diagnosis. Patient data were abstracted from the records of 37 acute care hospitals and 2 Veterans Affairs medical centers in Connecticut. A pathologist evaluated the original pathology slides without knowledge of the patients' outcomes. The patients' survival was compared with that of men in the general population by parametric

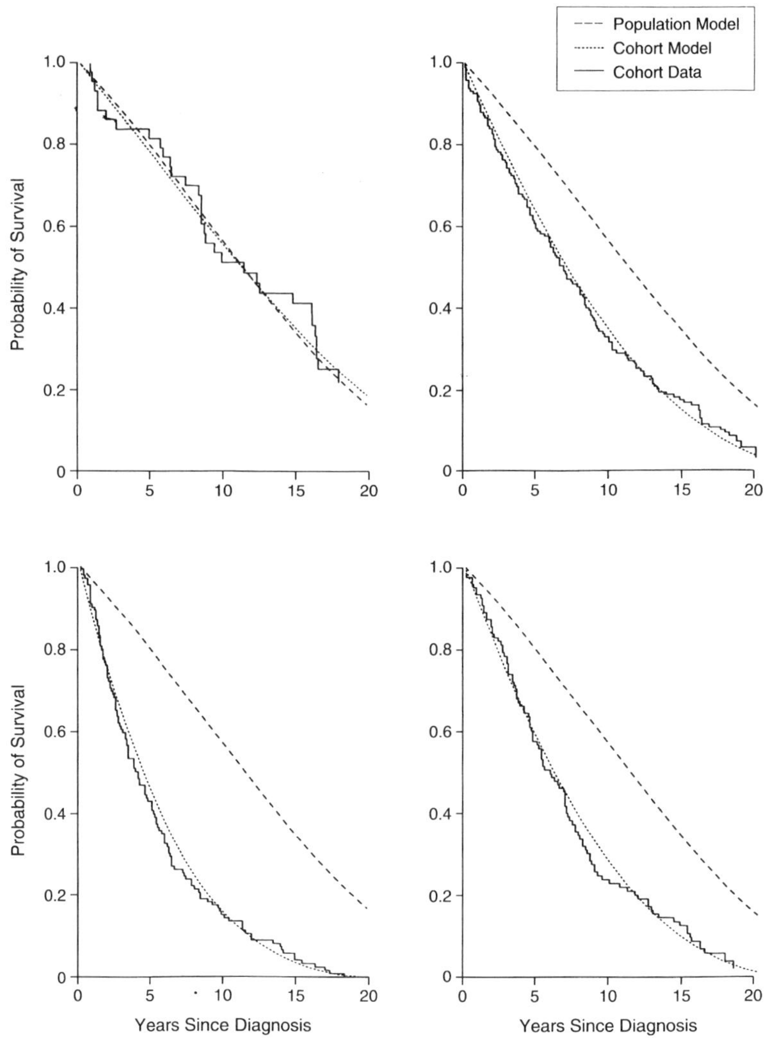

FIGURE 2.—Age-adjusted survival curves for low-, moderate-, and high-grade tumors. Observed cohort data are shown as Kaplan-Meier curves. Smooth curves are age-adjusted survival predicted for each group by the bivariate hazard model and by the general population model. **Top left graft** is for Gleason score 2–4 tumors (n = 44); **top right,** Gleason score 5–7 tumors (n = 160); **bottom left,** Gleason score 8–10 tumors (n = 130); and **bottom right,** Gleason score unknown (n = 117). (Courtesy of Albertson PC, Fryback DG, Storer BE, et al: Long-term survival among men with conservatively treated localized prostate cancer. *JAMA* 274:626–631, 1995. Copyright 1995, American Medical Association.)

proportional hazards models that took into account the tumor histologic findings, comorbidity, and age at diagnosis.

Results.—At a mean follow-up of 15.5 years, 9% of patients were alive at last contact, 34% had died of prostate cancer, 49% had died of other known causes, and 8% had died of unknown causes. The age-adjusted

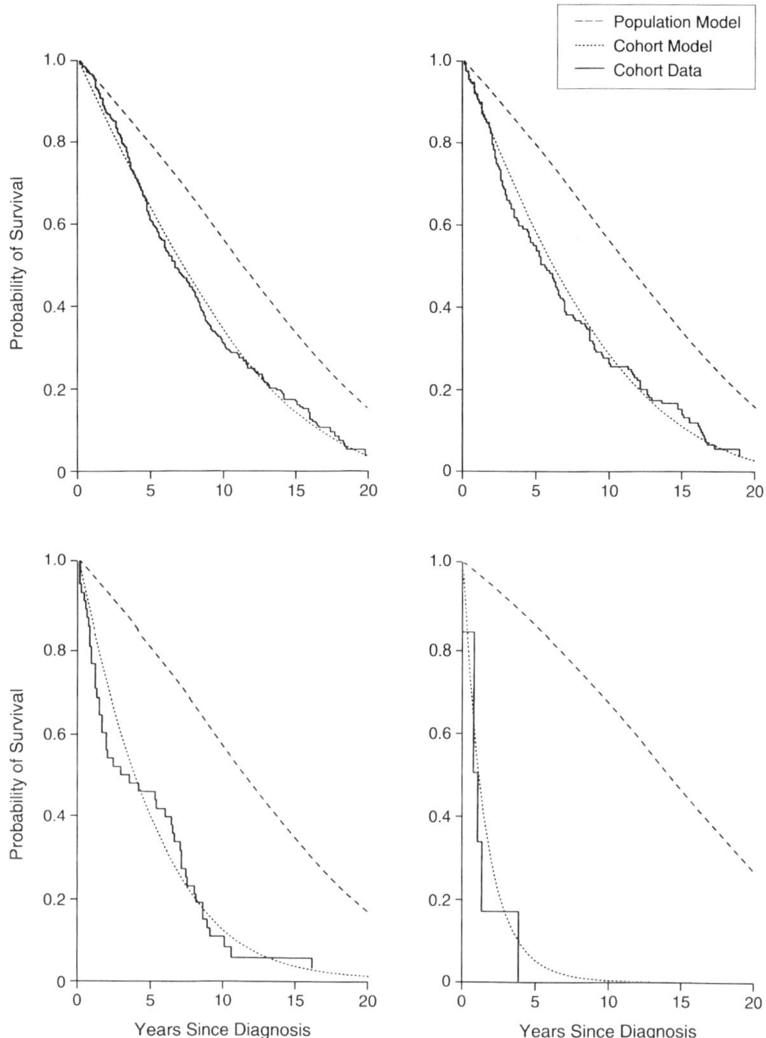

FIGURE 3.—Age-adjusted survival curves for levels of comorbidity indexed by the Index of Co-Existent Disease (*ICED*). Observed cohort data are shown as Kaplan-Meier curves. Smooth curves are age-adjusted survival predicted for each group by the bivariate hazard model and by the general population model. **Top left graft** is for ICED classification 0 ($n = 245$); **top right,** ICED classification 1 ($n = 150$); **bottom left,** ICED classification 2 ($n = 50$); and **bottom right,** ICED classification 3 ($n = 6$). (Courtesy of Albertson PC, Fryback DG, Storer BE, et al: Long-term survival among men with conservatively treated localized prostate cancer. *JAMA* 274:626–631, 1995. Copyright 1995, American Medical Association.)

survival of patients with Gleason score 2–4 tumors was not significantly different from that of men in the general population. Men with tumors of Gleason score 5–7 lost a maximum estimated life expectancy of 4–5 years, and those with tumors of Gleason score 8–10 lost no more than 6–8 years

(Fig 2). Survival was significantly and independently predicted by the tumor histologic findings and by the patients' comorbid illnesses (Fig 3).

Conclusions.—Men aged 65–75 years with conservatively treated low-grade prostate cancer showed no loss of life expectancy compared with the general population. As tumor grade increases, lost life expectancy increases progressively. Reports of survival and mortality for men with clinically localized prostate cancer must control for age, histologic findings, and comorbidity to avoid bias.

▶ Confusing recommendations regarding the proper treatment approach for older men with localized prostate cancer continue to appear. The frequency of radical prostatectomy has increased as a result of the increased frequency with which early disease is detected by prostate-specific antigen testing. Much data exist to suggest that deferred therapy of low- or intermediate-grade localized prostate cancer has minimal to no adverse impact on the survival of men older than 70 years of age. Who is right?

To some extent, probably both camps—those advocating treatment and those advocating deferred therapy have arguments with merit. The problem is selecting patients appropriately for each treatment approach. Albertsen et al. attempt to shed some light on this problem. The Connecticut Tumor Registry was used to identify 451 men with prostate cancer diagnosed between 1971 and 1976, who were aged 65–75 years at the time of diagnosis, and whose prostate cancer was confined to the gland. The patients were stratified by Gleason score and further analyzed for age-adjusted survival by comorbidity level. The first finding is certainly not unexpected: the higher the Gleason score, the more likely that survival would be impaired by deferred therapy (see Fig 2). However, for patients with Gleason 2–4 tumors, no impairment was noted. Using the Index of Co-Existent Disease, a similar decrement in survival was noted and was associated with higher comorbidity indices (see Fig 3).

It is evident that treatment decisions in older men with localized prostate cancer should take into account not only stage, but also Gleason score and associated comorbidities. Patient decisions that do not take into account the Gleason grade and associated comorbidities will be affected by selection bias and predisposed to an incorrect conclusion. The national randomized prostate cancer study comparing deferred therapy with intervention (PIVOT: Prostate Cancer Intervention versus Observation Trial) should begin to address some of these issues in a formal way, and the best recommendation is to refer patients for the PIVOT trial.

G.J. Bosl, M.D.

Detection of Circulating Tumor Cells in Patients With Localized and Metastatic Prostatic Carcinoma: Clinical Implications

Ghossein RA, Scher HI, Gerald WL, Kelly WK, Curley T, Amsterdam A, Zhang Z-F, Rosai J (Mem Sloan-Kettering Cancer Ctr, New York; Cornell Univ, New York)

J Clin Oncol 13:1195–1200, 1995

5–6

Background.—Recent reports have described the use of a reverse-transcriptase polymerase chain reaction (RT-PCR) technique to detect prostate-specific antigen (PSA)–positive cells in peripheral blood. These studies, however, were unable to determine the possible relationship between a positive RT-PCR assay and patient outcome. Combined with other clinical variables, the results of RT-PCR assays may help in selecting patients with prostate cancer for local treatment approaches, identifying progression at an early stage and defining disease-free status with greater precision. The frequency of detection of PSA-positive cells in the peripheral blood of patients with prostate cancer was studied.

Methods.—One hundred seven men with prostate cancer—representing different disease stages and different sensitivities to hormonal therapy—and 27 controls without prostate cancer were included. Peripheral blood samples from all subjects were studied by RT-PCR and Southern blotting to detect PSA messenger RNA (mRNA). The RT-PCR technique used has the potential for detecting circulating cells, even in patients with nonmeasurable serum PSA levels or from cancer cells that do not express the PSA protein. It was able to detect a single PSA-producing cell diluted into 1×10^6 blood mononuclear cells.

Results.—Sixteen percent of patients with T1 or T2 disease tested positive for PSA mRNA compared with 30% of those with T3, T4, or N-positive tumors and 35% of those with distant metastases. The test was negative in all control subjects. Positivity for PSA mRNA increased with increasing PSA levels. Of 73 patients with distant metastases, 16 had normal or undetectable PSA levels after hormonal therapy and 57 had androgen-independent disease. Positivity for PSA mRNA in these subgroups was 38% and 37%, respectively.

Conclusion.—The RT-PCR technique can detect PSA mRNA in peripheral blood cells of patients with prostate cancer. Positivity is more frequent with increasing tumor stage. The detection of PSA-positive cells in patients with no measurable PSA after hormonal therapy suggests that seeding of distant sites may be continuing in these patients. Further study of the relationships between continued seeding, disease progression, and survival is needed.

▶ Prostate-specific antigen is a highly tissue-specific marker. Its potential value in screening men for the presence of early prostate cancer has been well established. The gene encoding the protein has been cloned and can be identified by a variety of assays. Theoretically, circulating prostate cancer cells should be detectable by identifying cells in the peripheral blood that express PSA mRNA. In this study of 107 men with prostate cancer and 27 men without prostate cancer, PSA mRNA was detected in 28% of patients with serum PSA levels between 0 and 4 and in 56% of patients with serum PSA levels greater than 150. None of the control samples was positive. The frequency of positivity increased with tumor stage, but only 35% of patients with distant metastases had detection of PSA mRNA.

These data show that circulating tumor cells can be found in a proportion of patients with apparently localized disease. However, it is disappointing to find that only a minority of patients with proven distant metastases had evidence for circulating tumor cells. It should be noted that the lower limit of detection was 1 × 10⁶ cells. Further studies will need to be performed before we know whether this approach will have clinical applicability.

G.J. Bosl, M.D.

Immunocytochemical Detection of Isolated Tumour Cells in Bone Marrow of Patients With Untreated Stage C Prostatic Cancer

Pantel K, Aignherr C, Köllermann J, Caprano J, Riethmüller G, Köllermann MW (Universität München, Germany; Kliniken Wiesbaden Germany; Institut für Immunologie der Universitä at München, Germany)
Eur J Cancer 31A:1627–1632, 1995   5–7

Background.—Conventional diagnostic methods usually fail to identify the micrometastatic spread of tumor cells. However, such spread largely determines the prognosis of patients with primary epithelial cancers. Through the use of CK2, the monoclonal antibody to epithelial cytokeratin component number 18 (CK18), individual disseminated carcinoma cells can now be detected in the bone marrow of patients with cancer. This technique was applied to patients with stage C prostatic cancer.

Methods and Findings.—Forty-four untreated patients with clinical stage C adenocarcinoma of the prostate were included. One to 38 CK18-positive cells per sample of 2 × 10⁶ mononuclear cells were detected in the double-sided aspirates of the iliac bone marrow of 54.5% of the patients. In 13 of these 24 patients, CK-positive cells were found in only 1 of the 2 aspirates analyzed. This finding was not significantly correlated with established risk factors, such as primary tumor volume and histologic grade or the concentration of prostate-specific antigen and prostatic acid phosphatase in serum (Table 2).

Conclusion.—The finding of prostatic tumor cells in bone may indicate the metastatic capacity of a primary tumor. Thus, detecting these cells immunocytochemically may be useful for increasing the precision of current tumor staging and to monitor minimal residual cancer in individual patients. Although the follow-up in this study was too short to provide conclusive data on the prognostic significance of isolated CK18-positive cells in bone marrow, this has been shown recently in other types of primary epithelial cells.

TABLE 2.—Incidence of CK-Positive Cells in Bone Marrow of Patients With Stage C Prostatic Cancer

Risk factor	Cytokeratin positivity in bone marrow	
	Number of patients per group	Number of patients with ≥ 1 CK18$^+$ cells per sample* (%)
Total group	44	24 (54.5)
A. Tumor volume		
< 3 mL	23	13 (56.5)
$\geq$ 3 mL	16	8 (50.0)
B. Histological grade		
Gleason score <7	16	9 (56.2)
Gleason score $\geq$7	24	14 (58.3)
C. PSA level in serum		
< 40 ng/mL	34	20 (58.9)
$\geq$ 40 ng/mL	7	3 (42.9)
D. PAP level in serum		
< 5 ng/mL	25	14 (56.0)
$\geq$5 ng/mL	9	5 (55.5)

* Samples of 2×10^6 mononuclear cells aspirated from both sides of the upper iliac crest of each patient were stained with MAb CK2 using the alkaline phosphatase antialkaline phosphatase technique.

Abbreviations: PAP, prostatic acid phosphatase; *PSA*, prostate-specific antigen.

(Reprinted from *Eur J Cancer*, vol 31A, Pantel K, Aignherr C, Köllerman J, et al: Immuno-cytochemical detection of isolated tumour cells in bone marrow of patients with untreated stage C prostatic cancer, pp 1627–1632, 1995, with kind permission from Elsevier Science Ltd., The Boulevard, Langford Lane, Kidlington 0X5 1GB, UK.)

▶ Carcinoma of the prostate, as everyone knows, has a high probability of metastatic spread to bone. The authors of this study use a monoclonal antibody to epithelial cytokeratin to evaluate the bone marrow in patients who have previously untreated stage C carcinoma of the prostate. The majority of patients were able to demonstrate antibody-positive cells in the bone marrow. It is interesting to note that the risk factors one would usually anticipate—such as tumor volume, histologic grade, prostate-specific antigen, and prostatic acid phosphatase—were not especially useful in terms of correlations with positivity. We do know that the large majority of these patients will fail conventional surgical or radiation therapy. We also know that the majority of those failures will likely occur in the bone or bone marrow.

This paper is interesting in terms of its implications. It would be interesting to see a larger study of how this particular test correlates with other stages and, also, of how well it correlates with outcome.

E. Glatstein, M.D.

Prostate Specific Antigen Based Disease Control Following Ultrasound Guided ¹²⁵Iodine Implantation for Stage T1/T2 Prostatic Carcinoma

Blasko JC, Wallner K, Grimm PD, Ragde H (Northwest Tumor Inst, Seattle; Urology Resource Ctr, Seattle; Mem Sloan Kettering Cancer Ctr, New York)
J Urol 154:1096–1099, 1995   5–8

Introduction.—The Northwest Tumor Institute has developed and refined a technique of transrectal ultrasound-guided brachytherapy for patients with prostate cancer. There is increasing evidence that the posttreatment prostate-specific antigen (PSA) level can provide a sensitive, early indicator of persistent or recurrent tumor. Posttreatment PSA patterns were used to assess the intermediate-term efficacy of iodine-125 implantation for early-stage prostatic carcinoma.

Methods.—The study included 197 patients with clinical stage T1 or T2 prostatic carcinoma that was treated by outpatient ¹²⁵I seed implantation. All implantations were guided by transrectal ultrasound. The patients' mean age was 70 years. Before treatment, 70% of patients had a serum PSA level greater than 4 ng/mL. One hundred five tumors were well differentiated, with Gleason scores of 2–4; 87 were moderately differentiated, with Gleason scores of 5–6; and 5 were indeterminate. The minimum prescribed radiation dose to the prostate was 160 Gy; the median total implanted ¹²⁵I dose was 37 mCi. None of the patients received adjuvant hormonal therapy, and staging lymph node dissection and seminal vesicle biopsy were not routinely performed.

Results.—The PSA level normalized within 2 years of treatment in 98% of patients in whom it was increased before ¹²⁵I implantation. The PSA

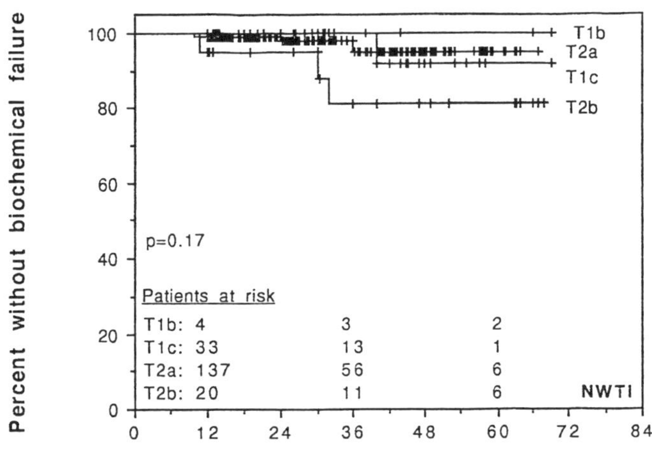

FIGURE 3.—Freedom from prostate-specific antigen-based disease progression by stage. *Abbreviation: NWTI,* Northwest Tumor Institute. (Courtesy of Blasko JC, Wallner K, Grimm PD, et al: Prostate specific antigen based disease control following ultrasound guided ¹²⁵iodine implantation for stage T1/T2 prostatic carcinoma. *J Urol* 154:1096–1099, 1995.)

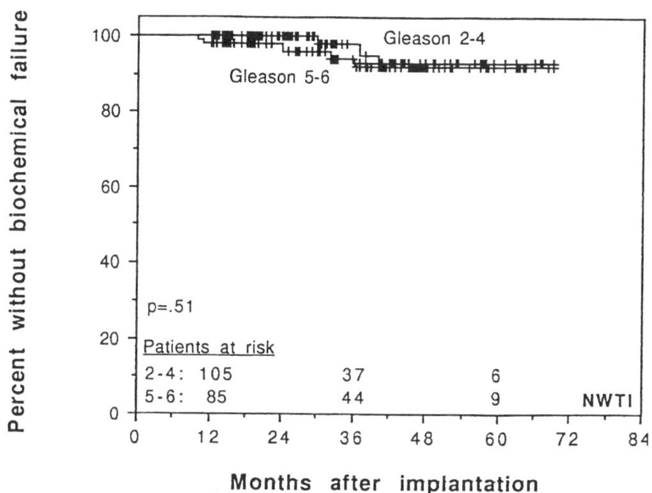

FIGURE 4.—Freedom from prostate-specific antigen-based disease progression by Gleason score. *Abbreviation: NWTI*, Northwest Tumor Institute. (Courtesy of Blasko JC, Wallner K, Grimm PD, et al: Prostate specific antigen based disease control following ultrasound guided ^{125}iodine implantation for stage T1/T2 prostatic carcinoma. *J Urol* 154:1096–1099, 1995.)

level decreased to less than 1 ng/mL by 24 months in 82% of patients and by 48 months in 97% of patients. The PSA level increased in 8 patients, 5 of whom also had clinically apparent treatment failure. The five-year actuarial rate of chemical failure—i.e., increasing PSA—or clinical failure was 7%. Fifteen patients were considered still at risk at 5 years. Failure

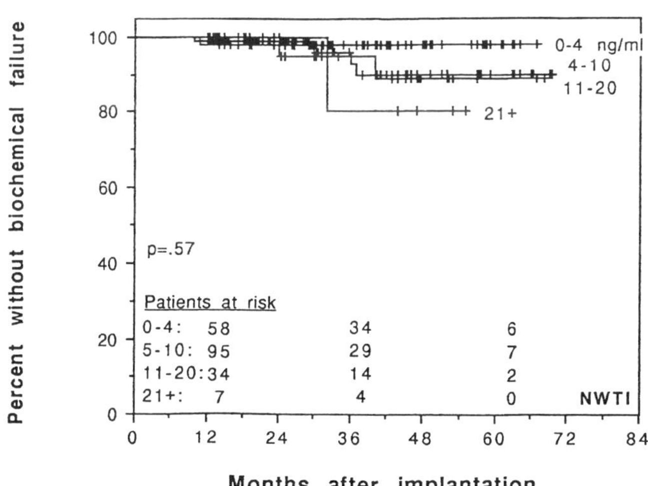

FIGURE 5.—Freedom from prostate-specific antigen-based disease progression by pretreatment PSA level. *Abbreviation: NWTI*, Northwest Tumor Institute. (Courtesy of Blasko JC, Wallner K, Grimm PD, et al: Prostate specific antigen based disease control following ultrasound guided ^{125}iodine implantation for stage T1/T2 prostatic carcinoma. *J Urol* 154:1096–1099, 1995.)

rates were nonsignificantly higher for patients with higher pretreatment PSA levels, Gleason scores of 5–6, and higher disease stage (Figs 3 –5).

Conclusions.—A low PSA-based failure rate was found in selected patients treated with ^{125}I implantation for early-stage prostatic carcinoma. The results compare favorably with those of prostatectomy. The good rates of clinical and chemical freedom from progression reported probably result from the combination of a highly effective treatment and careful patient selection.

▶ For the treatment of prostate cancer, the optimal treatment has yet to be defined. Advocates for surgery and external beam radiation therapy argue strenuously, but it is interesting that this paper shows an excellent case can be made for permanent ^{125}I seed implantation in T1 and T2 lesions. The follow-up after the first 7 years of this technique looks excellent. Permanent implants for prostate cancer have been done with either ^{125}I or palladium-103. Palladium is reported to have a higher relative biological effectiveness and may actually be the ideal isotope in the future. Both techniques have been pioneered by the Seattle group, using transrectal ultrasound for the placement of the radioactive sources. The technique is well described in this paper, and the results for T1 and T2 lesions are excellent.

The case for radiation therapy to the nodes is stronger on a theoretical basis, but it is very weak in terms of data that confirm its putative benefits. Therefore, the issue is how well the prostate itself is controlled, and these data appear excellent. Obviously, patient selection is a factor in achieving these kinds of results, and the authors imply that and do not try to extrapolate this treatment to every single patient. It is apparent from reading this paper that the technique itself is key to achieving these excellent results.

E. Glatstein, M.D.

Kinetics of Prostate-Specific Antigen After Manipulation of the Prostate
Bossens MMF, Van Straalen JP, de Reijke ThM, Kurth KH, Sanders GTB
(Academic Med Ctr, Amsterdam)
Eur J Cancer 31A:682–685, 1995
5–9

Background.—The effects of digital rectal examination (DRE) on prostate-specific antigen (PSA) levels are still debated (Table 1). The precise time at which peak levels of PSA occur after DRE is unknown. Serial measurements were performed to address this question.

Methods and Findings.—The kinetics of PSA were assessed after prostate manipulation in 8 patients treated with DRE and in 7 patients after needle biopsy. Seven of the patients in the first group had PSA baseline values less than 10 ng/mL. After DRE, blood samples were obtained at 1 and 30 minutes and at 1, 3, 6, 12, and 24 hours. Further monitoring was done in some patients. After DRE, the levels of PSA were significantly increased, with a maximum of 70%. In most patients, peak levels occurred

TABLE 1.—Summary of Previous Reports on the Effect of DRE, Prostate Massage, or TRUS on PSA Values

Author	No. of patients	Manipulation	Time of blood sampling	Effect on PSA levels
Stamey	16	Massage	1 min	Increase (mean, 2-fold)
Brawer	24	DRE	5–30 min	No effect
Hughes	85	TRUS	30 min	Increase (mean, 1.3-fold) if low baseline level
Adjiman	27	DRE by nonurologist	1, 12, 24, 72 hr	No effect
	13	DRE by urologist	1, 12, 24, 72 hr	Mostly increase (mean, 4.7-fold)
El-Shirbiny	13	Massage	1 hr	No effect
Crawford	2754	DRE	5–20 min	Small increase when baseline level > 20 ng/mL
Yuan	43	DRE	5 or 90 min	Increase in 9% of patients
	23	Massage	5 or 90 min	Increase in 15% of patients
Chybowski	143	DRE	2–30 hr	Increase (median, 0.4 ng/mL)
Walz	11	Massage	10, 30, 60 min, 2, 3, 5, 10, 24 hr	No effect

Abbreviations: DRE, digital rectal examination; *PSA*, prostate-specific antigen; *TRUS*, transrectal ultrasound.

(Reprinted from *Eur J Cancer*, Vol. 31A, Bossens MMF, Van Straalen JP, de Reijke ThM, et al: Kinetics of prostate-specific antigen after manipulation of the prostate, pp 682–685, copyright 1995, with kind permission from Elsevier Science Ltd, The Boulevard, Langford Lane, Kidlington 0X5 1GB, UK.)

between 30 and 60 minutes after DRE. In the second group of patients, PSA sampling was done similarly to that in the first group. Prostate-specific antigen levels were increased in all patients after biopsy. In only 2 of the 7 patients in this group did PSA levels return to baseline after 5 days.

Conclusion.—Clinicians should wait 3 days after DRE before measuring PSA. Caution is needed when interpreting PSA values after prostate needle biopsy, because this procedure results in important, long-lasting PSA increases. In patients undergoing biopsy, initial PSA levels are not correlated with the level of increase 5 days after the procedure.

▶ In medical school, we were taught that DRE could alter the acid phosphatase levels and that manipulation of the prostate should be avoided before drawing blood for this test. Subsequently, PSA has become an important tool for screening and managing patients with known disease. In 1992, Crawford et al.[1] reported that only patients with initial PSA levels between 10 and 20 µg/L had increases in serum levels of PSA that showed a trend toward statistical significance. However, patients with PSA values of 0.1–4 and 4.1–10 were found not to have significant changes in serum PSA levels after DRE. The sample size in the 2 lowest PSA subgroups in the Crawford study was large (2,427 and 240, respectively).

The teaching of the old school no longer seemed to be important; however, Bossens et al. reported exactly the opposite result. They studied 8 patients with DRE and 7 patients with needle biopsy. As previously reported, needle biopsies caused a large increase in PSA, which was protracted. However, patients undergoing only DRE were also shown to have a highly significant increase in PSA.

What were the differences between these 2 studies? In the Crawford study, PSA levels after DRE were obtained 5–20 minutes after DRE. In the study by Bossens et al., samples were drawn at 1 and 30 minutes, and at 1, 3, 6, 12, and 24 hours after DRE. The peak PSA level was achieved between 30 and 60 minutes after DRE in 6 of the 8 patients and at 3 hours and 12 hours in the remaining 2. Therefore, the patients in the Crawford study may have had their PSA levels obtained too soon after DRE. This was probably also true in other studies examining the effect of DRE on PSA levels (see Table 1).

Given these results and the results of other studies, PSA determinations should be made before DRE and should not be repeated for at least 5 days. After needle biopsy, PSA will be elevated for a substantial period, and it is probably advisable to wait at least one month after prostate biopsy for the serum PSA level to return to that patient's baseline.

G.J. Bosl, M.D.

Reference

1. Crawford ED, Schutz MJ, Clejan S, et al: The effect of digital rectal examination on prostate-specific antigen levels. *JAMA* 267:2227–2228, 1992.

Prostate Specific Antigen After Radiotherapy for Prostate Cancer: A Reevaluation of Long-Term Biochemical Control and the Kinetics of Recurrence in Patients Treated at Stanford University

Hancock SL, Cox RS, Bagshaw MA (Stanford Univ, Calif)
J Urol 154:1412–1417, 1995
5–10

Background.—Measurements of serum prostate-specific antigen (PSA) levels are useful in detecting new, persistent, or recurrent disease in patients with prostate cancer. Most studies of patients treated with prostatic irradiation for large tumors have reported modest cure rates. However, 1 recent study showed a significantly diminished cure rate among such patients and suggested that irradiation adversely affects clinical outcome. Trends in PSA levels were therefore studied retrospectively in patients treated with prostatic irradiation.

Methods.—A group of 110 patients who had been treated with prostatic irradiation and for whom at least 3 PSA values were available were identified from clinical records. The patients were classified into 3 groups:

nonrelapse (stable PSA values at less than 1 ng/mL), normal (PSA values within the normal range but more than 1 ng/mL), or relapse (increasing PSA trends).

Results.—Of the 110 patients, 38% remained disease-free with stable, normal PSA values (average follow-up, 12.4 years), and 30% had stable PSA values of less than 1 ng/mL. When patients with known lymph node involvement were excluded, 42% of the study population remained disease-free with stable PSA values. The risk of biochemical relapse correlated with clinical stage, Gleason pattern score, and pretreatment PSA values. The PSA doubling time also correlated with clinical stage. The mean PSA doubling time was 13.2 months among patients with local relapse and 3.3 months among patients with distant metastatic recurrence.

Conclusions.—External beam irradiation for prostatic cancer had a significant benefit, inducing durable disease control in 38% of the patients. The direct relationship among advanced clinical stage, aggressive histopathologic characteristics, and a more virulent course is confirmed.

▶ The story of PSA continues to evolve. This study from Stanford looked at 110 patients who had more than 1 PSA measurement. Higher clinical stages or Gleason scores were significantly correlated with risk of PSA relapse, as did the pretreatment PSA level. Patients who had short PSA doubling times were more likely to have cancers disseminate than recur locally. On the other hand, the authors found that radiation controlled prostate cancer durably 38% of the time, and, as a consequence, it is no particular shock that the larger tumors did not do as well. This is a major issue in patient selection with respect to therapy. Smaller tumors are generally seen much more commonly in the surgical series than the larger tumors, which are the major population of the radiation series. I am not sure we will ever be able to unravel some of these intricate issues, but this kind of work should be of some help in the future.

E. Glatstein, M.D.

Androgen Deprivation With Radiation Therapy Compared With Radiation Therapy Alone for Locally Advanced Prostatic Carcinoma: A Randomized Comparative Trial of the Radiation Therapy Oncology Group
Pilepich MV, Sause WT, Shipley WU, Krall JM, Lawton CA, Grignon D, Al-Sarraf M, Abrams RA, Caplan R, John MJ, Rotman M, Cox JD, Doggett RLS, Rubin P (St Luke's Hosp, Bethlehem, Pa; Wayne State Univ, Detroit; Kaweah Delta Cancer Care Ctr, Visalia, Calif; et al)
Urology 45:616–623, 1995
5–11

Background.—In patients undergoing radiation therapy for carcinoma of the prostate, the probability of locoregional recurrence increases with increasing size of the primary tumor. For patients with disseminated carcinoma of the prostate, androgen deprivation therapy has a high response rate. It was hypothesized that adjuvant androgen deprivation therapy, by reducing tumor volume, might lead to better outcomes of radiation therapy. The effects of androgen deprivation therapy before and during radiation therapy were assessed in patients with locally advanced carcinomas of the prostate.

Methods.—The phase III trial included 471 patients with large T2, T3, or T4 prostatic carcinomas but no evidence of bony metastasis. The patients were randomly divided into 2 arms: Those in arm I received goserelin, 3.6 mg subcutaneously every 4 weeks, and flutamide, 250 mg orally 3 times daily, 2 months before and during radiation therapy; those in arm II received radiation therapy only. The radiation dose to the pelvis was 1.8–2 Gy/day, to a total of 45 Gy. This was followed by a radiation boost to the prostate target volume, for a total dose of 65–70 Gy. The 2 groups were compared for local tumor control, disease-free survival, and overall survival.

Results.—Four hundred fifty-six patients were assessable, with a median potential follow-up of 4.5 years. The cumulative incidence of local progression at this time was 46% in arm I vs. 71% in arm II (Fig 1). The incidence of distant metastasis was 34% in arm I and 41% in arm II (Fig 2). The 5-year progression-free survival rate—including normal levels of prostate-specific antigen, measured at least once in 396 patients—was 36% in arm I vs. 15% in arm II. There was no significant difference in overall survival at 5 years, however.

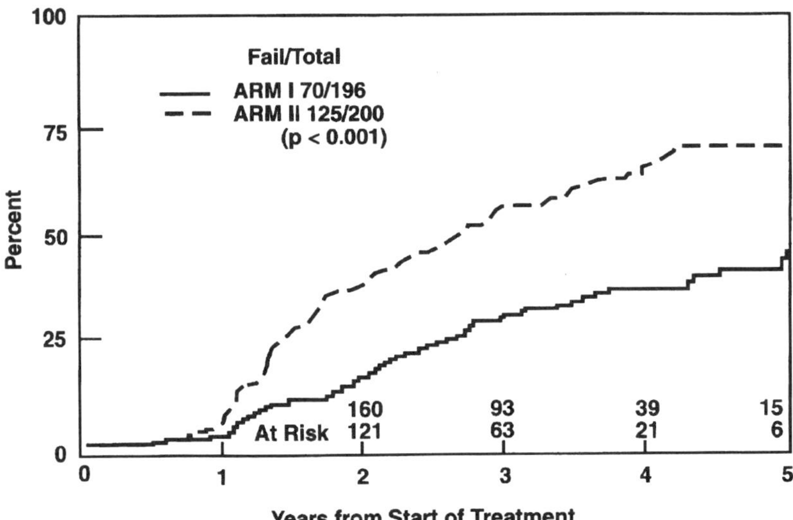

FIGURE 1.—Cumulative incidence of local progression by treatment group. Arm I is goserelin and flutamide plus radiation therapy. Arm II is radiation therapy alone. (Reprinted by permission of the publisher from Pilepich MV, Sause WT, Shipley WU, et al: Androgen deprivation with radiation therapy compared with radiation therapy alone for locally advanced prostatic carcinoma: A randomized comparative trial of the Radiation Therapy Oncology Group. *Urology* 45:616–623, Copyright 1995, by Excerpta Medica Inc.)

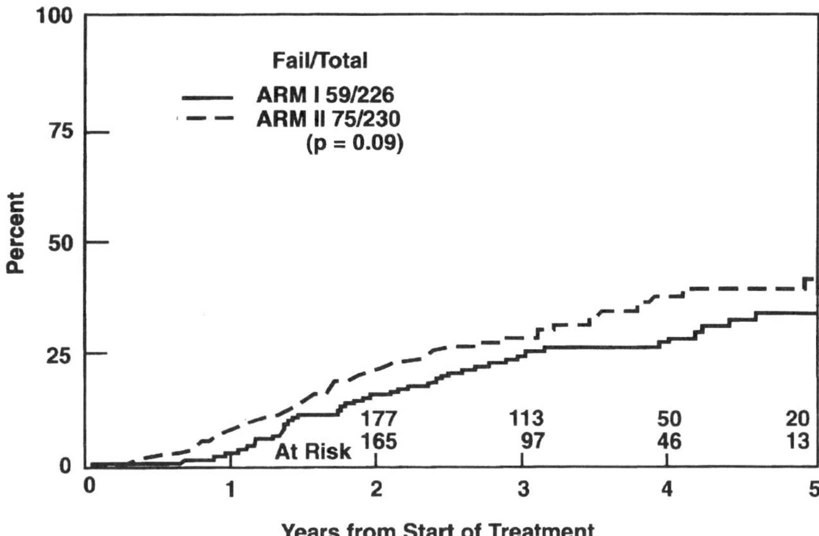

FIGURE 2.—Cumulative incidence of distant metastasis by treatment group. Arm I is goserelin and flutamide plus radiation therapy. Arm II is radiation therapy alone. (Reprinted by permission of the publisher from Pilepich MV, Sause WT, Shipley WU, et al: Androgen deprivation with radiation therapy compared with radiation therapy alone for locally advanced prostatic carcinoma: A randomized comparative trial of the Radiation Therapy Oncology Group. *Urology* 45:616–623, Copyright 1995, by Excerpta Medica Inc.)

Conclusion.—In patients with locally advanced carcinoma of the prostate, the addition of short-term androgen deprivation to radiation therapy yields significant increases in local control and disease-free survival. There is no associated increase in major toxicity. Longer follow-up will be needed to determine the effects of androgen deprivation on overall survival.

▶ Total androgen blockade has been shown to extend survival in patients with metastatic prostate cancer. The Radiation Therapy Oncology Group randomized 471 patients to receive either radiation therapy alone with standard treatment at relapse or radiation therapy plus androgen deprivation. The duration of androgen deprivation was only 3 months. All patients received goserelin acetate plus flutamide. Thirty-eight percent of the patients had abnormal serum acid phosphatase levels; serum prostate-specific antigen levels were not available. Seventy percent of the patients had T3–4 (stage C) disease. With a median follow-up of 4.5 years, the incidence of local progression was significantly decreased, whereas that of distant metastases was minimally decreased (see Figs 1 and 2). Progression-free survival was significantly improved ($P = 0.001$), but total survival was unaffected ($P = 0.7$).

Should short-term androgen deprivation be standard therapy after radiation therapy for patients with locally advanced prostate cancer? Progression-free survival is inadequate to evaluate this outcome. Although the follow-up is short, these data suggest that delayed therapy does not influence survival. It is very possible that treatment at the time of relapse will result in similar survival overall. Therefore, the routine use of androgen deprivation, either short-term or prolonged, after localized therapies is not standard therapy and remains a subject of controversy.

G.J. Bosl, M.D.

Advanced Prostate Cancer: The Results of a Randomized Comparative Trial of High Dose Irradiation Boosting With Conformal Protons Compared With Conventional Dose Irradiation Using Photons Alone
Shipley WU, Verhey LJ, Munzenrider JE, Suit HD, Urie MM, McManus PL, Young RH, Shipley JW, Zietman AL, Biggs PJ, Heney NM, Goitein M (Harvard Med School, Boston)
Int J Radiat Oncol Biol Phys 32:3–12, 1995   5–12

Purpose.—For men with advanced prostatic adenocarcinoma extending beyond the gland, long-term local recurrence is a common problem. As in tumors at many other sites, local prostate tumor control rates have improved with higher total radiation doses. In a previous phase I/II study, the feasibility of conformal external beam therapy delivered perineally by protons for men with advanced prostate cancer was established. A phase III trial of high- vs. conventional-dose external beam irradiation as monotherapy for patients with stage T3–T4 prostate cancer was examined.

Methods.—The study included 202 patients with stage T3–T4, Nx, N0-2, M0 prostate cancer. All received 50.4 Gy of radiation by 4-field photons. The patients were then randomized to receive either an additional 25.2 Cobalt Gray Equivalent by conformal protons (arm 1) or an additional 16.8 Gy by photons (arm 2). The total dose was 75.6 Cobalt Gray Equivalent in arm 1 and 67.2 Gy in arm 2. The 2 groups were compared for overall survival, disease-specific survival, total recurrence-free survival, and local control. Total recurrence-free survival was defined as clinical freedom from tumor, a prostate-specific antigen level of less than 4 ng/mL, and a negative prostate rebiopsy result (rebiopsy was done in 38 patients without evidence of disease). Local control was assessed by digital rectal examination and by rebiopsy.

Results.—Ninety percent of the patients and 97% of those in arm 2 completed their respective protocols. At a median follow-up of 61 months, 135 patients were alive, 67 had died of prostate cancer, and 20 had died of other causes. Grade 1 and 2 rectal bleeding and urethral stricture were more common in arm 1 (Fig 1). There were no significant differences in overall survival, disease-specific survival, total recurrence-free survival, or local control. For patients who completed their randomized treatment, the local control rates at 5 and 8 years were 92% and 77%, respectively, in arm 1, and 80% and 60%, respectively, in arm 2. Local control for poorly differentiated tumors (i.e., Gleason 4 or 5) at 5 and 8 years was 94% and 84%, respectively, in arm 1 vs. 64% and 19%, respectively, in arm 2 (Fig 6). The positive rebiopsy rate for patients whose digital examination normalized after treatment was lower in arm 1 vs. arm 2—28% vs. 45%—and for patients with well-differentiated and moderately differen-

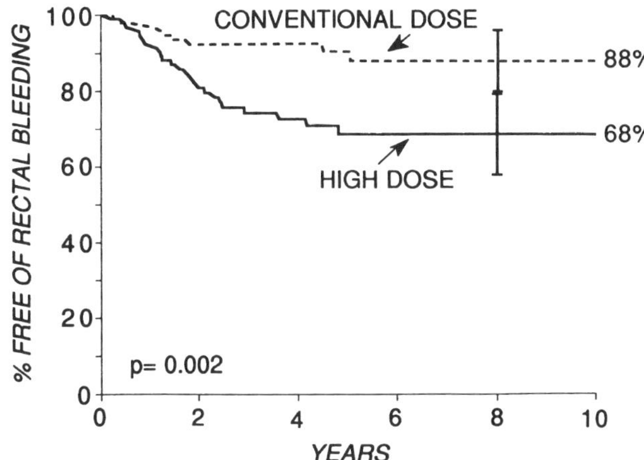

FIGURE 1.—Kaplan-Meier estimates of freedom from rectal bleeding for 189 patients completing a phase III trial of high-dose irradiation, boosting with conformal protons (93 patients, 75.6 Cobalt Gray Equivalent) compared with conventional-dose irradiation using photons alone (96 patients, 67.2 Gy). The *P* value is computed by the log-rank test. The 95% confidence limits are shown. (Reprinted from *Int J Radiat Oncol Biol Phys,* Vol. 32, Shipley WV, Verhey LJ, Munzenrider JE, et al: Advanced prostate cancer: The results of a randomized comparative trial of high dose irradiation boosting with conformal protons compared with conventional dose irradiation using photons alone, pp 3–12, Copyright 1995, with kind permission from Elsevier Science Ltd, The Boulevard, Langford Lane, Kidlington 0X5 1GB, UK.)

tiated tumors vs. poorly differentiated tumors—32% vs. 50% (Fig 7). These differences were not significant, however.

Conclusion.—Among patients with advanced prostate cancer, increasing the total tumor dose by 12.5% by a conformal proton boost signifi-

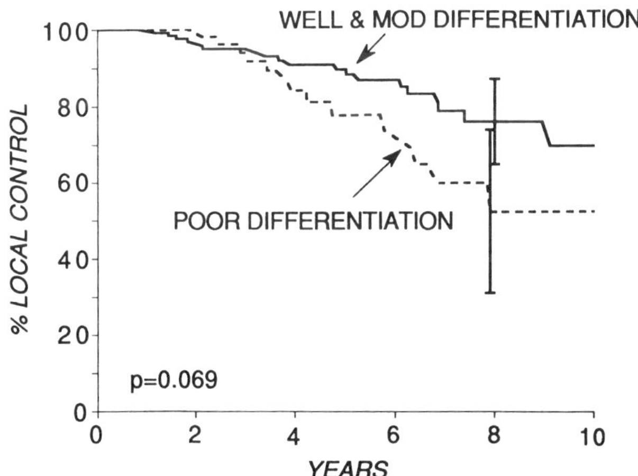

FIGURE 6.—Kaplan-Meier estimates of local control for the 189 patients completing the randomized comparative trial of radiation dose whose tumors were of well or moderate differentiation (Gleason Grades 1–3, 132 patients) or poorly differentiated (Gleason Grades 4 or 5, 57 patients). The *P* value is computed by the log-rank test. The 95% confidence limits are shown. (Reprinted from *Int J Radiat Oncol Biol Phys*, Vol. 32, Shipley WV, Verhey LJ, Munzenrider JE, et al: Advanced prostate cancer: The results of a randomized comparative trial of high dose irradiation boosting with conformal protons compared with conventional dose irradiation using photons alone, pp 3–12, Copyright 1995, with kind permission from Elsevier Science Ltd, The Boulevard, Langford Lane, Kidlington 0X5 1GB, UK.)

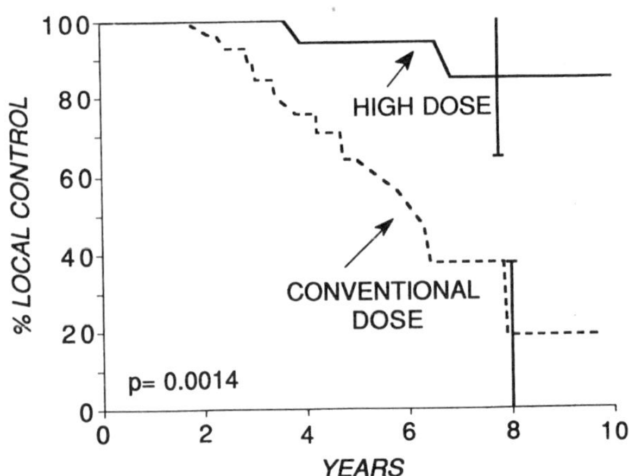

FIGURE 7.—Kaplan-Meier estimates of local control for the 57 patients with tumors of poor differentiation receiving, by randomized assignment, high-dose irradiation (boosting with conformal protons to 75.6 Cobalt Gray Equivalent, 26 patients) compared with conventional irradiation (photons alone to 67.2 Gy, 31 patients). The *P* value is computed by the log-rank test. The 95% confidence limits are shown. (Reprinted from *Int J Radiat Oncol Biol Phys*, Vol. 32, Shipley WV, Verhey LJ, Munzenrider JE, et al: Advanced prostate cancer: The results of a randomized comparative trial of high dose irradiation boosting with conformeal protons compared with conventional dose irradiation using photons alone, pp 3–12, Copyright 1995, with kind permission from Elsevier Science Ltd, The Boulevard, Langford Lane, Kidlington 0X5 1GB, UK.)

cantly improves local control only for patients with poorly differentiated tumors. The photon boost technique increases late radiation sequelae and, so far, has failed to improve overall, disease-specific, or total recurrence-free survival in any patient subgroup. The authors are conducting another phase III trial of the same proton boost technique in patients with T1, T2a, and T2b prostate tumors.

► For the past few years, proton therapy has been available for very restricted problems throughout the country as a whole. This is one of the first prospectively randomized studies reported, and it deals with stage T3–T4 prostate cancer. Patients received 4-field pelvic photon therapy and were then randomized to receive a boost either by conformal proton therapy or by photon therapy. The actual Cobalt Gray Equivalent for the proton therapy was slightly more than that administered by photons. Even so, for the total population treated, the survival, recurrence-free survival, and disease-specific survival, as well as local control, were not statistically different. There is a hint that there may be a modest benefit, but it is less than statistically significant. In certain subsets, perhaps, there may be more benefit associated with the proton therapy, but that remains to be seen because the numbers are small.

This is a well-performed study, and there is some basis for optimism in terms of some of the subgroups. On the other hand, I think it illustrates the difficulties of being able to document major gains with expensive treatments when we apply them to the common carcinomas, given their high predisposition to dissemination.

E. Glatstein, M.D.

Quality of Life: Radical Prostatectomy Versus Radiation Therapy for Prostate Cancer
Lim AJ, Brandon AH, Fiedler J, Brickman AL, Boyer CI, Raub WA Jr, Soloway MS (Univ of Miami, Fla)
J Urol 154:1420–1425, 1995

5–13

Introduction.—The efficacy of therapy in patients with prostate cancer is usually measured by patient survival, but greater emphasis has recently been placed on quality of life after treatment. The impacts of radical prostatectomy and external beam radiation therapy on the quality of life were compared.

Methods.—All patients with prostate cancer treated with either radical prostatectomy (136) or radiation therapy (60) were asked to complete a self-administered quality-of-life assessment questionnaire. Patient charts were reviewed to compare data on pretreatment disease stage, Gleason score, prostate-specific antigen (PSA) levels, posttreatment sexual dysfunction, bowel problems, and urinary incontinence between the patients who completed the questionnaire (responders) and those who did not (nonresponders).

Results.—Responders constituted 65% of the radical prostatectomy group and 77% of the radiotherapy group. There were no significant differences in the interval from treatment to last follow-up, pretreatment stage, Gleason score, serum PSA, or sociodemographic characteristics between responders and nonresponders. Problems with urinary incontinence (Table 2) and sexual dysfunction were significantly more common in the radical prostatectomy group, whereas problems with bowel function were more common in the radiotherapy group (Table 3). In both groups, the responders had significant associations between urinary incontinence, sexual dysfunction, and bowel complaints and depression, tension, and fatigue (Table 4). However, 91% of each group expressed satisfaction with their treatment, and 92% of the responders in the radical prostatectomy group and 87% of those who received radiotherapy stated they would undergo the treatment again.

Conclusions.—Although a substantial number of patients undergoing treatment for prostate cancer will experience significant morbidity, which

TABLE 2.—Perception of Incontinence As a Problem

	No. Pts. (%)	
	Radical Prostatectomy	Radiation Therapy
Is incontinence a problem for you?		
No/slight	75 (84)	37 (80)
Moderate	11 (12)	3 (7)
Big/extreme problem	3 (3)	6 (13)

Note: Nonresponders were excluded.
(Courtesy of Lim AJ, Brandon AH, Fiedler J, et al: Quality of life: Radical prostatectomy versus radiation therapy for prostate cancer. *J Urol* 154:1420–1425, 1995.)

TABLE 3.—Comparison of the Degree of Urinary Incontinence, Spontaneous Erections, and Bowel Complaints

	No. Radical Prostatectomy (%)		No. Radiation Therapy (%)	
	Responders (89 pts.)	Nonresponders (47 pts.)	Responders (56 pts.)	Nonresponders (14 pts.)
How often pads are worn due to wetness:				
Never	51 (57)	40 (85)	46 (100)	14 (100)
Almost never	24 (27)	2 (4)	0	0
Sometimes	7 (8)	0	0	0
Always	7 (8)	0	0	0
Spontaneous erections:				
Yes	2 (2)	3 (6)	21 (46)	14 (100)
No	97 (96)	44 (94)	25 (54)	0
Bowel complaints:				
Loose stools/diarrhea:				
Almost always	2 (2)	0	3 (7)	0
Sometimes	15 (17)	0	16 (35)	1 (7)
Almost never	72 (81)	47 (100)	27 (59)	13 (93)
Constant sensation to move bowels:				
Almost always	0	0	4 (9)	0
Sometimes	6 (7)	0	13 (28)	1 (7)
Almost never	83 (93)	47 (100)	29 (63)	13 (93)
Rectal bleeding:				
Sometimes	3 (3)	0	8 (17)	0
Never	86 (97)	47 (100)	38 (83)	14 (100)

(Courtesy of Lim AJ, Brandon AH, Fiedler J, et al: Quality of life: Radical prostatectomy versus radiation therapy for prostate cancer. *J Urol* 154:1420–1425, 1995.)

can impact on quality of life, the majority of patients would undergo the same treatment again, suggesting that patients are willing to accept some treatment complications to improve survival.

▶ There has been a long-term controversy concerning the impact of radiation therapy vs. that of radical prostatectomy on patients with prostate cancer. Each of the modalities has its strong advocates, and comparable objective data are hard to find. This study represents the results of a questionnaire surveying 136 patients who underwent radical prostatectomy vs. 60 who underwent external beam radiotherapy. When all the smoke clears, it appears as though both have similar impacts on quality of life, although there are some differences. The radical prostatectomy group had worse sexual function and worse urinary incontinence, whereas the external beam radiotherapy group had a worse bowel function.

It is worth noting that the technique of irradiation included whole pelvic radiation; many of us do not routinely treat pelvic nodes, because there are no data to show any objective benefit of such therapy. Thus, prostatic treatment only would be expected to virtually eliminate the possibility of bowel injury. In any event, most of the patients who were treated would undergo similar treatment the second time. The data from this survey suggest that the controversy will continue for quite a while.

E. Glatstein, M.D.

TABLE 4.—Comparison of Quality-of-Life Measures Between Radical Prostatectomy and Radiation Therapy

| | Mean Score | | |
	Radical Prostatectomy	Radiation Therapy	*P* Value
Emotional measures:			
Anger	4.41	5.68	Not significant
Depression	5.30	5.97	Not significant
Tension	4.71	5.67	Not significant
Vigor	22.54	21.3	Not significant
Fatigue	5.02	6.51	Not significant
Confusion	6.24	6.57	Not significant
Symptoms:			
Voiding	16.52	17.21	Not significant
Incontinence	10.4	7.75	0.001
Sexual function	8.12	9.74	0.0073
Bowel problems	7.01	8.22	0.012
Functional measures:			
Physical well-being	26.56	27.55	Not significant
Psychological state	28.53	28.58	Not significant
Hardship	13.77	13.84	Not significant
Sociability	13.22	12.75	Not significant
Functional Living Index: Cancer Score	84.06	83.98	Not significant

(Courtesy of Lim AJ, Brandon AH, Fiedler J, et al: Quality of life: Radical prostatectomy versus radiation therapy for prostate cancer. *J Urol* 154:1420–1425, 1995.)

Randomized Prospective Study Comparing Radical Prostatectomy Alone Versus Radical Prostatectomy Preceded by Androgen Blockade in Clinical Stage B2 (T2bNxM0) Prostate Cancer

Soloway MS, for the Lupron Depot Neoadjuvant Prostate Cancer Study Group (Univ of Miami, Fla)
J Urol 154:424–428, 1995

5–14

Objective.—For men undergoing radical prostatectomy, a positive surgical margin is a negative prognostic factor. It has been suggested that giving androgen deprivation therapy before surgery might decrease the chances of positive surgical margins in patients with clinically localized prostate cancer; however, the only evidence for this has come from non-randomized clinical trials. In a multicenter randomized trial, the ability of preoperative androgen deprivation to decrease the incidence of postoperative margins at radical prostatectomy was examined.

Methods.—The trial included 303 patients with stage cT2bNxM0 prostate cancer from 27 participating centers. One hundred forty-nine patients were assigned to receive 3 months of androgen deprivation therapy with 7.5 mg of leuprolide plus the antiandrogen flutamide, and 154 were assigned to surgery alone. Of 144 patients who underwent surgery, all had pelvic node dissection and 138 had prostatectomy.

Results.—The 2 groups were similar in terms of operating time, blood loss, need for transfusion, postoperative morbidity, and the length of hospital stay. The prostate-specific antigen level decreased to 2 ng/mL or less in all pretreated patients. In the surgery-only group, 4 patients had rectal injuries and 2 had ureteral injuries; these complications did not occur in the pretreatment group. The rate of capsule penetration by tumor was 47% in the patients who received preoperative androgen deprivation compared with 78% in the surgery-only group. The incidence of positive surgical margins was 18% vs. 48%. Six percent of the pretreated patients had tumor at the urethral margin compared with 17% of those who had surgery only.

Conclusion.—In men with clinical stage B2 prostate cancer, preoperative androgen deprivation therapy can reduce the rate of positive surgery margins, normalize prostate-specific antigen levels, and reduce prostate size. The ultimate value of preoperative androgen deprivation will depend on its impact on interval to relapse, clinical progression, and survival.

▶ The use of neoadjuvant androgen deprivation as treatment for patients with clinically localized prostate cancer is popular. Its use has been encouraged by early detection strategies with protein-specific antigen screening; most of the increase in the incidence in prostate cancer during the past 5 years is the result of the detection of localized, previously undetected disease. In addition, positive surgical margins are frequent in patients with stage B (T2) disease. This study by Soloway et al. seems to confirm that neoadjuvant androgen blockade is beneficial. Significantly reduced rates of capsule penetration, positive surgical margins, and tumor at the urethral margin appear to support the value of this approach.

Is this now the standard of care? In my opinion, no. Only with long-term follow-up can an improvement in survival be identified. With surgery alone, this group of patients will have a median disease-free survival of more than 5 years and an overall survival approaching 10 years. The use of adjuvant chemotherapy in the management of breast cancer has been supported by numerous randomized clinical trials conducted in more than 100,000 patients over the past 20+ years. On the other hand, the use of neoadjuvant chemotherapy in the management of cancer of the larynx has not improved survival, although it has improved the quality of life by permitting a proportion of patients to retain the larynx. In that case, preservation of function dominates over survival.

Neither function nor survival can be evaluated in this or other studies of neoadjuvant therapy in prostate cancer. The concept is intriguing (as it is in almost every other cancer responsive to a specific therapy), and the data to support its use are good (or else no one would conduct the experiment). However, the data do not support the use of neoadjuvant androgen deprivation/blockade as part of the routine management of patients with clinically localized prostate cancer.

G.J. Bosl, M.D.

The Antiandrogen Withdrawal Syndrome: Experience in a Large Cohort of Unselected Patients With Advanced Prostate Cancer
Small EJ, Srinivas S (Univ of California, San Francisco)
Cancer 76:1428–1434, 1995   5–15

Objective.—Discontinuing flutamide has proven effective in some patients with hormone-resistant prostatic cancer. This study examined the results of withdrawing flutamide in 107 consecutive men with metastatic prostatic cancer in whom progressive disease developed while the men were receiving the drug. In addition to antiandrogen therapy, the patients had undergone orchiectomy or received a luteinizing hormone–releasing hormone agonist.

Observations.—Three of the 82 evaluable patients had at least an 80% decrease in serum levels of prostate-specific antigen (PSA), and 9 others had a >50% decrease, for an overall response rate of 15%. The median duration of response was 3.5 months, although some patients responded for longer than 1 year. Whether concomitant treatment was given did not influence the response to withdrawal of flutamide. Patients who responded had received flutamide for a longer time than nonresponders (21.5 vs. 12 months), but the difference was not statistically significant. Patients who responded to drug withdrawal lived longer after the start of treatment for metastatic disease (44.5 vs. 35 months), but this difference also was not significant.

Implication.—Antiandrogen withdrawal should be tried before treatment is started for hormone-resistant prostatic cancer.

▶ By now, most oncologists know that withdrawal of antiandrogen can cause responses in patients with prostate cancer being managed with combined androgen blockage. In this series, the largest report to date, approximately 15% of patients had a greater-than-50% decrease in PSA level. The authors considered several pretreatment characteristics that might identify those patients who were more likely or less likely to respond to antiandrogen withdrawal. There appeared to be no direct relationship with the level of PSA at the time of antiandrogen withdrawal, and whether the patient was receiving the antiandrogen after bilateral orchiectomy or with a luteinizing hormone–releasing factor agonist did not appear to be influential. However, consonant with the clinical impression of many, prior response to hormone therapy did seem to make some difference; the median duration of response to previous treatment with flutamide was 21.5 months in responders and only 12 months in nonresponders. However, this did not reach statistical significance.

Any patient who has been treated with a combined androgen blockade and is progressing is a candidate for antiandrogen withdrawal. Both symptomatic and asymptomatic patients may respond. It appears to be somewhat more likely that a prior response—particularly a lengthy one—to combined androgen blockade will predict the quality of response to antiandrogen withdrawal. However, failure to respond should not exclude such patients from an attempt at antiandrogen withdrawal, provided that the clinical situation warrants it.

The antiandrogen withdrawal syndrome is an important treatment option in management of prostate cancer. As in breast cancer, secondary and tertiary hormone maneuvers may help a well-defined proportion of patients and may avoid adding the use of chemotherapy.

G.J. Bosl, M.D.

Estimating the Cost Effectiveness of Total Androgen Blockade With Flutamide in M1 Prostate Cancer

Hillner BE, McLeod DG, Crawford ED, Bennett CL (Virginia Commonwealth Univ, Richmond; Uniformed Services Univ of the Health Sciences, Bethesda, Md; Univ of Colorado, Denver; et al)
Urology 45:633–640, 1995
5–16

Purpose.—In patients with advanced prostate cancer, surgical or medical castration plus combined androgen blockade with flutamide is of proven therapeutic effectiveness. However, controversy continues regarding the cost-effectiveness of this approach; cost may be a major barrier to the addition of an antiandrogen. Decision analysis techniques were used to estimate the cost-effectiveness of flutamide added to surgical or medical castration in patients with M1 prostate cancer.

Methods.—The decision analysis model considered hypothetical cohorts of 70-year-old men with minimal and severe M1 prostate cancer and good

TABLE 2.—Baseline Analyses

| | Severe Disease | | Minimal Disease | | |
End point	Orch/LHRH + Flutamide	Orch or LHRH	Orch/LHRH + Flutamide	Orch/LHRH + Flutamide	Orch or LHRH
Flutamide efficacy (%)	25†	0	25†	50†	0
Median survival (mo)	34.3 (+4.8)	29.5	49.4 (+7.1)	60.9 (+18.6)	42.3
Average survival (mo)	39.2 (+4.9)	34.3	56.9 (+6.9)	66.1 (+16.1)	50.0
Discounted benefit* (mo)	4.0	NA	5.2	12.0	NA
Cost to progression					
If orchiectomy ($)	10,280	3,560	15,030	17,660	4,130
If goserelin ($)	15,770	7,370	25,640	31,110	12,640
If leuprolide ($)	19,150	10,100	31,090	37,700	18,180
Lifetime costs, if orch	22,900	17,340	30,300	29,800	21,600
Cost per life-year gained*					
If orchiectomy ($)	20,000	NA	25,300	13,700	NA
If goserelin ($)	25,000	NA	30,200	18,600	NA
If leuprolide ($)	26,900	NA	32,200	20,500	NA

* Costs and survival benefits discounted at a 5% annual rate. Costs rounded to nearest $10 for progression or $100 for cost per life-year. Benefits to the nearest tenth of a month. Time horizon was 7 years for severe disease and 10 years for minimal disease.

† Baseline efficacy of flutamide range for severe disease is from randomized trials. Trials for patients with minimal disease are in progress. The best case estimate for minimal disease is from a subgroup analysis.

Abbreviations: LHRH, luteinizing hormone-releasing hormone; *orch,* orchiectomy; *NA,* not applicable.

(Reprinted by permission of the publisher from Hillner BE, McLeod DG, Crawford ED, et al: Estimating the cost effectiveness of total androgen blockade with flutamide in M1 prostate cancer. *Urology* 45:633–640, Copyright 1995 by Excerpta Medica Inc.)

performance status. A societal perspective was used to calculate anticipated survival and incremental cost per life-year gained with flutamide plus orchiectomy or luteinizing hormone–releasing hormone (LHRH) agonists vs. orchiectomy or LHRH agonists alone. Data from the Intergroup 0036 trial were used for time to progression and survival rate. Treatment costs were based on Medicare data and wholesale drug prices. The estimated reduction in relative risk of progression attributed to flutamide was 25%. Costs and survival benefits were discounted at a rate of 5% per year.

Results.—In minimal disease, the use of flutamide was estimated to increase median survival from 42.3 to 49.4 months and average survival by 5.2 months. The incremental cost per life-year gained was $25,300. When the efficacy of flutamide was increased to 50%, the benefit was 12 months at a cost of $13,700 per life-year gained. When efficacy was decreased to 10%, the benefit decreased to 1.9 months, at a cost of $60,900 per life-year gained. In severe disease, the estimated median survival increased from 29.5 to 34.3 months with flutamide, and average survival increased by 4 months. The incremental cost per life-year gained was $20,000. When the efficacy of flutamide was decreased to 10%, the benefit was less than 2 months, at an incremental cost of $47,500 per life-year gained. In patients with severe disease, total costs were similar for treatment with orchiectomy plus flutamide compared with leuprolide alone. In patients with minimal disease, orchiectomy plus flutamide actually reduced costs (Table 2).

Conclusion.—In patients with metastatic prostate cancer, the incremental cost-effectiveness of flutamide is better than that of most accepted therapies (Table 4). If drug costs are covered in the reformed health care system, flutamide therapy should be initiated and covered for all patients with M1 prostate cancer and good performance status. Clinicians should encourage their patients to take part in clinical trials and lobby third-party payers to cover the costs of care received in comparative phase III trials.

▶ Total androgen blockade, accomplished through either medical or surgical castration plus flutamide, has gained widespread acceptance because survival has been prolonged in a randomized trial. The overall improvement in survival was relatively short when all patients were taken into consideration, but the difference was quite pronounced among patients with a low tumor burden. How cost-effective is such therapy? Hillner and colleagues undertook a cost-effectiveness study approach to estimating the societal value of the addition of flutamide to castration. They identified the difference between severe (extensive) and minimal (low-burden) disease.

Cost estimates were based on 1993 Medicare reimbursements for orchiectomy and on the 1994 average wholesale price of the various drugs used. In the analysis, it was assumed that (1) at progression, flutamide would be stopped, and (2) orchiectomy and LHRH analogues were equally effective. Using a baseline flutamide efficacy of 25%, the total costs to progression of disease in those receiving flutamide plus orchiectomy were

TABLE 4.—Cost-Effectiveness of Other Medical Interventions

Intervention	Cost per Life-Year (1992 $)
Liver transplantation	237,000
Mammography for women <50	232,000
Zidovudine for early HIV infection	8,200–88,500
Dialysis for end-stage renal disease	40,000–50,000
Flutamide in early metastatic prostate cancer	13,800–29,200
Hydrochlorothiazide for hypertension	23,500
Chemotherapy in node negative breast cancer	16,000–20,000
Lovastatin in secondary prevention of coronary artery disease	1,600–30,000
Universal hepatitis B vaccination of newborns	3,300
Smoking cessation counseling	3,000

Note: Primary source of each intervention's cost-effectiveness is available in a recent review (Smith TJ, Hillner BE, Desch CE: *J Natl Cancer Inst* 85:1460–1474, 1993.)

(Reprinted by permission of the publisher from Hillner BE, McLeod DG, Crawford ED, et al: Estimating the cost effectiveness of total androgen blockade with flutamide in M1 prostate cancer. *Urology* 45:633–640, Copyright 1995 by Excerpta Medica Inc.)

similar to the costs of leuprolide alone in severe disease, and they were *lower* by $3,000 in patients with minimal disease. The incremental cost of the administration of an LHRH analogue was always higher than that of orchiectomy because the analogue must be continued at the time of progression. Nonetheless, the cost per additional life-year ranged from $13,700 to $25,300 if surgical castration was performed and from $18,600 to $22,200 if an LHRH analogue (medical castration) was used (see Table 2).

The level of cost-effectiveness is quite similar to that of other medical interventions (see Table 4). This analysis strongly supports the use of flutamide as part of total androgen blockade in patients with prostate cancer with good performance, and it parallels the survival advantage identified in randomized trials.

G.J. Bosl, M.D.

High Failure Rate Associated With Long-Term Follow-Up of Neoadjuvant Androgen Deprivation Followed by Radical Prostatectomy for Stage C Prostatic Cancer
Cher ML, Shinohara K, Breslin S, Vapnek J, Carroll PR (Univ of California, San Francisco; UCSF/Mt Zion Cancer Ctr San Francisco, Calif)
Br J Urol 75:771–777, 1995   5–17

Background.—Authorities continue to disagree on the best management for patients with stage C prostatic carcinoma. Some suggest that cancer excision may be more complete when neoadjuvant androgen deprivation is given before radical prostatectomy. The goals of this treatment would be to decrease tumor stage, improve surgical margins, and effect salutary changes in long-term recurrence rates of local and distant cancers. A phase II trial was designed to determine whether neoadjuvant androgen deprivation may induce tumor stage reduction in patients with stage C prostatic cancer.

Methods.—Thirty men (age, 52–74 years) were given luteinizing hormone–releasing hormone agonist and an antiandrogen before radical prostatectomy. Twenty-six had radical prostatectomy with pelvic lymphadenectomy, 2 had pelvic lymphadenectomy only, and 1 had pelvic lymphadenectomy with radiotherapy. One patient refused additional therapy even though he had significant decreases in tumor volume and serum prostate-specific antigen (PSA) during androgen deprivation.

Findings.—Treatment toxicity was low. All patients had significant mean decreases in prostatic volume (35%), tumor volume (50%), and PSA concentration (96%). The maximum reductions were documented in the first 2 months of androgen deprivation. However, tumor stage was decreased in only 4 patients, despite significant physiologic changes in prostate and tumor volume. Forty-one percent of the patients who were surgically staged ultimately had more advanced disease. Twenty-one percent had lymph node metastases. After a mean 32.7-month follow-up, 72% of the patients showed evidence of disease recurrence, including detectable PSA. Local recurrence was documented in 19% of the 26 patients undergoing radical prostatectomy, distant recurrence in 4%, and both in 4%.

Conclusions.—Tumor stage reduction is uncommon in patients with stage C prostatic cancer treated with neoadjuvant androgen deprivation and radical prostatectomy. Local and distance recurrences and detectable PSA levels were frequently documented after such treatment in this series.

▶ Recently, Soloway and colleagues reported a small randomized trial comparing radical prostatectomy with neoadjuvant androgen blockade followed by radical prostatectomy (Abstract 5–14). The frequency of positive margins was decreased, but follow-up was short. This study by Cher et al. emphasizes the need to be cautious regarding the widespread use of neoadjuvant androgen deprivation in patients with organ-confined prostate cancer. This study was limited to patients with stage C prostate cancer. Androgen deprivation was maintained for 3 months, the same as in the Soloway study. The median time to recurrence was only 19 months, and 6 of 26 patients (23%) had a local recurrence. Most disturbing was the relatively infrequent occurrence of down staging (see Table 3 in the original article).

Neoadjuvant androgen deprivation is a reasonable research idea, not a form of standard care.

G.J. Bosl, M.D.

Phase I Study of Suramin Given by Intermittent Infusion Without Adaptive Control in Patients With Advanced Cancer
Kobayashi K, Vokes EE, Vogelzang NJ, Janisch L, Soliven B, Ratain MJ (Univ of Chicago)
J Clin Oncol 13:2196–2207, 1995   5–18

Background.—Although suramin has been found to be promising in the treatment of hormone-refractory metastatic prostate cancer, questions have been raised about the association of severe neurotoxicity to sustained peak plasma levels exceeding 300 µg/mL. Thus, the safe administration of suramin may require adaptive control. This approach, however, is time-consuming and difficult to do in most clinical settings. Results of a phase I study of a fixed dosing scheme that did not rely on adaptive control were evaluated.

Methods.—Fifty-four patients with hormone-refractory metastatic prostate cancer and 9 with other solid tumors were enrolled in the study. After an escalated day-1 dose, gradually declining doses of suramin were given to 63 patients on days 2, 8, and 9 of a 28-day cycle.

Findings.—On the first day, the doses administered ranged from 400 mg/m² to 2,080 mg/m². After the loading dose of 1,730 mg/m² was administered, the mean peak plasma concentration was 620 µg/mL. The mean trough concentration was 89.5 µg/mL on the first day of cycle 2. Five of 13 patients receiving a dose of 1,730 mg/m² had dose-limiting toxicities (DLTs), including malaise, neurotoxicity, pericardial effusion, and coagulopathy. Three of 5 patients had DLTs at 2,080 mg/m². Two patients receiving this dose level died during the study, 1 of a subdural hematoma sustained in a fall and 1 of respiratory failure resulting from classic suramin neurotoxicity. The former patient had a prolonged prothrombin time at the time of his death. The latter patient did not wish to be intubated. The occurrence of neurotoxicity was not significantly correlated with peak or trough concentrations during cycles 1 or 2.

Conclusions.—These findings demonstrate that suramin can be administered without adaptive control. Suramin given according to this schedule may have significant activity against hormone-refractory metastatic prostate cancer. Considering toxicity alone, a day-1 dose of 1,440 mg/m² is recommended for use in subsequent clinical trials. The maximum number of cycles recommended is 3. The optimal empiric dosing regimen has yet to be established.

Phase I and Clinical Evaluation of a Pharmacologically Guided Regimen of Suramin in Patients With Hormone-Refractory Prostate Cancer
Eisenberger MA, Sinibaldi VJ, Reyno LM, Sridhara R, Jodrell DI, Zuhowski EG, Tkaczuk KH, Lowitt MH, Hemady RK, Jacobs SC, VanEcho D, Egorin MJ
(Univ of Maryland, Baltimore)
J Clin Oncol 13:2174–2186, 1995   5–19

Background.—Suramin has been found to have antitumor activity in patients with hormone-refractory cancer of the prostate. However, suramin treatment has also been associated with a wide range of toxicities as well as clinical and laboratory changes. The overall and dose-limiting toxicity (DLT) of suramin given in intermittent short IV infusions until DLT or disease progression, the ability of an adaptive control with feedback (ACF) dosing strategy to maintain plasma levels of suramin in a preselected range, and preliminary evidence of antitumor activity were documented in a phase I trial. In addition, a population model of suramin pharmacokinetics was developed.

Methods.—Seventy-three patients with advanced, incurable, solid tumors were given a 5- to 7-day daily loading treatment, followed by intermittent infusions determined individually by ACF. A Bayesian algorithm and population models of suramin pharmacokinetics were used. Three cohorts received treatment based on target plasma suramin concentration ranges. The 27 patients in cohort 1 received 175–300 µg/mL; the 23 in cohort 2, 150–250 µg/mL; and the 23 in cohort 3, 100–200 µg/mL.

Findings.—Dose-limiting toxicity occurred most often in cohort 1. It manifested as a syndrome of malaise and fatigue, weight loss, anorexia, and changes in taste. Reversible neurologic, renal, cutaneous, and ophthalmologic toxicities, as well as edema, lymphopenia and anemia, and alopecia, also occurred. Of 67 assessable patients, 40 (60%) had a 50% decrease and 25 (37%) had a 75% decrease in prostate-specific antigen levels. These reductions lasted more than 4 weeks. Forty percent of 18 patients had measurable responses, and 49% of 37 had major improvements in pain. The overall time to disease progression was 170 days, and overall survival was 492 days.

Conclusions.—The incidence of grade 3–4 neurologic abnormalities was relatively low in these suramin-treated patients, especially in those given 100–250 µg/mL. All 3 cohorts studied showed evidence of significant and durable antitumor activity.

Prospective Evaluation of Hydrocortisone and Suramin in Patients With Androgen-Independent Prostate Cancer

Kelly WK, Curley T, Leibertz C, Dnistrian A, Schwartz M, Scher HI (Mem Sloan-Kettering Cancer Ctr, New York; Cornell Univ, New York)
J Clin Oncol 13:2208–2213, 1995   5–20

Background.—A number of schedules of hydrocortisone and suramin have been studied in patients with advanced prostate cancer. The results have been inconsistent. The efficacy of intermittent infusion of suramin was investigated in patients with androgen-independent prostate cancer whose disease progressed while they received hydrocortisone.

Methods.—Patients with previously untreated progressive androgen-independent prostate cancer received 40 mg of hydrocortisone per day. Treatment effects were monitored, and suramin was given on a pharmacokinetically derived, 2-week dosing schedule at the time of disease progression.

Findings.—Hydrocortisone was administered to 30 patients with a median Karnofsky performance status (KPS) of 90%. Twelve patients had measurable disease, and 29 had abnormal bone scans. All 30 patients had an increasing prostate-specific antigen (PSA) level before therapy. Six, or 20%, had a more than 50% decrease in PSA from the baseline value for a median of 16 weeks. In 28 patients, disease progressed after a median of 7 weeks. Two patients continued to receive hydrocortisone. Hydrocortisone and suramin were administered to those 28 patients whose disease progressed while receiving hydrocortisone alone. The median levels of suramin were 97–170 µg/mL for 4 weeks. There were no effects on measurable disease and no improvements in bone scans. Five patients, or 18%, had a greater than 50% decrease in PSA levels from baseline. Three of those patients had previously responded to hydrocortisone. Only 2 of 24 patients with no decrease in PSA after hydrocortisone treatment had a decrease in PSA levels with the addition of suramin. The toxicity profiles of each agent were acceptable, although a greater proportion of patients had hematologic, cardiac, and neurologic events after the addition of suramin.

Conclusions.—Patients with androgen-independent prostate cancer and disease progression after hydrocortisone therapy receive limited benefit from suramin treatment.

▶ New agents against prostate cancer certainly are needed. Suramin was first reported to have activity against hormone-refractory prostate cancer in 1988. It seems that we still can not figure out whether it is active. Initial trials were complicated by a number of unusual toxicities, including a coagulopathy, a significant rash, and a Guillian-Barré syndrome. When suramin was administered by continuous infusion, peak plasma concentrations were associated with the neuropathy, and a variety of alternate dosing schemes were developed to avoid excessively high serum concentrations.

Kobayashi and colleagues (Abstract 5–18) show that suramin can be administered without complicated pharmacokinetic modeling without neurotoxicity. This method of administration is easier than those previously reported, and the maximum tolerated dose was established. Responses were seen in patients with prostate cancer. However, none of these responses were seen in patients receiving the maximum tolerated dose.

Eisenberger and colleagues (Abstract 5–19) used a pharmacologically guided dosing schedule. Grade 3 and 4 toxicities encompassing anorexia, malaise or fatigue, paresthesias, motor weakness, and rash were observed in 5.5% to 38% of patients. Responses, measured by a 50% reduction in PSA, occurred in 60% and of 18 patients with bidimensionally measurable disease, 40% showed evidence of response.

Kelly and colleagues (Abstract 5–20) had previously reported that flutamide withdrawal and hydrocortisone treatment both resulted in significant reductions in PSA, improvement in bone pain, and reduction in measurable disease in patients with hormone-refractory prostate cancer. In an attempt to clarify this confusion, they studied a cohort of patients who received hydrocortisone before they were given suramin. Hydrocortisone alone caused a 50% decline in PSA in 20% of patients. After disease progression on hydrocortisone, a 50% decline in PSA was seen in only 5 of 28 (18%) of patients receiving suramin. Eisenberger and colleagues attempted to control for this phenomenon retrospectively.

Is suramin active or not? There probably is sufficient evidence to support a response rate of approximately 20%, as measured by a 50% decrease in PSA levels. Is it time to stop testing suramin? In the absence of very well-controlled randomized trials, further study of suramin probably is not warranted, given the low level of responsiveness, the difficulty of administering the drug, and the associated toxicities.

G.J. Bosl, M.D.

6 Genitourinary Cancer

Ultrasonographic Evaluation and Clinical Correlation of Intratesticular Lesions: A Series of 39 Cases
Coret A, Leibovitch I, Heyman Z, Goldwasser B, Itzchak Y (Tel Aviv Univ, Israel)
Br J Urol 76:216–219, 1995   6–1

Background.—Most patients with testicular neoplasms initially have a painless testicular mass or diffuse testicular enlargement clinically. However, swelling and hydrocele, tenderness after minor trauma, or a painful and tender scrotum with epididymo-orchitis have also been noted. Because the clinical presentation and assessment of patients with testicular tumors can be nonspecific and nondiagnostic, the accuracy of ultrasonography (US) in diagnosing testicular tumors was investigated.

Methods and Findings.—Thirty-nine patients referred because of pain, tenderness, and the appearance of a mass in the scrotum or scrotal swelling after trauma underwent US. The patients ranged in age from 3 to 61 years, with a mean age of 20.3 years. In 35 patients, intratesticular lesions were found on US. The remaining 4 patients had no suspicious findings after surgical exploration of the scrotum based on clinical findings only. Findings on US were consistent with neoplasm in 5 patients, but no tumor was discovered at surgery or on follow-up. In 1 patient, in whom the US findings suggested inflammation, an embryonal cell carcinoma was found on exploration 3 weeks later (Tables 1 and 2).

Conclusion.—Although US is very sensitive in differentiating an intratesticular from an extratesticular lesion and in excluding a testicular tumor,

TABLE 1.—Correlation Between Ultrasonography and Clinical or
Surgical Diagnosis

| | Diagnosis | | |
Ultrasonography	Positive	Negative	Total
Positive	29	5	34
Negative	1	4*	5
Total	30	9	39

* Includes only explorations with no pathologic findings. Cases with negative ultrasonography examinations and negative clinical examination are not included in the study.

(Courtesy of Coret A, Leibovitch I, Heyman Z, et al: Ultrasonographic evaluation and clinical correlation of intratesticular lesions: A series of 39 cases. *Br J Urol* 76:216–219, 1995.)

TABLE 2.—Results of the Ultrasonographic Evaluation of
Intratesticular Lesions

	%
Sensitivity	96.6
Specificity	44.4
Accuracy	84.6
Positive predictive value	85.3
Negative predictive value	80

(Courtesy of Coret A, Leibovitch I, Heyman Z, et al: Ultrasonographic evaluation and clinical correlation of intratesticular lesions: A series of 39 cases. *Br J Urol* 76:216–219, 1995.)

the patterns of different benign processes on US may be similar to those of tumors. Ultrasonography had a sensitivity of 96.6% and a specificity of 44.4% in diagnosing testicular lesions. Its positive predictive value and accuracy were 85.3% and 84.6%, respectively, indicating that exploration is needed when an intratesticular lesion is found on US, even when there is no clinical suspicion of such a neoplasm.

▶ Delay in the diagnosis of testicular tumors impacts on stage and survival. Components of physician delay in making a diagnosis are usually the result of either prolonged treatment for presumptive epididymitis or orchitis, or failure to follow up after an initial visit for testicular pain and treatment with antibiotics. Contrary to what is often written in textbooks, painful swelling of the testis is a very common initial presentation of testicular cancer. If treatment with antibiotics for presumptive infection does not result in the testis returning to normal within 2–4 weeks, US should be performed and the patient should be referred to a urologist.

How accurate is US? This simple study shows that testicular US is very successful at differentiating intratesticular from extratesticular tumors. It cannot, of course, distinguish between benign and malignant tumors. The high positive predictive value and accuracy (see Tables 1 and 2) strongly support the notion that an intratesticular lesion on US should be pursued by exploration through an inguinal approach. In my experience, testicular US is very accurate in identifying germ cell tumors (and, rarely, other less common tumors) in young men. Because second primary tumors occur in 2% of all men with testicular cancer, US is not only occasionally necessary for a variety of scrotal or testicular symptoms, but it is also reliable as a diagnostic tool.

G.J. Bosl, M.D.

The Role of Retroperitoneal Lymphadenectomy in Clinical Stage B Testis Cancer: The Indiana University Experience (1965 to 1989)

Donohue JP, Thornhill JA, Foster RS, Bihrle R, Rowland RG, Einhorn LH
(Indiana Univ Med Ctr, Indianapolis)
J Urol 153:85–89, 1995   6–2

Background.—Patients with clinical stage B testis cancer have undergone treatment with several methods. An experience with primary surgery in patients with clinical stage B cancer treated between 1965 and 1989 was reported.

Patients and Findings.—A total of 1,180 patients underwent retroperitoneal lymph node dissection for nonseminomatous germ cell testis cancer during this 25-year period; primary dissection was done in 638. One hundred seventy-four were thought to have clinical stage B disease preoperatively; surgery showed that 41 patients actually had pathologic stage A disease. Despite advances in clinical staging methods, this nonspecificity in clinical staging was consistent during the study. Sixty-five percent of the patients with pathologic stage B cancer were cured by retroperitoneal lymph node dissection alone, indicating that primary surgery for low-stage metastatic nonseminomatous germ cell testis cancer has both diagnostic and therapeutic value. Moreover, this cure rate was accomplished within an average of 4 hours. In the postcisplatin era (1979–1989), 140 patients with clinical stage B disease underwent primary retroperitoneal lymph node dissection. Of these, 32 had pathologic stage A cancer and 2 of them relapsed; both are presently disease-free with subsequent chemotherapy. Forty-nine of the remaining 108 patients with pathologic stage B disease did not receive adjuvant chemotherapy, whereas 59 were given cisplatin-based adjuvant chemotherapy. Eighteen of the 49 patients who were not given chemotherapy relapsed, and 2 died. None of the patients who were

TABLE 1.—Primary Retroperitoneal Lymph Node Dissection in Clinical Stage B Disease

Pathological Disease Extent	No. Pts. (%)	No. Relapse (%)	% Survival	No. Deaths
Early results, 1965 to 1978				
Stage A	9 (26)	0	100	0
Stage B, no adjuvant therapy	5 (15)	1 (20)	100	0
Stage B plus adjuvant therapy	20 (59)	11 (55)	75	4
All cases	34 (100)	12 (35)	88	4
Results, 1979 to 1989				
Stage A	32 (23)	2 (6)	100	0
Stage B, no adjuvant therapy	49 (35)	18 (37)	96	2
Stabe B plus adjuvant therapy	59 (42)	0	98.3	1
All cases	140 (100)	20 (14)	98	3*

* The 3 deaths were caused by cancer, postoperative complications, and septic chemotherapy complications, respectively.

(Courtesy of Donohue JP, Thornhill JA, Foster RS, et al: The role of retroperitoneal lymphadenectomy in clinical stage B testis cancer: The Indiana University Experience (1965 to 1989). *J Urol* 153:85–89, 1995.)

given postoperative cisplatin-based adjuvant chemotherapy relapsed. The overall survival in these 140 patients was 98%; 3 deaths occurred, 1 of which was caused by cancer (Table 1).

Conclusions.—Retroperitoneal lymph node dissection as monotherapy is curative in two thirds of selected patients with stage II disease, whereas the remaining one third with progression to clinical relapse can be reliably saved by chemotherapy. Risk-benefit, cost-benefit, and quality-of-life issues will be future considerations in selecting therapy for clinical stage II nonseminomatus germ cell testis cancer.

▶ The role of retroperitoneal lymphadenectomy in patients with clinical stage B germ cell tumors of the testis has been questioned because of the efficacy of chemotherapy. It is important to keep in prospective the value of this potentially curative operation. A total of 174 patients with clinical stage B tumors (i.e., patients with suspected retroperitoneal lymph node metastases with clinical staging) were retrospectively evaluated. There were several important findings.

First, 41 of 174 patients (24%) were found to have pathologic stage A disease, that is, no disease was found. Because 86% of the patients had CTs of the abdomen, the accuracy of clinical staging must be considered. Of these 41 patients, 32 (78%) were treated between 1979 and 1989. The only missing data are the preoperative levels of α-fetoprotein and human chorionic gonadotropin.

Second, among patients with pathologic stage II disease, 18 of 49 patients (37%) who received no adjuvant-based chemotherapy relapsed. Of patients with pathologic stage B disease who did not receive cisplatin-based adjuvant chemotherapy, 26% of patients with pathologic stage B1 disease relapsed, as did 55% of patients with stage B2 disease. This indicates the group of patients most likely to benefit from observation with treatment only at relapse.

Third, of the patients with pathologic stage II disease who received cisplatin-based adjuvant chemotherapy, none relapsed (see Table 1). The one observed death in the group was the result of neutropenic sepsis. Although this constitutes an important risk from systemic chemotherapy, the absence of relapse indicates the value of carefully administered adjuvant chemotherapy in this group of patients.

Therefore, the indications for treatment in pathologic stage II disease have not changed significantly in the past decade. Patients with relatively localized and small-volume disease should undergo modified bilateral retroperitoneal lymphadenectomy. Patients with disease of 5 cm or more, or who have multiple areas of ipsilateral or bilateral lymph node involvement should undergo initial chemotherapy. For the remainder, retroperitoneal lymph node dissection remains the standard, with adjuvant chemotherapy administered to patients with pathologic stage IIB disease.

G.J. Bosl, M.D.

Detection of Recurrence in Patients With Clinical Stage I Nonsemi-nomatous Testicular Germ Cell Tumors and Consequences for Further Follow-Up: A Single-Center 10-Year Experience

Gels ME, Hoekstra HJ, Sleijfer DTh, Marrink J, de Bruijn HWA, Molenaar WM, Freling NJM, Droste JHJ, Koops HS (Univ Hosp Groningen, The Netherlands)

J Clin Oncol 13:1188–1194, 1995

6–3

Objective.—The introduction of cisplatin-based chemotherapy significantly improved the prognosis for patients with disseminated nonseminomatous testicular germ cell tumors (NSTGCTs). Because of this and other advances, some institutions have adopted a "wait-and-see" policy, in which patients with clinical stage I NSTGCTs and no evidence of metastases are monitored at regular intervals after orchidectomy. Most relapses have occurred in the first year, and disease-free survival after treatment for relapse has ranged from 92% to 100%. A prospective 10-year experience with the wait-and-see approach to patients with stage I NSTGCTs was described.

Methods.—One hundred fifty-four such patients were treated from 1982 to 1992. The median patient age was 29 years. All patients underwent orchidectomy, followed by regular follow-up evaluations. These included α-fetoprotein and β-human choriogonadotropin levels, chest radiographs, and abdominal and thoracic CT scans. The frequency and time of recurrence, the detection of recurrence, and the presence of unfavorable prognostic factors, which were identified by multivariate logistic regression analyses were examined. The median follow-up was 7 years.

Results.—The recurrence rate was 27%. Ninety percent of recurrences were detected within the first year after orchidectomy, and all were detected within the first 2 years. Sixty-nine percent of the recurrences were detected in the abdominal lymph nodes, 21% in the retroperitoneum and mediastinum and/or lungs, and 10% in the mediastinum or lungs only. Tumor markers and CT scans detected 98% of the recurrences. Factors related to recurrence were the presence of vascular invasion, embryonal carcinoma, an elevated preoperative β-human choriogonadotropin level, and the absence of mature teratoma. The only independent risk factor was vascular invasion. Patients with recurrence were treated with polychemotherapy. Only 2 patients died, 1 of whom refused chemotherapy for recurrence. The overall disease-free survival rate was 99%.

Conclusion.—This prospective study supports the use of a wait-and-see policy in the management of patients with clinical stage I NSTGCTs. Follow-up monitoring to detect possible recurrence is appropriate, even in patients with unfavorable prognostic factors. The results suggest that chest radiographs might be omitted from the follow-up protocol and that follow-up might be discontinued after 5 years.

▶ Debate continues as to whether patients with clinical stage I NSTGCTs that do not show vascular/lymphatic invasion within the testis can be followed without retroperitoneal lymph node dissection (RPLND). Proponents of the "observation" approach point to the low death rate and low relapse rate, implying that most patients can avoid RPLND. Proponents of RPLND (via a nerve-sparing approach) cite lower relapse rates and frequently spared fertility.

In this study by Gels and colleagues, 154 patients with clinical stage I NSTGCTs were followed after orchiectomy. Because the study was initiated in 1982, tumors showing vascular/lymphatic invasion were included. Recurrence was proven in 42 of 154 patients (27.3%). The median time to relapse was 4 months (range, 2–24 months), and 90% of the recurrences were detected within 1 year. Of those patients who relapsed, 27 of 42 (64%) had retroperitoneal lymph node metastases. Recurrence was not predicted on the basis of preoperatively increased levels of α-fetoprotein (AFP) or human chorionic gonadotropin (hCG). The presence of vascular invasion was highly associated with the likelihood of recurrence. Computed tomography scans of the abdomen and tumor marker levels were simultaneously elevated at recurrence in 17 patients, whereas the diagnosis of recurrence was made in 8 patients based upon elevated serum tumor markers only. Of the 42 patients who had a relapse, 40 achieved a disease-free status after chemotherapy with or without resection of residual disease, and 2 patients died of recurrence. One patient who had recurrence refused all chemotherapy. The only prognostic factor independently associated with the likelihood of recurrence was vascular invasion. Specifically, the presence of embryonal carcinoma did not statistically increase the likelihood of recurrence.

The results of this study support prior conclusions that an observation policy is a safe approach to managing patients with clinical stage I NSTGCTs. Strict adherence to a follow-up policy is required on the part of both the patient and the physician. Consideration of observation as an alternative to RPLND can be given in the following circumstances: a patient with an NSTGCT, a T1 primary tumor without vascular or lymphatic invasion, serum tumor marker levels (AFP and hCG) that have fallen to normal or that are regressing at the expected half-life and are observed to fall to normal, and a normal radiographic evaluation of the chest and abdomen by CT.

G.J. Bosl, M.D.

Testicular Lymphoma: Late Relapses and Poor Outcome Despite Doxorubicin-Based Therapy
Touroutoglou N, Dimopoulos MA, Younes A, Hess M, Pugh W, Cox J, Cabanillas F, Sarris AH (Univ of Texas MD Anderson Cancer Ctr, Houston)
J Clin Oncol 13:1361–1367, 1995   6–4

Background.—Over the years, several prognostic models have been proposed for patients with intermediate-grade lymphoma. The International Prognostic Index (IPI) was recently introduced to predict outcomes and facilitate comparisons of outcomes among different patient populations. The value of the IPI in adults with testicular lymphoma treated with doxorubicin-based regimens was investigated.

Methods.—The cases of all untreated adults with testicular lymphoma seen at 1 center between 1969 and 1993 were reviewed in this retrospective analysis. Twenty-two patients were included—21 with intermediate-grade and 1 with high-grade lymphoma.

Findings.—Ten patients had an IPI score of 1 or less, and 12 had an IPI of more than 1. All those in the former group had Ann Arbor stage I disease, whereas all those in the latter group had Ann Arbor stages II–IV. Seventy-three percent of the patients attained complete remission (CR). At 153 months, 22% of complete responders remained in CR, including 40% of those with IPI scores of 1 or less and none of those with scores exceeding 1. The 153-month failure-free (FFS) rate was 16% for all patients, including 32% of those with IPI scores of 1 or less and 0% of those with scores of more than 1. All treatment nonresponders had CNS or contralateral testis involvement. Half of those relapsing from CR also had such involvement.

Conclusion.—Patients with testicular lymphoma have a poor prognosis despite treatment with doxorubicin-based chemotherapy. Prophylactic intrathecal chemotherapy and scrotal radiotherapy are recommended for all patients. Those with IPI scores of 1 or less can be given conventional doxorubicin-based treatments. Those with higher scores, however, should be considered for investigational systemic therapy.

▶ Testicular masses in patients older than 50 years of age should be considered to be lymphoma until proved otherwise. Testicular lymphoma is rare, and meaningful information can be obtained only through retrospective reviews. Retrospective reviews demonstrate a high systemic failure rate among patients whose presentation of lymphoma is that of testicular enlargement. This study supports and extends those observations. Whether the patient is seen with "clinical stage I" disease, the overwhelming majority have disseminated disease and should receive doxorubicin-based intensive therapy.

This series provides support for prophylactic CNS therapy and radiation therapy of the contralateral testis because relapses at these 2 sites occurred in 9 of 22 (41%) and 7 of 22 (32%) patients. Relapses continued to occur beyond 5 years. When the International Prognostic Index (IPI) is used, patients with IPI scores greater than 1 should be considered for clinical trials of more intensive therapy because of the short survival of this subgroup.

G.J. Bosl, M.D.

Adult Primary Pure Teratoma of the Testis: The Indiana Experience
Leibovitch I, Foster RS, Ulbright TM, Donohue JP (Indiana Univ, Indianapolis)
Cancer 75:2244–2250, 1995   6–5

Introduction.—Pure testicular teratoma in men is a relatively rare malignancy that can be invasive and metastatic. Compared with other types of germ cell tumor, the pure teratoma is generally thought to be less aggressive, less likely to progress, to present in less-advanced stages, and to have a better survival rate. For patients with clinical stage A pure testicular teratoma, surveillance has, therefore, been generally regarded as the best management approach. A 28-year series of patients with pure testicular teratoma was reviewed.

Patients.—During the period studied, 41 patients whose orchiectomy specimen showed pure teratoma were treated. Eighteen patients had clinical stage A disease; 4 patients had clinical stage A to B1 disease, based on questionable CT findings; 3 patients had clinical stage B1 disease; and 16 patients had advanced disease, stage B3 to C. The average age was 29 years, and the mean follow-up was 6.5 years.

Results—For patients in the first 3 groups—those with low-stage pure testicular teratoma—the overall risk of lymph node metastasis in the retroperitoneal lymph node dissection (RPLND) specimen was 40%. The risk of relapse after RPLND for these patients was 16%. For the patients with clinical stage A disease, the risk of retroperitoneal metastasis was 17% and the relapse rate was 11%. Of the patients seen with advanced-stage disease, 12.5% relapsed after chemotherapy and postchemotherapy RPLND. Thirty-seven percent of patients referred with pure teratoma had advanced disease at presentation.

Conclusion.—As previous studies have indicated, pure testicular teratoma does have metastatic potential. For adults with clinical stage A primary pure teratoma of the testis, management should not necessarily differ from that of any other type of nonseminomatous testicular tumor. The histologic diagnosis of pure teratoma does not mandate surveillance. Like other patients with clinical stage I nonseminomas, these patients should receive adequate information regarding their treatment options.

▶ Mature teratoma is a cell type of nonseminomatous germ cell tumor composed of tissue elements from different germinal layers. Mature teratomas contain well-differentiated tissues that are histologically similar to those found in the adult. They are usually found as part of a mixed germ cell tumor but are rarely found as the only element in a newly diagnosed testicular tumor. What is the origin and what are the implications for patient management?

Leibovitch and colleagues reviewed the experience at Indiana University. Forty-one patients were found to have had pure teratoma in the orchiectomy specimen. If these were benign tumors, then no metastases should be found. However, 19 of 41 patients (46%) were found to have clinical stage B/C disease, and 7 of 22 (32%) who were thought to have clinical stage A or, possibly, early stage B disease were found to have metastases at RPLND. Therefore, regional or distant metastases were found in 26 of 41 patients (63%).

The origin of mature teratoma and the metastases can be better understood in light of the biology of germ cell tumors. Mature teratomas have been shown to contain the chromosomal marker i(12p) just as do embryonal carcinomas and all other cell types. Therefore, they share a genetic origin with other cell types. Embryonal carcinoma is totipotential and has been demonstrated to differentiate in vitro, it has been presumed to do so in vivo based on the simultaneous presence of embryonal carcinoma with mature teratoma in mixed histology tumors. The genetic "switches" that regulate the differentiation of embryonal carcinoma cells are not known. However, the presence of mature teratoma in a germ cell tumor implies that embryonal carcinoma either is or has been present. Therefore, metastases can and, as this paper shows, often *do* develop. Therefore, adult patients with apparently pure mature teratoma must be managed as having a fully malignant germ cell tumor. There is an important difference between "mature" teratoma and "benign" teratoma; the latter does not exist, and the phrase should not be used in patient management.

G.J. Bosl, M.D.

Importance of Bleomycin in Favorable-Prognosis Disseminated Germ Cell Tumors: An Eastern Cooperative Oncology Group Trial
Loehrer PJ Sr, Johnson D, Elson P, Einhorn LH, Trump D (Indiana Univ, Indianapolis; Walther Cancer Inst, Indianapolis, Ind; Vanderbilt Univ, Nashville, Tenn; et al)
J Clin Oncol 13:470–476, 1995   6–6

Objective.—A prospective trial was done in 178 patients having minimal- or moderate-stage testicular or extratesticular germ cell tumors. Three cycles of cisplatin/etoposide (PVP_{16}) were compared with 3 cycles of cisplatin/etoposide/bleomycin ($PVR_{16}B$).

Treatment.—Cisplatin was given in a dose of 20 mg/m^2 on days 1 to 5, and etoposide on the same days in a dose of 100 mg/m^2. Bleomycin was given in a weekly dose of 30 IU for 9 consecutive weeks. If residual disease remained after 3 cycles of chemotherapy, it was resected; if persistent carcinoma was confirmed, 2 further courses were administered.

Results.—Severe nonhematologic toxicity occurred in 8% to 9% of patients in the 2 groups. Among 171 fully evaluable patients, 77% of those given PVP_{16} B had complete remission with chemotherapy alone, and 15

TABLE 3.—Unfavorable Outcome Variables

Variable	$PVP_{16}B$ ($n = 86$)	PVP_{16} ($n = 85$)
Primary treatment failure (n)	3	9
Drug-related death or drug intolerance (n)	2	1
Residual carcinoma (n)	2	8
Relapse (n)	8	17
Total		
No.	15	32
%	17	38*

* Three patients with completely resected residual carcinoma relapsed with cancer.
(Courtesy of Loehrer PJ Sr, Johnson D, Elson P, et al: Importance of bleomycin in favorable-prognosis disseminated germ cell tumors: An Eastern Cooperative Oncology Group trial. *J Clin Oncol* 13:470–476, 1995.)

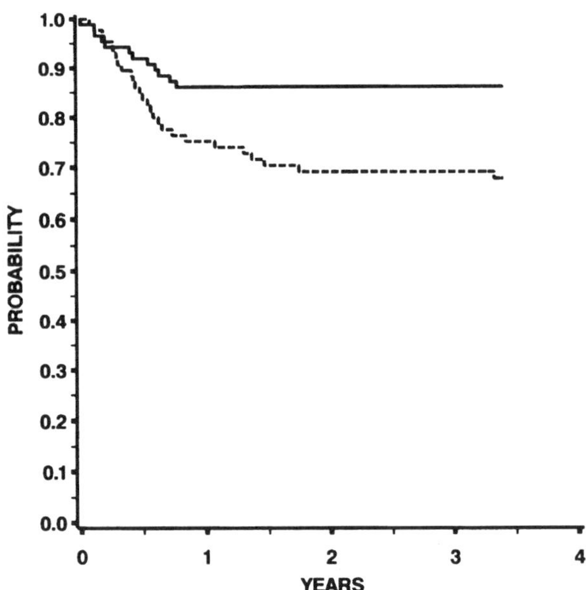

FIGURE 1.—Failure-free survival of all eligible patients. *Solid line,* treatment with 3 cycles of PVP$_{16}$B (cisplatin, etoposide, and bleomycin) (n = 86): 13 failures, 86% failure-free survival rate at 3 years. *Dashed line,* treatment with 3 cycles of cisplatin plus etoposide (PVP$_{16}$) (n = 85): 27 failures, 69% failure-free survival rate at 3 years (P = .01). (Courtesy of Loehrer PJ Sr, Johnson D, Elson P, et al: Importance of bleomycin in favorable-prognosis disseminated germ cell tumors: An Eastern Cooperative Oncology Group trial. *J Clin Oncol* 13:470–476, 1995.)

others were disease-free after persistent disease was resected, for an overall response of 94%. The overall response rate for patients not receiving bleomycin was 88%. Initial treatment failure and persistent carcinoma were both more frequent in the PVP$_{16}$ group (Table 3). More bleomycin-treated patients were continuously disease-free at 3 years (Fig 1). Overall survival at 3 years was 95% in this group and 86% in patients not given bleomycin, a significant difference.

Conclusion.—Bleomycin, as used in the PVP$_{16}$ B regimen, is a useful element of chemotherapy for patients with minimal- and moderate-stage germ cell tumors.

▶ During the past decade, the management of germ cell tumors has been influenced by the allocation of patients with advanced disease to clinical trials emphasizing good or poor risk status. In the "good-risk" category, the principal concern was maintenance of efficacy with acceptable toxicity. Because bleomycin was associated with both acute and chronic toxicity, nearly all efforts were directed at either reducing the dose of bleomycin or eliminating its use altogether. The Eastern Cooperative Oncology Group (ECOG) had previously shown that 3 cycles of cisplatin, bleomycin, and etoposide (PVP$_{16}$B) was equivalent to 4 cycles of the same regimen in patients considered to be "good risk" according to Indiana University criteria. The Memorial Sloan-Kettering Cancer Center had reported that the

2-drug regimen of etoposide and cisplatin (PVP$_{16}$) was equivalent to a 5-drug regimen that included bleomycin (so-called VAB-6) and was associated with considerably less toxicity. In this paper, Loehrer et al. report on the ECOP's attempt to eliminate the use of bleomycin when only 3 cycles of therapy were delivered and to establish the lower boundary for the number of cycles of therapy when bleomycin is included.

The proportion of patients with primary treatment failure and relapse was greater in the 2-drug arm ($n = 26$) compared with the 3-drug arm ($n = 11$). In addition, the presence of residual carcinoma in completely resected specimens after chemotherapy was more frequent in patients undergoing the two-drug treatment arm than in those receiving the 3-drug treatment arm (see Table 3). The failure-free survival of patients receiving 3 cycles of 2 drugs was inferior to that of patients receiving 3 cycles of 3 drugs (see Fig 1). The reduced efficacy observed in this trial is paralleled by a similar observation made when carboplatin was substituted for cisplatin in a separate study. In that trial, reported by Bajorin et al.,[1] the number of "events" (incomplete responses plus relapses) was approximately 2 times greater in patients receiving carboplatin compared with those receiving cisplatin.

What is the current recommended therapy for "good-risk" patients with germ cell tumors? There appear to be two equal options. Three cycles of PVP$_{16}$ B or 4 cycles of PVP$_{16}$ appear to have equivalent cure rates. The choice is dependent upon the physician's views regarding bleomycin toxicity. Bleomycin pulmonary toxicity is decreased when only 3 cycles of PVP$_{16}$ B are administered compared with 4 cycles. However, whatever toxicity is attributable to bleomycin will not occur if the drug is not administered.

This report by Loehrer et al. does not comment on Raynaud's phenomenon, but the patients who were receiving bleomycin experienced grade IV myelosuppression significantly more often than patients who did not (14% vs. 5%, respectively; $P = 0.06$). This is not the first time that the administration of bleomycin has been associated with higher rates of myelosuppression in patients with germ cell tumors. Whether this toxicity resulted in a greater proportion of patients requiring hospitalization for neutropenic fever is not reported. It can be argued that administration of hematopoietic growth factors can decrease the frequency of neutropenic fever. However, this observation must be taken in the context of the expense of the drug over all cycles of therapy. The cost differential between 4 cycles of 2 drugs and 3 cycles of 3 drugs will need to be studied. However, both regimens have equal efficacy; therefore, either may be chosen in the treatment of patients with germ cell tumors who meet good-risk criteria.

G.J. Bosl, M.D.

Reference

1. Bajorin DF, Sarosdy MF, Pfister DG, et al: Randomized trial of etoposide and cisplatin versus etoposide and carboplatin in patients with good-risk germ-cell tumors: A multi-institutional study. *J Clin Oncol* 11:598–606, 1993.

Adjuvant Polychemotherapy of Nonorgan-Confined Bladder Cancer After Radical Cystectomy Revisited: Long-Term Results of a Controlled Prospective Study and Further Clinical Experience

Stöckle M, Meyenburg W, Wellek S, Voges GE, Rossmann M, Gertenbach U, Thüroff JW, Huber C, Hohenfellner R (Univ of Mainz, Germany; Klinikum Barmen, Wuppertal, Germany)

J Urol 153:47–52, 1995   6–7

Background.—In 1992, the preliminary results of a controlled prospective study of treatment for locally advanced bladder cancer was published. The findings suggested that the addition of adjuvant chemotherapy after cystectomy significantly prolonged the progression-free interval in patients at high risk of progression. Follow-up at this time was, however, too short to determine whether longer relapse-free survival would lead to an improvement in long-term cure rate. The long-term results, as well as a further clinical experience, were reported.

Methods.—The analysis included 83 patients with nonorgan-confined bladder cancer with or without lymph node metastases (tumor stages pT3b, pT4a, and/or pN1, pN2). From 1987 to 1991, all 83 patients underwent radical cystectomy, and 38 received adjuvant polychemotherapy with methotrexate, vinblastine, and cisplatin plus doxorubicin (M-VAC) or epirubicin (M-VEC). Beginning in 1987, 49 patients were randomized to receive adjuvant treatment or no treatment. In 1990, an interim analysis found that patients receiving chemotherapy had a significant prognostic advantage, so recruitment was halted. Twenty-six patients were randomized to receive chemotherapy; 18 received M-VAC or M-VEC, 7 refused chemotherapy, and 1 received chemotherapy without cisplatin because of impaired renal function. Relapse-free and overall survival were evaluated in 1993.

Results.—The analysis continued to show that patients randomized to receive chemotherapy have significantly improved progression-free survival (Fig 1). At the time of this evaluation, follow-up of disease-free patients ranged from 38 to 78 months. The collective review of 83 patients included 38 who actually received M-VAC or M-VEC adjuvant chemotherapy—18 during the trial and 20 thereafter as routine therapy. The results in these patients were compared with those in 45 who did not receive adjuvant chemotherapy, either because of randomization, refusal, or other reasons. Again, patients treated with chemotherapy had a significant prognostic advantage (Fig 2).

Conclusions.—In patients with locally advanced transitional cell carcinoma of the bladder, adjuvant M-VAC or M-VEC chemotherapy significantly prolongs relapse-free survival. Definitive cure rates are improved as well. Methotrexate, vinblastine, epirubicin, and cisplatin will be compared prospectively with cisplatin plus methotrexate in an attempt to decrease toxicity.

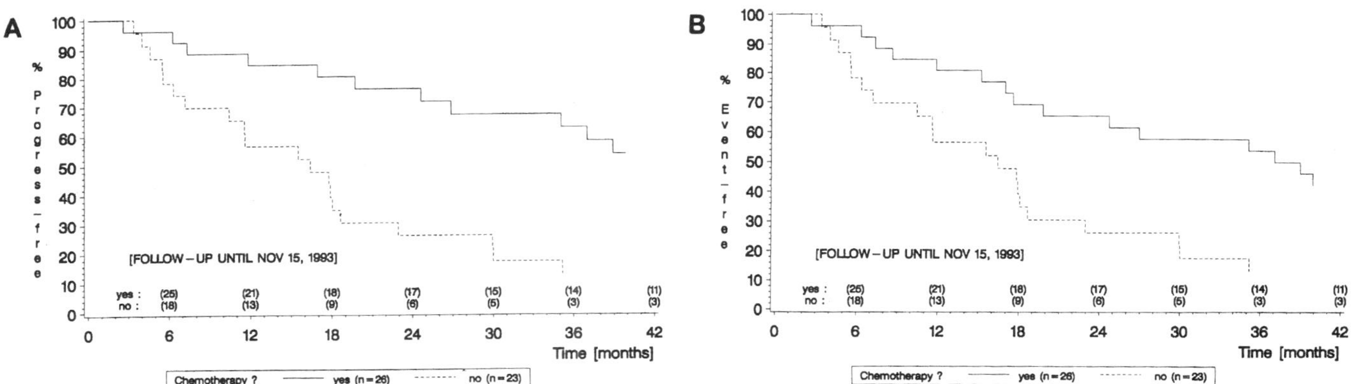

FIGURE 1.—Estimated Kaplan-Meier rates for treatment groups, as identified by randomization process (intent-to-treat analysis of prospective trial). A, progression-free patients. End point is tumor progression (P = .0005, log-rank). B, event-free patients (event defined as tumor progression or tumor-unrelated death). End point is tumor progression or death (P = .0055, log-rank). Numbers in parentheses indicate patients still at risk. (Courtesy of Stöckle M, Meyenburg W, Wellek S, et al: Adjuvant polychemotherapy of nonorgan-confined bladder cancer after radical cystectomy revisited: Long-term results of a controlled prospective study and further clinical experience. J Urol 153:47–52, 1995.)

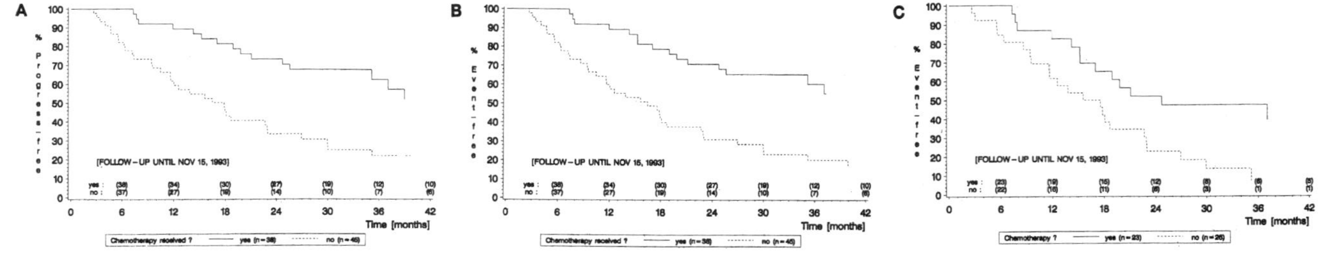

FIGURE 2.—Estimated Kaplan-Meier rates for treatment groups. **A,** progression-free patients among 38 actually treated with M-VAC/M-VEC and 45 who underwent surgical treatment only. End point is tumor progression (P = .0003, log-rank). **B,** event-free patients among same groups as noted in part **A.** End point is tumor progression or death (P = .0001, log-rank). **C,** event-free patients among 23 with positive lymph nodes actually treated with M-VAC/M-VEC compared with 26 with positive lymph nodes who underwent surgery only. End point is tumor progression or death (P = .0150, log-rank). *Numbers in parentheses* indicate patients still at risk. (Courtesy of Stöckle M, Meyenburg W, Wellek S, et al: Adjuvant polychemotherapy of nonorgan-confined bladder cancer after radical cystectomy revisited: Long-term results of a controlled prospective study and further clinical experience. *J Urol* 153:47–52, 1995.)

▶ There continues to be much discussion with regard to the value of neoadjuvant and adjuvant chemotherapy in patients with locally advanced bladder cancer with or without positive pelvic lymph nodes. Stöckle et al. report, for a second time and with extended survival data, their analysis of a randomized clinical trial of no adjuvant chemotherapy or adjuvant chemotherapy with methotrexate, vinblastine, cisplatin, and either doxorubicin (M-VAC) or epirubicin (M-VEC). They include in their analysis those patients treated with adjuvant therapy after the conclusion of the trial, as well as those who refused adjuvant therapy after cystectomy. The survival of patients receiving adjuvant chemotherapy was dramatically longer than that of patients who did not receive adjuvant chemotherapy (see Figs 1 and 2). These data support the use of cisplatin-based chemotherapy in the management of patients who have undergone cystectomy for locally advanced bladder cancer with or without regionally involved lymph nodes. Similar findings have been seen in data reported from a small randomized trial by Skinner and colleagues as well as in non-randomized data reported by Logothetis et al. It would appear that routine adjuvant chemotherapy is a reasonable treatment option for patients with pT_3b, pT_4a and/or pN_1 or pN_2 transitional cell carcinoma.

G.J. Bosl, M.D.

Analysis of Failure Following Definitive Radiotherapy for Invasive Transitional Cell Carcinoma of the Bladder

Mameghan H, Fisher R, Mameghan J, Brook S (Prince of Wales Hosp, Randwick, NSW, Australia)

Int J Radiat Oncol Biol Phys 31:247–254, 1995   6–8

Introduction.—The treatment of invasive bladder cancer remains controversial. Radical cystectomy and definitive radiotherapy followed by salvage cystectomy may or may not involve some neoadjuvant chemotherapy. It is important to be able to define the factors determining which patients should be advised about bladder salvage treatment methods. Identification of such factors would be of assistance to the clinician. In addition, it is possible that these factors might be predictive of distant failure.

Methods.—The records of patients with bladder cancer who received treatment in 1977 to 1990 were reviewed. Transitional cell carcinoma (TCC) had to have been confirmed histologically. Radiation therapy was 4–5 fractions per week at 1.8–2.5 Gy per fraction, for a total dose of 45–65 Gy. Chemotherapy included 100 mg/m² of IV cisplatin at 3-week intervals. A combination of cisplatin, methotrexate, and vinblastine was used in later patients. Bladder relapse was defined as a persistent tumor, local recurrence or a new TCC. Distant failure was defined as documented new metastases. The prognostic values of patient factors, treatment factors, and tumor factors were studied.

Results.—The sample was made up of 342 patients with a mean follow-up of 7.9 years. There were 159 cases of bladder relapse with a 5-year relapse rate of 55%. Significant prognostic factors were tumor multiplicity, ureteric obstruction, and higher T stage. The risks of bladder relapse were 91% for patients with multiple tumors and an obstructed ureter, 69% in patients with a single tumor and obstructed ureter, 68% in patients with multiple tumors without ureter obstruction. In patients with a single tumor without ureter obstruction, the risk depends on the tumor stage. There were 39 patients with distant failure, for a 5-year distant failure rate of 28%. Significant prognostic factors were ureteric obstruction and higher T stage.

Conclusion.—Distinct prognostic groups of patients with invasive bladder TCC were identified based on tumor multiplicity, T stage, and ureteric obstruction. The risk of bladder relapse ranged from 34% to 91%. These factors can aid physicians in selecting patients who will benefit from bladder preservation by definitive radiotherapy.

▶ For some reason, most urologists have concluded that bladder cancer represents a tumor for which radiotherapy has no role to play. It represents a difficult challenge, but this paper from Australia demonstrates that the majority of patients actually have their bladder cancer controlled after definitive radiation therapy. Obviously, patients do better with smaller tumors. Tumor multiplicity and ureteral obstruction also represent major prognostic factors. This paper contains a wealth of data that should be reviewed and discussed objectively by our urologic colleagues as well.

E. Glatstein, M.D.

Results of Treatment of 255 Patients With Metastatic Renal Cell Carcinoma Who Received High-Dose Recombinant Interleukin-2 Therapy

Fyfe G, Fisher RI, Rosenberg SA, Sznol M, Parkinson DR, Louie AC (Loyola Univ Med Ctr, Chicago; Natl Cancer Inst, Bethesda, Md; Pro-Neuron, Rockville, Md)
J Clin Oncol 13:688–696, 1995   6–9

Background.—More than 90% of patients with renal cell carcinoma eventually may have distant disease develop, which carries a 5-year mortality of 80% to 100%. Interferon-α has produced objective responses, but most of them have not proved durable. The T-cell growth factor interleukin-2 (IL-2) has also exhibited substantial activity against metastatic renal cell carcinoma.

Patients.—The effectiveness and safety of high-dose IL-2 treatment were determined in 255 adult patients with histologically documented metastatic renal cell carcinoma who were enrolled in 7 phase II clinical trials. Men predominated, and the median patient age was 52 years. The median interval from the time renal cell carcinoma was diagnosed to IL-2 treatment was 8.5 months.

Treatment.—The patients received Proleukin (aldes leukin) in a dose of 600,000 or 720,000 IU/kg given by IV infusion over 15 minutes at 8-hour intervals. Treatment continued for up to 14 doses over 5 days, as clinically tolerated. A second cycle of treatment was planned after 5–9 days of rest, and subsequently treatment could be repeated every 6–12 weeks in patients who responded or remained stable.

Efficacy.—The overall response rate was 14%, comprising 12 complete and 24 partial responses. The overall median duration of response was 20 months. It was projected that 78% of responders will continue in remission for 12 months, and 55% will continue for 18 months. Partial responses lasted a median of 19 months. The only factor predicting response was the baseline performance status. The median survival time for all patients was 16.3 months. In addition to performance status, previous nephrectomy and the interval from diagnosis to treatment predicted the survival time.

Toxicity.—Eleven patients (4%) died of treatment-related toxicity. Most of these deaths resulted from multiple medical problems, but much of the severe toxicity observed was in the form of capillary leak syndrome and resembled septic shock.

Conclusion.—High-dose treatment with IL-2 has produced durable remissions of renal cell carcinoma in patients with metastatic disease. Ways may someday be found to reduce the severe toxicity sometimes associated with this treatment.

▶ Patients with metastatic renal cell carcinoma have a particularly poor prognosis, because the disease is usually resistant to conventional therapeutic maneuvers, including radiotherapy, hormonal therapy, and chemotherapy. However, this is one malignancy for which biological response modifiers appear to have clinical potential. A number of preliminary studies involving small numbers of patients have consistently reported objective responses, either with interferon-α or IL-2. Fyfe and colleagues recently reported their results of using high-dose IL-2 therapy among a large cohort of patients with metastatic renal cell carcinoma. Although the overall objective response rate was modest at 14%, 12 patients (5%) achieved a complete response. Responses occurred in all sites of disease, including visceral metastases, and among patients with large tumor burden. Although the overall response rate was relatively low, the median duration of response for patients who *did* achieve a complete response has not been reached, and the median for patients achieving a partial response (24 patients, or 9%) was 19 months.

This study is important because it reports the results of a large cohort of patients who were given similar treatment. The results provide an impetus to continue the pursuit of biological-based approaches to patients with this disease, one in which we desperately need improved therapy. Severe, acute treatment-related toxicities were reported, and 4% of the patients died of adverse events. We will need to continue to carefully weigh the potential benefits and toxicities in future studies, when novel treatments such as IL-2 are pursued.

M.S. Tallman, M.D.

7 Gastrointestinal Cancer

Significant Prognostic Factors by Multivariate Analysis of 3926 Gastric Cancer Patients
Kim J-P, Kim Y-W, Yang H-K, Noh D-Y (Seoul Natl Univ, Korea)
World J Surg 18:872–878, 1994   7–1

Background.—Early detection and management of gastric cancer, the leading cause of cancer death, are primary goals. Significant prognostic factors, including sex, age, location of primary tumor, gross type, histologic type, depth of invasion, number of lymph node metastases, and type of treatment, were analyzed for their effect on 5-year survival.

Patients and Methods.—The medical records and pathologic reports of 3,926 selected patients with gastric cancer treated between 1981 and 1991 were retrospectively reviewed. The UICC TNM staging system was used. Prognostic factors were evaluated using univariate and multivariate analy-

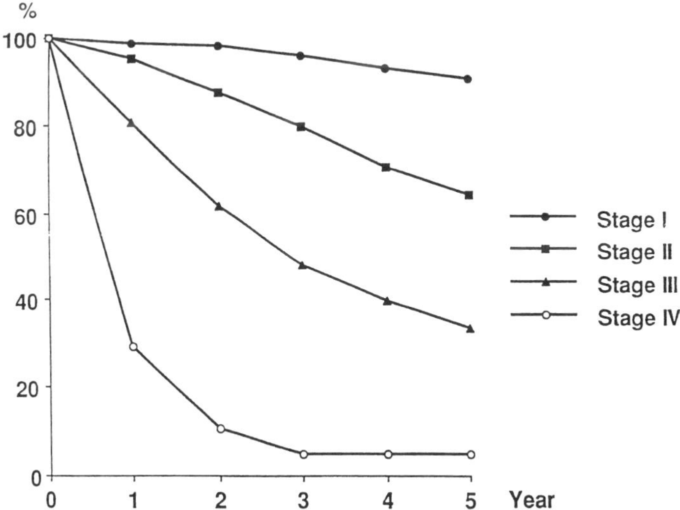

FIGURE 1.—Survival of the patients according to stage ($P < .05$). (Courtesy of Kim J-P, Kim Y-W, Yang H-K, et al: Significant prognostic factors by multivariate analysis of 3926 gastric cancer patients. *World J Surg* 18:872–878, Copyright 1994, Springer-Verlag.)

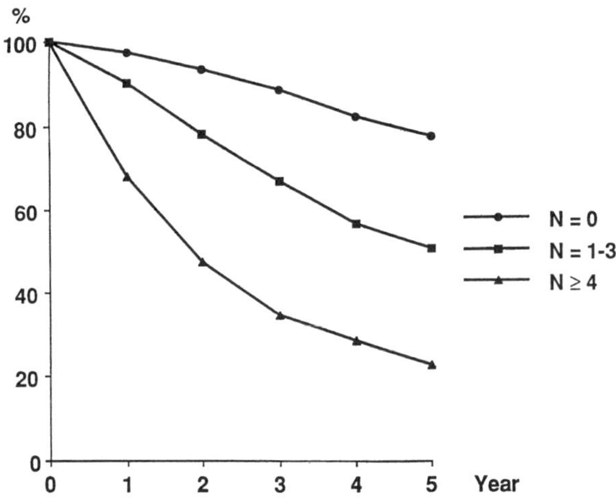

FIGURE 6.—Survival curves according to lymph node metastatis ($P < .0001$). (Courtesy of Kim J-P, Kim Y-W, Yang H-K, et al: Significant prognostic factors by multivariate analysis of 3926 gastric cancer patients. *World J Surg* 18:872–878, Copyright 1994, Springer-Verlag.)

ses. In addition, immunochemosurgery, postoperative chemotherapy, and surgery alone were assessed for their effect on survival in patients with stage III cancer.

Results.—The overall 5-year survival rate of patients with operable gastric cancer was 46.8%. The 5-year survival rates based on UICC clinical staging were 90.7% for stage I, 64.5% for stage II, 33.4% for stage III, and 4.9% for stage IV (Fig 1). After an analysis of the 5-year cumulative survival for each prognostic factor, univariate analysis showed some significance for age, depth of invasion, lymph node metastasis, location of primary tumor, histologic differentiation, and gross type. Multivariate analysis identified depth of invasion and lymph node metastasis as the most powerful prognostic factors (Fig 6). Additional significant factors included gross type, location, and histologic differentiation. With respect to postoperative treatment, significantly better survival rates were noted in patients with stage III cancer treated with immunochemosurgery compared with postoperative chemotherapy or surgery alone.

Conclusions.—The depth of invasion and the number of lymph node metastases are significant prognostic factors in gastric cancer. In patients with advanced gastric cancer, immunochemosurgery may prove to be beneficial after curative gastric resection.

▶ The authors' report is the largest single-institution experience in the treatment of gastric cancer, evaluating almost 4,000 patients in only a decade. The major value of this study is that it provides baseline information for future randomized therapeutic studies of the extent of operation and adjuvant therapy. As expected, the multivariate analysis demonstrated that the depth of invasion, lymph node metastasis, type of cancer, histologic differentiation and, to a lesser degree, location within the stomach impacted on survival. As demonstrated in the accompanying figures, node positivity could be dichotomized into 1 to 3 or 4 or more positive nodes with considerable impact on survival.

As with all such articles, prognostic studies should separate patient characteristics, tumor-related factors, surgical treatment–related prognostic factors, and adjuvant therapy factors. When analyzing the end results from multiple centers, the issue of "stage migration" must always be addressed, as recently demonstrated in the surgical resection study from The Netherlands.[1] Although the authors claim a benefit from chemoimmunotherapy in this article, such treatments remain investigational.

A.M. Cohen, M.D.

Reference

1. Bunt AM, Hermans J, Smit VT, et al: Surgical/pathologic-stage migration confounds comparisons of gastric cancer survival rates between Japan and Western countries. *J Clin Oncol* 13:19, 1995.

Primary Gastrointestinal Sarcomas: Analysis of Prognostic Variables
Conlon KC, Ephraim SC, Brennan MF (Mem Sloan-Kettering Cancer Ctr, New York)
Ann Surg Oncol 2:26–31, 1995   7–2

Introduction.—Primary malignant mesenchymal tumors of the gastrointestinal (GI) tract are relatively rare, accounting for 0.1% to 3.0% of all GI malignancies. The most frequent site of these sarcomas is the stomach, and the main histologic type is leiomyosarcoma. Because of their uncommon occurrence, the clinicopathologic determinants of survival in patients with primary GI sarcomas are uncertain. A 10-year experience with these tumors was reviewed to correlate their clinical presentation, pathologic findings, and treatment with their outcome.

Patients.—The review included 38 patients older than 16 years of age who were admitted with primary GI sarcoma from 1982 through 1991. The patients represented 2% of all adult patients with sarcoma admitted during that time. There were 26 men and 12 women (mean age, 59 years). Eighty-one percent of the patients had localized disease, whereas 16% had metachronous epithelial malignancies. Twenty tumors were found in the stomach, 9 in the small bowel, and 9 in the large bowel. Ninety-two percent of patients were symptomatic when they came to medical attention: 63% had abdominal pain, 45% had anorexia, 42% had weight loss, and 32% had fatigue.

Treatment and Outcome.—Twenty-seven patients had complete resection of their tumor, 7 had incomplete resection, and 3 had biopsy only. Nine patients underwent doxorubicin-containing chemotherapy. The histologic diagnosis was leiomyosarcoma in 35 patients; the other 3 patients

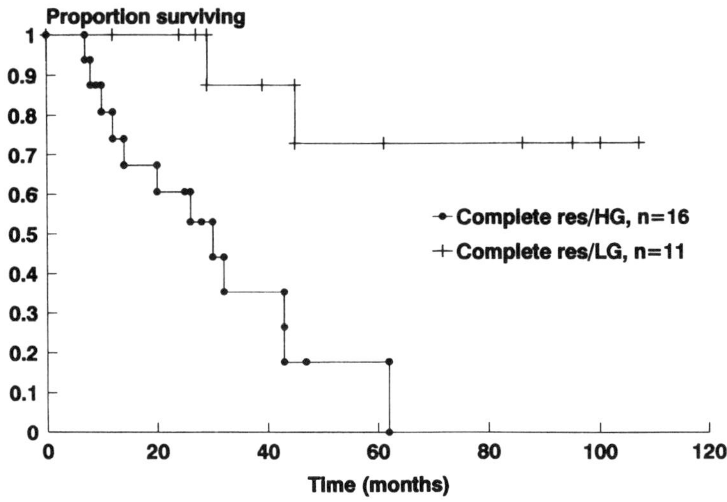

FIGURE 6.—Survival of patients undergoing a complete resection with either a high-grade (*HG*) or low-grade (*LG*) tumor (*P*=.002). (Courtesy of Conlon KC, Ephraim SC, Brennan MF: *Ann Surg Oncol* 2:26-31, 1995.)

had leiomyoblastoma, plexosarcoma, and synovial sarcoma. Sixty-eight percent of tumors were high-grade and 32% were low-grade; regional node involvement was present in 2 patients. At a median follow-up of 26 months, the actuarial 5-year survival was 28%. Forty-four percent of patients who underwent complete resection had tumor recurrence, the mean time of which was 9 months. The main sites of initial failure were hepatic metastases and local recurrence, each accounting for 42% of cases.

Prognostic Factors.—Weight loss and pain at presentation were adverse prognostic factors, and overall survival was significantly related to histologic grade, extent of resection, and a small bowel primary site. As long as the primary tumor was completely excised, resection of contiguous organs did not influence survival. Prognosis was unrelated to age, race, sex, previous surgery, tumor size, or adjuvant therapy. Among patients who underwent complete resection, 5-year survival was 72% for those with low-grade tumors vs. 18% for those with high-grade tumors (Fig 6).

Conclusions.—Primary GI sarcomas are uncommon tumors with a poor prognosis. Although complete surgical excision of the tumor is the optimal therapy, surgery alone appears to be inadequate for patients with high-grade tumors. Patients with high-grade primary GI sarcomas should therefore be considered for investigational adjuvant therapies.

▶ The authors analyze a recent experience with primary GI sarcomas, primarily leiomyosarcomas, seen at a major referral center during the past 12 years. Data are provided with regard to expected outcomes in the era of CT scanning. Two thirds of the patients were seen with pain rather then bowel obstruction, with 97% of 33 patients having an abnormal CT scan. Although prior studies—as well as this current report—indicate a 25% to 50% overall

5-year survival rate, this report provides important prognostic variable data. The figure provides impressive survival data comparing high-grade vs. low-grade tumors that are completely resected. Most of these lesions would not have been biopsied before resection.

Because almost half of the patients will have low-grade tumors with a long-term survival prognosis of more than 70%, these data support an aggressive approach toward complete resection by the initial operating surgeon.

A.M. Cohen, M.D.

Lymph-Node Metastases: Efficacy of Detection With Helical CT in Patients With Gastric Cancer

Fukuya T, Honda H, Hayashi T, Kaneko K, Tateshi Y, Ro T, Maehara Y, Tanaka M, Tsuneyoshi M, Masuda K (Kyushu Univ, Fukuoka, Japan)
Radiology 197:705–711, 1995   7–3

Background.—Helical CT may be more useful than conventional CT in identifying smaller lymph nodes. The value of helical CT in the detection of lymph nodes in patients with proved gastric cancer was investigated, and diagnostic criteria for differentiating between metastasis-positive and metastasis-negative nodes were sought.

Methods.—Fifty-eight patients with gastric cancer were included in the study. They were 39 men and 19 women with a mean age of 63.8 years. A total of 1,082 lymph nodes were resected. Of these, 138 were found to contain metastases. Helical CT findings were compared with those at resection.

Findings.—Helical CT was able to identify 1.1% of the 649 lymph nodes that were 1–4 mm in diameter, 45.1% of the 355 nodes of 5–9 mm, and 72% of the 78 nodes greater than 9 mm. For nodes of 5 mm or more, the sensitivity for identifying metastatic nodes was greater than for identifying nonmetastatic nodes, with those values being 75.2% and 41.8%, respectively. Significant differences were noted between positive and negative nodes in CT attenuation and short-to-long axis ratios.

Conclusion.—Helical CT is better than conventional CT in detecting lymph nodes in patients with gastric cancer. However, helical CT has a limited ability to detect lymph nodes in patients with little perigastric fat or nodes located in specific anatomical regions. The sensitivity of helical CT for identifying lymph nodes with metastases was greater than for detecting lymph nodes without metastases.

▶ Computed tomography is gaining a major role in the preoperative staging of various neoplasms. However, when it comes to evaluation of nodes, the only real criterion that can be used for distinguishing neoplastic nodes from those without neoplasm is the size. This study looks at the helical CT scanner and its ability to detect lymph node metastates in patients with gastric cancers. Fifty-eight patients underwent helical CT scanning followed by surgery for detection of lymphadenopathy in patients with gastric cancer. Those 58 patients yielded a total of 1,082 lymph nodes, of which 138 were positive at the time of surgery. The authors of this study compared the surgical findings with the CT findings. Anyone who wants to use CT as the reliable way of picking up lymphadenopathy should look carefully at the tables accompanying the original article. The kind of detection of positivity based on size is very humbling and provides a relatively low yield.

E. Glatstein, M.D.

Reconstruction After Gastrectomy and Quality of Life
Buhl K, Lehnert T, Schlag P, Herfarth C (Univ of Heidelberg, Germany)
World J Surg 19:558–564, 1995   7–4

Background.—Patients with gastric cancer commonly undergo total gastrectomy to ensure adequate safety margins for a real hope of cure. Total gastrectomy has become more frequent because of the increasing number of tumors found in the upper third of the stomach or cardiac region. Such radical procedures result in sequelae that can negatively affect patients' quality of life. In an attempt to fully assess quality of life and functional outcomes after gastric cancer surgery, a multidimensional study of postoperative sequelae was performed.

Methods.—One hundred four patients with no evidence of disease at 12 months or more after surgery were studied. Fifty-nine patients had undergone total gastrectomy and jejunal pouch reconstruction according to Hunt-Lawrence-Rodino. Twenty-four patients had had restoration of the alimentary tract by simple esophagojejunostomy using the Roux-en-Y technique, and 21 had had distal subtotal gastrectomy.

Findings.—Postoperative symptoms of heartburn or dumping did not significantly differ between the group undergoing total gastrectomy with pouch reconstruction and the group having distal gastric resection. Patients undergoing total gastrectomy and restoration with esophagojejunostomy had both sequelae. Nutritional status was also decreased in the latter group. All instruments used to measure quality of life showed improvements in patients with pouch reconstruction and after distal gastrectomy; however, differences were not significant.

Conclusions.—Distal gastric resection has no advantage over total gastrectomy with pouch reconstruction in terms of functional outcomes or postoperative quality of life. Thus, performing less radical procedures in an attempt to improve such outcomes is not justified. Pouch reconstruction is the treatment of choice for reconstruction after total gastrectomy in patients with gastric cancer.

▶ The authors looked at both functional and psychological parameters in patients undergoing potentially curative resection for gastric cancer, free of recurrence and stable at least 12 months after the operation. Although this was not a randomized trial, a detailed comparison was performed. The determining factor in the use of a jejunal pouch reconstruction vs. a simple esophagojejunostomy was not provided. We do not know whether this was based on the personal preference of the surgeons involved or on some aspects of the patients' weight, body habitus, etc.

These authors ought to be congratulated for their attempt at multifactorial determination of the quality of life in such patients. The data suggest that pouch reconstruction after total gastrectomy is to be preferred, assuming this can be done for technical reasons and with minimal increased morbidity. Because the overall cure rate in gastric adenocarcinoma remains quite small, quality-of-life considerations are even more important, considering that the duration of life is frequently only several years.

A.M. Cohen, M.D.

Reconstruction of the Food Passage After Total Gastrectomy: Randomized Trial
Fuchs K-H, Thiede A, Engemann R, Deltz E, Stremme O, Hamelmann H (Univ of Würzburg, Germany; Friedrich-Ebert-Krankenhaus, Neumünster, Germany; Chirurgische Universitätsklinik, Kiel, Germany)
World J Surg 19:698–706, 1995   7–5

Background.—Surgeons continue to seek the best way of reconstructing the upper gastrointestinal tract after total gastrectomy to ensure the best possible quality of life. The importance of the duodenal food passage remains uncertain. There is evidence from both experimental and clinical studies that interposing jejunum between the esophagus and duodenum is advantageous. Some investigators, however, prefer the Roux-en-Y technique, a technically easier form of reconstruction.

Objective.—One hundred twenty patients seen over 5 years who required total gastrectomy for malignant disease were randomly assigned to undergo either jejunal interposition with a pouch (JIP) or the Roux-en-Y operation with a pouch (RYP). Excluding the 14 patients for whom only RYP was technically feasible, there were 53 patients in each group.

Results.—Two patients in the RYP group and 1 in the JIP group died of septic complications secondary to anastomotic leakage, peritonitis, and multiorgan failure. Twenty-eight RYP patients were alive at 3 years, 26 without evidence of recurrent disease. All but 1 of 21 JIP patients alive at 3 years were free of recurrence. Few patients who were free of recurrent disease had functional gastrointestinal problems. Reflux esophagitis developed postoperatively in only 3 patients. The 2 groups did not differ with respect to body weight or quality of life.

Conclusion.—The relatively undemanding Roux-en-Y reconstruction is as clinically effective and problem-free as provision of a duodenal food passage in patients requiring total gastrectomy for malignant disease.

▶ The majority of patients who undergo total gastrectomy for cancer succumb to their disease. However, those who experience long-term survival and those who are cured may have markedly reduced quality of life related to their total gastrectomy. This study is a randomized, prospective comparison of 2 types of technical reconstruction after total gastrectomy. Both use a pouch to increase the reservoir, and the comparison is between an anatomical reconstruction to the duodenum and the far simpler Roux-en-Y reconstruction to the jejunum. In addition to perioperative complications, at 3 years, studies of body weight, functional assessment, and quality-of-life determinants were undertaken prospectively. There were no significant differences between the 2 operative techniques. The study demonstrates the importance of separating facts from opinion in outcomes of surgical treatment and the importance of long-term functional and quality-of-life considerations for patients undergoing radical cancer surgery.

A.M. Cohen, M.D.

Randomised Comparison of Morbidity After D1 and D2 Dissection for Gastric Cancer in 996 Dutch Patients
Bonenkamp JJ, Songun I, Hermans J, Sasako M, Welvaart K, Plukker JTM, van Elk P, Obertop H, Gouma DJ, Taat CW, van Lanschot J, Meyer S, de Graaf PW, von Meyenfeldt MF, Tilanus H, van de Velde CJH (Univ of Leiden, The Netherlands; Natl Cancer Ctr Hosp, Tokyo; Univ of Groningen, The Netherlands; et al)
Lancet 345:745–748, 1995   7–6

Background.—For patients with gastric cancer, surgery is the only treatment that offers hope of cure. However, authorities disagree as to the extent of lymph node dissection needed. A prospective study was begun in 1989 in The Netherlands to determine whether extended lymphadenectomy would increase the survival times of patients with gastric cancer.

Methods.—This multicenter trial included 1,078 patients. The patients were assigned to groups of equal size that underwent lymph node dissection limited to the perigastric nodes (D1) or dissection extending to regional lymph nodes outside the perigastric area (D2). Twenty-six and 56 patients, respectively, were subsequently excluded from the trial because of failure to meet eligibility criteria.

Findings.—Among 711 patients judged to have curable lesions, the patients in the D2 group had a greater operative mortality rate than patients in the D1 group. These rates were 10% and 4%, respectively. Also, 43% of the patients undergoing dissection extending to the regional lymph nodes outside the perigastric region had complications compared with 25% of those undergoing dissection limited to the perigastric nodes. The length of hospitalization after surgery was a median of 25 days in the D2 group and 18 days in the D1 group. The differences in morbidity and mortality persisted in almost all the subgroups.

Conclusions.—Lymph node dissection extending to the regional lymph nodes outside the perigastric region should not be done as a standard treatment for patients with gastric cancer in Western countries, at least not until the survival results of this study are known. The discrepancy between these results and those of nonrandomized series indicates the effects of variability among surgeons in retrospective studies.

▶ For many years, it has been noted that in patients with gastric cancer, the end results of gastrectomy done in centers in Europe, England, and the United States are inferior to those obtained in Japanese centers. The basis for this difference remains unclear, but extended regional lymphadenectomy is the standard operative procedure in Japan, whereas a more "ulcer-oriented" gastrectomy is performed in Western countries.

Since recent studies indicated that the extent of lymphadenectomy does not result in an increase in postoperative complications, this ambitious randomised comparison of limited vs. more extended lymphadenectomy has accrued more than 700 patients. The median follow-up is inadequate to comment on survival differences; however, the analysis of morbidity is disconcerting. The mortality of the more extended lymph node dissection group was 2½ times greater (10% vs. 4%), complications almost doubled, and the length of stay was one week greater. These results were obtained by many surgeons in a multicenter trial, and they presumably represent a more realistic assessment of the operative complications associated with radical gastrectomy. Under these circumstances, except when carried out by experienced hands at major medical centers, the treatment of gastric cancer should involve a limited regional lymph node dissection pending clear overall survival benefits that will outweigh the increase in operative mortality.

A.M. Cohen, M.D.

Final Results of a Phase III Clinical Trial of Adjuvant Chemotherapy With the Modified Fluorouracil, Doxorubicin, and Mitomycin Regimen in Resectable Gastric Cancer
Lise M, Nitti D, Marchet A, Sahmoud T, Buyse M, Duez N, Fiorentino M, Dos Santos JG, Labianca R, Rougier P, Gignoux M (Università di Padova, Italy; Ospedale Civile di Padova, Italy; Ospedale S Carlo Borromeo, Milano, Italy; et al)
J Clin Oncol 13:2757–2763, 1995   7–7

Purpose.—Most studies of the use of adjuvant chemotherapy for gastric cancer have yielded disappointing results. Previous studies of patients with advanced gastric cancer have shown a response rate of 60% in patients receiving the FAM2 regimen, which consists of 5-fluorouracil, doxorubicin, and mitomycin. Adjuvant chemotherapy with FAM2 was compared with surgery alone in patients with gastric cancer in a European Organization for the Research and Treatment of Cancer randomized clinical trial.

Methods.—The trial included 314 patients who had undergone curative resection for stage II or III gastric adenocarcinoma. The patients were randomized to receive adjuvant FAM2 chemotherapy or no further treatment. The patients received 7 cycles of FAM2 chemotherapy, repeated every 43 days. The differences in overall survival, time to progression, and disease-free interval were assessed by the log-rank and the Cox model.

Results.—Twelve percent of patients assigned to the FAM2 group never started receiving chemotherapy. Those who did start received a median of 5 cycles. The incidence of grade 3 or 4 hematologic toxicity in patients who began adjuvant treatment was 6% to 9%. The incidence of severe nonhematologic toxicity was 1% to 29%. Approximately half the patients required dosage reduction because of toxicity. Five-year survival was 70% for patients with stage II disease and 32% for those with stage III disease, with there being no significant difference between the chemotherapy and control groups. Patients receiving FAM2 did have a significantly longer time to disease progression and a borderline significant increase in disease-free survival.

Conclusion.—The toxicity of the FAM2 chemotherapy regimen is too high for use as standard adjuvant treatment for gastric cancer. To determine the true benefit of adjuvant chemotherapy for gastric cancer will require large-scale clinical trials of more active, less toxic regimens. These studies should give serious consideration to the concept of minimal residual disease.

Adjuvant Chemotherapy With 5-FU, Adriamycin, and Mitomycin-C (FAM) Versus Surgery Alone for Patients With Locally Advanced Gastric Adenocarcinoma: A Southwest Oncology Group Study
Macdonald JS, Fleming TR, Peterson RF, Berenberg JL, McClure S, Chapman RA, Eyre HJ, Solanki D, Cruz AB Jr, Gagliano R, Estes NC, Tangen CM, Rivkin S (Temple Univ, Philadelphia; Southwest Oncology Group Statistical Ctr, Seattle; Scott & White Clinic/Texas A & M, Temple, Tex; et al)
Ann Surg Oncol 2:488–494, 1995   7–8

Background.—Patients undergoing curative resection of gastric cancer have a 5-year survival rate of only 25% to 40%. One reason for this is the high likelihood of relapse and death after gastrectomy in patients with locally advanced tumors. Adjuvant chemotherapy has been investigated to help prevent recurrent disease. The FAM chemotherapy regimen—consisting of 5-fluorouracil, doxorubicin, and mitomycin C—was evaluated as adjuvant therapy for patients with resected gastric carcinoma.

Methods.—The phase III Southwest Oncology Group study included 193 patients with resected TNM stage I, II, or III gastric adenocarcinoma. Patients were randomized to receive 6 cycles of postoperative FAM chemotherapy, amounting to 1 year of treatment, or observation only. The 2 groups were compared for survival and disease-free survival by log-rank analysis.

Results.—At a median follow-up of 9.5 years, there were no significant differences between the groups in disease-free or overall survival (Fig 2). Survival was influenced by the quality of surgical resection, regardless of whether the patients received adjuvant FAM. When curative resection was

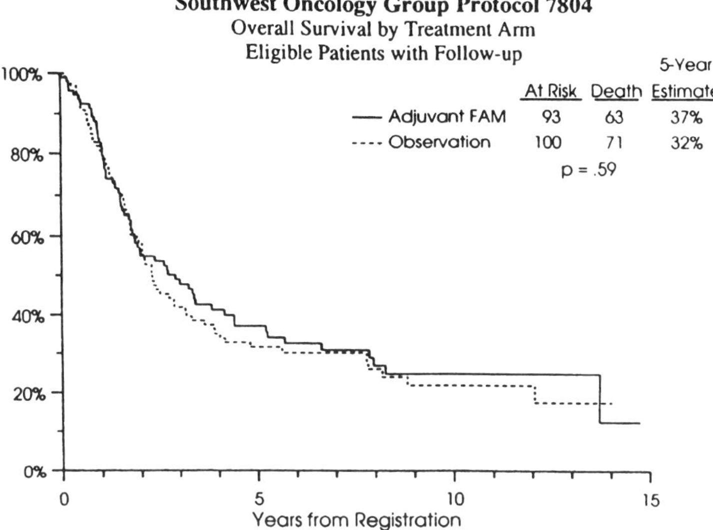

FIGURE 2.—Overall survival by treatment (eligible patients with follow-up). (Courtesy of Macdonald JS, Fleming TR, Peterson RF, et al: Adjuvant chemotherapy with 5-FU, Adriamycin, and mitomycin-C (FAM) versus surgery alone for patients with locally advanced gastric adenocarcinoma: A Southwest Oncology Group study. *Ann Surg Oncol* 2:488–494, 1995.)

achieved, i.e., there was no evidence of residual disease in the abdomen and tumor-free margins of greater than 1 cm, survival was significantly better. Six percent of patients receiving FAM had grade IV hematologic toxicity. Two patients died of apparent FAM-related toxicity, 1 of cardiomyopathy and 1 of hemolytic uremic syndrome.

Conclusion.—Adjuvant chemotherapy with FAM does not appear to improve survival for patients with resected gastric cancer. Prospective surgical quality control must be part of future studies of adjuvant therapy. Also, effective trials cannot be performed within a single cooperative group; the INT 0116 trial is under way, with participation of all cooperative groups in the United States.

▶ The previous 2 articles (Abstracts 7–7 and 7–8), combined with a prior randomized trial,[1] should convince all oncologists that adjuvant chemotherapy with combinations of 5-fluorouracil (5-FU), doxorubicin, and mitomycin-C is not effective in the treatment of gastric adenocarcinoma. The article by Lise et al. (Abstract 7–7), representing the European Organization for the Research and Treatment of Cancer clinical trial, shows that the use of a slightly increased dose of doxorubicin did produce a trend toward prolongation of disease-free survival (P value of 0.068), but this did not translate into any improvement in overall survival.

It is still possible that clinical trials using 5-FU, doxorubicin, and either methotrexate or cisplatin may be effective. It is quite clear that differences in surgical technique, as reported from major medical centers, vary greatly with regard to overall survival as well as technique. Whether these differences represent improved pathologic staging associated with more extensive lymph node dissection or an enhanced ability to clear the locoregional disease remains unclear. However, in light of these data, all clinical trials of adjuvant chemotherapy or chemoradiation therapy in gastric cancer must very carefully define and categorize the type of operative procedure performed.

A.M. Cohen, M.D.

Reference

1. Coombes RC, Schein PS, Chilvers C, et al: A randomized trial comparing adjuvant fluorouracil, doxorubicin and mitomycin with no treatment in operable gastric cancer. *J Clin Oncol* 8:1362–1369, 1990.

Epirubucin, Cisplatin, and Continuous Infusion 5-Fluorouracil Is an Active and Safe Regimen for Patients With Advanced Gastric Cancer: An Italian Group for the Study of Digestive Tract Cancer (GISCAD) Report
Zaniboni A, for the Italian Group for the Study of Digestive Tract Cancer (Brescia, Italy)
Cancer 76:1694–1699, 1995   7–9

Objective.—Patients with histologically documented gastric cancer that was either locally advanced or metastatic were entered in a multicenter trial intended to confirm the effectiveness of a regimen of epirubicin, cisplatin, and continuously infused 5-fluorouracil (ECF). Only patients younger than 70 years of age whose Eastern Cooperative Oncology Group performance status was 2 or less were admitted to the trial. Seven patients with locally advanced disease and 46 with metastatic cancer were evaluated.

Treatment.—A totally implanted venous port was used in most cases. Patients received epirubicin, 50 mg/m², by IV bolus injection and cisplatin, 60 mg/m² IV, for 1 hour at 3-week intervals for 8 cycles. They also received 5-fluorouracil, 200 mg/m² daily, by continuous infusion for 21 consecutive weeks, ceasing the day after the final injections of cisplatin and epirubicin.

Toxicity.—The patients received a median of 7 cycles of treatment. Five patients (9%) had neutropenic fever, and 11 (20%) had central venous catheter–related complications. There were no treatment-related deaths.

Efficacy.—Thirty of 53 patients (56%) had an objective response, and 8 patients (15%) had a complete response. Twelve patients remained stable, and 11 had progressive disease. In most cases, a peak response was observed after the fourth treatment cycle. Disease in the lymph nodes and liver responded most consistently. Five of the 7 patients with locally advanced disease had a partial response, and 3 of them underwent surgery with curative intent. Dysphagia improved significantly in 6 of 9 patients affected. The median duration of response was 10 months, and the overall median survival exceeded 9 months.

Conclusion.—The ECG regimen is an active and relatively safe protocol for patients with locally advanced or metastatic gastric cancer.

▶ Several reports have indicated high response rates for cisplatin-based combination chemotherapy in gastric cancer, but they have also noted considerable toxicity. A pilot protocol using prolonged IV infusional 5-fluorouracil (5-FU)-based chemotherapy produced a 71% response rate in a phase II trial. This report is of a multicenter phase II trial that used infusional 5-FU with bolus epirubucin and bolus cisplatin.

In this experience with 53 patients in a multicenter environment, the overall response rate was greater than half, with 8 patients having a complete response. Most important, the overall toxicity was quite mild and primarily hematologic, and only 3 patients required hospitalization for neutropenic fever. Prolonged infusion of 5-FU as a single agent has been used in advanced gastric cancer with a 31% response rate. If these response rates and the relatively low toxicity are further confirmed, a trial in an adjuvant setting will be warranted.

A.M. Cohen, M.D.

Prophylaxis With Intraoperative Chemohyperthermia Against Peritoneal Recurrence of Serosal Invasion-Positive Gastric Cancer

Yonemura Y, Ninomiya I, Kaji M, Sugiyama K, Fujimura K, Sawa T, Katayama K, Tanaka S, Hirono Y, Miwa K, Miyazaki I (Kanazawa Univ, Kanazawa City, Japan)

World J Surg 19:450–455, 1995

7–10

Introduction.—The peritoneum is the most frequent site of recurrence of gastric cancer. Trials of adjuvant systemic chemotherapy to control peritoneal dissemination have yielded disappointing results. A multidisciplinary approach to the treatment of peritoneal dissemination—combining surgery, intraperitoneal chemotherapy, and local hyperthermia—was evaluated.

Methods.—A new technique—continuous hyperthermic peritoneal perfusion (CHPP)—was developed for the study. It used a solution containing mitomycin-C, 30 mg, and cisplatin, 300 mg. A special closed-circuit CHPP device was used to perfuse this solution, warmed to 43.5°C, into the peritoneal cavity for 60 minutes. One hundred sixty patients with advanced gastric cancers who had undergone curative surgery were treated: 79 received CHPP and 81 received surgery only. All had macroscopic serosal invasion with no peritoneal metastases.

Results.—Survival was better for patients receiving CHPP. The difference was significant for those with pathologically confirmed serosal invasion-positive tumors, but not for those with serosal invasion-negative tumors (Fig 4). Patients with stage IV tumors also had a significant survival advantage with CHPP (Fig 5). Four patients in the CHPP group had

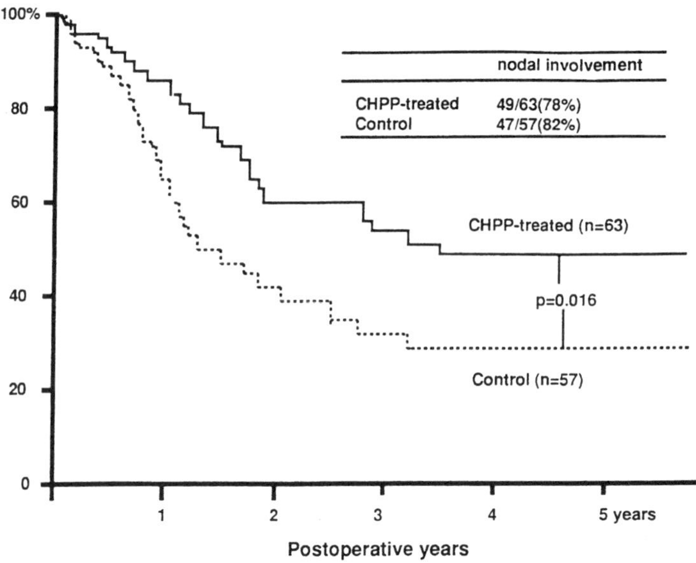

FIGURE 4.—Survival curves of patients with histologically proved serosal invasion-positive tumor, according to the treatment. (Courtesy of Yonemura Y, Ninomiya I, Kaji M, et al: Prophylaxis with intraoperative chemohyperthermia against peritoneal recurrence of serosal invasion-positive gastric cancer. *World J Surg* 19:450–455, Copyright 1995, Springer-Verlag.)

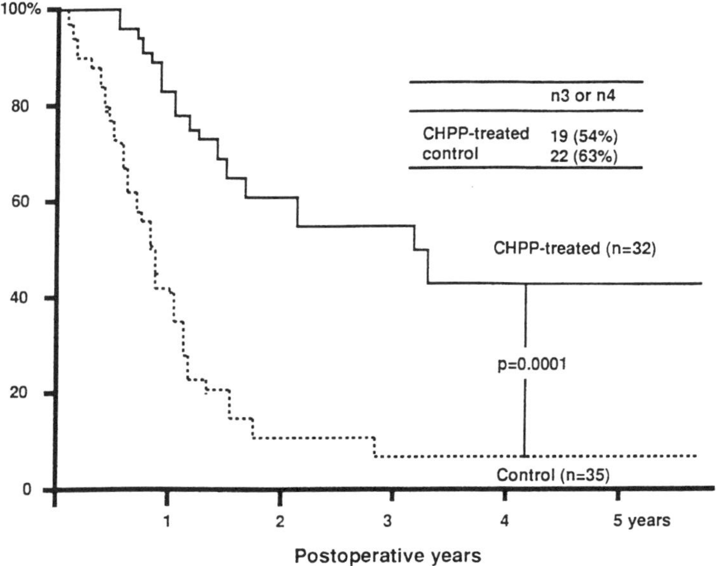

FIGURE 5.—Survival curves of patients with stage IV disease, according to the treatment. (Courtesy of Yonemura Y, Ninomiya I, Kaji M, et al: Prophylaxis with intraoperative chemohyperthermia against peritoneal recurrence of serosal invasion-positive gastric cancer. *World J Surg* 19:450–455, Copyright 1995, Springer-Verlag.)

adverse effects: 3 had transient hyperazotemia and 1 had severe bone marrow suppression. Mortality and morbidity were similar in the 2 groups.

Conclusion.—For patients who have undergone curative surgery for gastric cancer, CHPP appears to be a safe, simple, and readily available technique for the prevention of peritoneal recurrence. It should be evaluated for use in gynecologic malignancies, especially ovarian cancers, which also have frequent peritoneal dissemination.

▶ This nonrandomized trial of intraperitoneal adjuvant chemotherapy compares the treated group with a concurrent control group treated by surgery alone. The selection factors were not explained, but the 2 groups of patients were relatively similar with regard to the major prognostic factors. The adjuvant program involved intraoperative hyperthermic mitomycin-C and cisplatin perfused for 1 hour. The patients received oral fluorouracil analogue for 2–3 weeks after the operation. Of the 79 patients who received CHPP, there was only 1 postoperative death related to the chemotherapy, and there were 2 anastomotic leaks in each group.

The data suggested survival benefits in patients with transmural tumor penetration or stage IV disease. These data confirm the relative safety of this adjuvant strategy and provide a considerable incentive to proceed with a proper prospective randomized trial.

A.M. Cohen, M.D.

Cost-Effectiveness of Palliative Chemotherapy in Advanced Gastrointestinal Cancer

Glimelius B, Hoffman K, Graf W, Haglund U, Nyrén O, Påhlman L, Sjödén P-O (Univ of Uppsala, Sweden)
Ann Oncol 6:267–274, 1995   7–11

Background.—Although chemotherapy is widely used, the extent of its effects on cancer symptoms, quality of life, and survival in patients with advanced gastrointestinal cancer is uncertain. In addition, there has been no research regarding the costs involved. The cost-effectiveness of chemotherapy-induced gains in quantity and quality of life was investigated.

Methods.—Sixty-one patients with inoperable gastric, pancreatic, biliary, or colorectal cancer were randomly assigned to primary chemotherapy and best supportive care or to best supportive care alone. Patients in whom supportive measures alone did not provide adequate palliation were given chemotherapy.

Findings.—Improved or prolonged high quality of life was documented in 58% of the patients receiving primary chemotherapy and in 29% of those receiving supportive care alone. The primary chemotherapy group had significantly longer overall survival and quality-adjusted survival than did the group receiving supportive care only. Survival was significantly longer in patients with gastric cancer but not in those with colorectal or

TABLE 2.—Average Overall and Quality-of-Life-Adjusted Survival

| | Primary chemotherapy | | Best supportive care | | Incremental survival | |
	Overall	Quality-adjusted	Overall	Quality-adjusted	Overall	Quality-adjusted
				days (%)*		
Colorectal	396	292 (74)	247	128 (52)	149	164
Gastric	295	220 (75)	111	64 (58)	184	156
Pancreatic/ biliary	202	139 (69)	180	111 (62)	22	28
All	294	214 (73)	192	106 (55)	102	108

* Proportion of overall survival.
(Courtesy of Glimelius B, Hoffman K, Graf W, et al: *Ann Oncol* 6:267–274, 1995. Reprinted by permission of Kluwer Academic Publishers.)

pancreatic-biliary cancer (Table 2). The mean cost for all medical care was approximately 50% higher in patients receiving primary chemotherapy, but the 2 groups had comparable average costs per day. In both groups, most of the cost was attributable to hospitalization. Incremental costs per gained year of life were $21,300; per gained quality-adjusted year of life they were, $20,200; and per quality of life–patient they were $20,600. Patients with gastric and colorectal cancer had much lower costs, and those with pancreatic-biliary cancer had much greater costs.

Conclusion.—Palliative chemotherapy in patients with advanced gastric and colorectal cancer appears to be cost-effective. Its survival and quality-of-life benefits to patients with gastric and pancreatic-biliary cancer are less clear.

▶ This very important paper addresses the question of whether it is financially, as well as medically, justified to give specific anticancer therapy with no chance of cure because the quality of life is sufficiently improved at a reasonable cost. The authors' conclusion is that the patients who were randomized to receive palliative primary chemotherapy were more likely to have an improved and/or prolonged quality of life than the group randomized to receive best supportive care without chemotherapy. However, it is extremely important to point out that most of the improvement was in patients with gastric cancer; no significant improvement was seen in patients with colorectal or pancreatic-biliary cancer.

Because of the number of patients and the subgroups of patients evaluated in this study, I am not confident of the authors' conclusions, although I applaud the general design of the study and the attempt to obtain some objective measures of success in palliative treatment. Society will have to decide whether a 3-month increment of survival is worth the cost. As usual, society at large is very ambivalent about this, with the answer to increased premiums for health care or increased taxes being "yes" when personalized and "no" when generalized.

J.V. Simone, M.D.

Intraoperative Radiation Therapy for Gastric Cancer

Abe M, Nishimura Y, Shibamoto Y (Kyoto Univ, Japan)

World J Surg 19:554–557, 1995

7–12

Purpose.—For patients with gastric cancer, intraoperative radiotherapy (IORT) may lead to more effective control of local disease and, thus, to better survival. The results of IORT for gastric cancer were compared with those of surgery alone.

Methods.—Histologic classification and survival analysis were performed for 94 of 115 patients with gastric cancer who were treated by IORT. The controls were 127 patients who were treated by operation alone during the same period, who also underwent histologic classification. Survival was compared in the 2 groups. Survival between groups was also compared according to the presence or absence of serosal invasion and the grade of lymph node metastasis. This analysis included 57 patients in the IORT group and 171 controls.

Results.—There was no difference in survival for patients with stage I disease. For those with more advanced gastric cancer, 5-year survival increased by 10% to 20% in the IORT group (Fig 1). For patients with lymph node metastases within the N1 group or without serosal invasion, IORT carried no survival advantage, However, IORT was associated with

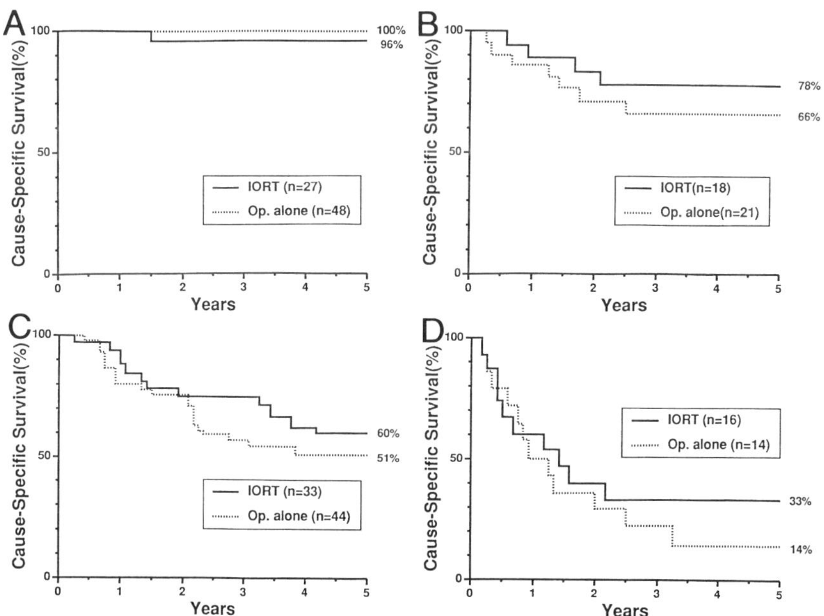

FIGURE 1.—Cause-specific survival curves of patients with gastric cancer treated by intraoperative radiation therapy (*IORT*) or by operation alone (*Op. alone*). **A,** survival rates with stage I gastric cancer. **B,** survival rates of stage II gastric cancer. **C,** survival rates with stage III gastric cancer. **D,** survival rates with stage IV gastric cancer. (Courtesy of Abe M, Nishimura Y, Shibamoto Y: Intraoperative radiation therapy for gastric cancer. *World J Surg* 19:554–557, Copyright 1995, Springer-Verlag.)

a 10% increase in 5-year survival for patients with serosal invasion and an 18% increase for those with N2 and N3 lymph node metastases.

Conclusions.—Intraoperative radiation therapy improves survival for some patients with gastric cancer, namely those with stage II–IV disease, those with serosal invasion, and those with N2 or N3 lymph node metastases. There were few significant complications of IORT.

▶ Abe and colleagues in Kyoto, Japan, have pioneered the use of intraoperative electron beam radiation therapy for the treatment of gastric and other cancers. Dr. Abe's work has led to the installation of intraoperative radiation therapy units in more than 20 centers in Japan. The comparison group in this report represents a concurrent group that underwent surgery at the same institution and in the same time frame but who did not receive intraoperative radiation based on the day of the scheduled operation.

The update from this seminal series suggests a small reduction in cancer-related mortality at 5 years. Although the authors consider this to be a positive trial, it is my perspective that benefits are minimal and are not justified by the expense and inconvenience of this complex combined-modality therapy strategy. It should be stressed that the intraoperative radiation dose was not given as a radiation boost, the strategy usually used in the United States for intraoperative radiation but, rather, represented a single dose of 28 Gy after a complete resection. Pattern-of-failure studies in gastric cancer would suggest that isolated retroperitoneal recurrence is unusual in gastric cancer, and it is still possible that intraoperative radiation therapy combined with an effective adjuvant chemotherapy strategy may impact long-term survival.

A.M. Cohen, M.D.

Long-Term Survival After Photodynamic Therapy for Esophageal Cancer

Sibille A, Lambert R, Souquet J-C, Sabben G, Descos F (Edouard Herriot Hosp, Lyon, France)
Gastroenterology 108:337–344, 1995

7–13

Background.—Several reports have described the use of photodynamic therapy (PDT) to destroy superficial esophageal and gastric cancers. However, because most reported series have been small and have had short follow-up, the efficacy of PDT remains unproven. The long-term results of using PDT in the treatment of small esophageal tumors in 123 patients were reviewed.

Methods.—The patients were treated from 1983 to 1991 on a PDT-based nonsurgical therapeutic protocol. The mean patient age was 66 years. One hundred four had squamous cell carcinoma, and 19 had adenocarcinoma. The tumors ranged in diameter from 0.5 to 4 cm and did not extend past the muscular layer or invade the adjacent organs. Eighty-eight more recent patients underwent endoscopic ultrasonography; staging was uT1 in 61 patients and uT2 in 27. The patients were injected with a hematoporphyrin derivative 72 hours before laser irradiation, which was delivered with a 630-nm dye laser. Fifty-six patients received PDT alone, including all of those with adenocarcinoma. The remaining 67 patients received other modes of therapy as well, i.e., radiotherapy or chemotherapy. Disease-specific survival was calculated by omitting patients who died of intercurrent disease that was unrelated to the esophageal tumor or its treatment.

Results.—Complete response rate at 6 months was 87%, although 36% of these patients had a local recurrence 12–18 months later. If detected at a superficial stage, the recurrent tumors responded to additional PDT. There was no significant difference in response rates for patients with squamous cell carcinoma versus adenocarcinoma, and additional modes of treatment had no apparent benefit. Overall actuarial 5-year survival was only 25%, but disease-specific survival was 74%. Relative 5-year survival was 95% for patients with uT1, N0 squamous cell cancers. Complications included nonsevere cutaneous photosensitization in 16 patients and esophageal stenosis requiring dilation in 43.

Conclusions.—Photodynamic therapy achieves effective local destruction of small flat or sessile esophageal tumors. The complete response rate and disease-specific survival are good. For patients with esophageal cancer who are not good candidates for surgery—particularly those with uT1, NO tumors—PDT may be a reasonable treatment alternative.

▶ Photodynamic therapy shows promise as an endoscopic treatment for pulmonary, urologic, and gynecologic tumors. Its use in the treatment of esophageal cancer has been similar to the use of Nd:YAG laser ablation as palliative treatment of locally advanced esophageal cancer with dysphagia. The authors report on the use of PDT as a potentially curative strategy for early esophageal cancer. In their very large experience of 123 patients, a complete response was obtained in 87% of the patients, although 36% of these patients subsequently had a recurrence. However, the actuarial survival in ultrasound stage T1 and T2 cancers indicated 5-year survival in one third of patients. Actuarial 5-year disease of specific survival occurred in more than three quarters of the patients. The side effects were minimal, although the patients had to avoid direct exposure to the sun for one month. The data suggest that PDT offers, with little risk, acceptable palliation and a cure for early cancer of the esophagus and appears to be an excellent alternative for patients who are medically unfit or unwilling to undergo esophagectomy.

A.M. Cohen, M.D.

Total Mesorectal Excision and Local Recurrence: A Study of Tumour Spread in the Mesorectum Distal to Rectal Cancer

Scott N, Jackson P, Al-Jaberi T, Dixon MF, Quirke P, Finan PJ (Centre for Digestive Diseases, The Gen Infirmary Leeds, England; United Leeds Teaching Hosps NHS Trust, Leeds, England)
Br J Surg 82:1031–1033, 1995   7–14

Background.—Evidence suggests that total mesorectal excision (TME) is associated with a decreased postoperative local recurrence rate in patients with rectal cancer. The frequency with which tumor can be found in mesorectum removed during TME was investigated, with special emphasis on mesorectal tissue below the tumor.

Methods and Findings.—Total mesorectal excision was performed in 20 patients with rectal cancer. Adenocarcinoma was discovered in the distal mesorectum in 4. Distal mesorectal spread commonly extended further than intramural spread. Carcinoma was detected at 1 and 3 cm distal to the main tumor mass in the 2 cases in which the lateral margin was clear but the distal mesorectum was not. At 4 years, the outcomes of patients with tumor in the distal mesorectum were worse. These patients had a greater risk of local recurrence and an increased frequency of distant metastasis.

Conclusions.—Distal tumor spread indicates poor prognosis in patients with rectal cancer. Incomplete excision of the mesorectum appears to contribute to local recurrence in some patients with rectal cancer, especially in those with tumors in the middle and lower third of the rectum.

▶ Total mesorectal excision has been championed by Heald and colleagues to maximize the lateral margins and also because of concerns about tumor distally within the mesorectum. This report addresses the latter point specifically. The data confirm that distal mesorectal spread, either in the lymph nodes, the lymphatics, or in the mesorectal nodules, does occur, although it usually is limited to within 3 cm of the gross luminal tumor. In operations for midrectal cancer, total mesorectal excision will be required to obtain a 3-cm mesorectal margin. These data support the importance of making a sharp-scissor or cautery dissection along the bony pelvis in patients with midrectal cancer and of avoiding shaving the distal mesorectum before placing a linear staple line across the rectum for a double-staple technique reconstruction, which is the most common operative approach at this time.

A.M. Cohen, M.D.

The Stockholm I Trial of Preoperative Short Term Radiotherapy in Operable Rectal Carcinoma: A Prospective Randomized Trial
Wilking N, for the Stockholm Colorectal Cancer Study Group (Karolinska Hosp, Stockholm)
Cancer 75:2269–2275, 1995   7–15

Introduction.—Even with "curative" resection, the 5-year survival rate for patients with rectal carcinoma is only about 50%. Many patients die solely as a result of uncontrolled locoregional disease. Randomized trials of adjuvant radiotherapy for patients with rectal cancer have yielded conflicting results. The final results of a randomized, multicenter trial of short-term preoperative radiotherapy for rectal cancer were evaluated.

Methods.—Eight hundred forty-nine patients with clinically resectable rectal adenocarcinoma were enrolled in the trial from 1980 to 1987. The patients were randomized to receive preoperative radiotherapy—25 Gy during the 5–7 days before surgery—or surgery alone. The study assessed the effects of preoperative radiotherapy on pelvic recurrence and whether improved local control increased survival.

Results.—The disease-free interval was longer in the preoperative irradiation group, largely because of a lower incidence of local recurrence. Six hundred eighty-four patients underwent "curative" operation. At a median follow-up of 107 months, the incidence of pelvic recurrence was significantly lower in curatively operated patients who also received preoperative radiotherapy. This was so for patients in all Dukes' stages. The treatment groups were similar in terms of frequency of distant metastases and overall survival, but time to local recurrence or distant metastases was significantly longer in the patients who received irradiation. The postoperative mortality rate was significantly higher in patients who received radiotherapy vs. those who had surgery only (8% vs. 2%).

Conclusion.—For patients with rectal cancer, preoperative short-term radiotherapy decreases the incidence of pelvic recurrence compared with surgery alone. Disease-free and overall survival are improved with preoperative irradiation among patients who undergo curative surgery. However, preoperative irradiation is associated with higher postoperative morbidity.

▶ This Scandinavian study has a large number of patients with excellent follow-up. The authors demonstrate that patients who receive 2,500 rad over 5–7 days preoperatively have a far lower likelihood of pelvic recurrence of rectal cancer than do patients who go directly to surgery. The results appear to be significant for all stages of the disease. Despite this improvement in the rate of recurrence of pelvic cancer, there was no significant improvement in overall survival.

This appears to have been a well-constructed study that has a positive result in terms of recurrence rates of pelvic cancer. In my own opinion, if the authors would just address their attention to the problem of recurrent lesions in the pelvis associated with major pain syndromes, they could probably make a stronger case. Every surgeon has had experience with some patients who have local recurrence with a tremendous pain syndrome that is virtually impossible to control. It is my opinion that preoperative or postoperative radiation has a high likelihood of preventing that particular problem from occurring. If that could be documented, the case for combined-modality treatment would be much stronger, even if it did not add a day to survival. Every physician who has ever had the misfortune of dealing with that particular pain syndrome knows exactly what I am talking about.

E. Glatstein, M.D.

Preoperative Infusional Chemoradiation Therapy for Stage T3 Rectal Cancer

Rich TA, Skibber JM, Ajani JA, Buchholz DJ, Cleary KR, Dubrow RA, Levin B, Lynch PM, Meterissian SH, Roubein LD, Ota DM (MD Anderson Cancer Ctr, Houston)

Int J Radiat Oncol Biol Phys 32:1025–1029, 1995   7–16

Background.—At the University of Texas M.D. Anderson Cancer Center, patients with operable rectal cancer have been treated with conservation surgery and postoperative adjuvant irradiation with or without chemotherapy since 1986. Patients with lesions greater than 3 cm and those with tumors extending beyond the bowel wall were found to have a high risk of local disease recurrence after local excision with or without adjuvant radiation therapy. Preoperative therapy was considered for patients undergoing local excision and postoperative irradiation was considered for stage T3 disease, because local disease recurred in 25% of patients. The results of preoperative infusional 5-fluorouracil (5-FU) chemoradiation therapy were reported.

Methods.—Seventy-seven patients with stage T3 rectal cancer were treated with preoperative infusions of 5-FU, 300 mg/m^2/day, plus daily radiation therapy, 45 Gy/25 fractions/5 weeks. Surgery was done about 6 weeks after chemoradiation therapy was completed. Twenty-five abdominoperineal resections and 52 anal sphincter–preserving procedures were performed. The median follow-up was 27 months.

Findings.—After treatment, tumor stages were T1–2, N0 in 35%; T3, N0 in 25%; and T1–3, N1 in 11%. Twenty-nine percent of the patients had no evidence of disease. Ninety-six percent had local tumor control after chemoradiation. Two patients had recurrent disease at the site of anastomosis, which was successfully treated with abdominoperineal resection. Overall, 99% of the patients achieved pelvic control. Patients without node involvement had greater survival rates after chemoradiation than did patients with node involvement. A greater number of patients with complete responses or microscopic foci only on pathologic assessment survived than did patients with gross residual tumor. The 3-year actuarial survival rate was 83%. Patients undergoing chemoradiation treatment did not have more acute, perioperative, or late complications than those treated with traditional radiation therapy alone.

Conclusion.—Excellent treatment responses enabled anal sphincter–sparing procedures to be performed in two thirds of these patients. The presence of gross residual disease in the resected specimen indicates a poor prognosis. Treatment that specifically targets these patients may further improve survival rates.

▶ Data from randomized clinical trials using postoperative chemoradiation therapy for rectal cancer demonstrated the benefit of infusions of 5-FU as an adjunct to the radiation therapy. These authors have used this strategy preoperatively in patients with resectable, but transmural, rectal cancer. A very impressive complete pathologic remission rate of 29% was obtained with a modest amount of nausea and diarrhea. A comparison was done of the continuous infusional 5-FU regimen vs. the bolus 5-FU/leucovorin program.[1] Chemoradiation therapy protocols will be important.

A.M. Cohen, M.D.

Reference

1. Minsky BD: Preoperative combined modality treatment for rectal cancer. *Oncology* 8:53–58, 1994.

Preoperative Infusional Chemoradiation and Surgery With or Without an Electron Beam Intraoperative Boost for Advanced Primary Rectal Cancer

Weinstein GD, Rich TA, Shumate CR, Skibber JM, Cleary KR, Ajani JA, Ota DM (MD Anderson Cancer Ctr, Houston)
Int J Radiat Oncol Biol Phys 32:197–204, 1995

7–17

Objective.—In patients with advanced rectal cancers that are tethered or fixed to the pelvic viscera or bones, pelvic tumor recurrence after surgery is correlated with the amount of residual disease. High-dose preoperative radiotherapy (preopXRT) has yielded resectability rates of up to 100% and local control rates of up to 84%. A new preoperative approach—protracted continuous-infusion chemotherapy given during the entire course of irradiation (preop-chemoXRT)—was evaluated in a pilot study.

Methods.—A total of 38 patients with tethered T3 or T4 primary rectal cancer were studied. All received 45 Gy of radiation given in 25 fractions over 5 weeks, plus infusional chemotherapy with cisplatin, 5-fluorouracil, or both. Surgical resection was performed in 37 patients; 13 had restorative surgery, whereas the rest had abdominoperineal resection or pelvic exenteration. In 11 patients with adherent pelvic tumors, electron beam intraoperative radiotherapy (EB-IORT), 10–20 Gy, was given as well. The results were compared with those in 36 historical control patients who had received preop-XRT. The radiation dose in this group was 45 Gy, and 93% had abdominoperineal resection or pelvic exenteration.

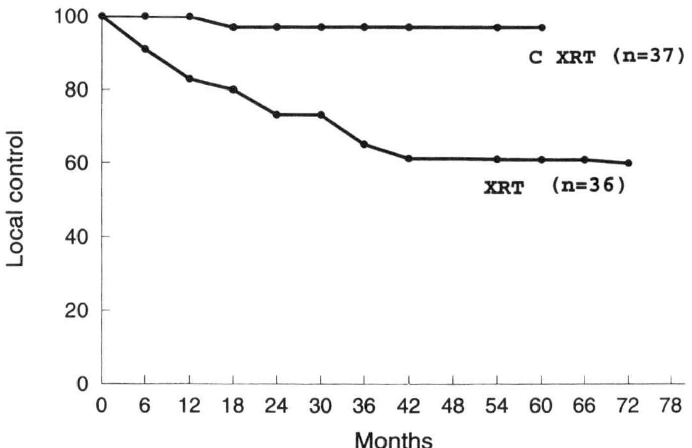

FIGURE 1.—Actuarial local control rates for preoperative chemoradiotherapy (*C XRT*) vs. preoperative radiotherapy (*XRT*, historical control group). The numbers of patients followed at each annual interval are shown. (Reprinted from *Int J Radiat Oncol Biol*, Vol. 32, Weinstein GD, Rich TA, Shurnate CR, et al: Preoperative infusional chemoradiation and surgery with or without an electron beam intraoperative boost for advanced primary rectal cancer, pp 197–204, Copyright 1995, with kind permission from Elsevier Science Ltd, The Boulevard, Langford Lane, Kidlington 0X5 1GB, UK.)

Results.—Patients treated with preop-chemoXRT had a local recurrence rate of only 3% compared with 33% for those treated with preopXRT (Fig 1). The 3-year survival rate was 82% with preop-chemoXRT plus resection, vs. 62% for the historical controls (Fig 2). Sixty-four percent of the

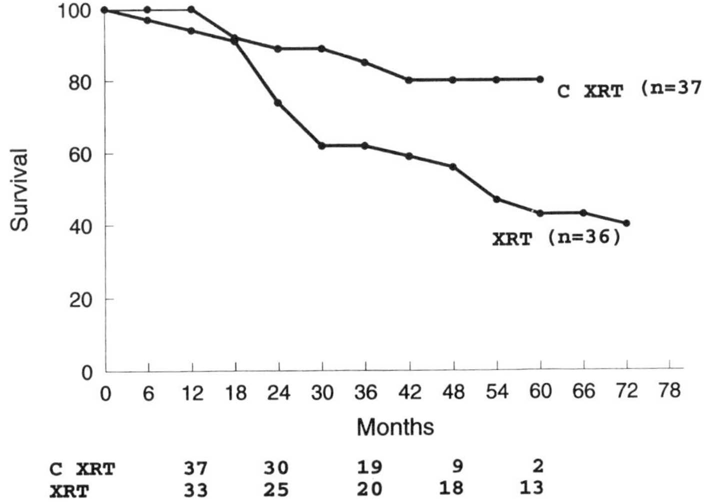

FIGURE 2.—Actuarial survival rates for preoperative chemoradiotherapy (*C XRT*) vs. preoperative radiotherapy (*XRT*). (Reprinted from *Int J Radiat Oncol Biol*, Vol. 32, Weinstein GD, Rich TA, Shurnate CR, et al: Preoperative infusional chemoradiation and surgery with or without an electron beam intraoperative boost for advanced primary rectal cancer, pp 197–204, Copyright 1995, with kind permission from Elsevier Science Ltd, The Boulevard, Langford Lane, Kidlington 0X5 1GB, UK.)

patients receiving EB-IORT had distant metastases compared with 19% of those who did not receive an intraoperative boost. The overall 3-year survival rate was 67% vs. 96% without EB-IORT. The preop-chemoXRT had acceptable acute and late toxicity.

Conclusion.—For patients with advanced primary rectal cancer, preop-chemoXRT offers important advantages over preopXRT alone. Control of pelvic disease and overall survival rates are better with preop-chemoXRT. Acute chemoradiation toxicity is increased, but late morbidity is unchanged. For patients with residual or clinically adherent disease, EB-IORT improves local control. However, survival is worse in these patients than in those who do not receive EB-IORT.

▶ This paper from the M.D. Anderson Cancer Center evaluates 37 patients with primary rectal carcinoma who underwent preopXRT to the pelvis with concomitant infusional chemotherapy, with or without an electron beam boost intraoperatively. The authors results, in terms of recurrence rates, were excellent and were compared with those in historical controls. The authors conclude that their treatment plan results in better local control of pelvic disease and better survival than preoperative therapy alone. The problem is that the patients for these studies came from different eras, and the follow-up on the historical controls is much longer. Thus, there are no late failures waiting to develop in the control population, whereas the follow-up of the experimental group is still short by comparison.

The simple truth is that there is no way to prove that this treatment is of major benefit without going through a randomized, prospective trial. Also, although I wish to believe that the intraoperative boost would add something, I cannot believe it until someone performs the prospectively randomized phase III study. Until that time, there are too many questions regarding selection that make interpreting these excellent results difficult. I hope that someone who has the capability is willing to perform that study soon. Then this issue can be put to rest one way or another.

E. Glatstein, M.D.

The Long-Term Effect of Adjuvant Postoperative Chemoradiotherapy for Rectal Carcinoma on Bowel Function

Kollmorgen CF, Meagher AP, Wolff BG, Pemberton JH, Martenson JA, Ilstrup DM (Mayo Clinic, Rochester, Minn)
Ann Surg 220:676–682, 1994   7–18

Background.—Adjuvant postoperative radiation therapy, frequently combined with chemotherapy, is increasingly being used in patients with rectal carcinoma. However, its long-term effects on bowel function have not been assessed.

Methods.—The medical records of patients undergoing anterior resection for rectal carcinoma in the preceding 2–5 years were reviewed. During this period, postoperative radiation therapy with chemotherapy was generally administered to patients with Astler-Coller stage B2 or C tumors but

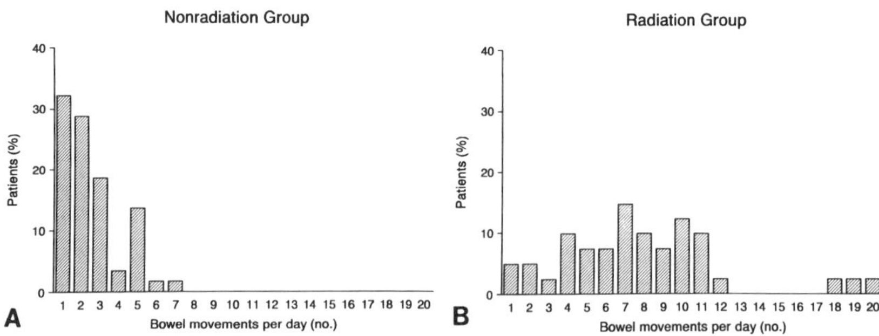

FIGURE 1.—Histograms comparing the number of bowel movements per day in the nonradiation and radiation groups. (Courtesy of Kollmorgen CF, Meagher AP, Wolff BG, et al: *Ann Surg* 220:676–682, 1994.)

not to those with earlier stage tumors. Extensive exclusion criteria were applied to minimize the possible confounding factors that may have been more common in the group receiving chemotherapy and that may affect bowel function. Forty-one patients who had postoperative chemoradiotherapy and 59 who did not were eligible. The groups were comparable in the ratio of males to females, the level of anastomosis, and the length of follow-up.

Findings.—Patients undergoing chemoradiotherapy had more bowel movements per day than those who did not have this adjuvant treatment. The median numbers were 7 and 2, respectively (Fig 1). The former group had bowel movement "clustering" more often, with those reports being 42% and 3%, respectively. Patients undergoing chemoradiotherapy also had more frequent nighttime bowel movements and were unable to defer defecation for more than 15 minutes more often; These respective findings were 46% vs. 14%, and 78% vs. 19%.

Conclusions.—Postoperative chemoradiotherapy has a major detrimental effect on long-term bowel function. Although the study was not prospective and randomized, it is unlikely that confounding variables were responsible for the substantially different results of the two groups.

▶ Multiple prospective randomized clinical trials have demonstrated the efficacy of postoperative chemoradiation therapy in the treatment of transmural and/or node-positive rectal cancer. The standard outcomes in such studies are local control and overall survival. Analyses and toxicity are focused on the acute effects of and patient tolerance to either postoperative radiation therapy alone or combined chemoradiation therapy. A multivariate analysis of the long-term functional results after coloanal anastomosis for rectal cancer, reported from the Memorial Sloan-Kettering Cancer Center, suggested that postoperative radiation therapy had a major adverse impact on late bowel function.

Dr. Kollmorgen and his associates at the Mayo Clinic have provided us with the best confirmatory data indicating a dramatic negative effect of postoperative chemoradiotherapy on bowel function. Appropriately, the authors waited a minimum of two years before auditing functional results, because it can take at least one year for acute toxicity to resolve. Not only did the median bowel movements increase by a factor of 3, but almost half of the patients in the chemoradiation group had clustering bowel movements and/or nighttime bowel movements, all of which significantly impact on the quality of life. What the study did not address is the potential adverse effects of such treatment on sexual function.

The mechanism of bowel dysfunction is unclear but is primarily related to loss of compliance of the neorectum. There may be some component of nerve damage as well. Anecdotal data with the use of preoperative radiation or chemoradiation suggest that functional loss is much less noticeable. This randomized, multicenter trial comparing preoperative chemoradiation with postoperative chemoradiation therapy is assessing not only the efficacy of cancer treatment but, also, the acute and long-term functional outcomes, as outlined in this paper.

A.M. Cohen, M.D.

Reference

1. Paty PB, Enker WE, Cohen AM, et al: Long-term functional results of coloanal anastomosis for rectal cancer. *Am J Surg* 167:90, 1994.

Adjuvant Preoperative Radiotherapy for Locally Advanced Rectal Carcinoma
Marsh PJ, James RD, Schofield PF (Christie Hosp Natl Health Service Trust, Manchester, England)
Dis Colon Rectum 37:1205–1214, 1994   7–19

Background.—Previous reports have suggested that adjuvant preoperative radiotherapy does not improve overall 5-year survival for patients with rectal carcinoma. However, these studies have used differing patient selection criteria, radiotherapy schedules and fields, and end points. Radiotherapy field extent may be especially important in terms of local recurrence. The results of adjuvant preoperative chemotherapy in patients with locally advanced rectal carcinoma were evaluated after a prospective, randomized trial.

Methods.—The study sample comprised 284 patients with tethered or fixed but operable carcinomas of the true rectum. Patients were randomized to receive either radiotherapy followed one week later by surgery, or surgery alone. The radiotherapy group received a 20-Gy dose of irradiation, in 4 daily fractions, to a $10 \times 10 \times 10$-cm volume in the posterior pelvis, centered on the tumor. All patients were followed up for at least 96 months.

Results.—The 2 groups had equal distribution of clinicopathologic variables. Preoperative radiotherapy had no marked effects in downstaging the irradiated tumors. The overall mortality was 70% in both groups; mortality related to rectal cancer was also similar, 66% with surgery alone and 61% with preoperative irradiation and surgery. Among patients who

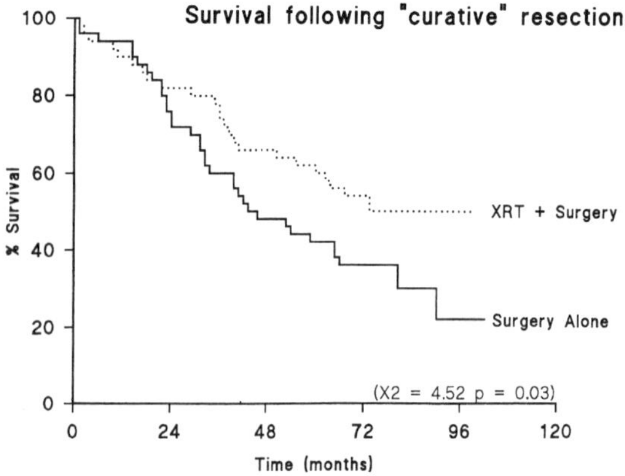

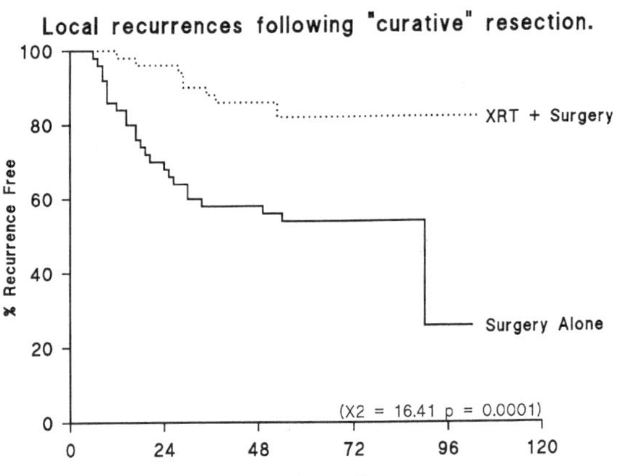

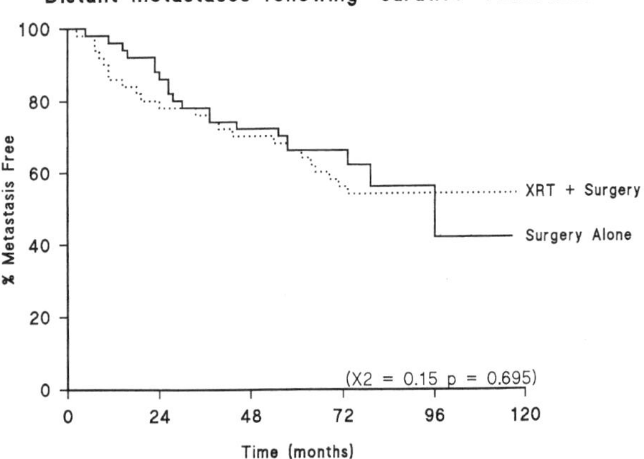

FIGURE 3.—Overall survival local recurrence-free, and metastasis-free survival curves for patients undergoing curative surgery in the Northwest of England Rectal Cancer Trial. *Abbreviation: XRT*, x-ray therapy. (Courtesy of Marsh PJ, James RD, Schofield PF: Adjuvant preoperative radiotherapy for locally advanced rectal carcinoma. *Dis Colon Rectum* 37:1205–1214, 1994.)

underwent curative surgery, patients assigned to preoperative radiotherapy had a significant reduction in mortality, 45% vs. 53%. The irradiated group had a highly significant reduction in local recurrence rate: 13% compared with 37% in the surgery group (Fig 3). Of 16 local recurrences in patients who received adequate radiotherapy, 10 occurred inside the radiotherapy field and 6 occurred outside the field. There were no significant differences in the rates of distant metastases.

Conclusions.—In patients with locally advanced rectal cancer, preoperative radiotherapy is associated with a highly significant reduction in the local recurrence rate. This form of adjuvant radiotherapy has no significant overall survival benefit, but it does for patients considered by the surgeon to have had a curative operation. The authors offer adjuvant preoperative radiotherapy to all patients with locally advanced rectal cancer who are scheduled to undergo radical surgery.

▶ This large randomized prospective clinical trial of a single-modality preoperative radiation therapy adds additional supporting data with regard to the efficacy of such treatments in reducing the risk of local recurrence. Although only representing a total of 2,000 cGy, the large fraction size (500 rads per fraction compared with 180–200 rads in "standard" fractionation) produces a reasonably high biological dose. The patient population was selected to be at high risk for local recurrence represented by clinical examination indicating either tethered or fixed cancers. Intrarectal ultrasound or scanning techniques were not used for patient selection.

As with all other studies using radiation therapy alone as the adjuvant modality, there is no impact on the overall 5-year survival rate. However, maximizing local control is a very important end point in the treatment of patients with rectal cancer, because uncontrolled local recurrence produces a highly morbid and poorly treated system complex.

There are considerable data that indicate that *postoperative* combined modality therapy with chemotherapy and radiation not only improves local control but increases the overall survival. Preliminary data with *preoperative* combined-modality therapy suggest even better local control and overall survival. An ongoing multicenter trial in North America, RTOG 94-01, will be comparing the preoperative vs. the postoperative efficacy of combined-modality therapy in terms of local control, functional outcome, and overall survival.

A.M. Cohen, M.D.

Reference

1. Minsky BD, et al: Preoperative 5-FU, low dose leucovorin and concurrent radiation therapy for rectal cancer. *Cancer* 73:273, 1994.

Intraoperative Irradiation After Palliative Surgery for Locally Recurrent Rectal Cancer

Suzuki K, Gunderson LL, Devine RM, Weaver AL, Dozois RR, Ilstrup DM, Martenson JA, O'Connell MJ (Mayo Clinic and Found, Rochester, Minn)
Cancer 75:939–952, 1995　　　　　　　　　　　　　　　　　　　　7–20

Introduction.—Surgery alone, or any other single treatment modality, is not likely to result in long-term disease control and survival for patients with locally recurrent rectal cancer. Previous reports have described the use of brachytherapy and intraoperative irradiation (IORT) combined with tolerable doses of external-beam irradiation (EBRT) in an attempt to minimize damage to normal tissues while safely increasing the total radiation dose to the tumor volume. The results of palliative reoperation for locally recurrent rectal cancer were reviewed, focusing on the roles of surgery, EBRT, IORT, and brachytherapy, alone or in combination.

Methods.—The analysis included 106 patients with proved locally recurrent rectal cancer who were treated with palliative resection from 1981 to 1988. None had signs of extrapelvic disease. Treatment included IORT in 42 patients. After maximal resection, 34 of the 42 patients who received IORT had gross residual disease, as did 61 of 64 patients who did not receive IORT. The dose of IORT was 15–20 Gy in 39 patients, and it was somewhat lower or higher in the other 3. Forty-one of those 42 patients received EBRT; the dose was 45 Gy or greater in 38 patients. Three- and 5-year survival rates were estimated by the Kaplan-Meier method.

Results.—For 12 patients receiving palliative resection alone, survival was 8% at 3 years and 0% at 5 years. On univariate analysis of all patients, the factors significantly affecting survival included microscopic vs. gross residual tumor, treatment method, IORT vs. no IORT, type of symptoms, type of fixation, and preoperative Eastern Cooperative Oncology Group status. With IORT, the 3-year survival rate was 44% for patients with gross residual tumor and 43% for those with pain at presentation. Extended vs. conventional resection, grade, age, and sex were not associated with survival on univariate analysis. At 3 years, the cumulative probability of distant metastasis was 60% in patients who received IORT and 54% in those who did not. The 3-year local relapse rates were 40% and 93%, respectively.

Conclusion.—For patients with locally recurrent rectal cancer, adding IORT to external irradiation and maximal surgical resection may improve local tumor control and survival. However, further treatment gains are needed. Rates of distant metastasis remain high; therefore, aggressive treatment should include more routine systemic therapy with 5-fluorouracil, leucovorin, and/or 5-fluorouracil levamisole. Even with IORT, patients with gross residual tumor after maximal resection have inadequate local tumor control. Studies to evaluate the use of radiation sensitizers or biological modifiers during external irradiation and IORT are recommended.

▶ The reader can either be encouraged or discouraged by this report from the Mayo Clinic. The addition of IORT in the multimodality treatment of patients with locally recurrent rectal cancer appears to improve local control and survival. However, despite this complicated, expensive, and morbid treatment approach, the local failure rate remained 40% and only 7 patients were alive without evidence of disease after a minimum follow-up of slightly more than 2½ years. The overall actuarial 5-year survival rate was less than 20%. The patterns of failure indicate that the majority of these patients ultimately have disseminated disease develop, despite initial recurrence limited to the pelvis.

Although this report suggests some improvement in local control and survival, further improvement will require even more complex multimodality therapy. The authors use intraoperative EBRT. In the presence of multifocal pelvic recurrence, a broader treatment field may be necessary, perhaps through high-dose-rate intraoperative brachytherapy strategies. The use of radiosensitizers such as infusional 5-fluorouracil may improve results. Most important, improved systemic "adjuvant" therapy will be necessary if this aggressive locoregional strategy is to be translated to include a greater 5-year survival.

A.M. Cohen, M.D.

Adenocarcinoma of the Rectum Treated by Radical External Radiation Therapy
Brierley JD, Cummings BJ, Wong CS, Keane TJ, O'Sullivan B, Catton CN, Goodman P (Princess Margaret Hosp, Toronto)
Int J Radiat Oncol Biol Phys 31:255–259, 1995   7–21

Background.—The overall 5-year survival rate for patients with rectal cancer who have an apparently complete resection has been reported to be 45% to 50%. However, not all patients are candidates for such resection. Treatment with radical external-beam radiation therapy has been described, suggesting a possible role for radiation therapy in patients who are not surgical candidates. The outcomes of 229 patients receiving primary radical external-beam radiotherapy for adenocarcinoma of the rectum were reviewed.

Methods.—The patients were treated at 1 center between 1978 and 1987. The patients were considered to have unresectable tumors, were medically unfit, and/or refused surgery. The dose range was 40 Gy given in 10 fractions by a split course during a 6-week period, to 60 Gy in 30 fractions in 6 weeks. Most commonly prescribed was a 52-Gy target absorbed dose given in 20 daily fractions over 4 weeks.

Findings.—Overall, the 5-year actuarial survival rate was 27%. This rate was 48% in patients with mobile tumors, 27% in those with partially fixed tumors, and 4% in patients with fixed tumors. Clinically complete tumor regression after radiation was achieved in 50% of the patients with mobile tumors, 30% of those with partially fixed tumors, and 9% of those

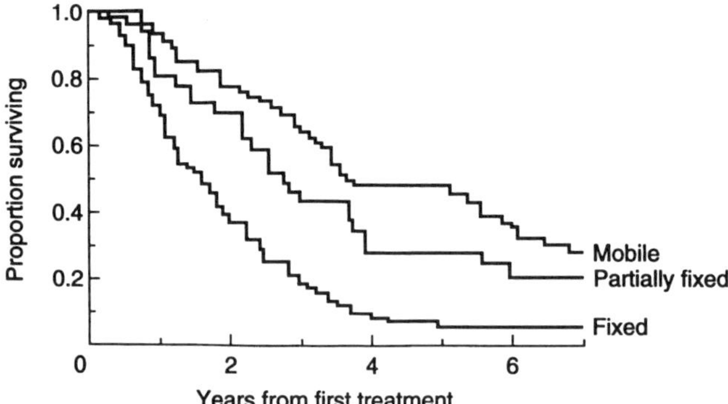

FIGURE 2.—Actuarial survival for 97 patients with mobile tumor, 37 with partially fixed, and 77 with fixed tumor. (Reprinted from *Int J Radiat Oncol Biol*, Vol. 31, Brierley JD, Cummings BJ, Wong CS, et al: Adenocarcinoma of the rectum treated by radical external radiation therapy, pp 255–259, Copyright 1995, with kind permission from Elsevier Science Ltd, The Boulevard, Langford Lane, Kidlington 0X5 1GB, UK.)

with fixed tumors. Local relapse later occurred in 18, 6, and 5 patients in these 3 groups, respectively. Fifty patients underwent salvage surgery after failing to attain complete remission or for local relapse. The 5-year actuarial survival rate from time of surgery among these patients was 42% (Figs 2 and 3).

Conclusion.—Radiation therapy can cure some patients with mobile or partially fixed rectal adenocarcinomas who are unsuitable for or refuse surgery. However, local control continues to be a problem. Salvage surgery may be necessary in patients who relapse or fail to achieve complete remission and who are fit for surgery. High-dose external-beam radiation should be a part of the planned preoperative regimen or should be palliative in patients with fixed rectal cancers.

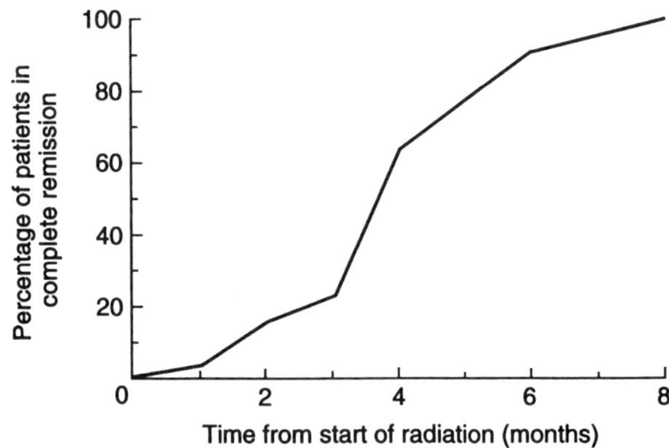

FIGURE 3.—Time to remission from the start of radiation for 66 patients, assessed clinically as having responded completely. (Reprinted from *Int J Radiat Oncol Biol*, Vol. 31, Brierley JD, Cummings BJ, Wong CS, et al: Adenocarcinoma of the rectum treated by radical external radiation therapy, pp 255–259, Copyright 1995, with kind permission from Elsevier Science Ltd, The Boulevard, Langford Lane, Kidlington 0X5 1GB, UK.)

▶ This very large experience (under the direction of Dr. Bernard Cummings) from the Princess Margaret Hospital is very important. The data represent a baseline with regard to what can be obtained in the treatment of primary cancer of the rectum by external-beam radiation therapy as a single modality for patients who did not undergo surgery because they were thought to represent an unacceptable risk either because of co-morbid medical conditions or because they had refused abdominoperineal resection. Although long-term survival is quite rare with fixed cancers, patients with mobile or partially fixed tumors fared remarkably well. One wonders whether results could have been improved further by combining external-beam radiation therapy with either intracavitary contact radiation or with a radiation implant.

The most important information provided in this study is the very slow regression of the tumor, as demonstrated in Figure 3. In patients who obtained complete remission, this rarely occurred within the first 3 months and, in general, it took between 4 and 6 months to completely regress. This important information should be applied to the use of preoperative radiation therapy for resectable rectal cancer, for which we have traditionally proceeded with an operation 4–6 weeks after the completion of radiation therapy. Although the surgical community is concerned about increasing fibrosis complicating the operation, continued delay of an operation by 6–8 weeks—or even longer—may be ultimately advantageous with regard to maximizing tumor regression.

A.M. Cohen, M.D.

Coloanal Anastomosis for Rectal Cancer: Long-Term Results at the Mayo and Cleveland Clinics
Cavaliere F, Pemberton JH, Cosimelli M, Fazio VW, Beart RW Jr (Mayo Clinic and Found, Rochester, Minn; Regina Elena Cancer Inst, Rome, Italy; Cleveland Clinic, Ohio; et al)
Dis Colon Rectum 38:807–812, 1995   7–22

Background.—In a previous report of 29 patients with rectal cancer, coloanal anastomosis was associated with acceptable mortality, morbidity, and survival, and adequate function. In a recent study, the short- and long-term complication rates, incidence of relapse, survival, and functional results of coloanal anastomosis were evaluated in a larger patient population.

Patients.—One hundred seventeen patients with rectal cancer who underwent coloanal anastomosis during a 10-year period were included. The median patient age was 59 years. A straight coloanal anastomosis was performed in the majority of patients, whereas 15% had a J-pouch. There were no diverting stomas in 38% of the patients. Endoscopic examination showed that the median distance from the anal verge to the lower edge of the tumor was 6.7 cm. Tumors were noted in the lower third of the rectum in 64% of the patients.

Results.—None of the patients died within 30 days after surgery. Early or late major or minor complications were experienced by 62%. Eighteen percent of the patients had anastomotic leakage, 21% had strictures, 15% had temporary urinary retention, and 14% experienced sexual dysfunction. A temporary stoma was required in 6 patients as a result of septic complications. Seventy-eight percent of the patients had satisfactory fecal continence. Frequent incontinence was not observed in any of the patients who had a J-pouch. Among individuals with a tumor of the lower third of the rectum, 79% had local recurrence and 16% had distant relapse. Median survival after relapse was 11 months. The 5-year disease-free actuarial survival was 69% for the entire patient population.

Conclusions.—Although the risks of complication after coloanal anastomosis are high, the long-term survival rates and functional outcomes are excellent. Coloanal anastomosis should therefore be considered a reasonable alternative to abdominoperineal resection.

▶ With increasing data indicating that the lateral, rather than the distal, margin is the most important determinant of local failure in the treatment of rectal cancer, it is clear that the treatment of patients with rectal cancer palpable on rectal examination does not always require an abdominal perineal resection. The widespread availability of intraluminal stapling devices combined with the "double-staple" technique allows for low colorectal anastomosis. However, for technical reasons, most commonly in a male with a large prostate, a per-anal approach, as originally described by Sir Alan Parks, has provided another technique for sphincter conservation. In such cases, a total proctectomy with upper anal mucosectomy and sutured anastomosis of the colon, either end-to-end or with a colon J-pouch with anastomosis to the dentale line, allows for a continent reconstruction.

In a combined report from the Mayo and Cleveland Clinics, excellent results were demonstrated with this approach used in selected patients. With a median follow-up of a little more than 4 years, only 7% of the patients have local regional recurrence with satisfactory functional results.

A.M. Cohen, M.D.

Response of Colon Cancer Cell Lines to the Introduction of *APC*, a Colon-Specific Tumor Suppressor Gene
Groden J, Joslyn G, Samowitz W, Jones D, Bhattacharyya N, Spirio L, Thliveris A, Robertson M, Egan S, Meuth M, White R (Univ of Utah, Salt Lake City; Whitehead Inst, Cambridge; Massachusetts Inst of Technology, Cambridge)
Cancer Res 55:1531–1539, 1995   7–23

Background.—Chromosome 5 inhibits the tumorigenicity of human colon carcinoma cell lines. Mutations in the tumor suppressor gene *APC* are responsible for adenomatous polyposis coli (*APC*), an inherited form of colon cancer.

Objective.—An attempt was made to obtain direct biological evidence that *APC* functions as a tumor suppressor and is responsible for the suppressive effects associated with transfer of the whole chromosome.

Methods.—A vector containing a full-length wild-type *APC* gene was introduced by transfection into 3 human colon carcinoma cell lines, each of which was characterized for mutations at the *APC* locus and for genomic instability.

Findings.—The response of each of the 3 cell lines to transfection by *APC* differed with the genotype of the particular cell line. Some of the cell clones derived from the transfected lines exhibited morphological alterations, including larger and flatter cells with relatively large, distinct nuclei. Micronuclei were frequently present, and many cells contained small granules or large vacuoles. Occasionally, numerous refractile vacuoles obscured the nucleus. In some instances, tumorigenicity was suppressed, as is evident from observations of cell growth in soft agar and of tumor formation in nude mice.

Conclusion.—These findings provide the first direct functional evidence that the *APC* gene may act as a tumor suppressor and may also have cytostatic and cytotoxic effects when overexpressed in colon cancer cell lines. Other observations suggest that *APC* helps maintain cell-cell interaction through adherens junctions.

▶ Many formidable obstacles remain before the use of gene therapy for solid tumors can be brought to clinical trial. However, colon cancer will be among the first solid tumors in which gene therapy will be evaluated based on elegant molecular studies, which have identified the role of many genes in the carcinogenesis and progression of colon cancer. The first step in identifying any potential candidate for gene therapy is to demonstrate that reintroduction of the gene into the malignant phenotype can, in appropriate model systems, reverse the manifestations of malignancy. It has already been demonstrated that inhibition of tumorigenicity by insertion of chromosome 5 can be achieved in human colon carcinoma cell lines.

Previous studies have suggested that the *APC* gene functions as a tumor suppressor in colon cancer cells. In this study, a wild-type *APC* gene was introduced by transfection into 3 human colon carcinoma cell lines, each of which had mutations at the *APC* locus. Two of the 3 cell lines could be stably transfected, and some of the cell clones derived from these transfections displayed altered morphologies and the suppression of tumorigenicity *in vitro* and in tumor formation in nude mice. The function of *APC* is, as yet, undetermined, although it has been postulated that it has a role in the maintenance of cell-cell interactions. This study suggests that APC may also have other unknown functions that control cell growth or cell death. Studies such as this one will be instrumental in the design of future gene therapies for colon cancer treatment.

R.F. Ozols, M.D., Ph.D.

Efficacy of Adjuvant Fluorouracil and Folinic Acid in Colon Cancer

Marsoni S, for the International Multicentre Pooled Analysis of Colon Cancer Trials (IMPACT) Investigators (Istituto Mario Negri, Milan, Italy)
Lancet 345:939–944, 1995

Background.—The role of adjuvant fluorouracil (FU) and folinic acid (FA) in the treatment of colon cancer is unclear. Three randomized trials were undertaken to determine the efficacy of FU and high-dose FA after surgery for Dukes' stage B and C colon cancer.

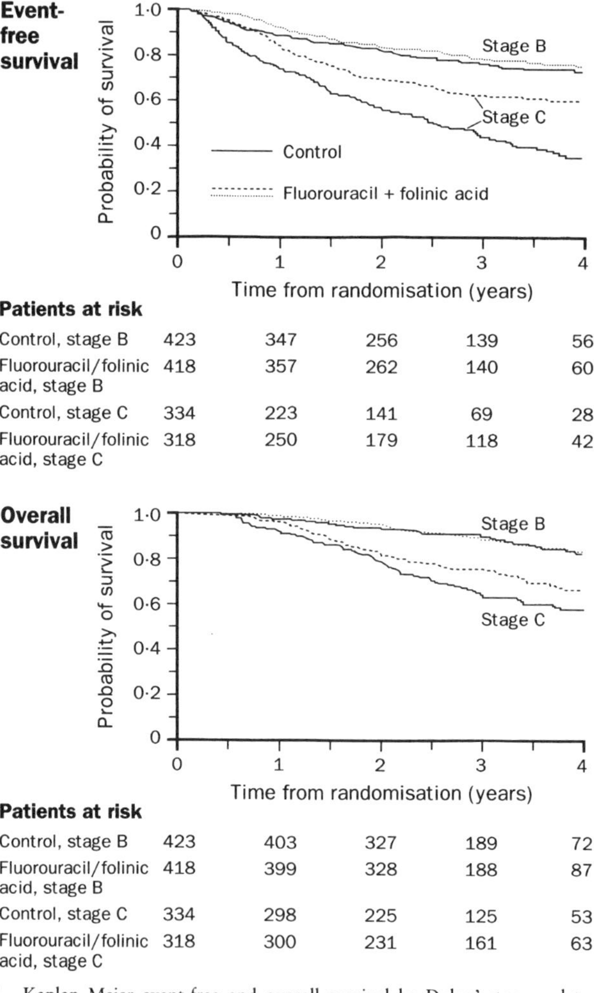

Patients at risk

Control, stage B	423	347	256	139	56
Fluorouracil/folinic acid, stage B	418	357	262	140	60
Control, stage C	334	223	141	69	28
Fluorouracil/folinic acid, stage C	318	250	179	118	42

Patients at risk

Control, stage B	423	403	327	189	72
Fluorouracil/folinic acid, stage B	418	399	328	188	87
Control, stage C	334	298	225	125	53
Fluorouracil/folinic acid, stage C	318	300	231	161	63

FIGURE 2.—Kaplan–Meier event-free and overall survival by Dukes' stage and treatment group. (Courtesy of Marsoni S, for the International Multicentre Pooled Analysis of Colon Cancer Trials Investigators: Efficacy of adjuvant fluorouracil and folinic acid in colon cancer. *Lancet* 345:939–944, 1995.)

Methods.—Data from studies by the Gruppo Interdisciplinare Valutazione Interventi Oncologia, the National Cancer Institute Canada Clinical Trials Group, and the Fondation Française de Cancerologie Digestive were pooled and analyzed. Each was a multicenter trial using the same treatment regimen: FU, 370–400 mg/m², plus FA, 200 mg/m², given daily for 5 days every 28 days for 6 cycles. A total of 1,493 patients were confirmed as eligible for the studies. Seven hundred thirty-six were assigned to treatment, and 757 were assigned to the control group.

Findings.—Fluorouracil/FA significantly decreased the mortality rate by 22% and events by 35%. The 3-year event-free survival was increased from 62% to 71%. The overall survival rate increased from 78% to 83% (Fig 2). Treatment compliance was good. More than 80% of the patients completed the treatment planned. Adverse effects were clinically acceptable, with only 1 death related to therapy. Gastrointestinal side effects were most common. Severe toxic effects occurred in fewer than 3% of patients.

Conclusion.—Fluorouracil plus high-dose FA is an effective, well-tolerated 6-month adjuvant regimen in the treatment of Dukes' stage B and C colon cancer. The antitumor activity obtained by the biochemical modulation of FU with FA can be achieved with different schedules, dosages, and durations of treatment.

▶ Studies appearing during the past decade have indicated that to avoid a false negative study, clinical trials exploring the efficacy of adjuvant therapies in common adult solid tumors should have a sample size in excess of 1,000 patients. The authors of this study combined 3 randomized clinical trials in colon cancer that had relatively identical entry criteria, a surgery-only control group, and an identical FU and FA regimen for the same duration. This has allowed a statistically significant benefit to be shown in the presence of almost 1,500 eligible patients. Although the median follow-up is just slightly more than 3 years, there is a highly statistically significant benefit, both in disease-free survival and overall survival. As with the FU and levamisole multicenter trial done in the United States,[1] the major benefit was seen in node-positive patients with multiple positive nodes. The authors claim benefit in patients with node-negative Dukes' stage B disease, but analyses of the figures do not support this claim.

These data indicate that we now have 2 effective adjuvant programs for node-positive colon cancer, 5FU/levamisole for 1 year or 5FU/FA (leucovorin) for 6 months. A multicenter trial comparing these 2 programs has been completed in the United States, and as these trials mature, a comparison of both efficacy and toxicity will be available. At present, adjuvant chemotherapy for node-negative colon cancer should be offered only to highly selected patients. Defining patients with high-risk node-negative colon cancer by clinical, molecular, or cell cycle characteristics is an ongoing effort by many groups.

A.M. Cohen, M.D.

Reference

1. Moertel CG, Fleming TR, Macdonald JS, et al: Levamisole and fluorouracil for adjuvant therapy of resected colon cancer. *N Engl J Med* 322:352–358, 1990.

Randomized, Double-Blinded, Placebo-Controlled Intervention Study With Supplemental Calcium in Families With Hereditary Nonpolyposis Colorectal Cancer

Cats A, Kleibeuker JH, van der Meer R, Kuipers F, Sluiter WJ, Hardonk MJ, Oremus EThHGJ, Mulder NH, de Vries EGE (Univ Hosp Groningen, The Netherlands; Netherlands Inst for Dairy Research, Ede)

J Natl Cancer Inst 87:598–603, 1995 7–25

Background.—Fat appears to promote colorectal cancer by increasing the levels of fatty and bile acids in the colon. These acids irritate and damage the epithelial cells of the colon, resulting in an increased rate of cellular proliferation. Some investigators have proposed the use of oral calcium supplementation as a dietary intervention for persons at high risk of colorectal cancer because it can reduce rectal epithelial cell proliferation through the binding of fatty and bile acids. However, placebo-controlled studies have yielded conflicting findings.

Methods.—Thirty subjects at high risk for hereditary nonpolyposis colorectal cancer were enrolled in a randomized, double-blinded, placebo-controlled trial to test oral calcium supplementation. By random assignment, equal numbers were given oral calcium carbonate supplements, 1.5 g, or placebo 3 times a day for 12 weeks.

Findings.—Compared with baseline values, the rectal whole-crypt labeling index was significantly reduced after calcium supplementation and placebo. There were no significant differences between the supplemental calcium and placebo groups in 3 bowel segments. During calcium supplementation, cytolytic activity was significantly decreased, whereas there was no change in the placebo group.

Conclusion.—In this group of first-degree relatives of patients with hereditary nonpolyposis colorectal cancer, oral calcium supplementation produced a minor, nonsignificant reduction in epithelial cell proliferation in the rectum compared with placebo. Such supplementation appears to have no effect on the same parameter in the sigmoid and descending colon.

▶ There is considerable interest in prevention trials for colorectal cancer because of the presence of measurable intermediate biomarkers as well as subgroups of patients with adenomatous polyps. A number of epidemiologic studies with confirmation in animal models suggest that calcium may play a protective role in the development of colorectal cancer. It appears that the mechanism of action is the binding of free fatty acids and bile acids within the colon.

The authors are to be congratulated in using a randomized, double-blind, placebo-controlled intervention trial with supplemental calcium. They chose a high-risk group of patients: individuals with a family history of hereditary nonpolyposis colorectal cancer (HNPCC). The calcium supplement was oral calcium carbonate, 1.5 g administered 3 times daily. The intermediate bio-marker was primarily labeling indices from biopsy specimens taken in the rectum, mid-sigmoid colon, and descending colon. The results indicate a slight but significant difference between the placebo and supplemental calcium with regard to reducing the labeling indices in the rectum. There were no effects in the colon. In addition, the benefit was in reduction in the labeling indices in the lumenal third of the crypts. The results indicate only a minor reduction of epithelial cell proliferation compared with placebo, and this benefit was limited to the rectum. This is of particular interest because patients with HNPCC are at increased propensity for colon cancer rather than rectal cancer.

A.M. Cohen, M.D.

Management and Survival of Patients With Adenocarcinoma of the Colon and Rectum: A National Survey of the Commission on Cancer
Beart RW, Steele GD Jr, Menck HR, Chmiel JS, Ocwieja KE, Winchester DP (Univ of Southern California, Los Angeles; Harvard Univ, Boston; American College of Surgeons, Chicago; et al)
J Am Coll Surg 181:225–236, 1995   7–26

Introduction.—The multidisciplinary Commission on Cancer (COC) of the American College of Surgeons develops criteria for periodic evaluation of the diagnosis, treatment, rehabilitation, and follow-up of patients with cancer. Each year, the COC conducts a nationwide survey of practices for several cancer sites. The management of patients with carcinoma of the colon or rectum was reviewed to identify current trends and changes in the pattern of care and survival since the last COC report on these sites.

Methods.—Detailed, field-tested data collection forms regarding carcinoma of the colon and rectum were sent to more than 1,200 approved cancer programs and 800 other facilities. Two different surveys were conducted: a long-term survey to evaluate 5-year survival rates and a short-term survey to assess current practices and trends. Specific information was sought regarding disease presentation, preoperative evaluation, surgical treatment, postoperative care, use of adjuvant therapy, and status at most recent follow-up.

Results.—The analysis included 39,502 reports from 943 hospitals, including 12,682 long-term and 16,527 short-term cases of colon carcinoma and 4,597 long-term and 5,696 short-term cases of rectal carcinoma. The anatomical distribution of the cases was consistent with a rightward migration of colon carcinoma. There was a 15% to 20% incidence of previous colorectal or other carcinoma. The mean patient age was 74 years, which is older than the age seen in most adjuvant therapy studies. Colorectal carcinomas were identified at a more advanced stage in African Americans than in other ethnic groups. The use of IV pyelography appeared to have decreased, whereas the use of CT scans had increased. Many patients had redundant positive results on both contrast studies and colonoscopy.

The tumors were fairly well differentiated, and they decreased in size slightly from 1983 to 1988. At the same time, the use of sphincter-sparing surgical approaches increased for patients with rectal carcinoma. The frequency of local treatment was low, and adjuvant therapy was not widely used. The liver was the most frequent site of tumor recurrence, and peritoneal recurrence was common as well. Survival was significantly related to both stage and grade. For patients with colon carcinoma, the 5-year relative survival rate was 74% for stage I, 63% for stage II, 46% for stage III, and 6% for stage IV. For those with rectal carcinoma, 5-year relative survival rates ranged from 72% for patients with stage I disease to 7% for those with stage IV disease. Survival was worse for older patients, men, and African Americans.

Conclusion.—There is some evidence of suboptimal use of diagnostic studies. More patients are receiving continence-preserving treatment. Survival is improving but varies among ethnic groups. The survival results are not as good as those recently reported from some individual centers.

▶ The COC is a multidisciplinary committee of the American College of Surgeons, one function of which is to review and approve cancer programs within hospitals. Twenty years ago, the Committee on Patient Care and Research established a program of patient care evaluation and required cancer committees at the approved hospitals to review patient treatments.

This study is a compilation of almost 40,000 patients with colorectal cancer reported from a total of 943 institutions. It represents approximately one sixth of all cases of colorectal cancer in the United States during the 1983 and 1988 reporting years. The time line antedated the National Institutes of Health Consensus Conference on the use of adjuvant chemotherapy for node-positive colon cancer and adjuvant chemoradiation therapy for transmural and/or node-positive rectal cancer. The original article contains detailed data presented in 11 tables and will be of interest to any physician looking after patients with colorectal cancer.

A.M. Cohen, M.D.

Radioimmunoguided Surgery in Primary Colorectal Carcinoma: An Intraoperative Prognostic Tool and Adjuvant to Traditional Staging
Arnold MW, Young DC, Hitchcock CL, Schneebaum S, Martin EW Jr (Ohio State Univ, Columbus)
Am J Surg 170:315–318, 1995

7–27

Rationale.—The Duke classification system has been used to predict survival in colorectal cancer for more than 6 decades but, despite advances

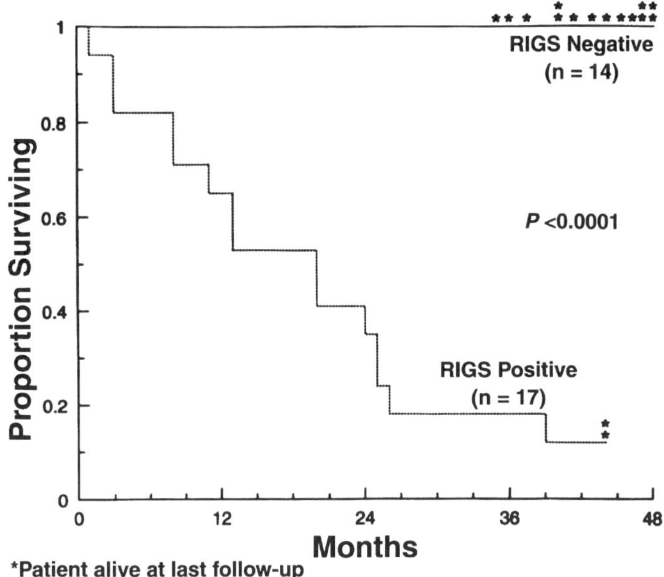

***Patient alive at last follow-up**

FIGURE 4.—Survival rates after primary resection of colorectal cancer as assessed by the presence (radioimmunoguided surgery *[RIGS]-positive*) or absence (*RIGS-negative*) of RIGS tissue. (Reprinted by permission of the publisher from Arnold MW, Young DC, Hitchcock CL, et al: Radioimmunoguided surgery in primary colorectal carcinoma: An intraoperative prognostic tool and adjuvant to traditional staging. *Am J Surg* 170:315–318, Copyright 1995, by Excerpta Medica Inc.)

in surgical technique and adjuvant chemotherapy, overall survival has not improved very much. Accurate staging by the conventional method requires adequate resection and lymph node sampling. In addition, traditional systems fail to take micrometastatic disease into account. Predictions of survival in individual cases remain very uncertain.

A New Approach.—Radioimmunoguided surgery (RIGS) was undertaken in 31 patients requiring primary resection of a colorectal tumor. The patients were injected with radioiodine-labeled CC49—a monoclonal antibody directed against the tumor-associated mucin glycoprotein TAG-072—approximately 3 weeks before resection. A RIGS examination was performed using a hand-held gamma detector, and the primary tumor was then resected together with any other RIGS-positive tissue identified with the probe. Patients were also staged using the tumor-node-metastases (TNM) system.

Results.—The patients were followed for 30–54 months after the resection of colon or rectal cancer. All patients had RIGS-positive tissue, including 2 who had no primary tumor left at the time of surgery. All but 4 of the 29 primary tumors were localized by the RIGS procedure. One hundred nine extraregional RIGS-positive sites were identified, averaging 3.5 sites per patient. Only 41% of these sites were identified by CT scanning. Seventeen of the 31 patients remained RIGS-positive at the end of surgery. These patients tended to have advanced-stage disease; no RIGS-negative patient had stage IV disease. All 14 RIGS-negative patients remained alive 2–4 years postoperatively. In contrast, 15 of the 17 RIGS-positive patients died of disease (Fig 4).

Conclusion.—The RIGS system is a useful supplement to conventional pathologic staging of colorectal cancer, and it provides immediate prognostic information.

▶ This is another in a series of articles from the group at Ohio State University that uses iodine-125–labeled monoclonal antibody and intraoperative radioimmunodetection with a hand-held gamma detecting probe. Most of the previous studies have involved patients with recurrent or metastatic disease. The focus of this article is the potential value of RIGS in patients who have primary colorectal cancer. The authors focus on removal, by surgical resection, of all localized radioactive material detected intraoperatively with the probe.

Previous studies have indicated that many of these areas did not detect cancer by routine histologic methods. Whether they represent areas of micrometastatic disease, soluble antigen only, or some other explanation, the data presented in this article suggest that extraregional sites of antibody localization were frequently found. Figure 4 indicates a dramatic survival advantage if such extraregional sites were removed. These data are very complex and represent a pilot experience. Further studies in such patients— ideally with a human antibody fragment—will be of great interest.

A.M. Cohen, M.D.

Randomised Trial of Monoclonal Antibody for Adjuvant Therapy of Resected Dukes' C Colorectal Carcinoma
Riethmüller G, Schneider-Gädicke E, Schlimok G, Schmiegel W, Raab R, Höffken K, Gruber R, Pichlmaier H, Hirche H, Pichlmayr R, Buggisch P, Witte J, and the German Cancer Aid 17-1A Study Group (Ludwig-Maximilians-Universität München,Germany; Zentralklinikum Augsburg, Germany; Chirurgische Klinik der Medizinisch Hochschule Hannover, Germany; et al)
Lancet 343:1177–1183, 1994   7–28

Background.—Various clinical trials involving patients with solid tumors have used monoclonal antibodies as treatment agents. However, no consistent pattern or response or improved survival has emerged. Antigenic heterogeneity and inadequate accessibility of cells in advanced tumors are possible explanations for these failures. A monoclonal antibody was used to target minimal residual disease in an early stage of tumor cell dissemination in patients with colorectal cancer.

Methods.—One hundred eighty-nine patients were enrolled. All had Dukes' stage C disease, had undergone curative surgery, and were free of manifest residual tumor. The patients were randomly assigned to an observation regimen or to postoperative treatment with 500 mg of 17-1A antibody, followed by four 100-mg infusions each month.

Findings.—At a median follow-up of 5 years, antibody treatment decreased the overall death rate by 30% and the recurrence rate by 27% (Fig 2). The effect of antibody was most marked in patients in whom distant metastasis was the first sign of a relapse. This effect was not observed for local relapses. The toxic effects of 17-1A antibody were infrequent and consisted primarily of mild constitutional and gastrointestinal symptoms. Four anaphylactic reactions occurred during 371 infusions. All were controlled by intravenous steroids. None necessitated hospital admission.

Conclusions.—In this series, postoperative 17-1A antibody treatment increased survival and reduced the rate of recurrence in patients with resected Dukes' C colorectal carcinoma. This therapy preferentially suppresses or delays the appearance of distant metastases without influencing the appearnce of local recurrences.

▶ Colorectal cancer remains refractory to many of the major chemotherapeutic agents. However, prospective randomized clinical trials in patients with transmural or node-positive *rectal* cancer indicate a benefit of 5-fluorouracil (5-FU) and pelvic radiation therapy. As a single agent, 5-FU has not shown benefit in *colon* cancer, but adjuvant 5-FU with levamisole and, likely, 5-FU with Leucovorin appear to produce a reduction of approximately 30% in the cancer death rate. This German cooperative group's report on the use of murine monoclonal antibody 17-1A suggests that a similar benefit can be obtained with passive immunotherapy.

The antibody used in this study is directed toward a cell surface glycoprotein. As opposed to carcinoembryonic antigen, this antigen is not shed from the cell membrane and cannot be detected in serum. Based on animal

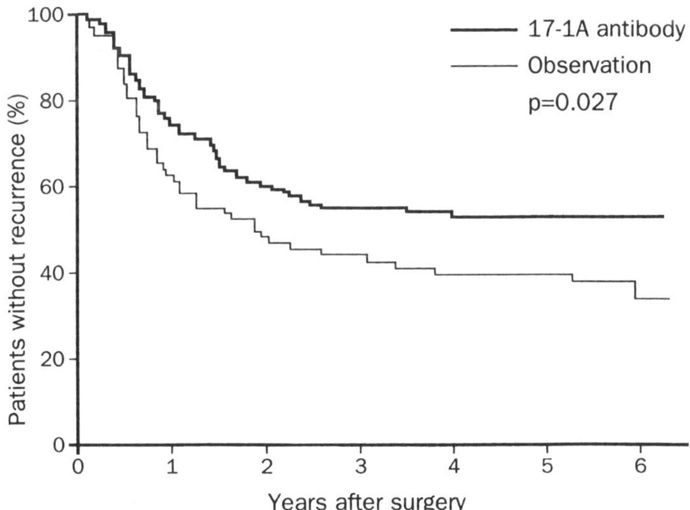

FIGURE 2.—Recurrence-free survival. The *P* value is adjusted with Cox's proportional hazard model. (Courtesy of Riethmüller G, Schneider-Gädicke E, Schlimok G, et al: Randomised trial of monoclonal antibody for adjuvant therapy of resected Dukes' C colorectal carcinoma. *Lancet* 343:1177-1183, Copyright by The Lancet Ltd, 1994.)

models of monoclonal antibody immunotherapy, the adjuvant setting is far more likely to be beneficial, particularly when the native antibody is used. Despite an origin in mice, this antibody induces a cellular immune response with human effector cells. Based on both the excellent tolerance in a phase I trial and the efficacy in nude mouse models, this study was undertaken.

Unfortunately, patients with both rectal and colon cancer were included in the trial. No patients received any chemotherapy, and none of the patients with rectal cancer received radiation therapy. Despite the integration of a number of different groups and a median follow-up of 5 years, this mature study shows improvement in disease-free survival and overall survival. As expected, the major benefit is with regard to distant metastasis-free survival.

These data on the use of murine antibody give considerable encouragement to future trials. Humanized or genetically engineered constructs should reduce the negative immune response to such therapy (human antimouse antibody). This will allow much longer term infusions of antibody. Also, such treatments can be combined with adjuvant chemotherapy. A prospective randomized clinical trial in patients with node-positive colon cancer has been proposed through the cooperative groups comparing adjuvant 5-fluorouracil/levamisole with or without 17-1A monoclonal antibody.

A.M. Cohen, M.D.

Failure of Orally Administered Dipyridamole to Enhance the Antineoplastic Activity of Fluorouracil in Combination With Leucovorin in Patients With Advanced Colorectal Cancer: A Prospective Randomized Trial

Köhne C-H, Hiddemann W, Schüller J, Weiss J, Lohrmann H-P, Schmitz-Hübner U, Bodenstein H, Schöber C, Wilke H, Grem J, Schmoll H-J (Hannover Med School, Germany; Hosp Rudolfsstiftung, Vienna; Georg-August-Univ, Göttingen, Germany; et al)

J Clin Oncol 13:1201–1208, 1995

7–29

Background.—Currently, fluorouracil (5-FU) is the most active antineoplastic agent used for the treatment of advanced colorectal cancer. Biochemical modulation with folinic acid (FA) improves response rates in advanced colorectal cancer. However, a recent meta-analysis of 9 randomized trials did not show a significant survival advantage. The ability of the nucleoside transport inhibitor dipyridamole (DP) to enhance the antitumor activity of 5-FU/FA was assessed in a randomized trial.

Methods.—By random assignment, 181 untreated patients with advanced colorectal cancer were given 5-FU, 600 mg/m^2, plus FA, 300 mg/m^2, on days 2–4 with or without DP, 75 mg given orally 3 times a day, on days 1–5. Every 3 weeks, cycles were repeated. All eligible patients had documented tumor progression. In 11 nonrandomized patients who were given paired cycles with or without DP, 5-FU pharmacokinetics were assessed using high-performance liquid chromatography.

Findings.—Toxicity and response could be assessed in 174 patients. Except for DP-related headache in 24% of the patients, there was no significant difference in toxicity between groups. The objective response rates for patients given 5-FU/FA and those given 5-FU/FA/DP were 15% and 13%, respectively. The dose intensity of 5-FU was significantly greater in the patients receiving DP. The pharmacokinetic parameters of 5-FU did not significantly differ, except that DP induced a prolonged half-life. The median times to progression and median survival were comparable in the 2 groups.

Conclusion.—In the dose and schedule used in this study, orally administered DP did not improve the antineoplastic activity of 5-FU/FA in patients with advanced colorectal cancer. The increase in 5-FU dose intensity that occurred in patients given FU/FA/DP was not clinically relevant.

▶ Considerable in vitro data support the use of DP as an additional modulating agent with 5-FU. 5-Fluorouracil modulated with FA has become the most commonly used regimen for patients with advanced colorectal cancer. In vitro data indicate that FA stabilizes the 5-FU anabolite FdUMP. This enhances the 5-FU–induced depletion of intracellular dTTP. Dipyridamole blocks the cellular uptake of nucleosides, which thereby blocks a critical salvage pathway.

The authors took these in vitro data to a prospective randomized trial. There were 90 patients in 1 arm and 84 patients in the other, and the overall response rates were low in both groups. Fifteen percent of the patients in the 5FU/FA group responded, and 13% of those with additive DP responded. As with all bimodulation studies, dose and timing are important. The authors used only a 3-day program of 5FU/FA rather than the more standard 5-day program. The lack of benefit may be related to the difficulty in getting adequate levels of DP into the needed intracellular position. There is great variability in DP absorption from the intestine, and a high degree of binding to plasma proteins. It is unlikely that adequate levels of intracellular DP were obtained. These data show the importance of continued studies of the mechanisms of drug action, but they also show the difficulty in such translational research.

A.M. Cohen, M.D.

Long-Term Results of Single Course of Adjuvant Intraportal Chemotherapy for Colorectal Cancer

Laffer UT, for the Swiss Group for Clinical Cancer Research (SAKK) (Surgical Clinic, Biel-Bienne, Switzerland)

Lancet 345:349–353, 1995   7–30

Objective.—Adjuvant chemotherapy after colorectal surgery has not had a significant effect on controlling metastatic disease. The results of a single course of portal infusion of mitomycin after surgery for colorectal cancer were assessed.

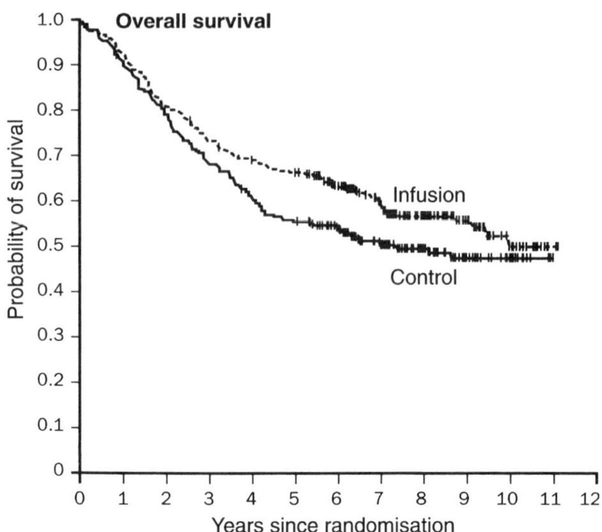

FIGURE.—Overall survival by treatment group. (Courtesy of Laffer UT, for the Swiss Group for Clinical Cancer Research (SAKK): Long-term results of single course of adjuvant intraportal chemotherapy for colorectal cancer. *Lancet* 345:349–353, copyright by The Lancet Ltd, 1995.)

Methods.—After curative resection of adenocarcinoma of the colon or rectum, 505 patients received either no adjuvant therapy or an immediate postoperative intraportal infusion of fluorouracil 500 mg/m² a day for 7 days, plus a single 10 mg/m² course of mitomycin.

Results.—At the median follow-up of 96 months, 235 patients, 108 of whom were in the infusion group, had died. The risk of relapse was reduced by 21% and the risk of death by 26% in the infusion group. The 5-year disease-free survival and 5-year overall survival rates were higher in the infusion group than in the control group (Fig). Node-negative, node-positive, rectal cancer and, especially, colon cancer infusion groups had fewer local relapses than did comparable control groups.

Conclusion.—A single course of portal chemotherapy after surgery for colorectal cancer increased survival by reducing the incidence of recurrences and metastases in all infusion groups.

▶ This article reports the long-term results (median follow-up, 8 years) of the Swiss Group for Clinical Cancer Research multicenter trial of perioperative intraportal adjuvant chemotherapy with fluorouracil and mitomycin. This relatively low-risk protocol reduced the risk of recurrence by one fifth and reduced the risk of death by one fourth. The major benefit was seen in node-positive patients and those with colon cancer.

The patterns of failure demonstrate that the efficacy was not isolated to the reduction in hepatic metastases, which was the initial hypothesis. The benefit appears to be that of systemic chemotherapy. Another consideration may be related to the perioperative use of the cytotoxic chemotherapy, which has a theoretical benefit. Traditional use of systemic chemotherapy is delayed for 4 to 6 weeks after the operation.

A trial that compares portal vs. systemic chemotherapy has recently been completed by the same clinical cancer research group. In the United States, there is an ongoing multicenter trial in node-positive/colon cancer patients, which examines the potential additive benefit of early postoperative systemic chemotherapy combined with the standard adjuvant program that begins at one month. The data from these 2 studies should provide important information with which to clarify and define appropriate adjuvant chemotherapy strategies in this very common disease.

A.M. Cohen, M.D.

Endoscopically Removed Malignant Colorectal Polyps: Clinicopathologic Correlations
Cooper HS, Deppisch LM, Gourley WK, Kahn EI, Lev R, Manley PN, Pascal RR, Qizilbash AH, Rickert RR, Silverman JF, Wirman JA (Fox Chase Cancer Ctr, Philadelphia; Western Reserve Care System, Youngstown, Ohio; Univ of Texas, Galveston; et al)
Gastroenterology 108:1657–1665, 1995   7–31

Background.—Malignant colorectal polyps are often removed by endoscopic polypectomy. Upon confirmation of malignancy, the clinician and patient must decide whether the polypectomy was adequate therapy or whether definitive surgical resection is required. At several institutions, endoscopically removed malignant colorectal polyps were examined to identify useful parameters for making this management decision.

Methods.—A total of 140 malignant colorectal polyps removed endoscopically with either 5-year conservative or resection follow-up were studied by 5 pathologists. Each polyp was evaluated for grade, status of the resection margin, distance between cancer tissue and the resection margin, lymphatic and/or venous invasion, and background adenoma or polypoid carcinoma. Cancer that was within 1 mm of the resection margin and/or grade III and/or with lymphatic and/or venous invasion was considered to have an unfavorable histologic parameter. The incidence of adverse outcomes (local and/or distant recurrence in patients treated with polypectomy alone or positive lymph nodes and/or residual local cancer in patients treated with surgical resection) was calculated.

Results.—Of the 140 polyps, 36 were managed with polypectomy only and 104 were managed with surgical resection. There were adverse outcomes in 16 patients, with an incidence of 5.5% in the polypectomy only group and 13.5% in the resection group (not a statistically significant difference). Only 2 of these patients did not have unfavorable histologic parameters (Table 1). An adverse outcome occurred in 21.4% of the patients with tumor tissue within 1 mm of the resection margin, 17.6% of the patients with lymphatic invasion, 18.2% of those with indefinite lymphatic invasion, 40% of the patients with venous invasion, 20% of

TABLE 1.—Outcome Related to Histologic Parameters

Unfavorable histology*	Adverse outcome (%)	No adverse outcome (%)	Total (%)
Present	14/71 (19.7)	57/71 (80.3)‖ ¶**	71/140 (50.7)
Indefinite	2/23 (8.6)†‡	21/23 (91.3)††	23/140 (16.4)
Absent	0/46 (0.0)	46/46 (100.0)	46/140 (32.8)
Total	16/140 (11.4)§	124/140 (88.6)	140/140 (100.0)

Note: Regarding adverse vs. no adverse outcome: present unfavorable vs. indefinite unfavorable, nonsignificant (*NS*); present unfavorable vs. absent unfavorable, $P < 0.0005$; indefinite unfavorable vs. absent unfavorable, NS; polypectomy only vs. polypectomy followed by resection, NS.

  * Unfavorable histology is tumor M+ and/or LI+ and/or VI+ and/or III+.

  † One patient with LI_i.

  ‡ One patient with LI_i, and colloid cancer.

  § Thirteen patients with lymph node metastases and 1 patient with local residual cancer in resection specimen (polypectomy followed by resection); 2 patients with distant and/or local recurrence (polypectomy only). Adverse outcome in polypectomy only cases, 5.5% (2 of 36). Adverse outcome in polypectomy followed by resection cases, 13.5% (14 of 104).

  ‖ One patient with negative resection (grade III signet cell cancer and M+) and distant metastases 4 years later.

  ¶ One patient with negative resection LI+, and liver metastases 23 years later.

  ** One patient with negative resection, LI+ and VI+, and liver metastases 7 years later.

  †† One patient with negative resection, III_i and LI_i, and liver metastases 2 years later.

  Abbreviations: M+, cancer at or near ($\leq$ 1.0 mm from) margin; *LI*+, lymphatic invasion present; LI_i, lymphatic invasion indefinite; *III*+, grade III cancer present; III_i, grade III cancer indefinite; *VI*+, venous invasion present.

  (Courtesy of Cooper HS, Deppisch LM, Gourley WK, et al: Endoscopically removed malignant colorectal polyps: clinicopathologic correlations. *Gastroenterology* 108:1657–1665, 1995.)

those with polypoid cancer, and 17.4% of those with indefinite polypoid cancer. Survival was similar in the polypectomy only and the resection groups.

Conclusion.—The feasibility of using histologic parameters to guide management decisions for patients with malignant colorectal polyps is supported by the findings. Definitive surgical resection is recommended when any of the following histologic features are present: cancer tissue within 1 mm of the resection margin, grade III cancer, lymphatic invasion, or venous invasion. Patients with polyps not having these histologic features may be safely treated with polypectomy only, subject to consideration of other patient factors.

▶ These authors present the largest study of endoscopically removed malignant colorectal polyps accrued from multiple medical centers. Some patients underwent postpolypectomy bowel resection, whereas others underwent polypectomy alone. Most importantly with regard to interpretation of the data, the patients who had polypectomy alone were all followed for a minimum of 5 years. The data and outcome analysis presented provide encouraging documentation for conservative therapy (polypectomy only) in a selected subset of patients. The criteria are histologic, and when all unfavorable histologic features were absent, no patient had recurrence or metastatic disease develop. There was a high interobserver correlation when 5 pathologists examined for margins, grade, and venous invasion. Reliability was lower regarding the presence of lymphatic invasion.

A.M. Cohen, M.D.

Survival After Curative Resection of Lymph Node Negative Colorectal Carcinoma: A Prospective Study of 910 Patients
Newland RC, Dent OF, Chapuis PH, Bokey L (Concord Hosp Sydney, Australia; Australian Natl Univ, Australian Capital Territory; Univ of Sydney, Concord, Australia)
Cancer 76:564–571, 1995   7–32

Background.—Nearly 50% of all patients undergoing bowel resection for colorectal carcinoma are without evidence of lymph node metastases or known residual tumor. The survival of these patients with clinicopathologic stage A and B tumors was compared with that of the general population and differences between groups were evaluated.

Patients and Methods.—Data prospectively collected for 910 patients from a single institution during a 21.5-year period were evaluated. The patients had been followed from 6 months to 21.5 years. Observed patient survival was compared with expected survival, based on age- and sex-matched data for the population of New South Wales. The "Survival" procedure developed by the Finnish Cancer Registry was used for this analysis.

Results.—Significantly poorer survival than anticipated was noted only for males with tumor spread beyond the muscularis propria (stage B). The decreased survival among these patients was associated with 5 independently acting variables, 4 of which were clinical and 1 of which was pathologic. The clinical variables included cardiovascular complication, permanent stoma, urgent operation, and respiratory complication. The pathologic variable was direct spread involving a free serosal surface.

Conclusions.—As predicted from the general population, survival of patients with clinicopathologic stage A or B tumors closely matched anticipated survival rates. The only exception was among males with stage B tumors. The significantly decreased survival for this group was largely the result of clinical, rather than pathologic, variables. The risk of occult metastases thus appears to be low for patients with stage A and B tumors, based on this classification.

▶ This article is one of a series of highly detailed analyses from the Colon and Rectal Unit at the University of Sydney, Australia, involving a prospected audit of a very large patient population. This report expands on the previous analysis, which indicated that in patients with stage B tumor, tumor penetration to involve the free serosal surface was relatively infrequent but reduced the 5-year survival by half. This appears to be the most important tumor pathology prognostic variable in node-negative patients, and it represents a distinction between a T3 and T4 cancer in the American Joint Comittee on Cancer Staging/International Union Against Cancer staging system. In patients with T3 cancer, tumor penetrates the muscularis propria into subserosal fat or pericolonic fat. Penetration to the serosa is also within the T3 category. However, if the tumor penetrates the free mesothelial surface, it is staged T4. Histologic determination of such transmural penetration may be difficult, and serosal cytology may play a role.[1]

A.M. Cohen, M.D.

Reference

1. Zeng Z, Cohen AM, et al: Serosal cytologic study to determine free mesothelial penetration of intraperitoneal colon cancer. *Cancer* 70:737–740, 1992.

Five-Year Prospective Study of DNA Tumor Ploidy and Colorectal Cancer Survival

Chapman MAS, Hardcastle JD, Armitage NCM (Univ Hosp, Nottingham, England)

Cancer 76:383–387, 1995
7–33

Background.—Numerous reports have suggested that DNA tumor content (ploidy) has an effect on recurrence and survival in colorectal cancer. In a previous prospective study of patients undergoing colorectal resections for carcinoma, individuals with aneuploid tumor had a significantly greater 2-year tumor recurrence rate than did those with diploid tumors. The 5-year survival rates of this cohort of patients were evaluated to determine the effects of tumor DNA ploidy on survival.

Patients and Methods.—Three hundred sixty-three patients were prospectively evaluated. All patients had undergone colorectal resections dur-

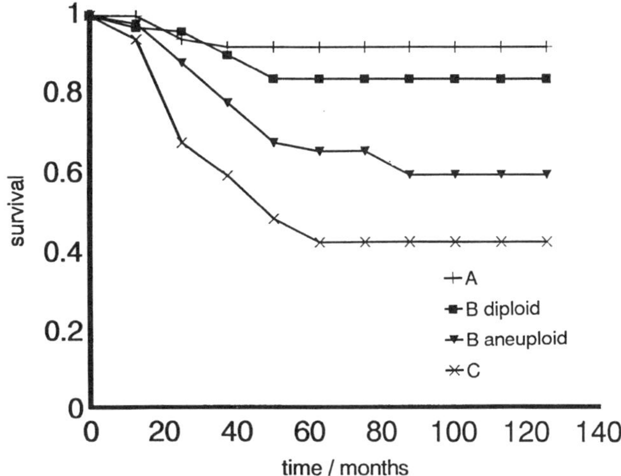

FIGURE 2.—Cumulative proportion of individuals surviving after curative resection vs. time in months for stage A and stage B diploid and aneuploid and stage C tumors. (Courtesy of Chapman MAS, Hardcastle JD, Armitage NCN: Five-year prospective study of DNA tumor ploidy and colorectal cancer survival. *Cancer* 76:383–387, 1995. Reprinted by permission of Wiley-Liss, Inc., a division of John Wiley & Sons, Inc.)

ing a 6-year period and were followed regularly for a minimum of 5 years or until death. Measurements of DNA tumor ploidy were obtained using fresh and paraffin embedded tissues.

Results.—Two patients were lost to follow-up. Of the tumors studied, 40% were diploid and the remainder were aneuploid. The 5-year survival rate among patients who had undergone curative resections was 76% for those with diploid tumors and 64% for those with aneuploid tumors. Subgroup analysis showed that the survival advantage associated with diploid tumors was limited to patients with stage B tumors (Fig 2). No associations between ploidy and sex, age of patient, stage, histologic grade, or tumor site were noted.

Conclusions.—The aggressiveness of stage B tumors can be objectively measured using ploidy, although these measurements are subject to sampling error. Patients with aneuploid stage B tumors may benefit from adjuvant therapy, given that such tumors are associated with unfavorable prognoses.

▶ For the past decade, investigators have attempted to use objective determinants of tumor DNA ploidy to determine prognosis. Direct determinations using flow cytometry from single-cell suspension nuclei, as well as monoclonal antibody techniques, have been used. Studies have primarily been retrospective on fixed tissues. Some studies have been prospective and have used fresh tissue. This report is the largest prospective study and has looked at ploidy from both fresh tissue and paraffin-embedded specimens. The data support the value of such studies as a prognostic determinant in node-negative colorectal cancer. This has considerable implications for defining a group of node-negative patients most likely to benefit from adjuvant chemotherapy. Technical issues with regard to sampling errors and discrepancy between fresh and fixed tissue must be resolved before widespread application of this technique is recommended.

A.M. Cohen, M.D.

Resection of Colorectal Liver Metastases

Scheele J, Stang R, Altendorf-Hofmann A, Paul M (Friedrich-Alexander Univ, Erlangen, Germany)
World J Surg 19:59–71, 1995   7–34

Background.—Resection of liver metastases from colorectal carcinoma cures a substantial proportion of patients. This procedure can result in a disease-free survival of 20 years or more. Research is now needed to determine the proportion of patients with resectable disease in unselected patient samples, the importance of early diagnosis through aggressive screening and its effect on treatment, reliable indicators of prognosis, the value of repeat resection when tumor recurs, and the best surgical technique.

Methods.—Between 1960 and 1992, 1,718 patients with liver metastases from colorectal cancer were seen at Erlangen University Hospital

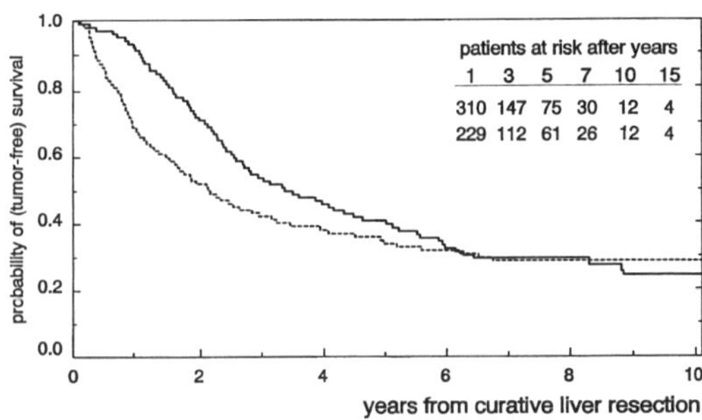

FIGURE 2.—Overall (*solid line*) and tumor-free (*broken line*) survival after potentially curative resection, with operative (30-day) mortality excluded. (Courtesy of Scheele J, Stang R, Altendorf-Hofmann A, et al: Resection of colorectal liver metastases. *World J Surg* 19:59–71, 1995, copyright Springer-Verlag.)

in Germany. Four hundred sixty-nine patients, or 27.3%, underwent hepatic resection. This surgery was performed with curative intent in 434 patients, or 25.3% (Fig 2).

Findings.—The operative mortality rate in the group undergoing curative resection was 4.4%. In the most recent 3 years, it was 1.8%. Significant morbidity was noted in 16% of the patients, with a reduction to 5% for the most recent 3 years. At the last follow-up, there were 350 patients with "potentially curative" resection and 65 with minimal macroscopic or microscopic disease. The latter group had a poor prognosis, with median and maximum survival times of 14.4 and 56 months, respectively. The patients with potentially curative resection had 5-, 10-, and 20-year actuarial survivals of 39.3%, 23.6%, and 17.7%, respectively. The 5-year tumor-free survival rate was 33.6%. Factors associated with reduced crude survival in a univariate analysis were the presence and extent of mesenteric lymph node involvement, grade III/IV primary tumor, synchronous diagnosis of metastases, satellite metastases, metastasis diameter of more than 5 cm, preoperative carcinoembryonic antigen elevation, limited resection margins, extrahepatic disease, and nonanatomical procedures. Patients with primary colon tumors had significantly better disease-free survival rates than did patients with rectal cancer. Resectability was adversely affected by the presence of 5 or more independent metastases. However, when a radical excision of all detectable disease was achieved, an increasing number of metastases had no significant predictive value for overall or disease-free survival. According to Cox multivariate regression analysis, factors that independently affected crude and tumor-free survival were the presence of satellite metastases, primary tumor grade, the time of metastasis diagnosis, diameter of the largest metastasis, anatomical vs. nonanatomical approach, year of resection, and mesenteric lymph node involvement.

▶ These authors present the largest single-institution experience in the area of potentially curative surgery for colorectal cancer hepatic metastases. A total of 350 patients underwent a potentially curative operation. The most important data are the actuarial overall 5-year survival rate of 39% and the actuarial disease-free survival of 33.6% at 5 years.

This study was done with a 30-day operative mortality of 4.4%, with a more recent mortality of 3.4% during the past 12 years. It is commonly stated that it is only worth resecting 1 or, at most, 2 lesions in the liver. The most important outcome in this study was the observation that as long as all the tumor could be removed, there was no significant negative predictive value associated with an increased number of metastases resected. Specifically, even in the 32 patients who had more than 4 metastases resected, an actuarial survival rate of 50% was obtained.

A.M. Cohen, M.D.

Anorectal Melanoma: A 64-Year Experience at Memorial Sloan-Kettering Cancer Center
Brady MS, Kavolius JP, Quan SHQ (Mem Sloan-Kettering Cancer Ctr, New York)
Dis Colon Rectum 38:146–151, 1995   7–35

Objective.—There is controversy regarding the surgical management of patients with the rare and deadly tumor anorectal melanoma. The prognosis is so poor that many surgeons believe that there is no need for abdominoperineal resection (APR). Toward better selection of patients for aggressive or conservative operative management, a large series of patients with anorectal melanoma was reviewed.

Methods.—The review included 85 patients with anorectal melanoma treated from 1929 to 1993 at 1 cancer center. There were 46 women and 39 men (median age, 60 years). The Kaplan-Meier product-limit method was used for graphic display of survival analyses and the log-rank test for comparison of survival distributions. Small patient groups were compared using Fisher's exact test.

Findings.—The 5-year survival rate was 17%, with a median survival of 19 months. Seventy-one patients had resectable disease: 43 underwent APR, 13 had wide local excision, and 15 had biopsy with or without fulguration. The 5-year disease-free survival distribution was 27% for patients who underwent APR vs. 5% for those who underwent local procedures only. This difference was not significant, but patients undergoing APR were more likely to have long-term survival. All 10 long-term survivors were women, and 9 had undergone APR (Fig 2). Patients with long-term survival after APR had a median primary tumor size of 2.5 cm, compared with 4 cm for patients who did not have long-term survival after APR.

Conclusion.—For selected patients with anorectal melanoma, APR is a reasonable approach to surgical management. It should be considered in patients with localized anorectal melanoma, especially those with smaller tumors and no evidence of nodal metastases. Survival after APR appears to be best for women with operable disease.

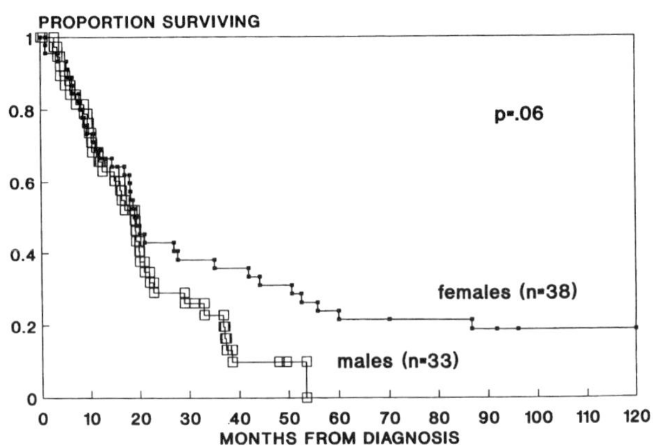

FIGURE 2.—Female patients had a more favorable survival distribution than male patients. The 5-year disease-free survival rate for patients with resectable disease at presentation was 29% vs. 0% ($P < .06$) for women compared with men, respectively. (Courtesy of Brady MS, Kavolius JP, Quan SHQ, et al: Anorectal melanoma: A 64-year experience at Memorial Sloan-Kettering Cancer Center. *Dis Colon Rectum* 38:146–151, 1995.)

▶ Anorectal melanoma is a rare and usually fatal disease. These tumors probably are not inherently more virulent, but the poor end results are likely related to the size of the tumor at presentation. Most patients are seen with bleeding, and some are seen with a mass. A small percentage had melanoma discovered incidentally on review of hemorrhoidectomy specimens.

There is considerable debate as to the appropriate treatment for such patients. Philosophically, one is reluctant to perform an APR with a permanent colostomy for a group of patients with a median survival of less than 2 years. However, as Figure 2 indicates, all long-term survivors in this series were female. Although this did not reach statistical significance, 9 of 10 of the long-term female survivors had been treated with APR as opposed to local excision. The data would suggest that a relatively favorable, small anorectal melanoma in a woman should be aggressively treated by APR, which will produce a median survival of 3 years. However, a "tail on the curve" of approximately 1 in 4 patients can be expected to survive 5 years.

A.M. Cohen, M.D.

Epidermoid Carcinoma of the Anal Margin: 17 Cases Treated With Curative-Intent Radiation Therapy

Touboul E, Schlienger M, Buffat L, Lefkopoulos D, Yao XG, Parc R, Tiret E, Gallot D, Malafosse M, Laugier A (Hôpital Tenon, Paris; Hôpital Saint-Antoine, Paris; Hôpital Rothschild, Paris)
Radiother Oncol 34:195–202, 1995

7–36

Objective.—Fewer than 10% of cancers arising from the anal canal are epidermoid lesions, and few long-term trials of radiotherapy are available. Curative radiotherapy was given to 17 patients with such tumors and no evidence of distant spread. Fifteen patients were followed for 7.4 years on average.

Treatment.—Nine patients were treated solely by a perineal electron beam of 9–17 MeV or, in 1 instance, by cobalt teletherapy. An initial course of 40–45 Gy, delivered in 4.5–5 weeks, was followed after a 3- to 4-week interval by a second course of 20–25 Gy via a reduced field. Seven patients received pelvic radiation using a 4-field technique to deliver a total dose of 40–45 Gy in 4.5–5 weeks. One patient received interstitial brachytherapy alone to the primary tumor. Seven of the 17 patients received inguinal irradiation, most often at the same time as the pelvis was treated.

Results.—Cancer-specific survival rates were 86% at 5 years and 77.5% at 10 years. On univariate analysis, the only factor influencing cancer-specific survival was tumor size (Table 5). Two patients relapsed locally. Inguinal lymph nodes were controlled in all but 1 of 13 patients. Complications included single cases of marked perianal ulceration, moderate anal stenosis, and severe anal/perianal necrosis. The sphincter was preserved in 82% of patients who were cured.

Conclusion.—External irradiation is an effective approach to early epidermoid cancers of the anal margin and usually preserves the sphincter.

TABLE 5.—Influence of Prognostic Factors on Outcome: Univariate Analysis (17 Cases)

| | | Cancer-specific survival | | | | |
| | | At 5 years | | At 10 years | | |
Factors	n	%	Patients at risk (n)	%	Patients at risk (n)	p-value
Sex						
Male	7	100	(9)	85.7 ± 13	(5)	0.22
Female	10	62.5 ± 21	(3)	62.5 ± 21	(1)	
Age (years)						
≤ 54	8	100	(6)	100	(4)	0.11
> 54	9	76.2 ± 15	(6)	61 ± 18	(2)	
Histologic finding						
Squamous grade 1	14	91.7 ± 8	(10)	80.2 ± 12.8	(4)	0.60
Squamous grade 2 or 3	3	66.7 ± 27	(2)	66.7 ± 27	(2)	
Tumor size						
≤ 2 cm	9	100	(8)	100	(5)	0.003
> 2 cm	8	66.7 ± 19	(4)	50 ± 20	(1)	
T-stage (UICC 1987)						
T1	9	100	(8)	100	(5)	0.016
T2	6	60 ± 22	(3)	40 ± 22	(1)	
T3–4	2	100	(1)	100	(1)	
Inguinal node status						
N0	15	92.3 ± 7.4	(11)	82 ± 12	(5)	0.29
N1–N3	2	50 ± 35	(1)	50 ± 35	(1)	
Circumferential invasion						
≤ 1/4	13	92.3 ± 7.4	(11)	82 ± 12	(5)	0.29
> 1/4	4	50 ± 35	(1)	50 ± 35	(1)	
Treatment						
Pelvic RT and perineal boost	7	80 ± 18	(4)	80 ± 18	(3)	0.89
Perineal irradiation alone	10	90 ± 9.5	(8)	75 ± 16	(3)	

(Reprinted from *Radiother Oncol*, Vol. 34, Touboul E, Schlienger M, Buffat L, et al: Epidermoid carcinoma of the anal margin: 17 cases treated with curative-intent radiation therapy, pp 195–202, 1995, with kind permission of Elsevier Science—NL, Sara Burgerhartstraat 25, 1055 KV Amsterdam, The Netherlands.)

Adjuvant chemotherapy and radiotherapy may be indicated for locally advanced tumors.

▶ In this country, the teaching is that carcinoma of the anus is a disease best approached by a combination of chemotherapy and radiation therapy. Data from Toronto have challenged this teaching, and this series from France also raises questions about such an approach. This abstract represents a relatively small series of 17 patients without obvious evidence of distant metastases who were treated with curative-intent radiation therapy alone. Documented nodal involvement was relatively infrequent. The dose of radiation was relatively high (6,000–7,000 rad), and the 5- and 10-year survival rates were really quite good. Local control was excellent in the T1 group, although the falloff was noticeable with more advanced disease.

The typical patient was able to have the sphincter preserved, but the major prognostic factor appeared to be the size of the primary tumor. This should not be a surprise, and it may explain some of the differences of opinion that exist regarding anal carcinomas. It may well be that small primary lesions are adequately treated with radiation alone. However, the typical patient treated in this country has a lesion greater than 2 cm, and I think that, for most patients, combined-modality treatment will still be the appropriate way to go. However, for the selected patient who has a truly small lesion, radiation alone may be adequate. It remains important, of course, to try to preserve the sphincter and to avoid a colostomy if possible. Even then, the larger the lesion, the more difficult this is to achieve.

E. Glatstein, M.D.

Results of Combined Modality Therapy for Patients With Anal Cancer (E7283): An Eastern Cooperative Oncology Group Study
Martenson JA, Lipsitz SR, Lefkopoulou M, Engstrom PF, Dayal YY, Cobau CD, Oken MM, Haller DG (Mayo Clinic and Found, Rochester, Minn; Dana Farber Cancer Inst, Boston; Fox Chase Cancer Ctr, Philadelphia; et al)
Cancer 76:1731–1736, 1995   7–37

Objective.—Combined radiotherapy and multiagent chemotherapy were evaluated in 50 patients who had histologically documented invasive squamous cell carcinoma of the anal canal. The median patient age was 59 years.

Treatment.—Patients initially received 4,000 cGy of external-beam megavoltage therapy, given over 4–5 weeks, to the pelvis, anal sphincter, and the entire perineum. After a 2- to 3-week interval, a boost of 1,000–1,300 cGy was delivered at a depth of 5 cm through a direct perineal field. At the same time, patients received 5-fluorouracil (5-FU), 1,000 mg/m^2, IV each day for 4 days. On the second day, a rapid infusion of mitomycin-C, 10 mg/m^2, was delivered. A second course of 5-FU was administered after 28 days. An anal biopsy specimen was obtained 6–8 weeks after radiotherapy ended. If residual disease was present, abdominal-perineal resection was performed.

Results.—Disease was eliminated in 34 of 46 evaluable patients (74%), and 11 others had a partial response. Only 1 patient failed to respond. The response was confirmed histologically in 40 patients, 31 of whom were entirely free of disease. One patient who was thought to have a partial response also had negative biopsy results. Seven patients in all had tumor resection. The overall survival rate at 7 years was 58%, at which time 53% of partial responders remained alive. Fifty-three percent of the patients were free of disease progression at 7 years. More than one third of the patients had severe toxicity, and 2 patients had life-threatening hematologic toxicity, but there were no treatment-related deaths.

Conclusion.—Multimodality treatment is an effective approach to patients with anal cancer, but it most likely can be improved.

▶ Since the original report by Nigro and colleagues first appeared 20 years ago, suggesting that a combination of 5-FU, mitomycin-C, and external beam radiation therapy could cure many patients with anal squamous cell carcinoma and obviate abdominal perineal resection, there have been a large number of publications using variations of the original treatment protocol. Cure rates as high as 90% have been reported, but the length of follow-up for many of these studies is only 3–4 years. In this report of a multicenter trial, the Eastern Cooperative Oncology Group used one of the most common treatment schedules and doses and provided direct survival data at 7 years. Although a local control rate of 80% was obtained, the 7-year survival rate was only 58%.

There are many reports of the use of radiation therapy alone or combinations of chemoradiation therapy and cisplatin treatment, and almost all reports push the radiation dose to 55–60 Gy. It remains unclear as to whether these higher doses of radiation therapy—with or without more complex chemotherapy—will improve local control and overall survival yet preserve functional outcome.

A.M. Cohen, M.D.

The Whipple Resection for Cancer in U.S. Department of Veterans Affairs Hospitals
Wade TP, El-Ghazzawy AG, Virgo KS, Johnson FE (John Cochran VA Hosp, St Louis, Mo; St Louis Univ, Mo)
Ann Surg 221:241–248, 1995   7–38

Background.—Resecting tumors in the pancreatic head is technically difficult and dangerous, because any delay in primary healing can produce life-threatening complications. Pancreaticoduodenectomy, or the Whipple procedure, was studied in a large series of patients with periampullary adenocarcinomas.

Methods.—Computerized hospital and death benefits records were analzyed for patients undergoing Whipple resection between 1987 and 1991 in the United States Department of Veterans Affairs hospitals. Patients with lymphomas and neuroendocrine tumors were excluded. In 45% of the cancers, institutional tumor registrar reports permitted tumor/node/metastases (TNM) staging.

Findings.—Whipple resection were done in 252 patients with pancreatic cancer and in 117 patients with other periampullar cancers. Thirty-seven percent of the patients had complications. The 30-day operative mortality rate was 8%. The operative mortality rate associated with postoperative sepsis was higher. Among patients with staged tumors, only those without lymph node involvement were able to survive for 5 years or more.

Conclusions.—When tumor does not invade the lymph nodes, cancer that is in or near the head of the pancreas can be cured by Whipple resection. Almost 40% of the patients have complications. Operative mortality is associated with the mean age of the patient population.

▶ This report from highly experienced centers and individuals suggests that Whipple resection for periampullary cancer can be done with an extreme low mortality rate and a 5-year survival rate of approximately 20%. This very large multicenter report from the Department of Veterans Affairs Hospitals represents the end results from 159 hospitals, covering the recent period from 1987 to 1991. These data are probably more representative of what can be expected throughout the United States. The actuarial 5-year survival for pancreatic ductal cancer was only 9%, compared with 36% for those patients with bile duct and periampullary cancers. There were no 5-year survivors among node-positive patients with pancreatic cancer.

In sum, these data have shown a dramatic reduction in the mortality associated with pancreaticoduodenectomy when the operation is performed by experienced, but not specialized, surgeons within the Veterans Affairs hospital system. The data indicate that prolonged survival occurs but 5-year survivors are rare. They also indicate that in most centers, the Whipple resection is a palliative procedure, except for the subset of periampullary or bile duct cancers. As long as the morbidity and mortality are minimized, resection in selected patients continues to offer the best chance for long-term survival.

A.M. Cohen, M.D.

Pancreaticoduodenectomy for Cancer of the Head of the Pancreas: 201 Patients

Yeo CJ, Cameron JL, Lillemoe KD, Sitzmann JV, Hruban RH, Goodman SN, Dooley WC, Coleman J, Pitt HA (Johns Hopkins Med Insts, Baltimore, Md)
Ann Surg 221:721–733, 1995   7–39

Background.—Pancreaticoduodenectomy for pancreatic adenocarcinoma has recently been shown to reduce the morbidity and mortality associated with this disease. Some centers have reported 5-year survival rates of approximately 20%, although the factors influencing these improved rates have not been determined. All patients undergoing pancreaticoduodenal resection for adenocarcinoma of the pancreatic head at the Johns Hopkins Hospital from 1970 to April 1994 were, therefore, evaluated in an effort to identify the factors affecting long-term survival. The resultant report constitutes the largest single institution experience described in the literature thus far.

Patients and Findings.—Two hundred one patients (mean age, 63 years) with pathologically proven adenocarcinoma of the head of the pancreas were included. Pancreaticoduodenectomy was performed over 24 years, with the last 100 resections undertaken between 1991 and 1994. The median follow-up was 12 months. Overall, the postoperative in-hospital mortality rate was 5%. In the most recent 149 patients, however, mortality has been 0.7%. The actuarial 1-, 3-, and 5-year survival rates were 57%, 26%, and 21%, respectively, for all 201 patients (Fig 1). The median survival was 15.5 months. At 5 years, 11 patients were alive. Of the 143 patients with negative margins (curative resections), the actuarial 5-year survival rate was 26%; the median survival was 18 months. Actuarial and median survival rates were significantly worse among the 58 patients with positive margins (palliative resections), at 8% and 10 months, respectively. Improvement in survival has been observed over the study period, with a 14% 3-year actuarial survival rate noted in the 1970s, 21% in the 1980s,

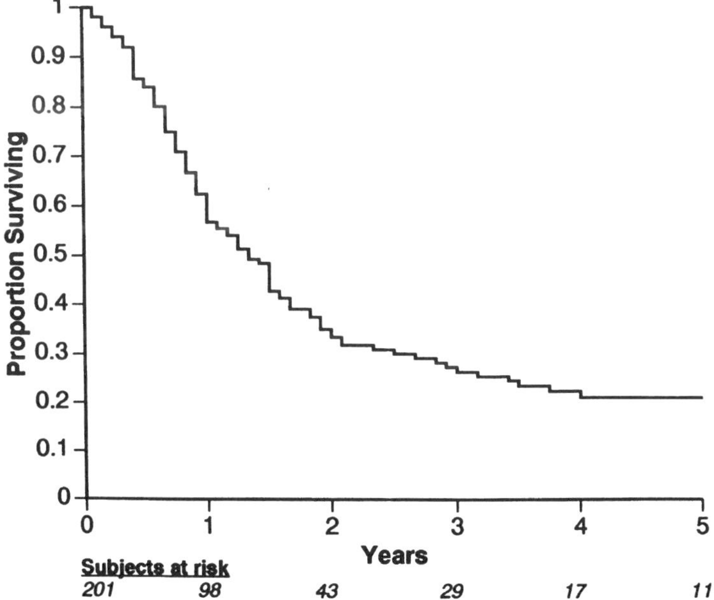

FIGURE 1.—Actuarial survival curve (Kaplan-Meier) for 201 patients undergoing pancreaticoduodenectomy for pancreatic adenocarcinoma. (Courtesy of Yeo CJ, Cameron JL, Lillemoe KD, et al: Pancreaticoduodenectomy for cancer of the head of the pancreas: 201 patients. *Ann Surg* 221:721–733, 1995.)

and 36% in the 1990s. As factors favoring long-term survival, univariate analysis identified tumor diameter of less than 3 cm, negative nodal status, diploid tumor DNA content, tumor S-phase fraction of less than 18%, pylorus-preserving resection, less than 800 mL of intraoperative blood loss, less than 2 units of blood transfused, negative resection margins, and use of postoperative adjuvant chemotherapy and radiation therapy. Diploid tumor DNA content, tumor diameter less than 3 cm, negative nodal status, negative resection margins, and decade of resection were found to be the strongest predictors of long-term survival on multivariate analysis.

Conclusion.—The survival rates in patients with pancreatic adenocarcinomas undergoing pancreaticoduodenectomy are increasing. The factors that are most predictive of outcome include DNA content, tumor diameter, and nodal and margin status, although postoperative combined modality chemoradiation also appears to influence long-term survival rates. The development of improved adjuvant therapy, such as strategies that combine chemoradiation with immunotherapy, may help to further increase survival in these patients.

▶ These authors report the largest single-institution study of pancreaticoduodenectomy for pancreatic adenocarcinoma, representing the experience with 201 patients at the Johns Hopkins Hospital over 24 years. They demonstrate an ongoing reduction in the in-hospital mortality rate, now less than 1% in the last 149 patients. The overall actuarial survival rate at 5 years was 21%. Tumor size was important, with a doubling in the survival rate for patients with tumors less than 3 cm. The survival rate for node-negative patients was 2.5-fold greater than that for those with positive nodes. Dr. Cameron and his colleagues at John Hopkins have demonstrated that, in expert hands, pancreaticoduodenectomy for cancer of the head of the pancreas offers palliation with a low mortality rate and a modest likelihood for cure. These data present an excellent baseline for the development of adjuvant therapies in this highly lethal disease.

A.M. Cohen, M.D.

Relation of Perioperative Deaths to Hospital Volume Among Patients Undergoing Pancreatic Resection for Malignancy
Lieberman MD, Kilburn H, Lindsey M, Brennan MF (Mem Sloan-Kettering Cancer Ctr, New York; Dept of Health Care Research and Information Services, Albany, NY)
Ann Surg 222:638–645, 1995   7–40

Objective.—Reported improvements in the operative mortality associated with major pancreatic resection, along with the lack of other treatments, support the use of such resections in patients with pancreatic cancer. However, individual surgeons or centers can have only limited experience with these operations, which raises questions as to whether the results achieved by specialized centers can be extrapolated to less experienced hospitals. The number of pancreatic resections performed by hospitals and surgeons was evaluated for its impact on perioperative mortality.

Methods.—The analysis included discharge abstracts of 1,972 patients who underwent pancreaticoduodenectomy or total pancreatotomy for cancer in New York State from 1984 to 1991. The possible associations of hospital and surgeon experience with perioperative outcome were assessed by logistic regression analysis. Hospitals were classified according to the minimal number of such resections performed in a given year: less than 10 cases, minimal volume; 10–50 cases, low volume; 51–80 cases, medium volume; and 81 or more cases, high volume. Surgeons were classified as low volume if they had less than 9 cases; medium volume, 9–41 cases; and high volume, more than 41 cases.

Results.—More than three fourths of patients were treated at minimal- or low-volume centers. These 2 groups of hospitals made up 98% of the institutions treating peripancreatic cancer. There were only 2 high-volume hospitals, which had a perioperative mortality rate of 4%. This was significantly lower than the 22% mortality rate at minimal-volume hospitals and the 12% mortality rate at low-volume hospitals (Fig 2).

Patients who underwent surgery performed by low-volume surgeons had a perioperative mortality rate of 16% compared with a rate of 5% for surgery done by high-volume surgeons. Perioperative death was significantly related to hospital volume of pancreatic resections on logistic regression analysis. After control for hospital volume, surgeon experience was not significantly related to mortality.

Conclusion.—Hospital experience with pancreatic resection has a major impact on perioperative mortality after such procedures. The results suggest that some defined minimal hospital experience should be observed for

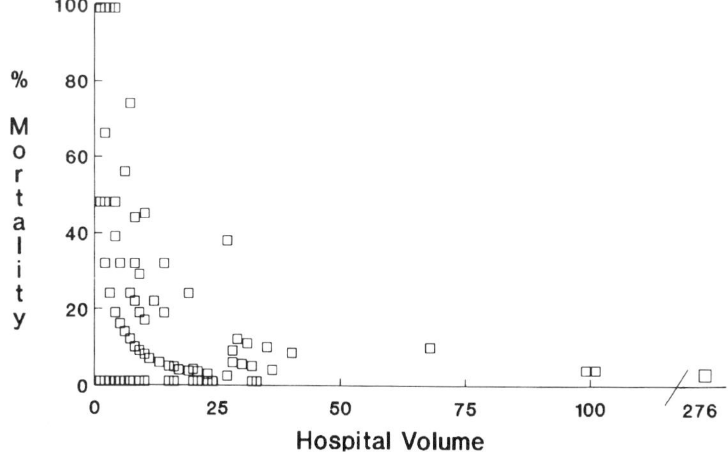

FIGURE 2.—Scattergram of crude in-hospital mortality rates according to hospital volume. (Courtesy of Lieberman MD, Kilburn H, Lindsey M, et al: Relation of perioperative deaths to hospital volume among patients undergoing pancreatic resection for malignancy. *Ann Surg* 222:638–645, 1995.)

elective pancreatotomy. The data represent a first step in efforts to include outcome information in cost-effectiveness analysis.

▶ This New York State–wide analysis of the mortality associated with radical pancreaticoduodenectomy (Whipple procedure) or total pancreatectomy in the time frame of 1984–1991 supports the marked reduction in operative mortality by both surgeons as well as institutions that performed such procedures on a frequent basis. Figure 2 demonstrates graphically the mortality differences.

It will be interesting to see just how generic such data are. Are there marked differences in mortality in relation to hospital or surgical volume for esophagogastrectomy, major hepatic resection, major rectal resection, radical prostatectomy, cystectomy, etc.? Radical pancreatic resection is associated with a low mortality rate in experienced hands and at high-volume institutions. However, there remains a very high morbidity rate associated with such procedures. Management of morbidity to avoid a subsequent mortality is a very important part of patient management.

A.M. Cohen, M.D.

Long-Term Survival After Resection for Ductal Adenocarcinoma of the Pancreas: Is It Really Improving?

Nitecki SS, Sarr MG, Colby TV, van Heerden JA (Mayo Clinic, Rochester, Minn)
Ann Surg 221:59–66, 1995   7–41

Objective.—Ductile pancreatic adenocarcinoma is almost always fatal. Even after surgical resection, the 5-year survival rate is less than 10%. However, at some centers, increased 5-year survival rates have been reported in selected patients undergoing curative resection. These reports prompted a retrospective review of a 10-year experience.

Methods.—The medical records were reviewed of 174 patients with ductile adenocarcinoma (aged, 34–82 years) who underwent curative resection. The average follow-up after surgery was 22 months. Specimens from the 31 three-year survivors were reexamined histologically.

Results.—Operative procedures included 123 (71%) pancreatoduodenectomies, total pancreatectomies in 20% of patients, and pancreaticoduodenectomies in 9%. Incomplete resections accounted for 16%. Fifty-six percent of patients had lymph node involvement, 21% had duodenal invasion, and 12% had perineural invasion. The operative mortality rate was 3%. Morbidity was 33%. The overall 5-year survival was 6.8%, and median survival was 17.5 months (Fig 2). Patients without nodal metastases had a significantly greater 5-year survival advantage than did node-positive patients. Also, patients with smaller tumors had a significantly greater 5-year survival advantage than did patients with large tumors (Fig 5). In the 40% of patients who had complete resections, no lymph node involvement, and no tumor invasion, the 5-year survival rate

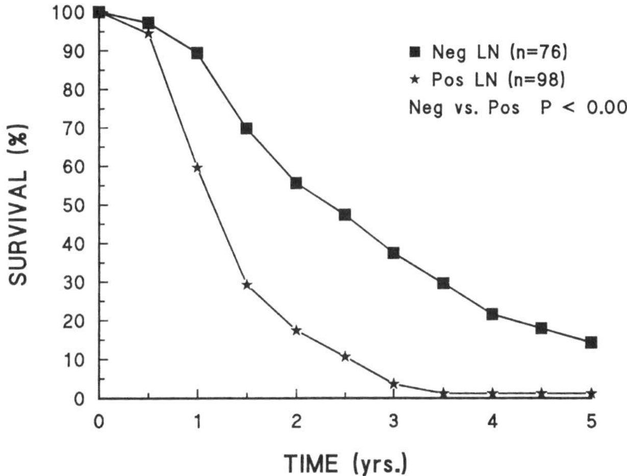

FIGURE 2.—Actuarial 5-year survival rate, according to lymph node involvement. (Courtesy of Nitecki SS, Sarr MG, Colby TV, et al: Long-term survival after resection for ductal adenocarcinoma of the pancreas: Is it really improving? *Ann Surg* 221:59–66, 1995.)

was 23%. Twelve patients who were originally excluded because they did not have pancreatic cancer had a mean survival of 53 months compared with patients with pancreatic cancer, whose mean survival was 17.5 months.

Conclusion.—The overall 5-year survival rate was 7% for patients in this study. In patients with negative nodes and no invasive tumors, the

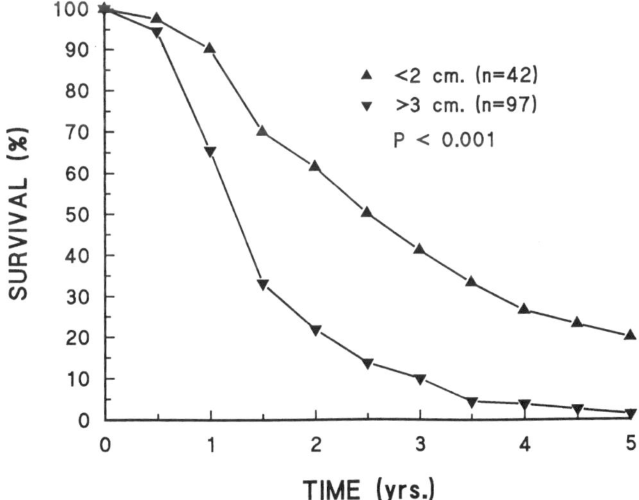

FIGURE 5.—Actuarial 5-year survival according to tumor size. (Courtesy of Nitecki SS, Sarr MG, Colby TV, et al: Long-term survival after resection for ductal adenocarcinoma of the pancreas: Is it really improving? *Ann Surg* 221:59–66, 1995.)

5-year survival rate was 23%. Tumor staging is an important prognostic indicator. Pathologic re-review is very important.

▶ This article presents the long-term survival data from a major medical center's extensive contemporary experience with resection of ductal adenocarcinoma of the pancreas. The authors noted that a number of recent reports have indicated that as many as one quarter of patients undergoing resection achieve long-term survival. Because that did not seem to be the experience at their center, they undertook a "re-review" of their experience.

On additional study, a number of patients who were originally characterized as having ductal adenocarcinoma were found to have either islet cell tumors, ampullary carcinoma, or other nonductal cancers and, therefore, were excluded. Despite a hospital mortality of only 3%, the overall actuarial 5-year survival was only approximately 7%. Very few node-positive patients or patients with cancers larger than 3 cm survived more then 3 years.

These data indicate that, except for the relatively uncommon, small, node-negative ductal adenocarcinoma of the head of the pancreas, most patients cannot be cured of their disease by radical surgery. However, in experienced hands with a low mortality, radical resection likely offers both excellent palliation and a small chance for cure for the patient with obstructive jaundice. It is likely that major improvements in survival will depend on an adjuvant chemotherapy program that is effective, which is something that does not exist at this time.

A.M. Cohen, M.D.

Hepatocellular Carcinoma and Cirrhosis in 746 Patients: Long-Term Results of Percutaneous Ethanol Injection

Livraghi T, Giorgio A, Marin G, Salmi A, de Sio I, Bolondi L, Pompili M, Brunello F, Lazzaroni S, Torzilli G, Zucchi A (Ospedale Civile, Milan, Italy; Ospedale Cotugno, Naples, Italy; Ospedale Monoblocco, Padua, Italy; et al)
Radiology 197:101–108, 1995   7–42

Background.—Percutaneous injection of ethanol (PEI) has become a widely used treatment for cirrhosis of the liver and relatively early hepatocellular carcinoma (HCC). However, there have been no large, sufficiently stratified reports of long-term survival after this treatment. The indications for PEI were assessed in a long-term follow-up study.

Methods.—The study included 746 patients who underwent PEI from 1985 to 1993 at 9 Italian centers. There were 567 men and 179 women (mean age, 64 years). The Child cirrhosis class was A in 458 patients, B in 234, C in 41, and unknown in 13. Four hundred seventy patients had a single HCC measuring 5 cm or less, 204 had multiple tumors, and 22 had advanced tumors. Seven hundred ten patients received conventional, multisession ultrasonography-guided PEI on an outpatient basis. The other 36

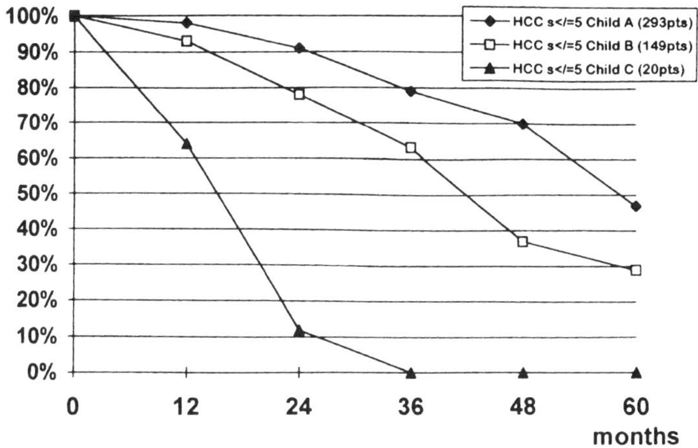

Months	0		12		24		36		48		60	
Stage HCC - Child	% Cum Survival	Pts	% Cum Survival	Pts	% Cum Survival	Pts	% Cum Survival	Pts	% Cum Survival	Pts	% Cum Survival	Pts
s</=5 - Child A	100	293	98	260	91	179	79	117	70	77	47	20
s</=5 - Child B	100	149	93	125	78	75	63	40	37	12	29	5
s</=5 - Child C	100	20	64	12	12	1	0	0	0	0	0	0

FIGURE 2.—Five-year cumulative survival curves for patients with single hepatocellular carcinomas (HCCs) 5 cm or smaller in diameter stratified according to Child class. (Courtesy of Livraghi T, Giorgio A, Marin G, et al: Hepatocellular carcinoma and cirrhosis in 746 patients: Long-term results of percutaneous ethanol injection. *Radiology* 197:101–108, 1995. Radiological Society of North America.)

patients had multiple injections of PEI in a single session. The patients were followed for a mean of 36 months.

Results.—For patients with Child class A cirrhosis and a single HCC measuring 5 cm or smaller, survival was 79% at 3 years and 47% at 5 years. Survival was 63% at 3 years and 29% at 5 years for patients with Child class B and a single small HCC; it was 0% for both time periods for those with Child class C and the same HCC characteristics (Fig 2). Among patients with Child class A cirrhosis, the 3-year survival rate was 47% for multiple HCCs, 53% for single HCCs larger than 5 cm, and 16% for advanced HCC. Survival figures at 5 years for these groups were 26%, 30%, and 0%, respectively. The PEI treatment carried a severe complication rate of 1.7% and a mortality rate of 0.1%.

Conclusion.—For patients with cirrhosis and HCC, PEI is a safe, effective, repeatable, and inexpensive procedure. The resulting survival rate is similar to that of surgery. Although randomized studies are lacking, PEI is recommended as the treatment of choice for most patients recruited at ultrasonography screening, except for those who are candidates for orthotopic liver transplantation and surgical resection.

▶ The major treatment options for HCC in patients with cirrhosis include surgical resection, cryosurgery, arterial chemoembolization, orthotopic liver transplantation, and PEI. Readers are referred to the original article for an excellent and detailed analysis not only of the PEI technique but, also, the results achieved with other treatment modalities. Patients with HCC and Child class C cirrhosis will likely die within 2 years of their cirrhosis. The major cause of death for patients with HCC with either Child class A or B cirrhosis is progression of cancer. The PEI data presented in this article demonstrate survival rates comparable to those of surgical resection with a very safe and repeatable modality at low cost. The more recent use of multiple side-hold needles and multiple planes of injection may further improve the local control with PEI.

A.M. Cohen, M.D.

Hepatic Resection for Metastic Neuroendocrine Carcinomas
Que FG, Nagorney DM, Batts KP, Linz LJ, Kvols LK (Mayo Clinic and Found, Rochester, Minn)
Am J Surg 169:36–43, 1995   7–43

Objective.—Hepatic resection for metastatic neuroendocrine malignancy is appealing because the course of the disease is long, complete resection is possible, and severity of disease is related to tumor volume. The safe and effective use of this procedure as primary treatment for symptomatic patients in whom complete resection was possible was documented in a retrospective study.

Methods.—Hepatic resections, including right, left, and extended hepatectomies and nonanatomical resections, were performed on 74 patients (age, 25–77 years) between 1984 and 1992. Tumor type and grade were established. Patient outcomes were assessed.

Results.—There were 50 carcinoid tumors, 8 glucagonomas, 7 multi-hormonal islet cell carcinomas, 5 nonfunctioning islet cell carcinomas, 2 gastrinomas, and 1 insulinoma. One patient's tumor was classified as a neuroendocrine malignancy. The resections that were performed included 22 right or left hepatectomies, 7 right or left hepatectomies with anatomical extensions, 7 right or left hepatectomies with nonanatomical extensions, and 38 nonanatomical resections. Primary tumors were concurrently resected in 37 patients. The postoperative mortality rate was 2.7%, and morbidity was 24%. The overall survival rate was 73% at 4 years, and the mean follow-up was 2.2 years. Twelve patients died with evidence of tumor progression. There was no significant difference in survival between patients who had curative surgery and those who had palliative surgery. Fourteen of 23 symptomatic patients remained asymptomatic after surgery. Intent of resection, tumor grade, and tumor type were not significantly associated with survival.

Conclusion.—Hepatic resection for metastatic neuroendocrine malignancy is safe and appears to prolong survival.

▶ These authors report an extensive experience with a highly controversial operative procedure. Most, but not all, of the patients were highly symptomatic. Patients had recurrent symptoms develop between 8 and 58 months after liver resection, at a mean interval of 20 months. The authors provide no quality-of-life data. In their institution, they have a large referral practice for neuroendocrine tumors metastatic to the liver. Many of these tumors have been treated by a long-acting somatostatin analogue, acute or intermittent hepatic artery occlusion, and/or systemic chemotherapy. They provide no comparative data regarding the use total or subtotal hepatic resection of all metastatic diseases of the liver compared with the use of other modalities. However, because their pattern of practice is such that patients generally have not been referred unless they are refractory to other approaches, it is likely that surgical resection plays a role in highly selective symptomatic patients.

As the authors stress and I strongly agree, an aggressive preoperative evaluation and analysis should indicate that at least 90% of the tumor should be resectable. Ideally, the patient should undergo resection only if all the tumor in the liver can be eradicated. These patients appear to be an ideal group to consider for subtotal resection and cryosurgical ablation of the remaining tumor to treat all disease within the liver. Further studies should provide more detailed analyses of prior treatment to assess the sequential treatment strategy of the various modalities, such as chemotherapy, hepatic artery embolization, hepatic artery ligation, cryosurgery, somatostatin, and subsequent resection.

A.M. Cohen, M.D.

Hepatic Resection for Hepatocellular Carcinoma: An Audit of 343 Patients
Lai ECS, Fan S-T, Lo C-M, Chu K-M, Liu C-L, Wong J (Univ of Hong Kong)
Ann Surg 221:291–298, 1995   7–44

Background.—Hepatic resection has generally been viewed as the only treatment option that offers a chance of long-term survival for patients with hepatocellular carcinoma (HCC). Because of early detection of cancer and technologic advances, strategies for the surgical treatment of patients with primary liver cancer have continuously evolved. A 22-year experience with hepatectomy for HCC was reviewed.

Methods.—The analysis included 343 patients with HCC who were undergoing hepatic resection at a Hong Kong hospital. One hundred forty-nine patients were treated from 1972 to 1987, 128 from 1987 to 1991, and 66 from 1992 to the present; these periods reflected changes in perioperative management. For survival analysis, the patients were stratified into 2 categories: before or after 1987. Seventy-eight percent of the patients had large tumors, 73% had cirrhosis, and 73% had a major hepatectomy. The results were assessed both in the perioperative period and during subsequent follow-up.

TABLE 6.—Long-Term Outcome of Patients With Hepatocellular Carcinoma Who Had Hepatectomy Between 1972 and 1994

	Survival†		Disease-Free Survival		Survival After Recurrence†	
Survival	Before 1987	After 1987	Before 1987	After 1987	Before 1987	After 1987
1 yr (%)	48	68	34.7	35.9	18.3	45.6
3 yr (%)	21	44	14.9	22.8	7.9	16.5
5 yr (%)	14	35	8.9	22.8	6.6	NA
Median (mo)	12.3	25.9	7.8	4.7	3.5	10.3

† $P < .001$.

(Courtesy of Lai ECS, Fan S-T, Lo C-M, et al: Hepatic resection for hepatocellular carcinoma: An audit of 343 patients. *Ann Surg* 221:291–298, 1995.)

Results.—The resectability rate improved from 14% at the beginning of the study to 23% at the end. The morbidity rate decreased significantly (from 73% to 32%), and the hospital mortality rate decreased from 21.5% to 6%. The 30-day mortality rate decreased nonsignificantly, from 14% to 4.5%. The surgical approach used in the latter part of the series was a significant contributor to the reduced hospital mortality rate. Survival was significantly better for patients treated after 1987; survival rates at 1, 3, and 5 years were 68%, 44%, and 35%, respectively, for the more recently treated patients (Table 6). The improvement in prognosis was attributed to early detection and effective treatment for recurrences.

Conclusion.—Technologic advances and newer management strategies have improved the results of hepatic resection for patients with HCC. The newer surgical techniques used include a bilateral subcostal incision, meticulous attention to guard against bleeding and bile leakage, and use of an ultrasonic dissector to transect the hepatic parenchyma. Further improvements in prognosis might be possible through prevention of the frequent recurrences; because of socioeconomic obstacles, liver transplantation is not a viable option for patients with HCC in Asia.

▶ This report from Queen Mary Hospital in Hong Kong describes an extensive experience with resection for HCC. The authors compared 3 intervals at their institution from the perspective of morbidity, mortality, and end results. Three quarters of their patients had cirrhosis, and more than 80% were positive for hepatitis B surface antigen. Their major complication rate has decreased from 73% to 32%, and the mortality rate has decreased from 14% to 4.5%. The overall in-hospital mortality rate in the most recent time frame (the last 66 patients) was 6%. One third of the patients will survive 5 years.

It is important to keep these data for comparison purposes when other modalities are selected for treatment of such patients. Small tumors that are less than several centimeters, particularly tumors detected by ultrasound or α-fetoprotein screening programs, may be effectively treated by percutaneous injection of ethanol. Larger tumors, multifocal tumors, or those in patients with end-stage cirrhosis have been treated by transplantation. This report documents the appropriateness of resective surgery with a relatively low acceptable morbidity, minimal mortality, and very acceptable long-term survival.

A.M. Cohen, M.D.

Factors Affecting Long-Term Outcome After Hepatic Resection for Hepatocellular Carcinoma
Vauthey J-N, Klimstra D, Franceschi D, Tao Y, Fortner J, Blumgart L, Brennan M (Mem Sloan-Kettering Cancer Ctr, New York; Univ of Florida, Gainesville)
Am J Surg 169:28–35, 1995   7–45

Background.—Experience with hepatocellular carcinoma (HCC) is limited in the West. The factors influencing outcome after resection are not clearly defined. A large series of patients who underwent complete resection for HCC was reviewed.

Patients and Findings.—One hundred six patients underwent hepatic resection between 1970 and 1992 for HCC at Memorial Sloan-Kettering Cancer Center. Thirty-three percent had cirrhosis. Ninety-five percent were Child-Pugh A. The overall operative mortality was 6% to 14% in patients with cirrhosis and 1% in patients without cirrhosis. Compared with whites, Asians had a greater prevalence of cirrhosis and smaller tumors. The overall survival was 41% at 5 years and 32% at 10 years. In a univariate analysis, greater survival rates were associated with the absence of vascular invasion, absence of symptoms, solitary tumor, negative margins, small tumor, and the presence of tumor capsule. Survival was unaffected by ethnic origin, cirrhosis, necrosis, or grade. According to a multivariate analysis, only vascular invasion predicted outcome.

Conclusions.—One third of the patients with HCC undergoing resection can be expected to survive in the long term. There were no major histopathologic or prognostic differences between Asians and whites undergoing resection, aside from a greater incidence of cirrhosis in Asians. Survival was not adversely affected by early cirrhosis. Long-term outcome was predicted by vascular invasion.

▶ These authors present an analysis of a retrospective review of patients undergoing hepatic resection over 22 years at a single institution. Almost all the patients were symptomatic, and 95% were Child-Pugh class A. Only one third had frank cirrhosis. A great deal of univariate analysis data are provided. Vascular invasion, the presence of a single tumor vs. multiple tumors, impacted on survival. It is of interest that there was no difference as to ethnic origin (Asian or white), whether they had cirrhosis, were hepatitis B–positive, or had elevation in their α-fetoprotein level. In a multivariate analysis, the absence of vascular invasion predicted long-term outcome.

Most importantly, these patients underwent resection with an operative mortality of only 6% overall. Kaplan-Meier survival at 5 years is 41%, which is very encouraging. Between 5 and 10 years, there was continued mortality related to second primary, late recurrences, or liver failure. The data support an aggressive approach in the resection of selected patients with hepato-cellular carcinoma.

A.M. Cohen, M.D.

Hepatic Cryosurgery in Treating Colorectal Metastases
Weaver ML, Atkinson D, Zemel R (Allegheny Gen Hosp, Pittsburgh, Pa)
Cancer 76:210–214, 1995   7–46

Background.—In patients with hepatic metastases from colorectal ad-enocarcinoma, adding cryosurgical ablation to surgical resection may im-prove disease-free survival. A preliminary analysis of 47 patients treated between November 1987 and February 1992 was reported.

Methods.—The patients were 31 men and 16 women (age, 31–75 years). Documented metastases limited to the liver from colorectal adenocarci-noma were treated with cryosurgery with or without resection. Follow-up ranged from 24 to 57 months, with a median of 26 months. The lesions were mapped and cryoprobes were placed under the guidance of intraop-erative ultrasonography. Each lesion was frozen to $-196°C$ for 15 min-utes, thawed for 10 minutes, and frozen again for 15 minutes. Follow-up CT scans were obtained before patients were discharged from the hospital and 6 months and 1 year after cryosurgery. Carcinoembryonic antigen concentrations were determined every month.

Findings.—The median length of hospitalization was 10 days. Actual 24-month survival was 62%. At a median of 30 months, 11% of the patients had no evidence of disease. Complications of treatment included myoglobinuria, coagulopathy, pleural effusions, and bile duct injuries. Two patients (4%) died of multisystem organ failure with irreversible coagulopathies.

Conclusion.—The number of patients with liver metastases who may become free of disease is increased by cryosurgical ablation. Studies with longer follow-ups are needed to determine the effect on overall survival.

▶ Cryosurgery for hepatic tumors, particularly colorectal metastases, is currently being widely performed because of the general availability of the technology. Both the cryosurgical equipment and intraoperative ultrasound are necessary to define the extent of tumor freezing. This report from one of the major centers with experience in using this technique has a median follow-up of just more than 2 years. It puts into perspective the expected benefits in terms of control of tumor in the liver in comparison with rather considerable complications, including a 4% mortality rate. As a result of animal data, the authors have doubly frozen and thawed each lesion to maximize benefit. The data suggest that cryosurgery will ultimately play some role in the control of hepatic cancer, but such treatment is complex, expensive, and associated with considerable morbidity and mortality. As is the case with surgical resection, long-term survival will await more effective "adjuvant" chemotherapy after cryoablation.

A.M. Cohen, M.D.

Superior Staging of Liver Tumors With Laparoscopy and Laparoscopic Ultrasound

John TG, Greig JD, Crosbie JL, Miles WFA, Garden OJ (Univ of Edinburgh, Scotland)
Ann Surg 220:711–719, 1994   7–47

Background.—Laparoscopy may be useful for selecting patients with intra-abdominal malignancies to undergo surgical intervention. Laparoscopic ultrasonography, a new technique that combines the principles of high resolution intraoperative contact ultrasonography with those of the laparoscopic assessment, enables laparoscopists to make detailed assessments of the liver. Laparoscopic contact ultrasonography was compared with staging laparoscopy in the preoperative evaluation of patients with liver tumors. The impact of laparoscopic ultrasonography on patient selection for hepatic resection with curative intent was also determined.

Methods.—A cohort of 50 patients with a diagnosis of potentially resectable liver tumors was analyzed. Staging laparoscopy was successful in all patients. Laparoscopic ultrasonography was done in 43 patients.

Findings.—In 46% of the patients, laparoscopy identified factors that precluded curative resection. In 33%, laparoscopic ultrasonography showed liver tumors that were not visible during laparoscopy. It provided additional staging information for 42% of the patients (Fig 3). The resectability rate among patients undergoing laparoscopic staging was 93%, which is significantly higher than the rate of 58% achieved with operative assessment without laparoscopy.

Conclusions.—Patient selection for curative liver resection is optimized by staging laparoscopy with laparoscopic ultrasonography. More prospec-

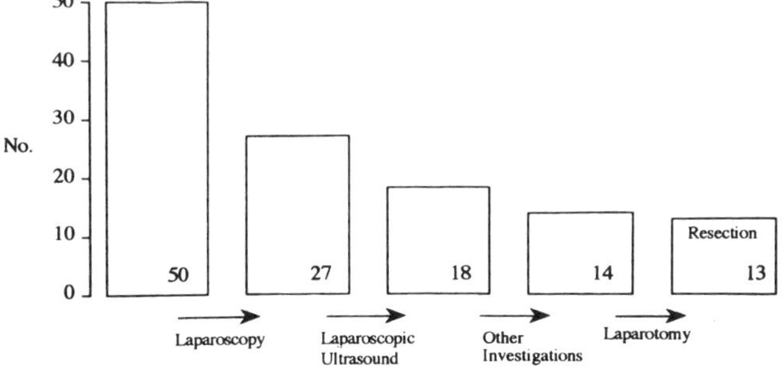

FIGURE 3.—Schematic diagram to illustrate patient selection for operative assessment of the resectability of liver tumors in 50 consecutive patients in whom laparoscopy with laparoscopic ultrasonography was undertaken. (Courtesy of John TG, Greig JD, Crosbie JL, et al: Superior staging of liver tumors with laparoscopy and laparoscopic ultrasound. *Ann Surg* 220:711–719, 1994.)

tive comparisons of laparoscopic ultrasonography with existing imaging modalities are needed to further clarify the exact role of this rapidly evolving method.

▶ Small subsets of patients with primary liver cancer or hepatic metastases from other primary sites can be cured by surgical resection. From a quality-of-life perspective as well as a cost-consideration analysis, "exploratory laparotomy" without resection should be minimized. The existing extent of disease evaluation is quite effective in ruling out extra-abdominal tumors. However, although the hepatic extent of disease evaluation by CT/MRI is quite accurate, intraoperative ultrasound appears to have the highest resolution in detecting lesions at the 5-mm level. In addition, CT scanning is unreliable with regard to the portal lymph nodes and peritoneal seeding.

Figure 3 demonstrates the value of laparoscopy in the determination of the resectability of both hepatic and extrahepatic disease. It also shows that the incremental benefit of laparoscopic ultrasound results in a resectability rate greater than 90%.

Not all of the patients underwent CT portography, which is currently the most accurate method of determining the extent of disease in the liver with the use of CT. None of the patients underwent MRI, however, when considering cost as well as efficacy, it appears that patients with potential resectable liver tumors should have the abdomen assessed by abdominal CT (plus or minus pelvic CT), subsequent CT portography followed by laparoscopy with laparoscopic ultrasound prior to attempted resection.

A.M. Cohen, M.D.

Percutaneous Hepatic Vein Isolation and High-Dose Hepatic Arterial Infusion Chemotherapy for Unresectable Liver Tumors

Ravikumar TS, Pizzorno G, Bodden W, Marsh J, Strair R, Pollack J, Hendler R, Hanna J, D'Andrea E (Yale School of Medicine, New Haven, Conn)
J Clin Oncol 12:2723–2736, 1994   7–48

Background.—Primary and metastatic liver tumors are significant contributors to cancer-related mortality. Because hepatic tumors do not respond significantly to systemic treatment, regional chemotherapy has been attempted. A percutaneous isolated chemotherapy perfusion approach for treating advanced primary and metastatic liver tumors was evaluated in a prospective, nonrandomized trial.

Methods.—Twenty-three patients were initially enrolled in the study. Chemotherapy was delivered through a hepatic artery catheter. Hepatic venous blood was isolated by a novel percutaneous double-balloon inferior vena cava catheter passed through a detoxification/filtration cartridge in a venovenous bypass circuit. A total of 58 procedures were performed on 21 patients. Twelve received fluorouracil (5-FU) dose escalations, and 9 received doxorubicin dose escalations. All were given 2 treatments every 3 weeks. Additional treatments were given when stabilization or response was noted.

Findings.—Dose was directly correlated with the peak concentration of drug entering the hepatic veins. The system functioned efficiently throughout the dose range. Extraction efficiencies ranged from 64% to 91%. The hepatic vein drug levels demonstrated a sixfold increase in 5-FU, with dose escalation from 1,000 to 5,000 mg/m^2. There was a twofold increase in doxorubicin, with dose escalations of 50 to 120 mg/m^2. Treatment required only an overnight hospital stay. There were no treatment-related deaths. The most common toxicity associated with treatment was transient hypotension, caused by catecholamine depletion by the filter. Dose-limiting toxicity was noted in patients given 5-FU at a dose of 5,000 mg/m^2 and doxorubicin at a dose of 120 mg/m^2. Two patients receiving doxorubicin at doses of 90 mg/m^2 and 120 mg/m^2 had significant tumor responses.

Conclusions.—The use of a double-balloon catheter to isolate and detoxify hepatic venous blood during intra-arterial treatment is safe and technically practicable. This procedure allows large doses of intrahepatic chemotherapy to be administered at short intervals. It should also permit new dose-intensification strategies to enhance tumor responses in primary and metastatic liver tumors.

▶ In the majority of patients with primary liver cancer, the cancer is unresectable because of the presence of cirrhosis or because of the extent of the cancer. Overall, one third of patients with colon cancer hepatic metastases die with tumor limited only to the liver. An additional one third of patients die with liver-predominant recurrence. In a small subset of patients with primary or metastatic liver cancer, resection and cure are possible. In patients who are not able to undergo resection, alternatives such as alcohol injection, arterial embolization, cryosurgery, and regional chemotherapy may be partially effective. Unfortunately, many of these tumors are relatively resistant to systemic chemotherapy or hepatic artery infusional chemotherapy.

The concept of isolation perfusion is an extremely attractive strategy for delivering high-dose-rate chemotherapy only to the organ of interest. However, surgical isolation perfusion is a complex operative procedure, and it is quite difficult to provide repeated treatments. In addition, the presence of "leakage" outside the regional system can produce systemic toxicity. This paper describes an exciting advance in regional treatment of unresectable liver tumors by combining a percutaneous isolation perfusion system with a charcoal detoxification to minimize systemic effects. The study is primarily a phase I trial demonstrating impressive improvements in the AUC (the pharmacokinetic area under the curve). Even within the phase I study, there were several dramatic regressions in patients who received doxorubicin.

The treatment program is complicated and involves a multidisciplinary approach with surgeons, medical oncologists, interventional radiologists, and anesthesiologists. However, the logistics appear solvable, and this may represent a useful strategy for patients with liver cancer.

A.M. Cohen, M.D.

Postoperative Prophylactic Lipiodolization Reduces the Intrahepatic Recurrence of Hepatocellular Carcinoma

Takenaka K, Yoshida K, Nishizaki T, Korenaga D, Hiroshige K, Ikeda T, Sugimachi K (Fukuoka City Hosp, Japan; Kyushu Univ, Fukuoka, Japan)
Am J Surg 169:400–405, 1995   7–49

Introduction.—Despite early detection of hepatocellular carcinoma (HCC), the recurrence rates after resection are still high, and regional prophylactic chemotherapy of the remnant liver increases the disease-free survival rate. Little is known about postoperative adjuvant chemotherapy for HCC in patients with liver cirrhosis. The effectiveness of orally administered systemic chemotherapy was compared with that of prophylactic lipiodolization to determine the most promising postoperative adjuvant chemotherapy for suppressing the recurrence of HCC in patients with cirrhosis. The term lipiodolization refers to the administration of chemotherapeutic agents suspended in an oily contrast medium (ethyl ester of fatty acid from poppy seed oil) and given through feeder arteries.

Methods.—From 1989 to 1992, 48 patients who had hepatic resection were divided into 3 groups: 12 were given orally administered chemotherapy (300 to 400 mg of 5-fluorouracil (5-FU) derivatives daily, either l-hexylcarbamoyl-5-FU or uracil and tegafur; 17 were given prophylactic lipiodolization, 1.8 times on average, using a 44-mg mean dose of epirubicin per treatment; and 19 controls were not given chemotherapy.

Results.—In the 48 patients, recurrence was found in 23 remnant livers. The 3-year, disease-free survival rate was 15% for the controls, 50% for the patients given orally administered chemotherapy, and 86% for the prophylactic lipiodolization patients (Fig 3). Compared with the controls and the patients given orally administered chemotherapy, the patients

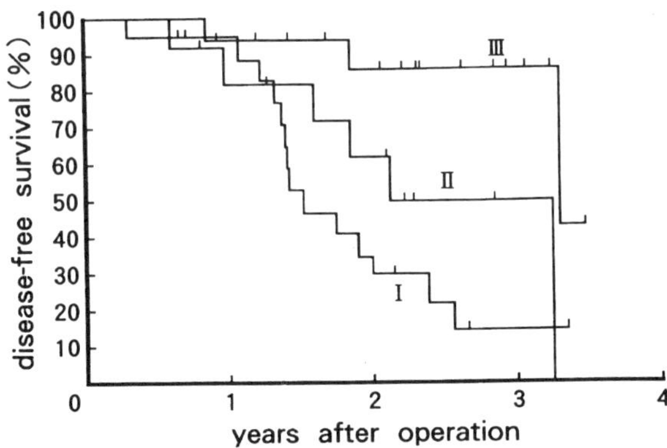

FIGURE 3.—The crude disease-free survival rate of patients with hepatocellular carcinoma divided into 3 groups according to postoperative chemotherapy. The control group (1) received no chemotherapy (*n* = 19); the OC group (II) received 30 to 400 mg of oral 5-fluorouracil derivatives daily (*n* = 12); the PL group (III) underwent prophylactic lipiodolization 1.8 times on average, using a 44-mg mean dose of epirubicin per treatment (*n* = 17). The *P* values from comparisons of the curves were: I vs. II, .249; II vs. III, .025; I vs. III, .001, respectively, as analyzed by the log rank test. (Courtesy of Takenaka K, Yoshida K, Nishizaki T, et al: Postoperative prophylactic lipiodolization reduces the intrahepatic recurrence of hepatocellular carcinoma. *Am J Surg* 169:400–405, Copyright 1995 by Excerpta Medica Inc.)

given the prophylactic lipiodolization had a significantly higher disease-free survival curve. As a background analysis, 25 variables were studied, such as tumor size, number of tumors, and hours for operative procedures; no statistical differences were found, nor were any differences found in the survival curves of the 3 groups.

Conclusion.—For reducing intrahepatic recurrence after resection, prophylactic lipiodolization was found to be an effective treatment for patients with HCC. By performing lipiodolization once or twice during the year after resection with a small dose of anticancer agents, intrahepatic recurrence can be reduced; however, to more fully evaluate the effectiveness of this procedure, a further randomized, prospective study using more patients with a sufficient liver function or a good performance status is necessary.

▶ The authors present a nonrandomized comparison of surgery alone, oral chemotherapy, and hepatic artery chemotherapy using intermittent epirubicin dissolved in lipid contrast medium after potentially curable resection of HCC. The trial design makes any definitive comments with regard to efficacy unrealistic. However, the groups are quite comparable, particularly with regard to liver function and the presence of cirrhosis. These obviously are highly selected patients, because in all groups, the actuarial 3-year survival rate exceeded 80%. However, there was a dramatic reduction in hepatic recurrence in the adjuvant lipid contrast chemotherapy group.

With our increasing ability to achieve ablation of HCC in the patient who has cirrhosis by using either segmental resection, cryosurgery, or injection of ethanol, an effective adjuvant therapy for this often multifocal disease is warranted. The data presented are adequate to justify a randomized clinical trial of such adjuvant therapy stratified by the method of ablating the primary tumor.

A.M. Cohen, M.D.

Treatment of Hepatocellular Carcinoma With Combined Suppression and Inhibition of Sex Hormones: A Randomized, Controlled Trial
Manesis EK, Giannoulis G, Zoumboulis P, Vafiadou I, Hadziyannis SJ
(Hippokration Gen Hosp, Athens, Greece)
Hepatology 21:1535–1542, 1995   7–50

Background.—Several lines of evidence have shown that hepatocellular carcinoma (HCC), a frequent complication of chronic liver disease, is associated with sex hormones and that endogenous androgens and, possibly, estrogens play a role in hepatic carcinogenesis and tumor growth via a receptor-mediated process. The effects on survival of treatment with combined suppression and inhibition of sex hormones in patients with HCC were investigated.

Patients and Methods.—Eighty-five patients (mean age, 62 years) with advanced, unresectable disease were evaluated. Of these, 33 patients were randomly assigned to undergo treatment with the luteinizing hormone–releasing hormone analogue triptorelin and the antiestrogen tamoxifen (TMX), 23 to triptorelin and the antiandrogen flutamide, and 29 to placebo only. Survival rates were compared between groups, and covariate factors predictive of survival were evaluated.

Results.—Age, sex, tumor extension, underlying cirrhosis, and biochemical parameters were similar among groups. Significantly longer survival times were noted for patients in the TMX group at 282 days compared with 112 days for the flutamide group and 127 days for the placebo group. Among patients in the TMX group, those in the upper quartile survived for 384 days or longer; 57.1% of these patients were women. The corresponding figures for the flutamide and placebo groups were 134 days (33.3% women) and 170 days (16.7% women), respectively. The patients receiving TMX also had a significantly higher tumor volume doubling time: 296 days vs. 101 days for the flutamide group and 99 days for the placebo group. The covariates that were found to be predictive of survival on a Cox proportional hazards model included TMX treatment, baseline Okuda's HCC stage, hepatitis B surface antigen, portal vein diameter, carcinoembryonic antigen, and a self-assessment quality-of-life score. Although the degree of serum sex hormone suppression was not a significant predictor of survival, the interaction of female sex and TMX treatment was significantly associated with longer survival.

Conclusion.—Tamoxifen treatment leads to significant increases in survival and the tumor volume doubling time in patients with inoperable HCC. The effect is most notable in females and is not associated with sex hormone suppression.

▶ There are considerable anecdotal data suggesting that HCC can occur in association with androgen or estrogen use. Hence, in the absence of highly effective cytotoxic therapy for HCC, antiandrogenic and/or antiestrogenic drugs were explored in a randomized trial. The use of TMX, particularly in women with HCC, appeared to increase the likelihood of long-term survival. Although the authors of this paper did not provide any data on hormone receptors, other studies have demonstrated increased androgen receptor and suppression of estrogen receptors in HCC. This makes it difficult to accept that the mechanism of action of TMX in this trial is its antiestrogenic effect. Additional studies that explore the mechanism of action in these circumstances will be of great interest and may provide a strategy for further clinical trials.

A.M. Cohen, M.D.

Milan Multicenter Experience in Liver Transplantation for Hepatocellular Carcinoma

Mazzaferro V, Rondinara GF, Rossi G, Regalia E, De Carlis L, Caccamo L, Doci R, Sansalone CV, Belli LS, Armiraglio E, Montalto F, Galmarini D, Belli L, Gennari L (Natl Cancer Inst, Milan, Italy; Niguarda Ca'Granda Hosp, Milan, Italy; IRCCS Maggiore Hosp, Milan, Italy)
Transplant Proc 26:3557–3560, 1994   7–51

Objective.—Patients with hepatocellular carcinoma (HCC) experience a high recurrence rate, even after orthotopic liver transplantation (OLT), and patient survival is significantly associated with tumor stage. In a retrospective 3-center study, the outcome of patients with HCC and, some of the predictive factors relating to recurrence were determined, and treatment guidelines and criteria for patient selection were established.

Methods.—Between April 1984 and September 1993, 103 patients received OLT. The 23 patients who died within 3 months were excluded from the study. Of the remaining 80 patients aged 14–60 years, 85% were male and 78 had cirrhosis. All patients received cyclosporine. The influence of patient variables, tumor characteristics, and pre- and post-treatments on recurrence was evaluated.

Results.—Actuarial tumor-free survival at 5 years was 70%, whereas actual survival was 65% (Fig 1). No patient-related variables were significantly correlated to recurrence. The alpha-fetoprotein level, tumor and node stage, number of nodules, presence of capsule, and vascular invasion were significantly related to recurrence (Fig 2). Patients without vascular invasion had a significantly higher 3-year survival rate than did patients with vascular invasion. Pretransplant treatment did not affect survival. Patients receiving posttransplant immunosuppression plus steroids had lower tumor-free survival rate than patients receiving immunosuppressant therapy only.

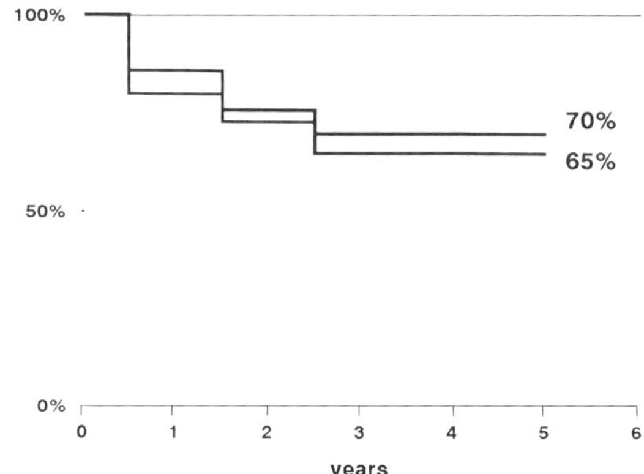

FIGURE 1.—Five-year overall (65%) and tumor-free (70%) survival of 80 patients who underwent orthotopic liver transplantation for hepatocellular carcinoma. The median follow-up was 19 months. (Courtesy of Mazzaferro V, Rondinara GF, Rossi G, et al: Milan multicenter experience in liver transplantation for hepatocellular carcinoma. *Transplant Proc* 26:3557–3560, 1994. Reprinted by permission of Appleton & Lange, Inc.)

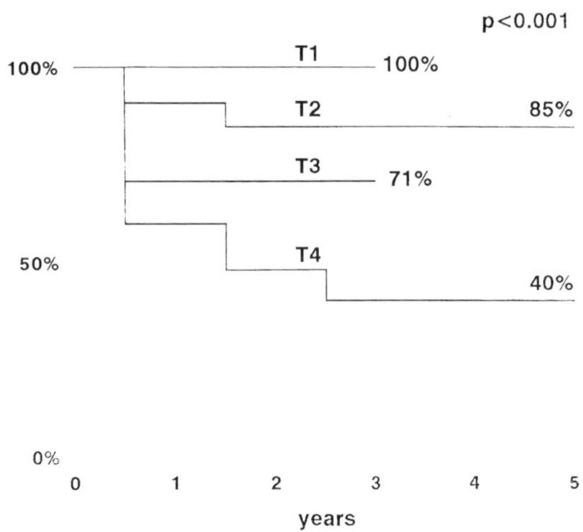

FIGURE 2.—Disease-free survival by tumor stage (T) at the time of transplantation (*T1*, 20 patients; *T2*, 24 patients; *T3*, 15 patients; *T4*, 19 patients). T1–T2 vs. T3–T4 curves: *P* < .001. (Courtesy of Mazzaferro V, Rondinara GF, Rossi G, et al: Milan multicenter experience in liver transplantation for hepatocellular carcinoma. *Transplant Proc* 26:3557–3560, 1994. Reprinted by permission of Appleton & Lange, Inc.)

Conclusion.—Tumor stage, vascular invasion, and degree of immunosuppression were significantly related to cancer-free survival. Nonetheless, recurrence rates of HCC after OLT are high.

▶ This retrospective review from 3 liver transplant centers in Milan suggests that long-term survival is possible after OLT in the treatment of patients with early stage of HCC. The data from this study are far more optimistic then those from the large series from the University of Pittsburgh.

Several important caveats are presented. First, the median follow-up of the entire patient population is only 19 months. This indicates that the life-table 5-year projections may be misleading. In addition, the authors do not tell us how many of these tumors were incidental findings. It is likely that the majority of patients were undergoing liver transplantation for cirrhosis-associated liver failure, and the findings of cancer were noted only on pathologic review of the resected specimen. A final caveat is the lack of comparison with straightforward surgical resection of the early lesions. Such surgical resection can frequently be performed safely in patients with cirrhosis, with similar results being obtained.

In the multivariate analysis, adverse features predicated a very poor outcome, and transplantation, with its "wider margins," was not thought to impact on overall survival. The failure patterns in such patients generally are systemic. Orthotopic liver transplantation for HCC requires further investigation and probably is not a realistic and appropriate use of limited donor resources.

A.M. Cohen, M.D.

Randomised Trial of Endoscopic Stenting Versus Surgical Bypass in Malignant Low Bileduct Obstruction
Smith AC, Dowsett JF, Russell RCG, Hatfield ARW, Cotton PB (Middlesex Hosp, London)
Lancet 344:1655–1660, 1994
7–52

Objective.—Most patients with pancreatic cancer are treated palliatively, and the main symptom requiring treatment is jaundice resulting from extrahepatic biliary obstruction. Nonsurgical approaches for the management of malignant low bile duct obstruction are now available, including percutaneous and endoscopic stenting. These procedures raise questions about the best way of relieving jaundice, particularly for patients who are fit for surgery and are expected to live more than a few weeks. The benefits of surgical and endoscopic procedures for the relief of malignant low bile duct obstruction were compared in a prospective, randomized trial.

Methods.—The study included 204 patients with low common bile duct obstruction resulting from probable primary carcinoma of the pancreas, the ampulla of Vater, or the bile duct. None had endoscopic evidence of duodenal invasion likely to cause gastric outlet obstruction, and none were candidates for curative surgical resection. The patients were randomized to undergo either endoscopic stent insertion or surgical biliary bypass. In the endoscopic group, no more than 3 attempts at stent insertion (including a combined endoscopic-radiologic procedure) were permitted. After the exclusion of 3 patients who proved to have benign disease, 101 surgical and 100 stented patients were available for assessment.

Results.—There were 7 failures in the surgical group and 5 in the stenting group; of the latter patients, 4 went on to have bypass surgery. Of the 94 patients successfully treated by surgery, 36 had choledochoduodenostomy, 28 had choledochojejunostomy, and 30 had cholecystenterostomy. The complication, success, and long-term survival rates were unaffected by the type of procedure performed, the center in which it was done, or whether a consultant or trainee performed the operation. Forty-five patients underwent gastroenterostomy during the initial surgery, including 2 who did not have biliary bypass. Of the 95 patients who had successful stenting, 64 required just 1 attempt, 22 needed 2 attempts, and 9 needed 3 attempts. Nineteen patients required a combined percutaneous transhepatic-endoscopic procedure.

Among patients with technical success, the therapeutic success rates were 98% in the surgical group and 97% in the stenting group. The complication rates were 29% and 11%, respectively. The complication rate was 38% in patients having prophylactic gastroenterostomy vs. 21% in those having no gastric drainage, but this difference did not affect 30-day mortality, procedure-related mortality, or length of hospital stay. Of 17 procedure-related deaths, 14 occurred in the surgical group vs. only 3 in the stented group; there was no difference in 30-day mortality. Patients in the surgical group had a median hospital stay of 26 days vs. 19

days in the stenting group. Thirty-six patients in the stenting group had recurrent obstructive jaundice resulting from stent blockage, as did 1 patient in the surgical group who was treated by stenting. Death occurred within 1 week of stent placement in 3 patients. Stent replacement was necessary in 27 patients, 10 of whom needed 2 or more stent changes. Eighteen percent of the patients in the surgical group who did not have initial gastroenterostomy had late gastric outlet obstruction develop. Ten of 56 patients in the stenting group who had gastric outlet obstruction develop subsequently underwent gastroenterostomy. There was no significant difference in median survival: 26 weeks in the surgical group, and 21 weeks in the stenting group.

Conclusions.—For patients with malignant low bile duct obstruction, endoscopic stenting and surgery are both effective palliative procedures. Endoscopic stenting is associated with fewer early complications and surgery with fewer late complications. Gastric outlet obstruction is the main drawback to stent placement. Successful endoscopic stenting relies on the exclusion of patients who are candidates for potentially curative resection. Imaging techniques and sound judgment are accurate in this regard, as suggested by the finding that only 1 patient in the surgical group underwent such resection.

▶ This is the largest prospective randomized trial of operative bypass vs. endoscopic stenting for bile duct obstruction resulting from cancer of the distal bile duct, the ampulla of Vater or the pancreas. It is important to stress that these patients were seen without imminent gastric outlet obstruction, and that none were considered candidates for potential curative resection either by imaging technique or because of their overall medical status. The selection was accurate in that only one of the operative patients at exploration was deemed to have resectable disease and underwent pancreaticoduodenectomy. The authors are to be commended for their very high rate of successful endoscopic stenting (95 of 100 patients). However, 22 patients required 2 attempts and 9 required 3 attempts. Also, 19 patients required a combined transhepatic and endoscopic procedure to obtain a successful bypass.

The data indicate significantly more major complications associated with operative bypass as well as procedure-related mortality. However, there was no statistical difference in a 30-day mortality. As would be expected, many of the patients with stents required replacement of the stent for recurrent jaundice. Data in regard to the prevalence of serious late cholangitis are not provided. Ten percent of the patients in the stent group eventually required an operation for gastric outlet obstruction.

Although the authors did not provide quality-of-life or cost analyses, these are important additional considerations.

This clinical trial provides justification for stenting patients who are not suitable for potentially curative surgical resection. With the increasing use of spiral CT, laparoscopic staging, and laparoscopic ultrasound, resectability rates covering more than 90% of patients explored are to be expected.

Assuming the institution has the technical expertise, endoscopic stenting would appear to be the appropriate approach for the remainder of patients. With the increasing use of laparoscopic bypass, late gastric outlet obstruction can be treated with either an intestinal stent or a laparoscopically performed gastrojejunostomy.

A.M. Cohen, M.D.

Assessment of Five-Year Experience With Abdominal Organ Cluster Transplantation

Alessiani M, Tzakis A, Todo S, Demetris AJ, Fung JJ, Starzl TE (Univ of Pittsburgh Med Ctr, Pa)
J Am Coll Surg 180:1–9, 1995   7–53

Background.—Cluster exenteration, one of the more radical oncologic surgeries, has been used to treat patients with otherwise unresectable malignancies of the upper abdominal tract. A 5-year experience with exenteration in 57 patients treated with variations of resectional and transplant reconstructive methods was retrospectively reviewed.

Patients and Methods.—Patient diagnoses included cholangiocarcinoma in 20; hepatocellular carcinoma in 12; endocrine neoplasms in 14; sarcoma in 6; and adenocarcinoma of the pancreas in 2, colon in 2, and gallbladder in 1. Sixty-one transplantations were performed, using 3 different organ replacement techniques: liver-pancreas-duodenum en bloc (original procedure), liver only (modified procedure), and liver plus pancreatic islets. Survival and tumor recurrence analyses were stratified by procedure, tumor type and extent, and immunosuppression.

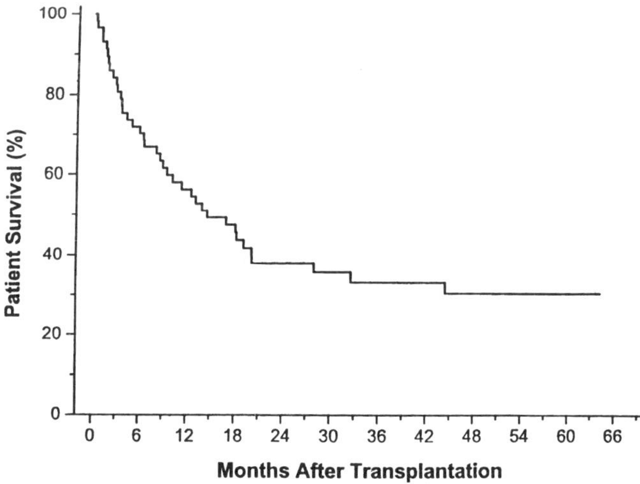

FIGURE 2.—The overall actuarial patient survival rate curve. (Courtesy of Alessiani M, Tzakis A, Todo S, et al: Assessment of five-year experience with abdominal organ cluster transplantation. *J Am Coll Surg* 180:1-9, 1995. By permission of the Journal of the American College of Surgeons.)

Findings.—At 3 months, actuarial survival was 82%. At 1 year, actuarial survival was 56%; at 2 years, 38%; at 3 years, 33%; and at 5 years, 30% (Fig 2). Eighteen of the 57 patients have survived between 17 and 61 months, and 12 are free of tumors. No significant differences were noted for actuarial survival rates stratified by transplantation procedure, immunosuppression, and tumor diagnosis and extent. A better 3-year survival rate was observed for endocrine tumors, at 64%, compared with 44% for sarcoma, 25% for hepatocellular carcinoma, 20% for cholangiocarcinoma, and 20% for other adenocarcinomas. Tumor recurrence resulted in the deaths of 23 patients. Eleven patients with no lymph node involvement, no vascular invasion, and liver metastasis only had the lowest incidence of recurrence, at 27% vs. 73.5%.

Conclusions.—Abdominal organ cluster transplantation is beneficial in patients with unresectable endocrine neoplasms, fibrolamellar hepatocellular carcinoma, and selected cholangiocarcinoma restricted to the liver. Patients with sarcoma can achieve long-term survival, although high recurrence rates have been noted in these individuals.

▶ This report by Starzl and colleagues of the University of Pittsburgh updates their 5-year experience with upper abdominal exenteration and transplantation. This is one of the most heroic and expensive strategies in the treatment of patients with cancer, and the histologic subtypes must be analyzed and ascertained as to the potential value of such an approach. Although seemingly impractical, the accompanying figures demonstrate that one can produce a modest number of long-term survivors.

Despite the heroic surgical procedure, all patients survived the operation; however, 4 of the 57 patients required urgent retransplantation. More than 80% of the patients were alive at 3 months. The data were presented primarily as overall survival data (not disease-free), with the best results occurring for endocrine tumors (64%) compared with cholangiocarcinoma and other adenocarcinoma (20%). One of 3 patients who were alive had recurrent cancer.

This experience should be perceived as an early report of a pilot project. However, highly selected young patients with otherwise unresectable cancer may be cured or at least provided with several years of survival with such multiorgan transplantation.

A.M. Cohen, M.D.

Management of Retroperitoneal Sarcomas: Does Dose Escalation Impact on Locoregional Control?
Fein DA, Corn BW, Lanciano RM, Herbert SH, Hoffman JP, Coia LR (Fox Chase Cancer Center, Philadelphia)
Int J Radiat Oncol Biol Phys 31:129–134, 1995   7–54

Background.—Only half the patients with retroperitoneal sarcomas undergo complete resection. Of these, nearly half have local tumor recurrence develop. The role of radiotherapy in patients with retroperitoneal sarcomas has not been definitively established. One experience with adjuvant radiotherapy in the treatment of retroperitoneal sarcomas was analyzed to determine whether irradiation with dose escalation improves locoregional control.

Methods.—Twenty-one patients were treated surgically with curative intent and radiotherapy between 1965 and 1992. The patients were followed up from 14 to 340 months. Radiotherapy was delivered postoperatively in 19 patients and preoperatively in 2. Radiation doses ranged from 36 to 90 Gy.

Findings.—At 2 years, the local rate of control was 72% and the survival rate was 69%. Local control was unaffected by tumor size, stage, grade, and histology. Of 8 patients receiving a total dose exceeding 55.2 Gy, 25% had local failure compared with 38% of 13 patients receiving 55.2 Gy or less. The only serious complication was a small bowel obstruction requiring surgery in one patient.

Conclusions.—Because of the high likelihood of local recurrence, postoperative radiotherapy at doses exceeding 55 Gy is recommended for patients with retroperitoneal sarcomas after surgical resection. Clinicians should consider innovative adjuvant radiation methods for escalating doses to more than 55 Gy, including intraoperative radiotherapy, brachytherapy, or the use of small bowel exclusion devices to decrease small bowel toxicity.

▶ Retroperitoneal sarcomas represent a major challenge in terms of the enormous volume that needs to be treated, which is in basic conflict with a variety of intra-abdominal organs whose tolerance is exceedingly dose-limited (e.g., the bowel, kidney, and liver).

This paper attempts to address the problem retrospectively. Unfortunately, the number of patients is small and the follow-up on these patients is relatively brief. One needs *at least 5 years* of follow-up to be confident that one can interpret the outcome. Even 5 years may not be long enough, but it is at least a pretty good indication of long-term local control. The authors conclude that they should treat such patients with a dose in excess of 55 Gy. Actually, their data do not support such a conclusion, because there is no significant difference in the outcome of patients who had a dose of 55 Gy or higher compared with patients who had only 50 Gy. With the small number of patients, a short follow-up, and a conclusion that does not give any information about morbidities, I think this paper should have been placed in someone's desk drawer for a couple of years and then been looked at again and updated. If there had been a minimum of at least 5 years of follow-up on every patient, perhaps one could have reached some kind of conclusion even with these small numbers.

E. Glatstein, M.D.

Peritonectomy Procedures

Sugarbaker PH (Washington Hosp Ctr, Washington, DC)
Ann Surg 221:29–42, 1995   7–55

Objective.—A new strategy for the treatment of colorectal tumor, designed to prevent peritoneal carcinomatosis, involves the cytoreductive approach, which combines surgery and intraperitoneal chemotherapy. Six peritonectomy techniques for treating peritoneal surface malignancies have been developed.

Methods.—The procedures performed include a greater omentectomy-splenectomy, left upper quadrant peritonectomy, right upper quadrant peritonectomy, lesser omentectomy-cholecystectomy with stripping of the omental bursa, pelvic peritonectomy with sleeve resection of the sigmoid color, and antrectomy. Tubes and drains were placed into the abdomen for postoperative intraperitoneal chemotherapy (Fig 16).

Summary.—These procedures result in maximal surgical cytoreduction coupled with maximal chemotherapeutic cytoreduction. Early postoperative intraperitoneal chemotherapeutic treatment of peritoneal surface malignancies has resulted in long-term, disease-free survival in selected patients.

▶ This surgical technique paper describes in eloquent detail the complex surgical strategy necessary to adequately perform cytoreductive surgery for patients with low-grade carcinomatosis. This approach is recommended when it is combined with early postoperative intraperitoneal chemotherapy. The author has achieved impressive long-term survival with a very large experience by using this combined modality approach in patients with pseudomyxoma peritonei and similar low-grade malignancies.

The surgical procedures are heroic, both for the patient and the surgeon. Most surgeons have attempted rather modest "debulking" approaches that

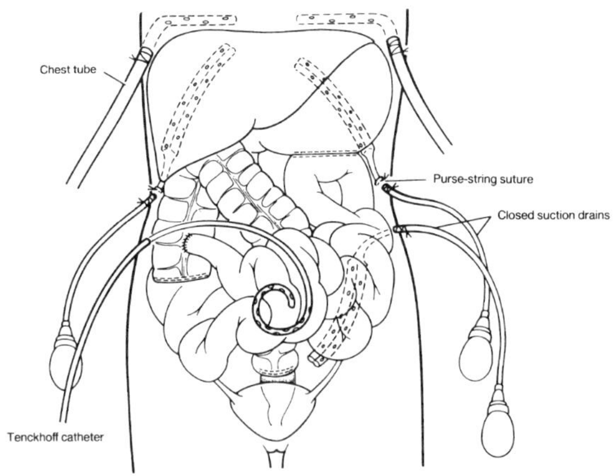

FIGURE 16.—Tubes and drains required for early postoperative intraperitoneal chemotherapy. (Courtesy of Sugarbaker PH: Peritonectomy procedures. *Ann Surg* 221:29–42, 1995.)

still leave a significant amount of tumor within the abdomen. Reports of the morbidity and mortality of this approach, as well as long-term survival, will be necessary to ascertain the value of such an aggressive approach.

A.M. Cohen, M.D.

Pseudomyxoma Peritonei

Costa MJ (Univ of California-Davis Med Ctr, Sacramento)
Arch Pathol Lab Med 118:1215–1219, 1994   7–56

Background.—Extracellular mucin in the peritoneal cavity is the unifying diagnostic feature in pseudomyxoma peritonei. The clinicopathologic characteristics of patients with peritoneal implants showing a predominance of extracellular mucin were analyzed to determine both the primary site compared with a control group of nonpseudomyxomatous peritoneal implants and the histologic predictors of survival.

Methods and Findings.—Thirty-five patients with pseudomyxomatous peritoneal implants and 90 consecutive patients with peritoneal implants without extracellular mucin were studied. The histologic patterns of the nonpseudomyxomatous implants were glandular in 43%, serous in 21%, signet ring in 20%, solid in 13%, and clear cell in 2%. The pseudomyxomatous implants originated from a mucinous epithelial tumor of the appendix in 31%, compared with 1% for the nonpseudomyxomatous implants. Other primary sites gave rise to pseudomyxomatous and nonpseudomyxomatous implants with comparable frequencies. These sites were the colon for 26% and 30%, respectively; ovary, 23% and 16%; stomach, 11% and 10%; small intestine, 3% and 1%; urinary bladder, 3% and 1%; endometrium, 0 and 10%; prostate gland, 0 and 6%. Twenty-nine patients with extracellular mucin in their implants and 71 without extracellular mucin were followed up for 3 years. Three-year survival rates in the 2 groups were 24% and 4%, respectively. Three-year follow-up data were also available for 90 of 110 and 10 of 15 patients with and without invasion in the primary tumor or its peritoneal implants, respectively. In these 2 groups, the 3-year survival rates were 80% and 4%, respectively (Fig 4). Primary tumor or implant invasion was present in 21 of 35 pseudomyxomatous implants and eliminated any improvement in survival related to the presence of extracellular mucin. Increased survival in patients with pseudomyxoma peritonei was associated with the histologic findings of noninvasive implants resulting from mucinous epithelial tumors with low malignant potential histologically.

Conclusions.—The clinical outcome of patients with pseudomyxoma peritonei depends on the invasiveness of the related mucinous neoplasm. Thus, any assessment of treatment and prognosis must include histopathologic classification into invasive and low malignant potential subtypes.

▶ Pseudomyxoma peritonei is a clinical term used in the presence of intraperitoneal neoplasms that produce gross gelatinous mucinous collec-

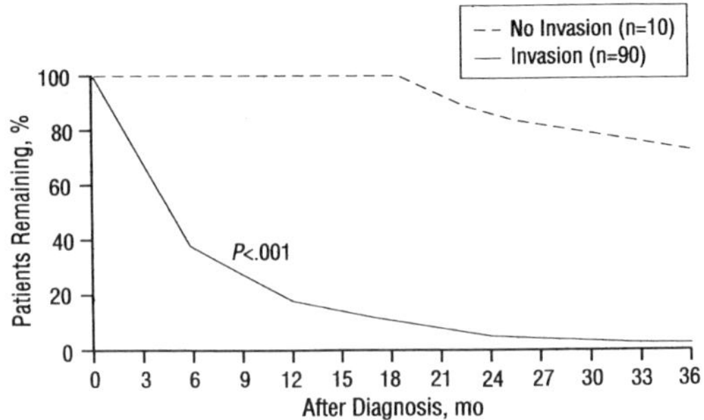

FIGURE 4.—Clinical follow-up: invasive vs. noninvasive implants. *Patients Remaining* indicates percentage with follow-up and who are alive as a function of months after the diagnosis; *Invasion*, patients with invasive tumors; and *No Invasion*, noninvasive, low malignant potential-type tumors. (Courtesy of Costa MJ: Pseudomyxoma peritonei. *Arch Pathol Lab Med* 118:1215-1219, 1994.)

tions. The sites of origin, the histology, and the clinical outcomes are extremely heterogenous. There is a broad spectrum of treatment options. At some centers, the disease is considered quite indolent, and moderate debulking with subsequent further debulking based on symptoms and deferral of chemotherapy is the standard approach. Other groups consider such patients to have aggressive cancer and are treated with systemic chemotherapy. At other centers, an aggressive debulking with peritonectomy followed by intraperitoneal chemotherapy is favored. Interpretation of outcomes has been complicated by the heterogenous nature of the patients treated.

In this clinical pathologic analysis, 35 patients with clinical features of pseudomyxomatous implants were compared with patients with carcinomatosis without extracellular mucin. The most important data define the histopathologic correlates of indolent disease. As shown in Figure 4, patients with noninvasive implants have a biologically favorable outcome and presumably can be managed by multiple debulking operative procedures. In addition, as suggested by Sugarbaker and colleagues,[1] a potentially curative strategy combining radical resection with intraperitoneal chemotherapy may be feasible.

A.M. Cohen, M.D.

Reference

1. Sugarbaker PH, et al: Peritoneal carcinomatosis from appendiceal cancer: Results in 69 patients treated by cytoreductive surgery and intraperitoneal chemotherapy. *Dis Colon Rectum* 36:323–329, 1993.

8   Adult Leukemia

Myeloid Markers in Adult Acute Lymphocytic Leukemia: Correlations With Patient and Disease Characteristics and With Prognosis
Preti HA, Huh YO, O'Brien SM, Andreeff M, Pierce ST, Keating M, Kantarjian HM (MD Anderson Cancer Ctr, Houston)
Cancer 76:1564–1570, 1995   8–1

Objective.—Because the expression of myeloid markers on lymphoblasts has been associated with a relatively poor outcome in patients with acute lymphocytic leukemia (ALL), the treatment response and outcome were reviewed in 162 adults with newly diagnosed ALL, 64 of whom (40%) had myeloid marker (MY)–positive disease.

Study Population.—All patients were 15 years of age or older and had not been previously treated. The MY-positive and MY-negative patients were similar with regard to performance status, organ enlargement, and peripheral blastosis. Myeloid marker–positive disease was significantly more prevalent in patients with null-cell ALL and was less frequent in those with mature B-cell disease. Burkitt's translocations were more frequent in patients with MY-negative disease.

Management.—Patients received varying dose regimens of vincristine-doxorubicin-dexamethasone (VAD) therapy. Some high-risk patients underwent autologous bone marrow transplantation within 2 months of achieving a complete response.

Results.—A complete response was achieved by induction treatment in 64% of patients with MY-positive disease and 78% of patients with MY-negative disease. The respective rates of resistant disease were 20% and 12%. There were no marked differences in duration of remission or survival during a median follow-up of 45 months. The 3-year survival rates were 26% and 31%, respectively, for the MY-negative and MY-positive patient groups. Neither the duration of remission nor survival could be correlated with individual myeloid-associated antigens or the expression of CD34.

Conclusion.—The presence of MYs on lymphoblasts of ALL is a manifestation of lineage heterogeneity, but it had no significant prognostic influence in VAD-treated adults with ALL.

▶ The clinical relevance of expression of MY in adult ALL has been a controversial topic. In this study, the authors have shown no significant difference in the prognosis of patients with MY-positive ALL treated with VAD regimens compared with patients with MY-negative ALL treated similarly. This is in contrast to the findings of some studies in which MY-positive ALL in adults has been associated with poor response to therapy and shortened survival.

There are several possible reasons for the lack of consensus in the literature regarding the significance of MY expression in ALL. As the authors suggest, one reason is that some of the previously reported cases may be better classified as minimally differentiated acute myeloid leukemia (AML-M_0). Furthermore, definitions vary as to which acute leukemias qualify as MY-positive ALL. Perhaps the most important reason, however, is that surface antigen expression, or lineage assignment, may not be the best way to define certain leukemias. For instance, Philadelphia chromosome–positive ALL represents a distinct entity, which is best defined by the molecular genetic BCR-ABL fusion, with production of a BCR-ABL fusion protein (P190 or P210).

Although myeloid antigen expression is common in these cases of ALL, perhaps they should not be equated with more generic cases of MY-positive ALL. Similarly, MY-positive, therapy-induced ALL associated with structural abnormalities of chromosome 11q23 could be considered a separate disease, defined not only by myeloid antigen expression but by rearrangement of the mixed lineage leukemia gene on chromosome 11. Absence of CALLA (CD10) expression with concomitant present of CD15 expression has been shown to be a potent predictor of structural 11q23 abnormalities in cases of ALL. One could argue, therefore, that CALLA-negative, CD15-positive ALL should be considered distinct from the more general pool of MY-positive ALL.

Failure to establish consensus regarding the clinical status of MY-positive ALL may be remedied if morphologic and immunophenotypic findings are interpreted in light of genotypic and clinical data. Although myeloid antigen expression alone may not define distinct ALL variants, initial decisions regarding therapy heavily rely on the rapid assignment of cell lineage characteristics to individual cases of acute leukemia. With that in mind, Preti and co-workers have added a carefully performed and valuable study to the body of literature regarding MY-positive ALL.

W.G. Finn, M.D.

A Five-Drug Remission Induction Regimen With Intensive Consolidation for Adults With Acute Lymphoblastic Leukemia: Cancer and Leukemia Group B Study 8811

Larson RA, Dodge RK, Burns CP, Lee EJ, Stone RM, Schulman P, Duggan D, Davey FR, Sobol RE, Frankel SR, Hooberman AL, Westbrook CA, Arthur DC, George SL, Bloomfield CD, Schiffer CA (Univ of Chicago; CALGB Statistical Ctr, Durham, NC; Univ of Iowa, Iowa City; et al)

Blood 85:2025–2037, 1995   8–2

Objective.—Although most adults with acute lymphoblastic leukemia (ALL) achieve complete remission, the remissions do not last very long. Recent studies have emphasized the use of more and more intensive multiple chemotherapy regimens and the identification of prognostic factors to tailor therapy to the individual patient. The phase II Cancer and Leukemia Group B Study 8811 was conducted to assess the results of a new intensive chemotherapy regimen and to identify clinical and biological prognostic factors.

Methods.—The analysis included 197 adult patients (median age, 32 years) with ALL. The induction course included cyclophosphamide, daunorubicin, vincristine, L-asparaginase, and prednisone. That course was followed by an early intensification course of cyclophosphamide, cytarabine, 6-mercaptopurine (6-MP), vincristine, and L-asparaginase; a third course consisting of cranial irradiation and methotrexate and 6-MP; a late intensification course; and then prolonged maintenance treatment with 6-MP, methotrexate, vincristine, and prednisone. The treatment period totaled 2 years.

Results.—The complete response rate was 85%; 7% of patients had refractory ALL, and 9% died during induction. The complete response rate was 94% for patients younger than 30 years of age and 85% for those aged 30–59 years compared with 39% for those aged 60 years or older. Patients who had a mediastinal mass or blasts with a T-cell immunophenotype also had a better complete response rate. The response rate and duration were unaffected by co-expression of myeloid antigens. The complete response rate was 70% for patients with evidence of the Philadelphia chromosome vs. 84% for those without such evidence.

At a median follow-up of 43 months, median survival for the total sample was 36 months. For the 167 patients who achieved a complete response, the median duration of remission was 29 months. Favorable prognostic factors in terms of remission duration and survival included younger age, a white blood cell count of less than 30,000/µL, L1 morphology, T or TMy immunophenotype, and absence of the Philadelphia chromosome. The estimated 3-year survival rate was 69% for patients younger than 30 years of age, 39% for those aged 30–59 years, 89% for those with a mediastinal mass, 59% for those with a white blood cell count of less than 30,000/µL, 63% for those with L1 morphology, 69% for those with T or TMy antigen expression, and 62% for those without the Philadelphia chromosome. There were 15 patients with no adverse prognostic factors; their estimated 5-year survival rate was 100%.

Conclusion.—A new, intensive chemotherapy regimen for adults with ALL yields a high complete response rate and a high percentage of durable remissions. For patients less than 30 years of age, the results are similar to those in high-risk childhood ALL. Outcomes are especially good for patients with a mediastinal mass or a TMy immunophenotype. The poor prognostic factors identified warrant validation in other studies. Innovative treatment approaches are needed for patients with adverse prognostic factors, particularly older age and adverse cytogenetic or molecular biological features.

▶ The outcome for adults with ALL remains poor despite complete remission rates comparable to those achieved among patients with acute myeloid leukemia. The major cause of treatment failure remains relapse of disease. Recently, attention has focused on increasing the intensity of remission induction in postremission treatment with multiagent chemotherapy. Larson and colleagues from the Cancer and Leukemia Group B (CALGB) Study report more encouraging results in adults with ALL with a regimen consisting of 5 courses of therapy including induction, early intensification, CNS prophylaxis and interim maintenance, late intensification, and prolonged maintenance that continues for 21 months from diagnosis.

This study, CALGB 8811, included 197 patients between the ages of 16 and 80 years (median age, 32 years), of whom 167 patients (85%) achieved a complete response. The toxic death rate during induction was 9%. The median follow-up was 43 months, the median survival for all patients was 36 months, and the median remission duration for the 167 patients achieving a complete response was 29 months. The proportion of patients surviving at 3 years varied with age. For those patients younger than 30 years of age, estimates of a 3-year survival rate are 69%, and for those patients 30–59 years of age, 39%. Pretreatment characteristics that predicted a favorable remission duration or survival include a younger age, the presence of a mediastinal mass or lymphadenopathy, a white blood cell count of $<30/\mu L$, L1 morphology, T or TMy immunophenotype, and the absence of the Philadelphia chromosome. For a small cohort of 15 patients with no unfavorable prognostic factors, the estimated probability of survival at 5 years is 100%. These investigators had planned to achieve initial cytoreduction as rapidly as possible during the induction course and, subsequently, to administer intensive chemotherapy. For this reason, no delays in treatment or dose reductions were permitted because of pancytopenia, as long as the patient had no fever or obvious infection.

This study is important because it suggests that we are making progress in this disease. The outcome for certain subsets of patients appears considerably more favorable than previous studies had estimated. Furthermore, pretreatment characteristics may provide significant prognostic information. Therefore, future studies directed at individualizing therapy based on such prognostic factors will be important.

M.S. Tallman, M.D.

Long-Term Follow-Up of Adults With Acute Lymphoblastic Leukemia in First Remission Treated With Chemotherapy or Bone Marrow Transplantation
Horowitz MM, for the Acute Lymphoblastic Leukemia Working Committee (Med College of Wisconsin, Milwaukee)
Ann Intern Med 123:428–431, 1995   8–3

Background.—Research conducted in 1991 demonstrated that leukemia-free survival rates were similar in adults with acute lymphoblastic leukemia (ALL) in first remission treated with chemotherapy or HLA-identical sibling bone marrow transplantation. Whether these results were still valid after an additional 4 years of follow-up was determined.

Methods.—Four hundred eighty-four consecutive patients with ALL in first remission were treated with chemotherapy in 44 German hospitals. A second cohort of 234 consecutive patients received HLA-identical sibling bone marrow transplants for ALL in first remission in 98 centers worldwide. The median follow-up was 7.5 years.

Findings.—The actuarial 9-year relapse probabilities were 66% for the patients given chemotherapy and 30% for those undergoing transplantation. The patients in the chemotherapy group had a 9-year leukemia-free survival rate of 32% compared with 34% for those in the transplantation group.

Conclusions.—These findings confirm those of the earlier analysis of these cohorts. Fewer relapses but more treatment-related deaths occur among patients undergoing transplantation than in those treated with chemotherapy. Therefore, leukemia-free survival rates were similar among patients receiving these different treatments for ALL in first remission.

▶ Although the optimal postremission therapy for patients with acute myeloid leukemia has not been determined, results of a number of studies have suggested that histocompatible-matched sibling bone marrow transplantation may offer the most favorable outcome for younger patients. The optimal postremission strategy for adults with ALL in first remission has not been established. In this paper, Horowitz and colleagues retrospectively compared chemotherapy and bone marrow transplantation in cohorts of 484 and 234 consecutive patients with ALL in first remission.

Although HLA-identical sibling transplantation was associated with fewer relapses than chemotherapy in adults with ALL in first remission, the 9-year leukemia-free survival rate was similar to the rates for those who received chemotherapy alone. This observation holds for patients in low- and high-risk groups, as defined by white blood cells at diagnosis, immunophenotype, and time to achieve first remission.

These studies show that, although late relapses were less common in the patients treated with transplantation, this potential benefit was insufficient to overcome the increased treatment-related mortality seen with transplantation. This study showed fewer relapses but more treatment-related mortality with bone marrow transplantation than with chemotherapy. Therefore, leukemia-free survival rates, the ultimate end point, were similar with both treatment strategies. It stands to reason that, with further improvement in transplantation techniques and its supportive care, a leukemia-free benefit may emerge among the transplantation cohort. However, at present, the optimal therapy for adults with ALL in first complete remission will require further studies.

M.S. Tallman, M.D.

Allogeneic Bone Marrow Transplantation in Adult Acute Lymphoblastic Leukemia in First Complete Remission: A Comparative Study
Sebban C, for the French Group of Therapy of Adult Acute Lymphoblastic Leukemia (Hôpital Edouard Herriot, Lyon, France)
J Clin Oncol 12:2580–2587, 1994   8–4

Introduction.—Intensive chemotherapy has produced high rates of complete remission in adults with acute lymphoblastic leukemia (ALL), but the long-term results are disappointing. The best form of postremission management remains uncertain.

Objective.—The efficacy of allogeneic bone marrow transplantation (BMT) was compared with that of both chemotherapy and autologous marrow transplantation in a multicenter series of 257 patients with ALL.

Patients.—Patients 15–40 years of age who had had a complete response to induction or salvage treatment, and who had at least one potential sibling bone marrow donor, were eligible. Patients without a sibling donor were randomly assigned to autologous BMT or chemotherapy. There were 116 patients allocated to undergo allogeneic BMT and 141 to serve as control patients.

Results.—There were no significant differences in overall or disease-free survival rates between the study and control groups. Considering only the 96 patients believed to have high-risk ALL, median disease-free survival time was 21 months for the patients having allogeneic BMT and 9 months for controls, a significant difference. There also was a significant difference in overall survival. No differences in overall or disease-free survival were found among standard-risk patients according to allocation arm.

Conclusions.—Allogeneic BMT is worthwhile for adult patients having high-risk ALL in first complete remission. If standard-risk leukemia is present, allogeneic BMT is indicated only in those patients who relapse.

▶ The results of BMT therapy for ALL have been less successful than those in myeloid leukemias. This French study underscores the problem. A large number of adults with ALL were entered into the study and were treated either with allogeneic BMT, if a suitable donor was available, or, if not, given chemotherapy or autologous transplantation. The authors found that there was a significantly better outcome for patients receiving BMT only when poor-risk patients were considered, as described in the abstract. When patients with so-called standard-risk features were considered, survival was not significantly different.

The conclusion of this paper, that allogeneic transplantation should be reserved for patients with poor-risk adult ALL, parallels the conclusion for cases of childhood ALL. Chemotherapy is as effective as marrow transplantation for most patients with childhood ALL, and the latter is thus reserved for those with features indicating an extremely poor prognosis.

J.V. Simone, M.D.

2-Chlorodeoxyadenosine Activity in Patients With Untreated Chronic Lymphocytic Leukemia

Saven A, Lemon RH, Kosty M, Beutler E, Piro LD (Ida M and Cecil H Green Cancer Ctr, La Jolla, Calif; Scripps Clinic and Research Found, La Jolla, Calif)
J Clin Oncol 13:570–574, 1995
8–5

Introduction.—Chronic lymphocytic leukemia (CLL) is caused by the clonal proliferation of B lymphocytes. The purine analog 2-chlorodeoxyadenosine (2Cd-A) has activity in patients with CLL who do not respond to alkylator therapy. A phase II trial of 2-CdA in patients with previously untreated CLL was reported.

Methods.—The analysis included 20 previously untreated patients with CLL. All received 2-Cda in a 0.1 mg/kg/day 7-day continuous IV infusion every 4 to 5 weeks. Treatment continued until the maximum response was achieved or until prohibitive toxicity occurred.

Results.—The median number of courses administered was 4. The complete response rate was 25% and the partial response rate was 60%, for an overall response rate of 85%. The responses lasted for a median of more than 8 months. The main form of toxicity was myelosuppression. Grade III or IV thrombocytopenia occurred in 20% of patients. Opportunistic infections developed a median of 19 months after cessation of 2-CdA therapy in 3 patients, all of whom received corticosteroids.

Conclusions.—Major activity of 2-CdA was documented in patients with previously untreated CLL. The response rates are lower in previously treated patients, perhaps in part because of poor marrow reserve related to previous therapy. Randomized studies are needed to compare the efficacy of 2-CdA, fludarabine, and chlorambucil in the treatment of CLL.

▶ Chronic lymphocytic leukemia (CLL), the most common leukemia in the Western world, is not curable with currently available chemotherapeutic agents. Although the disease is generally indolent, progression in most patients eventually precipitates treatment. Conventional treatment for patients with Rai stages I and II who require therapy is a single alkylating agent with or without prednisone. Patients with Rai stages III and IV have a poor prognosis, with a median duration of survival of less than 2 years. In this population of patients, there is no advantage to using aggressive combination chemotherapy compared with single alkylating agents and prednisone. Recently, fludarabine, a purine nucleoside analog, has been shown to be equally—if not more—effective than alkylating agents in the setting of advanced disease.

2-Chlorodeoxyadenosine is another synthetic purine nucleoside analog that is resistant to degradation by adenosine deaminase, an enzyme critical to purine and deoxypurine metabolism. The phosphorylated drug accumulates in cells such as lymphocytes and monocytes that are rich in the phosphorylating enzyme deoxycytidine kinase, but low in the dephosphorylating enzyme 5-nucleotidase. The phosphorylated metabolite does not readily exit the cell, and it causes DNA strand breaks in both dividing and nondividing lymphocytes; this important fact distinguishes this class of agents from conventional cytotoxic chemotherapy. It also results in apoptosis or programmed cell death. In previously treated patients with CLL, complete remission rates are low, but partial remission rates of approximately 30% to 45% indicate significant biological activity in this setting.

Saven and colleagues from the Scripps Clinic and Research Foundation now report, for the first time, the activity of the 2-CdA purine necleoside analog in patients with previously untreated CLL. The authors have shown what was anticipated, namely that patients who have not been exposed to prior alkylating-agent chemotherapy and who are early in the natural history of their disease respond significantly better to this agent than do those who were heavily pretreated. Five of 20 patients (25%) achieved a complete response, and 12 (60%) achieved a partial response with a median duration of response of more than 8 months (range, 3–27 months).

Although the purine nucleoside analogs are known to cause prolonged suppression of CD4 cells, T-cell subsets were not followed in this study. Such analyses will be important in future studies to evaluate the contribution of of exposure 2-CdA to the inherent risk of infection in this patient population. Although sophisticated molecular studies to document complete eradication of the malignant clone also were not done in this particular study, the high response rates are extremely encouraging in a disease in which complete remission is rarely achieved.

The importance of this study lies in the demonstration that a novel nontoxic agent can induce impressive complete and partial response rates in a common but, as yet, incurable disease. Further understanding of perturbations in *bcl-2* and other putative oncogenes (such as Rb) that purportedly are involved in the pathogenesis of the disease, will provide insights into the mechanisms of apoptosis. These studies, together with the application of sophisticated techniques to detect minimal residual disease, may make cure an achievable goal in patients with this most common leukemia.

M.S. Tallman, M.D.

Improved Survival for Patients With Acute Myelogenous Leukemia

Mitus AJ, Miller KB, Schenkein DP, Ryan HF, Parsons SK, Wheeler C, Antin JH (Brigham and Women's Hosp, Boston; New England Med Ctr, Boston; Beth Israel Hosp, Boston; Children's Hosp, Boston)

J Clin Oncol 13:560–569, 1995   8–6

Objective.—Despite advances in chemotherapy and supportive care, the overall survival for patients with acute myelogenous leukemia (AML) is still poor. Cure rates are no higher than 25% to 30%. A multicenter trial designed to improve survival in patients with AML by improving the induction and consolidation phases of therapy was initiated in 1987. The results in 94 patients were reported.

Methods.—In an attempt to increase the rate of remission, the standard 3+7 chemotherapy protocol of daunorubicin and cytarabine was modified with high-dose cytarabine on days 8 through 10 to create a 3+7+3 regimen. Toward decreasing the rate of leukemia relapse, all patients who entered complete remission (CR) were offered allogeneic or autologous bone marrow transplantation (BMT). Ninety-four patients were enrolled from 1987 to 1993; the results were analyzed by intention to treat.

Results.—The complete response rate was 89%. The remission rate was so high that previously identified outcome predictors—including cytogenetic findings, white blood cell count, French-American-British classification, age, and sex—were not prognostically useful. The 5-year survival rate was 55% overall. Bone marrow transplantation was performed in 60% of all patients who had CR. Five-year event-free survival was 56% in patients receiving allogeneic BMT and 45% in those receiving autologous BMT, a nonsignificant difference.

Conclusions.—This new approach to therapy for AML—using 3+7+3 chemotherapy to increase the remission rate and BMT to decrease the rate of leukemic relapse—yields excellent long-term disease-free survival. The improvement over historical data probably results from the very high rate of induced remission and the effectiveness of consolidation therapy. This new approach offers the possibility of cure to many patients with AML.

▶ The optimal therapy for patients with AML who achieve CR is not known. Although intensive chemoradiotherapy followed by HLA-matched allogeneic BMT results in long-term disease-free survival in 45% to 60% of cases, the results achieved with reinfusion of autologous bone marrow after consolidation chemotherapy are similarly encouraging. Despite the obvious potential of reinfusing clonogeneic leukemic cells and the absence of the potentially beneficial graft-vs.-leukemia effect, this approach has a number of advantages, including the lack of need for a matched donor, the absence of graft-vs.-host disease and, generally, a lower morbidity and mortality. The increasing ability to deliver effective intensive postremission chemotherapy without transplantation has made this dilemma even more complicated.

Mitus and colleagues now report an approach to the treatment of patients younger than 65 years of age who have newly diagnosed AML. These investigators modify what has become the standard induction chemotherapy regimen of an anthracycline antibiotic (either daunorubicin or idarubicin) and cytosine arabinoside, with the addition of high-dose cytosine arabinoside given for 3 days on days 8–10 of induction. Three cycles of consolidation chemotherapy were administered, and then allogeneic or autologous BMT was offered to all patients who achieved CR. In recent years, the treatment of AML has focused on postremission therapy, partly because physicians have been relatively satisfied with the 65% to 70% CR rate that is achieved with standard induction chemotherapy and partly because of the enthusiasm for high-dose chemoradiotherapy with BMT.

This study addresses two important issues. First, although the standard induction chemotherapy is satisfying, effective in the majority of patients with de novo AML, there is room for substantial improvement. The authors suggest that this is possible in that CR were achieved in 84 of 94 patients (89%). The Australian Leukemia Study Group[1] has also addressed this issue by adding etoposide to standard induction chemotherapy, and although the CR rate achieved was no different than that attained with conventional chemotherapy, the duration of remission may be improved. The second issue addressed in this study is whether BMT given as intensive consolidation to all patients who achieve a CR improves disease-free survival. A unique feature of this study is that all patients received both the identical induction program and consolidation program before transplantation. In addition, the data were analyzed by an intent-to-treat analysis in an effort to eliminate bias by not excluding patients who relapsed before transplantation. There was no significant difference in the event-free survival at 5 years among patients undergoing allogeneic BMT compared with those receiving autologous BMT (56 vs. 45%, respectively, $P = 54$). The major causes of death among patients undergoing allogeneic BMT were clearly related to the toxicities of the procedure itself and with a low relapse rate, whereas the major causes for treatment failure among patients undergoing autologous transplantation were relapsed.

Although this was not a prospective randomized trial comparing one induction program vs. another or allogeneic transplantation vs. autologous transplantation, the results are important because they refocus our attention on improving induction chemotherapy. In addition, this study suggests that the approach presented results in improved disease-free survival compared with previous historical data, and that either postremission approach (matched allogeneic BMT or autologous BMT) is effective. The induction program requires confirmation perhaps in the cooperative group setting. Future directions will include identifying better ways to diminish the toxicities of the allogeneic transplant procedure itself and to prevent relapse after autologous BMT.

M.S. Tallman, M.D.

Reference

1. Bishop JF, Lowenthal RM, Joshua D, et al: Etoposide in acute nonlymphocytic leukemia: The Australian Leukemia Study Group. *Blood* 75:27–32, 1990.

Change in Karyotype Between Diagnosis and First Relapse in Acute Myelogenous Leukemia

Estey E, Keating MJ, Pierce S, Stass S (MD Anderson Cancer Ctr, Houston)
Leukemia 9:972–976, 1995   8–7

Background.—The prognostic significance of a change in the leukemia cell karyotype between first diagnosis and relapse was evaluated in a retrospective review of patients with acute myelogenous leukemia. In addition, the incidence and type of change and the duration of remission were evaluated in terms of the likelihood of change.

Methods.—More than 200 cases of acute myelogenous leukemia seen between 1975 and 1994 at the M.D. Anderson Cancer Center were evaluated retrospectively. The karyotype was determined according to the International System of Human Cytogenetic Nomenclature and the 4th International Workshop on Chromosomes in Leukemia. A clone was defined as 2 or 3 cells having the same abnormality based on specific criteria. Clones were defined as cells that had undergone clonal evolution (CE) or clonal devolution (CD). They could also be considered unrelated clones. Patients were subjected to various regimens of principal and postremission induction chemotherapy. Data were evaluated with χ^2, Fisher's exact test, or the log-rank test.

Results.—In 38% of the 212 case subjects, the karyotype at diagnosis and relapse was the same. At initial diagnosis, 40% of the patients had a normal karyotype; in 56% of these subjects, the karyotype was normal at relapse. Of those with an abnormal karyotype at diagnosis, 30% had the same karyotype at relapse, whereas 61% underwent a change between presentation and relapse. The majority of changes were the result of CE, CD, or both. Karyotype was a relatively stable characteristic. Insufficient metaphases were determined to be an artifact because repetition of this finding was found in only 6% of cases at relapse. There was no difference in the length of remission in those with an unchanged normal karyotype and those with a karyotype that changed from normal to abnormal. Moreover, a change in the cytogenetic pattern had little effect on the outcome of therapy.

Discussion.—A change in karyotype has no effect on the duration of remission; the duration of remission does not predict the likelihood of change in karyotype at relapse. Clonal evolution is not necessarily associated with a poor prognosis.

▶ It is well known that leukemic cell karyotype at the time of diagnosis in patients with acute myelogenous leukemia has prognostic importance. Data have emerged that suggest that patients with certain specific chromosomal abnormalities have either particularly favorable or unfavorable outlooks. However, both the frequency of the change in karyotype between the time of diagnosis and the time of relapse and the prognostic importance of such a change are unknown.

To address these issues, investigators at the M.D. Andersen Cancer Center retrospectively reviewed the cases of 212 patients with acute myelogenous leukemia seen between 1975 and 1994. They found that the karyotypes at diagnosis and relapse were identical in 38% of patients. A change in karyotype between these time points occurred in 61% of 101 patients who were seen with an abnormal karyotype and had sufficient metaphases at relapse for analysis. Karyotype changes included CE, CD (regression), or both. In general, a change in karyotype between the time of diagnosis and relapse had no significant influence on duration of remission. Furthermore, the investigators found no relationship between the length of a preceding remission and the likelihood of change in the cytogenetic pattern at first relapse. They also reported that a change in karyotype at first relapse did not influence the outcome of therapy in the great majority of patients, with the possible exception of a small number of patients who were seen with a karyotype other than inv(16), t(15;17), or t(8;21), but in whom only 10 or more normal metaphases were found at first relapse.

Although the number of patients in subgroups with certain karyotypes was small, this study suggests that the appearance of CE does not necessarily imply a uniformly fatal outcome. Further studies will need to be done to determine the molecular mechanisms by which karyotypes change and the mechanisms that lead to leukemic relapse.

M.S. Tallman, M.D.

Karyotype in Acute Myeloblastic Leukemia: Prognostic Significance in a Prospective Study Assessing Bone Marrow Transplantation in First Remission

Ferrant A, Doyen C, Delannoy A, Straetmans N, Martiat P, Mineur P, Bosly A, Van Den Berghe H, Michaux JL (Université Catholique de Louvain, Brussels, Belgium; Katholieke Universiteit Leuven, Belgium)
Bone Marrow Transplant 15:685–690, 1995   8–8

Background.—Prognostic indicators may be of great benefit to patients undergoing autologous or allogeneic bone marrow transplant (BMT) to prevent them from experiencing the toxic effects associated with certain therapies. In this prospective study, patients with acute myeloblastic leukemia (AML) in their first remission (CR1) were followed to determine the prognostic value of the karyotype.

Methods.—Patients younger than 56 years of age who received a diagnosis of AML formed the cohort of this study. Cytogenetic analysis and karyotyping were performed on 134 subjects; normal and abnormal clones were defined. The patients underwent induction with cytosine arabinoside, 100 mg/m² day, for 7 days, coupled with daunorubicin, 50 mg/m² day, for 3 days. After CR1 was achieved, a consolidation course was prescribed; patients not attaining CR1 received a different therapy. Graft-vs.-host disease was prevented with a combination of cyclosporine and methotrexate. Allografts or autografts were then performed. Data were interpreted using the Kaplan-Meier product-limit method, the Cox regression model, and the chi-square statistic.

Results.—A CR was achieved in 88% of patients, and all but 1 normalized their karyotype. The median delay between CR1 and allogeneic BMT was 73 days; for autologous BMT, the delay averaged 99 days. Cytogenic classification revealed the following karyotype information: 10 favorable, 49 intermediate risk, 44 unfavorable. Of those patients undergoing an allograft, the karyotype prognosis predicted 4 good, 11 intermediate, and 5 poor prognoses. Patients with an unfavorable karyotype were less likely to undergo BMT than were those with an intermediate or favorable karyotype, especially if there were no HLA-matched siblings available. The 5-year survival probability was calculated as 29% for all patients. The relapse probability was 63%. Survival probabilities according to karyotype were favorable, 80%; intermediate, 32%; and unfavorable, 11%. Multivariate analysis of all prognostic factors indicated that cytogenetic factors had the strongest influence on prognosis.

Discussion.—Autologous BMT did not change the poor prognosis associated with an unfavorable karyotype. The biology of certain leukemias with an unfavorable karyotype cannot be transcended by aggressive antileukemic methods.

▶ It has become apparent that patients with certain characteristic karyotypes have unfavorable prognoses when undergoing conventional chemotherapy for AML. Although it is generally believed that patients with such unfavorable karyotypes at the time of diagnosis will require less intensive therapy to achieve prolonged disease-free survival, the overall benefits of autologous and allogeneic BMT in this setting are unclear.

In this report, 134 consecutive patients with newly diagnosed AML were studied to evaluate the prognostic importance of karyotype on the outcome after allogeneic or autologous BMT in CR1. All patients received conventional induction chemotherapy with cytosine arabinoside and daunorubicin. Upon the achievement of CR1, consolidation chemotherapy with the identical dose and schedule administered during induction was given. The preparative regimen for both allogeneic and autologous transplantation included high-dose cytosine arabinoside, cyclophosphamide, and total body irradiation. Cyclosporine and methotrexate were used for graft-vs.-host disease prophylaxis. No transplants were T-cell–depleted. Patients were grouped by either favorable karyotypes, including t(15;17) and inv (16); intermediate prognosis karyotypes, including normal, X, Y, and t(8:21); or unfavorable prognosis karyotypes including other abnormalities.

The 5-year leukemia-free survival rate for patients undergoing allogeneic transplantation was 62%, compared with that for patients undergoing autologous transplantation, which was 32%. The 5-year leukemia-free survival rate for patients with favorable karyotypes was 65% compared with 33% for patients with an intermediate karyotype and 11% for patients with an unfavorable karyotype. The respective relapse rates were 35% for patients with a favorable karyotype, 52% for patients with an intermediate karyotype, and 87% for patients with an unfavorable karyotype.

The major limitation of this study concerns the number of patients in subgroups. For example, only 4 patients with favorable karyotypes underwent allogeneic BMT, and only 2 patients with favorable karyotypes received an autologous BMT. Although the number of patients in certain categories was too small to permit confidence regarding results, this paper is important because it suggests that unfavorable karyotypes indicate that the biology of such leukemias is such that even the most intensive antileukemic approach routinely available may not be enough to eradicate such leukemic clones. Further studies to confirm these observations will be extremely important.

M.S. Tallman, M.D.

Timed Sequential Chemotherapy for Previously Treated Patients With Acute Myeloid Leukemia: Long-Term Follow-Up of the Etoposide, Mitoxantrone, and Cytarabine-86 Trial

Archimbaud E, Thomas X, Leblond V, Michallet M, Fenaux P, Cordonnier C, Dreyfus F, Troussard X, Jaubert J, Travade P, Troncy J, Assouline D, Fiere D (Hôpital Edouard Herriot, Lyon, France; Hôpital André Michallon, Grenoble, France; Hôpital Claude Huriez, Lille, France; et al)

J Clin Oncol 13:11–18, 1995

8–9

Background.—Timed sequential chemotherapy (TSC) is intended to maximize the number of leukemic cells killed by cytotoxic drugs by recruiting cells initially and administering a second sequence of cycle-active drugs when the cell numbers peak. This has proven to be effective as first-line treatment of acute myeloid leukemia (AML), and also in patients who relapse after conventional chemotherapy.

Objective.—A TSC regimen of mitoxantrone, etoposide, and cytarabine was evaluated in 133 patients with AML, 111 in relapse and 22 who had failed to respond to previous chemotherapy. All but 2 patients had a World Health Organization performance status of 2 or less at the outset.

Management.—Mitoxantrone was given on days 1 to 3, etoposide on days 8 to 10, and cytarabine at both intervals. A second course of induction therapy was allowed if there was no complete remission. Some patients received maintenance treatment with reduced drug doses for 6 months. The median follow-up was 40 months.

Results.—Complete remission was achieved in 60% of patients and in 76% of those who were in first elapse of AML. Twenty-nine percent of patients failed to respond to treatment. The projected 5-year disease-free survival rates for patients less than 60 years of age who achieved a complete response ranged from 20% to 46%. Previous resistance to treatment was the most prominent adverse prognostic factor for both complete response and survival. Eleven percent of patients died of toxic drug effects. More than half the patients became septic.

Conclusion.—Approximately 1 in 5 patients with treatment-resistant or relapsed AML can expect prolonged disease-free survival after receiving TSC.

▶ The basis of the approach reported in this study is that one can gain an advantage by giving chemotherapy in a sequence that is timed to maximize a theoretical number of leukemia cells killed by cytotoxic agents. The theory is that one may recruit leukemia cells into the S-phase of cell cycle, when they are more susceptible to a second chemotherapeutic agent. The results in this sizable population of patients who had AML refractory to initial conventional therapy or who had relapse develop while receiving conventional therapy, was surprisingly good. Sixty percent of the patients achieved a second remission, and about 20% became long-term survivors.

However, all is not well in the interpretation of this study. Despite the authors' conclusions, 13 patients (younger than 50 years of age) received an allogeneic bone marrow transplantation, and 12 patients received an autologous bone marrow transplantation. As shown in Figure 3 in the original article, those who received an allogenic bone marrow transplantation apparently had a better survival, although one cannot leap to that conclusion because there was a favorable age selection bias of patients who received such treatment.

I include this paper to warn the reader about interpreting at face value any data given by the authors. In fact, the only conclusion one can arrive at after reviewing this paper is that the timed sequential chemotherapy may indeed be effective in improving outcome, but the use of 3 different types of regimens after this initial therapy casts some doubt on its independent contribution to the overall results.

J.V. Simone, M.D.

Autologous or Allogeneic Bone Marrow Transplantation Compared With Intensive Chemotherapy in Acute Myelogenous Leukemia
Zittoun RA, for the European Organization (for Research and Treatment of Cancer (EORTC) and the Gruppo Italiano Malattie Ematologiche Maligne dell' Adulto (GIMEME) Leukemia Cooperative Groups) (Univ La Sapienza, Rome; Leiden Univ, The Netherlands; St Radboud Hosp, Nijmegen, The Netherlands; Univ di Firenze, Florence, Italy; Ospedale San Martino, Genoa, Italy)
N Engl J Med 332:217–223, 1995   8–10

Background.—The majority of patients with primary acute myelogenous leukemia who enter complete remission after induction therapy relapse in spite of various types of maintenance chemotherapy. In adult patients younger than 60 years of age, treatment after initial induction of remission has been intensified. More and more patients in complete remission are treated with allogeneic or autologous bone marrow transplantation. The results of bone marrow transplantation are often from single institutions or registries and may carry a selection bias. In a prospective trial, disease-free survival and overall survival were examined after 3 postremission treatments.

Methods.—Patients with untreated acute myelogenous leukemia underwent induction treatment with daunorubicin (45 mg per square meter of body surface area) and cytarabine (200 mg per square meter). Those in a complete remission received intensive consolidation chemotherapy of intermediate-dose cytarabine (1,000 mg per square meter) and amsacrine (120 mg per square meter). Patients with an HLA-identical sibling underwent allogeneic bone marrow transplantation; the others randomly underwent autologous bone marrow transplantation with unpurged bone marrow, or a second course of intensive chemotherapy of high-dose cytarabine (2 g per square meter) and daunorubicin (45 mg per square meter). Comparisons were made on the basis of intention to treat.

Results.—The median follow-up was 3.3 years. A complete remission was achieved in 623 patients; 576 of these had received the first course of intensive consolidation chemotherapy. Of the 623 patients in complete remission, 168 were assigned to undergo allogeneic bone marrow transplantation, and 254 were randomly assigned to either autologous bone marrow transplantation or a second course of intensive consolidation chemotherapy. Of the 623 patients, 343 completed the treatment assignment. The relapse rate was the highest in the group receiving intensive chemotherapy; it was the lowest in the group receiving allogeneic transplantation. The mortality rate was the highest in the group receiving allogeneic transplantation and the lowest in the group receiving intensive chemotherapy. Adverse prognostic factors were: FAB class other than M2 or M3, longer interval from diagnosis to complete remission, need for more than one course of induction chemotherapy to achieve a complete remission, poor or intermediate prognosis according to cytogenetic classification of Keating et al., a high white blood cell count, and an elevated serum lactate dehydrogenase concentration. The projected rates of disease-free survival at 4 years were 55% for allogeneic transplantation, 48% for autologous transplantation, and 30% for intensive chemotherapy. After complete remission, the overall survival was similar for the 3 groups because more patients who relapsed after a second course of intensive chemotherapy responded to subsequent autologous bone marrow transplantation. Hematopoietic recovery occurred later after autologous transplantation, and the duration of hospitalization was longer with bone marrow transplantation.

Conclusions.—Autologous and allogeneic bone marrow transplantation result in better disease-free survival than does intensive consolidation chemotherapy with cytarabine and daunorubicin during a first complete remission in acute myelogenous leukemia. Transplantation immediately after a relapse or during a second complete remission might also yield good results. Other prospective studies have reported different regimens of intensive consolidation chemotherapy to be either superior to conventional regimens or equivalent to bone marrow transplantation.

▶ This large Italian study is noteworthy because of the number of patients evaluated and because of its attempt to answer a long-standing question regarding leukemia therapy. In adult acute myelogenous leukemia (AML), is either allogeneic or autologous bone marrow transplantation superior to systemic chemotherapy? The authors conclude that either type of transplantation is superior, as shown in Figure 2 in the original article. With chemotherapy, a disease-free survival of only 30% was obtained compared with rates of 55% with allogeneic transplantation and 48% with autologous. However, there are a number of notes of caution to be observed in the interpretation of this study. First, as shown in Figure 3 in the original article, the *overall* survival of the 3 groups was not greatly different. The authors attribute this to the ability of getting patients who fail chemotherapy treatment into a prolonged disease-free interval, during which time autologous transplantation is done. Nearly all the patients in this study were between the ages of 15 and 45 years. This is certainly the most favorable group of adults in which to see a response to any form of therapy. Thus, the study does not completely resolve the issue. If one provided treatment with aggressive chemotherapy and used autologous bone marrow transplantation to treat the first relapse, survival was not significantly different from the result in those patients who received transplantation in initial remission.

A critical factor to keep in mind is that the figures represent patients who have already achieved remission and should not be misconstrued as a reflection of the overall survival of the initial population of patients. Complete remission was achieved in 66% of the patients who were entered into the study; they were eligible to undergo one of the courses of treatment during remission. Therefore, if one wishes to estimate the overall effectiveness of therapy for AML in adults from the disease-free survival and survival curves presented, one must multiply them by 0.66. Thus, disease-free survival from diagnosis is about 20% for patients receiving chemotherapy compared with about 36% for allogeneic and 32% for autologous transplantation. If one uses the same mathematics for overall survival, the range is a 30% to 40% overall survival rate, irrespective of treatment. These results are better than historical results, but they are nothing to brag about.

J.V. Simone, M.D.

Rapid Engraftment After Autologous Transplantation Utilizing Marrow and Recombinant Granulocyte Colony-Stimulating Factor-Mobilized Peripheral Blood Stem Cells in Patients With Acute Myelogenous Leukemia

Demirer T, Buckner CD, Appelbaum FR, Petersen FB, Rowley S, Weaver CH, Lilleby K, Sanders J, Chauncey T, Storb R, Schiffman K, Benyunes MC, Fefer A, Montgomery P, Bensinger WI (Fred Hutchinson Cancer Research Ctr, Seattle; Seattle VA Hosp; Univ of Washington, Seattle; et al)
Bone Marrow Transplant 15:915–922, 1995   8–11

Background.—Studies of patients with lymphoma and solid tumors have found that peripheral blood stem cells (PBSCs) collected after recombinant human granulocyte colony-stimulating factor (rhG-CSF) produce very rapid, sustained platelet recovery compared with bone marrow (BM). The effects of administering rhG-CSF to patients with AML in first or second remission to enhance PBSC collection were investigated.

Methods.—Twenty-six patients with AML were included in the study. Sixteen had BM harvested in first complete remission (CR) and 10 in second CR for cryopreservation. Twenty patients received rhG-CSF alone, and 6 received rhG-CSF after chemotherapy. Twenty-four of the patients had PBSCs collected at a median 7 days after marrow harvest. In 2 patients thought to be in second CR, PBSCs were not collected because of early relapse. Three patients in first CR, 8 in second CR, and 3 in first relapse then proceeded to autologous BM transplantation (BMT) using marrow plus PBSCs mobilized by rhG-CSF. A historical control group of 158 patients with AML who had received purged or unpurged autologous BMT without PBSCs was used for engraftment parameter comparison.

Findings.—All patients had a granulocyte level exceeding 0.5×10^9/L at a median of 13 days. Platelets were 20×10^9/L at a median of 14 days. Seventy-three of the 91 historical control patients receiving unpurged marrow alone had granulocyte levels of 0.5×10^9/L at a median 30 days, and 46 had platelets exceeding 20×10^9/L at a median 40 days.

Conclusions.—Engraftment in patients with AML receiving marrow and rhG-CSF–mobilized PBSCs was earlier than that observed previously in patients receiving purged or unpurged marrow. Whether the inclusion of marrow is needed for prompt and sustained engraftment is still not known.

Conclusions about the incidence of leukemic relapse after rhG-CSF administration cannot be drawn from these data.

▶ Although autologous BMT for patients with AML in first complete remission has become an attractive postremission strategy for patients with suitable sibling marrow donors, delayed engraftment, particularly as platelets, causes significant morbidity and mortality. The use of PBSCs as a source of hematopoietic reconstitution in patients with lymphoma and solid tumors has resulted in rapid and sustained platelet recovery compared with that after BM alone.

In this study, Demirer and colleagues used PBSCs mobilized with rhG-CSF in addition to BM as a source of hematopoietic reconstitution for patients undergoing autologous BMT for AML.

This study shows that the patients had earlier engraftment than previously observed. Whether the combination is necessary or whether peripheral blood-derived hematopoietic stem cells alone would be sufficient to provide a similar rapid engraftment will await further studies. It is important to know that little information is available regarding the impact of growth factor in this setting on the incidence of leukemic relapse.

M.S. Tallman, M.D.

Randomized Comparison of Interferon-α With Busulfan and Hydroxyurea in Chronic Myelogenous Leukemia

Hehlmann R, and the German CML Study Group (Universität Heidelberg, Mannheim, Germany)
Blood 84:4064–4077, 1994

8–12

Introduction.—Because curative bone marrow transplantation can be performed in few patients with chronic myelogenous leukemia (CML), most of these patients receive drug therapy. Historically, palliative treatment has been achieved mostly with either busulfan or hydroxyurea (HU). More recently, interferon-α (IFN) has been an effective palliative agent during the chronic phase and has also brought about complete cytogenetic remission and prolonged survival in some patients. In a randomized trial, the relative effects of busulfan, HU, and IFN on survival, hematologic and cytogenetic responses, toxicity, and the course of the disease were evaluated.

Methods.—Patients with newly diagnosed CML in the chronic phase were randomly assigned to receive either daily subcutaneous IFN, intermittent busulfan, or daily HU. The patients were followed up regularly to document drug resistance, adverse effects of therapy, diagnosis of blast crisis, and survival.

Results.—The patients achieved 5-year survival at the rate of 59% in the IFN group, 32% in the busulfan group, and 44% in the HU group. Survival was largely determined by the rate of progression to blast crisis, with longer survival being associated with slower progression. Survival was significantly reduced in patients in whom IFN therapy was discontinued compared with those who continued IFN therapy until blast crisis. There were no significant differences between the 3 groups in the rates of complete and partial hematologic remissions, but the median duration of hematologic response was longest in the IFN group. Cytogenetic response was significantly more common in the IFN group than in the busulfan or HU groups. Adverse reactions requiring discontinuation of therapy occurred in 18% of the IFN group, 10.2% of the busulfan group, and 0.5% of the HU group.

Discussion.—These results show a significant survival advantage associated with IFN therapy in patients with CML compared with therapy with a standard bisulfan regimen but not to therapy with HU. However, patients who achieve a complete cytogenetic response with IFN have a survival advantage over HU-treated patients. Nevertheless, IFN must be used with caution, because it is associated with a high rate of adverse drug effects, requires regular injections and good patient compliance, and is considerably more costly than other therapies.

▶ I included this study because it is large, well done, and addresses an important question about the management of CML. As shown in Figure 2 in the original article, the survival of patients treated with IFN was superior to that of patients who received busulfan but not to patients who received HU. Although IFN is more toxic than the other agents (sufficient to cause discontinuation of therapy in some patients), it was not as likely to cause prolonged myelosuppression. The authors' conclusion is that IFN and HU are of approximately equal effectiveness. This is at variance with other investigators' findings, which have found IFN to be more effective. The authors of this paper explain that difference by the fact that they use HU much more aggressively, i.e., they insist on reducing the leukocyte count to the normal range in contrast to a goal of less than 30,000, which is normal in many other studies.

One might ask whether a better result could be achieved for patients with CML if these two agents could be combined. Studies are under way in several centers to try to answer this question, because the end results are still quite dismal. Even though it might take years for all patients to succumb, there is no plateau in any of the survival curves indicating cures.

J.V. Simone, M.D.

Significant Reduction of Medical Costs by Differentiation Therapy With *all-trans* Retinoic Acid During Remission Induction of Newly Diagnosed Patients With Acute Promyelocytic Leukemia
Takeshita A, Sakamaki H, Miyawaki S, Kobayashi T, Kuriyama K, Yamada O, Oh H, Takenaka T, Asou N, Ohno R, and the Japan Adult Leukemia Study Group (Hamamatsu Univ, Japan; Tokyo Metropolitan Komagome Hosp; Gumma Univ, Maebashi, Japan; et al)
Cancer 76:602–608, 1995
8–13

Introduction.—Several studies have shown that differentiation therapy with all-*trans* retinoic acid (ATRA) induces an exceptionally high rate of complete remission with minimal complications in patients with acute promyelocytic leukemia (APL). Because the patients have fewer complications, they require less antibiotic treatment or platelet and erythrocyte infusions, which prompted a comparison of medical costs between patients treated with intensive chemotherapy and those treated with ATRA.

Methods.—The medical costs were calculated using monthly bills sent from the hospitals to the national health insurance for 76 patients with newly diagnosed APL, including 36 patients treated with standard intensive chemotherapy and 40 treated with ATRA therapy either alone or in combination with low-dose chemotherapy. Because the ATRA had been donated, the costs of all antileukemic drugs were excluded from the cost analysis.

Results.—Excluding the costs of antileukemic drugs, the medical costs during the 2 months after admission averaged $46,300 for the chemotherapy group and $32,300 for the ATRA group. The difference was mainly attributable to the increased need for antibiotics and for platelet and erythrocyte transfusions in the chemotherapy group. The cost of antibiotics averaged $7,200 in the chemotherapy group and $3,900 in the ATRA group. The cost of platelet and erythrocyte transfusions averaged $11,300 in the chemotherapy group and $7,000 in the ATRA group.

Conclusions.—Medical costs during remission induction therapy for APL were significantly lower for patients treated with ATRA than for those treated with standard intensive chemotherapy. This cost reduction, combined with the superior efficacy and diminished complication rate associated with ATRA therapy, argues for the incorporation of ATRA into the frontline therapy for APL.

▶ Multiple phase II studies have now shown that the vitamin A derivative ATRA induces high rates of complete remission in patients with APL through differentiation of the leukemic promyelocytes into mature neutrophils. A second potential major benefit of this approach compared with cytotoxic chemotherapy is the apparent rapid resolution of the life-threatening coagulopathy. Patients receiving ATRA pills may do so as outpatients once their conditions are otherwise stable.

The authors of this study report a retrospective comparison of the costs of remission induction with ATRA and conventional chemotherapy. They conclude that ATRA should be incorporated into the frontline therapy for patients with APL for medical and economic reasons. The cost savings are a significant benefit; however, a first prospective randomized comparison between ATRA plus chemotherapy and conventional chemotherapy alone showed a higher complete remission rate and improved event-free survival with the addition of ATRA. Further studies are under way to confirm this important initial observation. If these observations prove to be definitely true, then ATRA should be incorporated into the frontline therapy of patients, because overall outcome is significantly improved with the added benefit of cost reduction.

M.S. Tallman, M.D.

Effect of Aggressive Daunomycin Therapy on Survival in Acute Promyelocytic Leukemia

Head D, Kopecky KJ, Weick J, Files JC, Ryan D, Foucar K, Montiel M, Bickers J, Fishleder A, Miller M, Spier C, Hanson C, Bitter M, Braziel R, Mills G, Welborn J, Williams W, Hewlett J, Willman C, Appelbaum FR (St Jude Children's Research Hosp, Memphis, Tenn; Southwest Oncology Group Statistical Ctr, Seattle; Cleveland Clinic, Ohio; et al)
Blood 86:1717–1728, 1995   8–14

Background.—In the initial reports of the treatment of acute promyelocytic leukemia (APL), a morphological subtype of acute myeloblastic leukemia (AML), cytotoxic chemotherapy was associated with poor outcomes and a high frequency of early deaths from bleeding caused by coagulation abnormalities. However, subsequent studies of chemotherapy in patients with APL showed a survival similar to or slightly better than that achieved in patients with other AML variants. The effect of aggressive daunomycin treatment on survival in patients with APL was investigated by the Southwest Oncology Group (SWOG).

Methods and Findings.—The outcomes in patients with APL achieved from 1982 through 1986 were compared with those achieved from 1986 through 1991. Forty-five patients with APL treated from 1982 through 1986 had a median survival of 106 months and a disease-free survival of more than 105 months. The corresponding times for 417 other patients with AML were 6 and 14 months. These differences were not apparent between 1986 and 1991. In the 141 patients with APL treated from 1982 through 1991, greater doses of daunomycin during induction were significantly correlated with higher complete remission rates, longer survival, and longer disease-free survival, after adjustments were made for significant patient and disease characteristics. The outcomes of APL did not appear to be significantly affected by cytosine arabinoside (Ara-C) induction dose, the inclusion of other chemotherapeutic agents in induction, postremission treatment other than daunomycin, APL subtype, or patient age. However, high-dose Ara-C had a significant detrimental effect in consolidation. Other morphological AML subtypes were not associated with different outcomes.

Conclusions.—High-dose daunomycin selectively increases survival in patients with APL. Chemotherapy needs to be individualized for subtypes of AML. The treatment response in patients with APL is independent of age. Acute promyelocytic leukemia was the only morphological subclassification of AML that contributed important prognostic information.

▶ Although the emerging role of all-*trans* retinoic acid (ATRA) for patients with acute promyelocytic leukemia (APL) has received a great deal of attention recently because of the ability of this vitamin A derivative to induce high rates of complete remission with rapid amelioration of the coagulopathy, few data are available regarding the long-term outlook with this approach. It is well known that the cells from patients with APL appear particularly sensitive to anthracyclines.

Head and colleagues report the results of a retrospective analysis of the outcome with cytotoxic chemotherapy for patients with previously untreated APL. They found a statistically significant association with cumulative daunomycin dose during induction with survival and disease-free survival. Previous studies conducted by the Southwest Oncology Group and reports by others of patients treated with lower-dose anthracycline regimens do not show this marked survival advantage.

These data suggest that a combination of prolonged delivery and/or total daunomycin dose may be more important than the induction dose of this agent alone in providing patients with long-term disease-free survival. Although the biological reason for the apparent peculiar sensitivity of leukemic cells from patients with APL to anthracyclines is not known, this observation has been a consistent one.

These results are important because of the high rates of complete remission for patients with APL treated with ATRA. It is not yet clear whether these rates achieved with ATRA will translate into prolonged disease-free survival. Clearly, this can be achieved with high-dose daunorubicin. This study raises the question of incorporating high-dose anthracyclines for patients with APL in some combination with ATRA.

M.S. Tallman, M.D.

Graft-Versus-Leukemia Effect of Donor Lymphocyte Transfusions in Marrow Grafted Patients

Kolb H-J, for the European Group for Blood and Marrow Transplantation Working Party Chronic Leukemia (Univ of Munich, Germany)
Blood 86:2041–2050, 1995   8–15

Background.—The immune reactivity of allogeneic lymphocytes plays an important role in controlling leukemia after bone marrow transplantation (BMT). Chimerism and tolerance provide ideal conditions for adoptive immunotherapy with donor lymphocytes in patients with recurrent leukemia after BMT. The effect of donor lymphocyte transfusions on acute and chronic leukemia in patients with relapse after BMT was studied.

Methods.—Donor lymphocyte infusions were administered to 84 patients with chronic myeloid leukemia (CML), 23 with acute myeloid leukemia (AML), 22 with acute lymphoblastic leukemia (ALL), 5 with myelodysplastic syndrome (MDS), and 1 with polycythemia vera with osteomyelofibrosis (PCV). The polymerase chain reaction was used to monitor for *bcr/abl* messenger RNA transcripts and for the occurrence of graft-vs.-host disease (GVHD) and myelosuppression.

Findings.—Donor lymphocyte transfusions induced complete remissions in 73% of patients with CML, 29% of the patients with AML, in 1 patient with MDS, and in the patient with PCV. Adoptive immunotherapy with donor lymphocyte transfusions had no effect on ALL. Patients with CML in the chronic phase had durable remissions. Eighteen patients with ALL, AML, MDS, and transformed-phase CML in remission after chemotherapy also received lymphocyte transfusions but did not achieve durable remissions. Grade 2 or higher GVHD developed in 41% of the patients. Thirty-four percent of the patients had signs of myelosuppression. Of 17 patients dying without leukemia, 14 had GVHD and/or myelosuppression.

Conclusions.—Donor lymphocyte transfusion is an effective treatment of recurrent leukemia in patients with CML, PCV, AML, and MDS. Toxicity may be improved by strictly controlling GVHD and by infusing marrow or blood stem cells in patients with severe myelosuppression.

▶ In 1990, Kolb was the first investigator to report that lymphocyte infusions from the original marrow donor could induce remission in patients who have relapse after allogeneic BMT. Since then, several institutions have reported similar results in small numbers of patients. Appropriately, Kolb now reports on the largest number of patients treated to date with donor lymphocyte infusion for remission induction following relapse after allogeneic BMT.

Remissions were obtained in the majority of patients with CML (54 of 84), a minority of patients with AML (5 of 23), and no patient with ALL (0 of 22). For patients who have relapse with leukemia within 1 year of an allogeneic transplant, a second transplant is complicated by high mortality, whereas further chemotherapy is, at best, palliative. Immunotherapy using adoptive transfer of donor lymphocytes offers new hope for durable remissions in patients with CML and AML who relapse after an allogeneic BMT.

The importance of donor cell dose and the prevention of complications such as marrow aplasia and graft-vs.-host disease have yet to be unraveled for this new form of therapy.

R. Burt, M.D.

9 Adult Lymphoma

How Relevant Is Secondary Leukaemia for Initial Treatment Selection in Hodgkin's Disease?
Hess CF, Kortmann RD, Schmidberger H, Bamberg M (Universitätklinik, Göttingen, Germany)
Eur J Cancer 30A:1441–1447, 1994   9–1

Background.—Reported rates of secondary leukemia in patients cured of Hodgkin's disease (HD) vary widely, and there is much controversy as to whether the possibility of inducing leukemia should be taken into account when selecting initial treatment.

Objective and Methods.—The decision analysis approach was used to examine the influence of secondary leukemia in choosing the initial treatment for HD. The "expected utility" of alternative management strategies was determined, taking survival, relapse-free survival, and treatment-related leukemia into account.

Results.—It appears neessary, when considering initial treatment, to attempt to estimate all possible events that may follow initial treatment, including the risk of recurrence and the likelihood of salvage treatment succeeding. In patients with early or intermediate-stage HD, the minimal risk of leukemia after effective radiotherapy should be weighed against the increased risk should treatment fail and salvage therapy be necessary. The difference in leukemia risk between radiotherapy and combined-modality treatment is less than 4% for stage IIB HD, and nearly zero for stage IIIA cases. In advanced-stage HD, adding radiotherapy to chemotherapy does not compromise the expected utility of initial treatment. The results were not affected by taking quality-of-life matters (latency between treatment and leukemia; patient attitudes about the risk of leukemia) into account.

Implications.—Even small gains in survival outweigh the risk of treatment-related leukemia when selecting initial treatment for HD. There would appear to be no sound reason to administer less intense treatment to avoid inducing leukemia.

▶ This is an interesting but complex paper because it requires an appreciation of the moderately challenging mathematics that are used. The basic premise of the authors is that to assess whether the likelihood of a secondary leukemia should influence initial treatment, one must follow each cohort of patients through all likely outcomes. They also rightly insist that one must include all negative events, including the requirement for salvage therapy. One can summarize their findings in the following manner: For patients given initial radiotherapy alone, consideration of secondary leukemia becomes progressively more important, with increasing recurrence rates. This is a result of the increasing rates of leukemia after successful salvage chemotherapy on top of the initial radiation. On the contrary, for patients who are given initial chemotherapy without radiation, increasing recurrence rates have a minor effect on the subsequent occurrence of secondary leukemia.

The obvious conclusion is that there is no basis for reducing the intensity of the initial treatment for HD to avoid secondary leukemia. One must keep in mind, however, that the comparisons are between groups that received radiotherapy only vs. a group that received only chemotherapy as their sole initial treatment. Therefore, the likelihood of recurrence and the requirement for another round of treatment play a major role in the interpretation of the study. There is no substitute for a highly effective initial treatment.

J.V. Simone, M.D.

Etoposide, Vinblastine, and Doxorubicin: An Active Regimen for the Treatment of Hodgkin's Disease in Relapse Following MOPP
Canellos GP, for the Cancer and Leukemia Group B (Dana-Farber Cancer Inst, Boston)
J Clin Oncol 13:2005–2011, 1995

9–2

Background.—Of the variety of second-line regimens used to treat patients experiencing a first relapse of Hodgkin's disease (HD), one of the most common is doxorubicin, bleomycin, vinblastine, and dacarbazine (ABVD). However, pulmonary toxicity induced by bleomycin is a significant risk in patients with ABVD, as is nausea and vomiting associated with dacarbazine. A new regimen was developed to avoid both gastrointestinal and pulmonary complications: etoposide, vinblastine, and doxorubicin (EVA). The efficacy of EVA was evaluated in a clinical trial with patients who did not respond or relapsed after initial therapy with mechlorethamine, vincristine, procarbazine, and prednisone (MOPP).

Methods.—Patients older than 15 years of age with histologically proven, measurable HD in first relapse at least 4 weeks after a single prior MOPP regimen were eligible for study. All eligible patients were evaluated at baseline with chest x-ray studies, abdominal CT scans, electrocardiography, bone marrow aspirate or biopsy, complete blood cell counts, and liver and renal function chemistries. The EVA regimen was given as follows: etoposide on days 1, 2, and 3, and vinblastine and doxorubicin only on day 1. The regimen was repeated every 28 days for 4–6 cycles. Efficacy was assessed using measures of the time to complete response, the duration of complete response, survival, and the time to treatment failure (TTF).

Results.—Of the 45 evaluable patients, 40% had a complete response and 33% had a partial response. A complete response was not significantly predicted by sex, disease stage, extranodal involvement, prior response to

MOPP, or duration of prior response to MOPP. However, nodular sclerosis histology, B symptoms, and performance status ≥ 1 were all negatively correlated with a complete response. Overall, the median TTF was 10 months and the median survival was 3.2 years. Of the 18 patients with a complete response (followed for a median of 4.3 years), only 7 have relapsed, and the median duration of complete response has not been reached. Both TTF and survival were significantly longer in patients with an initial response of longer than 12 months and with an absence of B symptoms. Myelosuppression was the major toxicity in these patients, with no pulmonary toxicity observed, no nausea or vomiting in 25%, and only mild or moderate nausea and vomiting in 63%.

Conclusion.—The monthly EVA regimen is effective in inducing prolonged complete responses in patients with HD after relapse or no response to MOPP. This regimen may be especially appropriate in patients with compromised lung function.

▶ The outlook for patients with HD, whether limited or advanced, has improved remarkably, and the overwhelming majority of patients are now cured of their disease. Although combination chemotherapy with MOPP remains the time-honored gold standard, for patients who relapse after treatment with this regimen, ABVD induces second complete remissions in approximately 30% of patients, with some patients remaining relapse-free for prolonged periods. However, pulmonary toxicity, which is usually attributable to bleomycin associated with the latter regimen, is potentially fatal.

The authors report the results of the use of a novel regimen, EVA, for patients who have relapsed or have failed to respond to initial therapy with MOPP. This regimen was developed to eliminate the gastrointestinal toxicity of dacarbazine and to avoid bleomycin-associated pulmonary complications, particularly in patients treated with combined modality therapy conducted by the Cancer and Leukemia Group B. Patients can only have received 1 prior course of MOPP, either in relapse or in demonstrated progressive disease during treatment. The overall response rate was 73% among 45 patients treated, with a complete remission rate of 40% and a partial remission rate of 33%. With a median follow-up of 42 months, the median time to treatment failure was 10 months, with 31% of patients continuing progression-free. Among the 18 patients achieving a second complete remission, only 7 have recurred.

The failure-free survival and overall survival rates were significantly better in patients whose first remission induced with MOPP was longer than 12 months and who were free of B symptoms. Pulmonary toxicity was not observed. The primary toxicity was myelosuppression. This report is encouraging in that it demonstrates that this regimen may be useful in patients with bleomycin-related pulmonary complications or severe vinca alkaloid neuropathy during primary therapy.

M.S. Tallman, M.D.

Detection of Immunophenotypic Abnormalities in Paraffin-Embedded B-Lineage Non-Hodgkin's Lymphomas

Gelb AB, Rouse RV, Dorfman RF, Warnke RA (Stanford Univ, Calif; Univ of California, San Francisco; Veterans Affairs Med Ctr, Palo Alto, Calif)
Am J Clin Pathol 102:825–834, 1994   9–3

Introduction.—It is difficult to distinguish among the various types of malignant lymphomas and benign reactive proliferations. Immunophenotyping has shown promise as an adjunct technique in the diagnosis and classification of non-Hodgkin's lymphomas. The immunophenotypic abnormalities identified by paraffin-section immunohistochemistry was reported retrospectively.

Methods.—The records of 1,474 patients who were given a diagnosis of non-Hodgkin's lymphomas and classified by morphological criteria, including the results of paraffin- or frozen-section immunohistochemical analysis, were reviewed. Paraffin-section immunohistochemistry identified B-lineage. The abnormal immunophenotypic features were listed, and the proportion of patients with each feature was calculated.

Results.—Of the 1,474 sections, B-lineage was confirmed in 92% by CD20 reactivity, in 71% by CD45RA reactivity (especially in decalcified tissues), and in 22% by immunoglobulin (Ig) light chain restriction. Immunoglobulin light chain restriction was seen most frequently in association with plasmacytoid diffuse small lymphocytic lymphomas (67%) and next most frequently in mantle cell lymphomas (43%); it was more common in extranodal than in nodal sites (Table 2). Abnormal co-expression of CD43 in neoplastic B cells was the most common immunophenotypic abnormality and was seen most often in mantle-cell lymphomas (60%), followed by small lymphocytic lymphomas (39%), diffuse large-cell lymphomas (16%), and follicular lymphomas (5%) (Table 3). The overexpression of *bcl*-2 oncogenic protein occurred in 71% of follicular lymphomas but not in reactive follicular hyperplasias. It also was more common

TABLE 2.—Immunoglobulin Light Chain Restriction

| | Antigen Expression | | | | | |
| | Nodal Sites | | Extranodal Sites* | | Totals | |
Histologic Type	No. of Cases	No. Positive (%)	No. of Cases	No. Positive (%)	No. of Cases	No. Positive (%)
Small lymphocytic lymphomas						
Not otherwise specified	42	7 (17)	66	16 (24)	108	23 (21)
Plasmacytoid	17	12 (71)	45	30 (67)	61	41 (67)
Monocytoid B-cell/MALToma	15	5 (33)	36	13 (36)	51	18 (35)
Mantle cell lymphoma	27	11 (41)	15	7 (47)	42	18 (43)
Diffuse large-cell lymphoma	58	14 (24)	95	24 (25)	153	38 (25)
Immunoblastic plasmacytoid	10	1 (10)	10	5 (50)	20	6 (30)
Follicular lymphoma	63	18 (29)	34	9 (26)	97	27 (28)

* Includes biopsy specimens from extranodal sites in some patients with histories of nodal lymphomas.
(Courtesy of Gelb AB, Rouse RV, Dorfman RF, et al: Detection of immunophenotypic abnormalities in paraffin-embedded B-lineage non-Hodgkin's lymphomas. *Am J Clin Pathol* 102:825–834, 1994.)

TABLE 3.—Coexpression of CD43 (Leu–22)

| | Antigen Expression | | | | | |
| | Nodal Sites | | Extranodal Sites* | | Totals | |
Histologic Type	No. of Cases	No. Positive (%)	No. of Cases	No. Positive (%)	No. of Cases	No. Positive (%)
Small lymphocytic lymphomas						
Not otherwise specified	140	29 (21)	79	26 (33)	219	55 (25)
Plasmacytoid	13	2 (15)	39	7 (18)	52	9 (17)
Monocytoid B-cell/MALToma	11	1 (9)	28	10 (36)	39	11 (28)
Mantle cell	32	20 (62)	16	9 (56)	48	29 (60)
Diffuse large-cell lymphoma	189	33 (17)	327	51 (16)	516	84 (16)
Immunoblastic cell	70	9 (13)	68	13 (19)	138	22 (16)
Small noncleaved cell	13	5 (38)	11	3 (27)	24	8 (33)
Follicular lymphoma	104	4 (4)	46	4 (9)	150	8 (5)

* Includes biopsy specimens from extranodal sites in some patients with histories of nodal lymphomas.

(Courtesy of Gelb AB, Rouse RV, Dorfman RF, et al: Detection of immunophenotypic abnormalities in paraffin-embedded B-lineage non-Hodgkin's lymphomas. *Am J Clin Pathol* 102:825–834, 1994.)

with follicular small cleaved cell lymphoma than in follicular mixed small- and large-cell and large-cell lymphomas, respectively (Table 4). Combining 2 immunophenotypic criteria significantly improved the diagnostic value, especially when CD43 co-expression and Ig light chain restriction were used together (Table 5).

Discussion.—Common immunophenotypic abnormalities were identified that could be useful in diagnosing and classifying difficult cases, particularly when a panel of antibodies is used. However, immunophenotypic abnormalities must be interpreted within the context of other clinical and pathologic findings, because they may not be specific enough on their own.

▶ The subject of the classification of the non-Hodgkin's lymphomas is complex and has a lot of importance, not only for pathologists interested in a logical process of categorization, but also for clinicians who have to deal with this group of neoplasms, which are extraordinary in their range of biological activity. In the non-Hodgkin's category, a plethora of classification systems led to the retrospective analysis from the National Cancer Institute

TABLE 4.—Expression of bcl-2 in Follicular Lesions

| | Antigen Expression | |
Histologic Type	No. of Cases	% Positive
Reactive follicular hyperplasia	34	0
Follicular lymphomas (total)	96	71
Follicular small cleaved cell	23	83
Follicular mixed small- and large-cell	35	74
Follicular large-cell	38	61

Chi-square *P* value < .001.

(Courtesy of Gelb AB, Rouse RV, Dorfman RF, et al: Detection of immunophenotypic abnormalities in paraffin-embedded B-lineage non-Hodgkin's lymphomas. *Am J Clin Pathol* 102:825–834, 1994.)

TABLE 5.—Coexpression of CD43 vs. Immunoglobulin Light Chain Reaction

| | Antigen Expression | | | | | | | | | | |
| | Nodal Sites | | | Extranodal Sites* | | | Totals | | | | |
Histologic Type	No. Cases	No. Coexpressing CD43 (%)	No. Ig Restricted (%)	Either Criterion (%)	No. of Cases	No. Coexpressing CD43 (%)	No. Ig Restricted (%)	Either Criterion (%)	No. of Cases	No. Coexpressing CD43 (%)	No. Ig Restricted (%)	Either Criterion (%)
Small lymphocytic lymphomas												
Not otherwise specified	54	24 (44)	14 (26)	35 (65)	88	33 (38)	22 (25)	50 (57)	142	57 (40)	36 (25)	85 (60)
Plasmacytoid	11	5 (45)	7 (64)	(72)	38	10 (26)	23 (61)	28 (74)	49	15 (312)	30 (61)	36 (73)
Monocytoid B-cell/MALToma	10	1 (10)	2 (20)	3 (30)	24	7 (29)	10 (42)	12 (50)	34	8 (24)	12 (35)	15 (44)
Mantle cell lymphoma	18	10 (56)	6 (33)	10 (56)	12	4 (33)	4 (33)	6 (50)	30	14 (47)	10 (33)	16 (53)
Diffuse large-cell lymphoma	76	8 (11)	13 (17)	20 (26)	111	17 (15)	20 (18)	35 (32)	187	25 (13)	33 (18)	55 (29)
Follicular lymphoma	61	5 (8)	18 (30)	23 (38)	44	4 (9)	12 (27)	13 (30)	105	9 (9)	30 (29)	36 (34)

* Theoretically includes biopsy specimens from extranodal sites in some patients with nodal lymphomas but no history thereof provided.
(Courtesy of Gelb AB, Rouse RV, Dorfman RF, et al: Detection of immunophenotypic abnormalities in paraffin-embedded B-lineage non-Hodgkin's lymphomas. *Am J Clin Pathol* 102:825–834, 1994.)

Moving?

I'd like to receive my *Year Book of Oncology* without interruption.
Please note the following change of address, effective:

Name: _______________________________

New Address: _______________________________

City: _______________ State: _______ Zip: _______

Old Address: _______________________________

City: _______________ State: _______ Zip: _______

Reservation Card

Yes, I would like my own copy of *Year Book of Oncology*. Please begin my subscription with the current edition according to the terms described below.* I understand that I will have 30 days to examine each annual edition. If satisfied, I will pay just $77.95 plus sales tax, postage and handling (price subject to change without notice).

Name: _______________________________

Address: _______________________________

City: _______________ State: _______ Zip: _______

Method of Payment
○ Visa   ○ Mastercard   ○ AmEx   ○ Bill me   ○ Check (in US dollars, payable to Mosby, Inc.)

Card number: _______________ Exp date: _______________

Signature: _______________________________

LS-0909

Your Year Book Service Guarantee:

When you subscribe to the *Year Book*, we'll send you an advance notice of future volumes about two months before they publish. This automatic notice system is designed to take up as little of your time as possible. If you do not want the *Year Book*, the advance notice makes it quick and easy for you to let us know your decision, and you will always have at least 20 days to decide. If we don't hear from you, we'll send you the new volume as soon as it's available. And, of course, the *Year Book* is yours to examine free of charge for 30 days (postage, handling and applicable sales tax are added to each shipment.).

BUSINESS REPLY MAIL
FIRST CLASS MAIL   PERMIT No. 762   CHICAGO, IL

POSTAGE WILL BE PAID BY ADDRESSEE

Chris Hughes
Mosby-Year Book, Inc.
200 N. LaSalle Street
Suite 2600
Chicago, IL 60601-9981

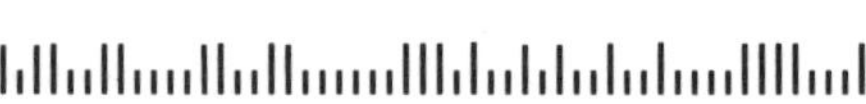

BUSINESS REPLY MAIL
FIRST CLASS MAIL   PERMIT No. 762   CHICAGO, IL

POSTAGE WILL BE PAID BY ADDRESSEE

Chris Hughes
Mosby-Year Book, Inc.
200 N. LaSalle Street
Suite 2600
Chicago, IL 60601-9981

that was published in the 1980s and that culminated in the "formulation." It was called a formulation because it was designed to serve as an intermediary among the different classification systems and was not planned to replace any of them. In addition, the formulation was published without anyone's name being associated with it.

It is obvious from the ongoing developments in immunology and molecular biology that we are in a transition period in which new technologies are developing almost daily. These technologies hopefully will be sufficiently accurate in the future to permit us to develop a new classification approach, which ultimately will not be based on classic morphology. The key is to be able to assess the adequacy of the science itself, which may thereby permit us to use a new gold standard. In my opinion, at the present time the gold standard is still morphology, even with all of the reservations that we have in terms of its inability to reproduce reliably with 90% accuracy.

This paper from Stanford evaluates immunophenotypic procedures in B-cell non-Hodgkin's lymphomas that have been imbedded in paraffin. This is an impressive paper not only for the work that was done, but also for the analysis and the pithy discussion that went into it. It is also impressive to look at the tables and see the percentages of expression of various immunophenotypic abnormalities. It is obvious that we have a long way to go before we can reliably trust the use of immunophenotypic procedures for routine classification. This is not to say that in the hands of experts we should have reservations. However, it does imply that these tests are subtle, are associated with their own probabilities of errors, and are not necessarily easy to reproduce reliably from one laboratory to another, although they appear to be reliable within any one laboratory. Even so, just as any other technology that is applied, the studies show that one can be fooled by false positivity or false negativity. Pathologists who wish to base everything on immunophenotyping have to demonstrate the reliability that these tests have, at least in comparison to morphology.

There are proposals for still another classification of lymphoid neoplasms.[1] This new classification system effectively is a modification of the working formulation that includes the addition of some recently described entities, such as the monocytoid B-cell lymphoma, maltoma, and mantle cell lymphomas, among others. This new classification system spends a lot of time describing the procedures that need to be done and what the expected outcome is (although it gives no information on probabilities of deviation). It is disappointing however, to see a complete absence of clinical pathologic correlation, and the only clinical information that is described represents generalizations that cannot be applied reliably to any single case.

All of us want to see a classification system that represents scientific validity as well as clinical usefulness. If these two aspects of classification are separated, it will defeat the purpose and welfare of patients and physicians alike. It is still disappointing to realize that true entities, such as composite lymphomas, still fail to be categorized by any of the classification systems.

Obviously, the mysteries of lymphoma are far more subtle than any of us fully appreciates. The discussion in this paper points out a variety of problems that make it difficult to interpret immunophenotyping. Aberrant co-expressions apparently are common among these different lymphoid neoplasms. There is some reason to believe that for at least some types of lymphoma, the expression of immunophenotyping may differ if the biopsy specimen is obtained from nodal, as opposed to extranodal, tissue. It is possible that the expression of immunophenotyping may vary throughout the course of disease, making the interpretation of the presence or absence of some of these reactions difficult.

This paper sheds light on what is otherwise a very confusing field at the present time. The data that the authors present need corroboration from other sources, but it is clear that immunophenotyping will continue and will ultimately prove to be a major source of data, from which clinical pathologic correlations should be made. I have some question as to whether this is reliable enough, at the present time, to serve as a routine classification system, although its value in difficult morphologic cases is already clear. It is somewhat disconcerting, however, to project a new classification system every time a new test appears to describe a pathologic entity.

E. Glatstein, M.D.

Reference

1. Harris NL, Jaffe ES, Stein H, et al: A revised European-American classification of lymphoid neoplasms: A proposal from the International Lymphoma Study Group. *Blood* 84:1361–1392, 1994.

Comparison of Autologous Bone Marrow Transplantation With Sequential Chemotherapy for Intermediate-Grade and High-Grade Non-Hodgkin's Lymphoma in First Complete Remission: A Study of 464 Patients
Haioun C, for the Groupe d'Etude des Lymphomes de l' Adulte (Hôpital Henri Mondor, Créteil, France)
J Clin Oncol 12:2543–2551, 1994   9–4

Objective.—Promising results have been achieved in treating partially responsive patients with aggressive non-Hodgkin's lymphoma (NHL) and treatment-sensitive patients in relapse by intensive chemotherapy, followed by autologous bone marrow transplantation. In a prospective, randomized study, this sequence was compared with a regimen of sequential chemotherapy for consolidation in patients younger than 55 years of age who were in first complete remission of intermediate- and high-grade NHL after receiving induction therapy.

Study Plan.—Two hundred thirty patients were randomized to receive high-dose combination chemotherapy that included cyclophosphamide, carmustine, and etoposide (CBV) and then to undergo autologous marrow transplantation. Another 234 patients received consolidative chemotherapy with a sequential regimen of ifosfamide, etoposide, asparaginase, and cytarabine. All patients had at least one adverse prognostic factor.

Results.—The median follow-up was 28 months. Patients given high-dose chemotherapy followed by marrow transplantation had a 3-year disease-free survival rate of 59% compared with 52% for those given sequential chemotherapy. There were 2 transplant-related deaths.

Conclusion.—There was failure to demonstrate an adantage for high-dose CBV treatment, followed by autologous marrow transplantation, compared with sequential chemotherapy in patients with poor-risk NHL.

► This large series from France shows no difference in outcome between the two regimens for this large subpopulation of patients with NHL. A cynic would say, "What did they expect?" Autologous transplantation is simply another name for describing aggressive chemotherapy with blood cell support. On the other hand, a supporter would say, "The use of autologous bone marrow transplantation is rampant and costly (although perhaps no more costly than aggressive multiagent chemotherapy) and, therefore, controlled studies like this are necessary." Previous studies have claimed an advantage for autologous transplantation, but the authors claim that no randomized study exists that controls for patient selection, induction regimen, and ablative therapy. My own personal bias is that there will be subpopulations of patients with lymphoma for whom autologous transplantation may be superior. The reason for this bias is that lymphoma is one of the diseases for which chemotherapy exerts a demonstrable dose-response relationship, so that any technique that can increase the tolerable total dose may be able to show an improvement in outcome.

J.V. Simone, M.D.

Treatment of Waldenström's Macroglobulinemia Resistant to Standard Therapy With 2-Chlorodeoxyadenosine: Identification of Prognostic Factors
Dimopoulos MA, Weber D, Delasalle KB, Keating M, Alexanian R (MD Anderson Cancer Ctr, Houston)
Ann Oncol 6:49–52, 1995   9–5

Background.—About half of all patients with Waldenström's macroglobulinemia respond to standard treatment with alkylating agents and steroids. 2-Chlorodeoxyadenosine (2CdA) has been effective for about 40% of patients who are resistant to treatment or experience relapse. A series of patients with resistant macroglobulinemia were followed to identify those most likely to benefit from 2CdA.

Methods.—The study included 46 consecutive patients with Waldenström's macroglobulinemia that had failed to respond to standard therapy. There were 25 women and 21 men (median age, 60 years). Most patients were treated because of progressive anemia, lymphadenopathy or organomegaly, or hyperviscosity syndrome. Twenty patients had primary resistance, 17 had refractory relapse, and 9 had a relapse while not receiving treatment. All received 2 courses of 2CdA on an outpatient basis. The dose was 0.1 mg/kg/day, given by 7-day continuous infusion with a portable pump via a central venous catheter.

Results.—A response to 2CdA was achieved in 43% of patients. The response rates were 78% in patients who relapsed while not receiving treatment and 57% in those with primary resistance within the first year compared with 22% for those in later stages of disease. Response was unrelated to patient age or sex, presence of lymphadenopathy or splenomegaly, pretreatment hemoglobin, severity of blood or marrow lymphocytosis, serum level of abnormal protein or β_2-microglobulin, or the pretreatment CD4+ or CD8+ lymphocyte count. For responders, the median survival after treatment was 28 months and the median progression-free survival was 12 months. Patients with primary refractory disease had a projected median survival of 36 months compared with a median survival of 13 months for patients with refractory relapse.

Conclusion.—For patients with macroglobulinemic lymphoma that is resistant to standard therapy, 2CdA is a potentially beneficial treatment. Response rates are best for patients who experience relapse while not receiving treatment or during their first year of primary refractory disease. For patients in later phases of resistant disease, 2CdA appears to be of little help. Alternative treatments should be given in this situation.

▶ Recently, several reports from the M.D. Anderson Cancer Center have suggested that the purine nucleoside analogue 2CdA is effective in patients with Waldenström's macroglobulinemia, an uncommon, relatively indolent lymphoproliferative disorder that is currently not curable with standard alkylating agents or even doxorubicin-based regimens.[1] The same investigators have now adopted a treatment philosophy whereby, to avoid prolonged pancytopenia, a limited number of cycles (usually 2 courses) of 2CdA are administered.[2]

The same investigators have now moved a step forward by attempting to identify the pretreatment characteristics that might identify those patients with resistant Waldenström's macroglobulinemia who would be most likely to benefit from 2CdA. Among a cohort of 46 consecutive patients resistant to alkylating agents and corticosteroid therapy, 20 (43%) responded. The median survival after treatment was 28 months, and the median progression-free survival of responding patients was 12 months. Those patients who fared best were those who had relapsed while not receiving prior therapy (78%) or those who had primary resistant disease treated with 2CdA within the first year (57%) compared with those in the later phases of their disease (22%). Interestingly enough, responses to 2CdA were seen in 3 of 4 patients who had previously responded to fludarabine but who had experienced a relapse while not receiving therapy compared with only 1 of 9 patients with disease resistant to fludarabine. Although the investigators studied patient age, the presence of adenopathy and splenomegaly, the pretreatment hemoglobin, the degree of blood or marrow lymphocytosis, the serum level of abnormal paraprotein or β-2 microglobulin, and the pretreatment number of CD4+ or CD8+ lymphocytes, only phase of disease was found to be an important pretreatment predicter of response.

This study confirms that a limited number of courses of 2CdA can induce durable, unmaintained remissions. Repeated cycles contribute to a marked and profound decrease in CD4+ lymphocyte counts, which may lead to opportunistic infections and, therefore, may not be necessary. Cross-resistance between the purine nucleoside analogues has been an area of importance, particularly in hairy cell leukemia (for those patients who have received prior 2-deoxycoformycin) and chronic lymphocytic leukemia (for those patients who have received prior fludarabine). The study by Dimopoulos and colleagues suggests that there is cross-resistance in patients with Waldenström's macroglobulinemia for patients resistant to fludarabine who then receive 2CdA.

M.S. Tallman, M.D.

References

1. Dimopoulos MA, Kantarjian H, Estey E, et al: Treatment of Waldenström macroglobulinemia with 2-chlorodeoxyadenosine. *Ann Intern Med* 118:195–198, 1993.
2. Dimopoulos MA, Kantarjian H, Weber D, et al: Primary therapy of Waldenström's macroglobulinemia with 2-chlorodeoxyadenosine. *J Clin Oncol* 12:2694–2698, 1994.

Mediastinal Large B-Cell Lymphoma: Clinical and Immunohistological Findings in 18 Patients Treated With Different Third-Generation Regimens
Falini B, Venturi S, Martelli M, Santucci A, Pileri S, Pescarmona E, Giovannini M, Mazza P, Martelli MF, Pasqualucci L, Ballatori E, Guglielmi C, Amadori S, Poggi S, Sabattini E, Gherlinzoni F, Zinzani PL, Baroni CD, Mandelli F, Tura S (Univ of Perugia, Italy; Univ of Bologna, Italy; Univ 'La Sapienza', Rome)
Br J Haematol 89:780–789, 1995   9–6

Introduction.—The histologic features of mediastinal large B-cell lymphoma (MLCL) include a diffuse proliferation of large cells with clear cytoplasm and the presence of a varying degree of sclerosis, which results in a typical pattern of compartmentalization. Most patients are young women who come to attention with a bulky, invasive mediastinal mass and symptoms of cough, chest pain, dyspnea, and superior vena cava syndrome. The MLCL subtype is relatively uncommon, so there are few data regarding its response to therapy. The immunophenotype, clinical features, and response to third-generation chemotherapy of 18 patients with MLCL were evaluated.

Methods.—The patients were drawn from a series of 286 patients with high-grade non-Hodgkin's lymphoma (HG-NHL) collected in 3 years. The patients all took part in a prospective, multicenter comparison of the MACOP-B and F-MACHOP chemotherapy regimens. The histologic, immunohistologic, and clinical findings of the 18 patients with MLCL were studied.

Results.—Approximately 60% of patients with MLCL had a previously unrecognized phenotype, one characterized by co-expression of B-cell–associated antigens—the CD19, CD20, and CD22 Ig-associated dimers—and activation-associated antigens, namely CD30 and CDw70. The phenotype was thought to result from the tumor's derivation from a subset of thymic-activated B cells. The activation-associated antigens CD25 and Ki-27, unclustered, were always negative.

The patients were 13 women and 5 men with a median age of 31 years. Seventy-two percent came to attention with a bulky mediastinal mass, and most had an associated mediastinal syndrome. Most patients had stage IIA disease when initially seen. Aggressive chemotherapy was given to all patients: 11 received F-MACHOP with a complete response rate of 18%, and 7 received MACOP-B, with a complete response rate of 57%. In contrast, the 135 patients with HG-NHL treated with F-MACHOP during the same study had a complete response rate of 69.6%. The difference in the F-MACHOP outcomes for patients with MLCL vs. those with HG-NHL remained significant, even after adjustment for poor prognostic factors, i.e., a mediastinal mass of greater than 10 cm plus an increased level of lactic dehydrogenase.

Conclusion.—Most patients with MLCL appear to have a previously unrecognized phenotype, one associated with co-expression of B-cell and activation-associated antigens. The results of this series suggest that F-MACHOP might not be the best form of chemotherapy for patients with MLCL associated with bulky mediastinal disease and increased LDH. The question of whether MACOP-B is a better treatment approach will have to be answered in randomized, multicenter trials.

▶ Mediastinal large B-cell lymphoma is a well-recognized, distinct clinical pathologic entity. Characteristic features include its occurrence mostly in young adult females seen with a bulky mediastinal mass that invades adjacent organs and structures. Because this physiologic subtype of malignant lymphoma is uncommon, this study was undertaken to address the response to chemotherapy.

The authors selected 18 cases from 286 patients seen between September 1988 and August 1991 for enrollment in a prospective, multicenter trial comparing MACOP-B and F-MACHOP chemotherapy. The immunophenotype was distinctive in that the authors observed coexpression of B-cell markers (CD19, CD20, CD22, and Ig-associated dimers) and activation-associated antigens (CD30 and CDw70) in approximately 60% of cases. In contrast, the activation-associated antigens CD25 and Ki-27 were consistently negative. This peculiar phenotype was believed to reflect derivation from a subset of phymic-activated B cells. The median age was 31 years, and 72% of patients were seen with a bulky mediastinal mass associated with mediastinal syndrome in more than 50% of cases. A complete response with MACOP-B was achieved in 57% of cases but in only 18% of cases treated with F-MACHOP. When the latter regimen was used to treat 135 patients with high-grade malignant lymphomas of other histologic types, the complete response rate was 70%. Two patients considered to be in partial response because of persistence of a mediastinal mass may well have been in complete response because there was no progression at 21+ and 29+ months of follow-up. In this case, the complete response rate with MACOP-B would be 85%.

Although this series does not establish MACOP-B as the optimal treatment for MLCLs, the results suggest that the disease is quite responsive to this third-generation regimen. In addition, we have gained additional information regarding the biology of the disease.

M.S. Tallman, M.D.

A Clinical Analysis of Two Indolent Lymphoma Entities: Mantle Cell Lymphoma and Marginal Zone Lymphoma (Including the Mucosa-Associated Lymphoid Tissue and Monocytoid B-Cell Subcategories): A Southwest Oncology Group Study
Fisher RI, Dahlberg S, Nathwani BN, Banks PM, Miller TP, Grogan TM (Loyola Univ, Maywood, Ill; Southwest Oncology Group Statistical Ctr, Seattle; Univ of Southern California, Los Angeles; et al)
Blood 85:1075–1082, 1995   9–7

Objectives.—The clinical and pathologic findings were reviewed in 376 previously untreated patients from 3 randomized clinical trials who had stage III or stage IV non-Hodgkin's lymphoma, and who received full-dose CHOP (cyclophosphamide, doxorubicin, vincristine, and prednisone), alone or combined with immunotherapy. Two newly recognized pathologic entities were sought: mantle-cell lymphoma (MCL) and marginal zone lymphoma (MZL), including the mucosa-associated lymphoid tissue (MALT) and monocytoid B-cell (MCBC) subtypes. They were evaluated to determine whether their clinical courses differ from that of the relatively indolent lymphomas with which they formerly were classified.

Findings.—Mantle-cell lymphoma was diagnosed in 36 patients (10% of the series), and MZL was diagnosed in 43 patients (11%). The cases of MCL were fairly evenly distributed among the nodular, diffuse, and blastic variants. The patients with MZL included 19 with MALT; 21 with MCBC; and 3 nonclassifiable cases. Thirteen of the 21 patients with the MCBC lymphoma and 7 of the 19 with MALT also had follicular lymphoma. The overall outcome for patients with MZL did not differ from that for the larger group of patients with non-Hodgkin's lymphoma, but patients with MCBC had better overall and failure-free survival rates than those with MALT lymphoma. Patients with MCL did significantly less well than did those in Working Formulation categories A through E.

Conclusion.—Mantle-cell lymphoma is not an indolent form of lymphoma; affected patients are candidates for innovative treatment measures.

▶ The Working Formulation for the classification of malignant lymphomas, published in 1982, accomplished a great deal by providing detailed clinical information on each of the 10 histologies of lymphoma and the mechanism of integrating previous classification systems. However, hematopathologists have identified several new entities that do not clearly fit into any one category. The first is MCL, which is associated with the characteristic chromosomal translocation t(11;14) and the *bcl*-1 oncogene that contributes to the overexpression of the PRAD1 gene. The second entity is marginal zone B-cell lymphoma, which includes low-grade B-cell lymphoma of MALT and MCBC. Not only do these entities fall outside of the Working Formulation classification, but their natural history and optimal therapy are unknown.

In this analysis, Fisher and colleagues have retrieved pathologic material and clinical data from patients with these diagnoses entered on 3 Southwest Oncology Group (SWOG) studies in an effort to determine the clinical presentation and natural history of these 2 histologic subtypes of malignant lymphoma. The authors report that each subtype constitutes approximately 10% of patients with advanced-stage disease previously classified as Working Formulation categories A–E. In addition, the authors report that (1) the failure-free survival and overall survival rates of patients with MCL are significantly worse than those of patients with lymphomas classified in the Working Formulation categories A–E; and (2) the failure-free survival and overall survival rates in patients with MZL are the same as those in patients with lymphomas categorized as Working Formulation A–E; and (3) the failure-free and overall survival rates of patients with MCBC are higher than those in patients with MALT lymphomas. Therefore, patients with advanced-stage MALT lymphomas may appear to have a more aggressive course.

In the 36 patients who had MCL, the MCLs were further subclassified into either nodular (39%), diffuse (28%), or blastic (33%) variants. Subclassification results in a statistically different failure-free and overall survival, although the failure-free 10-year survival estimates were all less than 10%. Because they are uncommon and newly described, their natural history has not been frequently studied.

The information provided by Fisher and colleagues significantly contributes to a more precise definition of each entity, as well as to our understanding of these entities' natural history and optimal therapy. The findings reported in this article may explain variable results in earlier studies, because patients with these histologic subtypes have been included among the indolent lymphomas. It is clear that MCL should not be considered indolent. In the future, the challenge will be to identify novel innovative therapeutic approaches for patients with this aggressive disease.

M.S. Tallman, M.D.

Long-Term Survival After Histologic Transformation of Low-Grade Follicular Lymphoma
Yuen AR, Kamel OW, Halpern J, Horning SJ (Stanford Univ, Calif)
J Clin Oncol 13:1726–1733, 1995   9–8

Background.—A major cause of morbidity and mortality among patients with low-grade follicular lymphoma is histologic transformation

(HT) of the malignancy to the intermediate- or high-grade level. To describe the progression of the disease, a retrospective review was conducted of patients given a diagnosis of low-grade follicular lymphoma between 1965 and 1988 who had undergone HT to a higher level.

Methods.—The subjects were categorized as having either extensive or limited disease. Information about the extent of the disease at the time of HT was elicited from medical records, radiology reports, physical examination, and biopsy records. In addition, demographic information, treatment (radiotherapy and chemotherapy), blood chemistries, pathologic and histologic information, and particulars about the location of the disease were collected. A complete response (CR) was defined as tumor regression coupled with normal radiographic findings. The overall survival and survival curves were calculated. Data were interpreted according to Kaplan and Meier methods and Cox multivariate regression.

Results.—Most of the 74 patients who were selected for evaluation were seen with advanced small cleaved-cell lymphoma, and nearly 50% had been treated with chemotherapy. The median time of HT was 5.5 years after the initial diagnosis (range, 7 months to 25 years). Most often, transformation was from follicular small cleaved-cell lymphoma to diffuse large-cell lymphoma. Most patients were younger than 60 years at HT; more than half of them had extensive involvement. Almost one third of these patients had received no chemotherapy. Those treated with radiotherapy alone experienced a higher CR than patients treated with chemotherapy regimens. The median survival was 9.75 years; the type of treatment delivered had no effect on survival. After HT, the median survival was 22 months (range, 1 day to 207 months). A CR, achieved as the result of radiotherapy alone, chemotherapy alone, or a combination of therapies, occurred in 30 patients after HT. Complete response was related to the extent of the disease at presentation and not to prior treatment: 66% of patients with limited disease and 20% of those with extensive disease achieved a CR. Twelve patients treated with radiotherapy had a good outcome. Overall survival did not differ between initially treated and untreated patients, but untreated patients had a longer median survival after transformation.

Discussion.—These findings indicate that patients with low-grade follicular lymphoma who undergo histologic transformation do not necessarily face a poor prognosis. In fact, some patients can survive for a long time. The factors that predict survival include a limited extent of the disease at presentation, no prior chemotherapy, and a CR after treatment. Treatment might be deferred in these patients to influence a favorable outcome.

▶ It is well known that patients with low-grade lymphomas can undergo HT to an intermediate- or high-grade lymphoma. Few large series have studied the natural history of patients undergoing HT. In this report, investigators from Stanford University analyzed the clinical course of 74 patients with low-grade lymphomas who underwent HT between 1965 and 1988. The median time from diagnosis to transformation was 66 months, and the median duration of survival after transformation was 22 months. The most favorable prognosis was seen in patients with limited disease with no prior chemotherapy.

Response to therapy was another important prognostic factor. Interestingly, patients who attained a complete remission after HT had an overall median duration of survival of 81 months (range, 10–208 months). In this particular subset of patients, the extent of disease was highly correlated with the achievement of complete remission. Sixty-six percent of the patients with limited disease at the time of HT achieved complete remission compared with only 20% of those with extensive disease.

This report is of great interest because it involves the largest collection of patients with low-grade lymphomas undergoing HT and documents that, although it is generally believed that such patients have uniformly poor prognosis, there is a subset of patients with a reasonably favorable outlook. It is possible to achieve a complete remission after HT, and such a complete remission may be durable. Although this particular study does not address the mechanisms by which low-grade lymphomas undergo HT, other reports have suggested that genetic mutations such as the *t53* tumor-suppressive gene may promote such evolution. Finally, this report further emphasizes that the optimal therapy for patients with indolent lymphomas has not been established.

M.S. Tallman, M.D.

Randomized Trial of Interferon Maintenance in Multiple Myeloma: A Study of the National Cancer Institute of Canada Clinical Trials Group

Browman GP, Bergsagel D, Sicheri D, O'Reilly S, Wilson KS, Rubin S, Belch A, Shustik C, Barr R, Walker I, James K, Zee B, Johnston D (Queen's Univ, Kingston, Canada)
J Clin Oncol 13:2354–2360, 1995

9–9

Background.—Studies of the benefit of interferon (IFN) maintenance in patients with myeloma have yielded conflicting results. The National Cancer Institute of Canada Clinical Trials Group (NCIC CTG) initiated a randomized trial in 1987 comparing IFN maintenance with observation in patients with myeloma who had responded to melphalan-prednisone (MP) induction treatment.

Methods.—Of 402 patients enrolled in the study, 176 responded to MP and were randomly assigned to the IFN or control groups. All patients had symptomatic clinical stage I, II, or III multiple myeloma. Melphalan-prednisone was stopped after a stable response plateau of the monoclonal protein was achieved. Interferon was continued to relapse and restarted on subsequent MP response. Eighty-five patients received IFN maintenance, and 91 were observed. The median follow-up was 43 months.

Findings.—The median duration of survival was 43 months for patients receiving IFN and 35 months for those in the control group. After adjustment for chance imbalances in baseline prognostic factors, primarily performance status, the median survival durations were 44 months for the IFN-treated group and 33 months for controls. Patients given IFN also had a better progression-free survival from randomization to first relapse. Fifty-eight percent of the patients had to decrease their IFN dose because of toxicity. Eighty-four percent of those patients were able to return to their initial dose, and 14% had to discontinue IFN therapy.

Conclusions.—In patients with multiple myeloma who respond to MP, IFN maintenance treatment improves progression-free and overall survival. However, the toxicity is substantial. Patients must weigh this disadvantage against the potential benefits in response duration and survival.

▶ Despite several studies exploring the potential benefits of IFN in patients with multiple myeloma, no definitive role has been established. Browman and colleagues report a multicenter trial of 402 patients with symptomatic clinical stages I, II, and III myeloma who received MP.

Although this trial does not firmly establish a definitive role for maintenance IFN therapy in responding patients with myeloma, it provides yet another study with a large number of patients addressing this important issue. Once a plateau in the paraprotein occurs, there is no established role for any kind of maintenance therapy. A study clearly establishing the benefits of maintenance IFN in this disease would be welcome. However, although an important one, this study does not establish such a role. Although there were marginally statistically significant improvements for overall survival, IFN was associated with significant toxicity and had to be reduced because of side effects in more than 60% of patients.

One interesting aspect of this study was that patients who had relapse subsequently had reinduction, with melphalan or prednisone and then either received IFN or were observed during the maintenance phase, as they had been with previous randomization. The benefits reported in this study for maintenance IFN must be carefully considered, given the degree of toxicity of the IFN. Although these data are certainly provocative, the results reported, taken together with the results of several other reported trials, still fail to provide convincing evidence that all patients responding to conventional alkylating agent chemotherapy should receive maintenance IFN.

M.S. Tallman, M.D.

Toxoplasmosis and Primary Central Nervous System Lymphoma in HIV Infection: Diagnosis With MR Spectroscopy
Chinn RJS, Wilkinson ID, Hall-Craggs MA, Paley MNJ, Miller RF, Kendall BE, Newman SP, Harrison MJG (University College London Hosps Trust; Reta Lila Weston Inst of Neurological Studies, London; University College, London)
Radiology 197:649–654, 1995   9–10

Background.—Because the signs and symptoms of neurologic disease are often nonspecific in HIV-positive patients, neuroradiologic assessment is important in the differential diagnosis of any neurologic abnormality. Magnetic resonance imaging abnormalities often indicate specific diagnoses, especially in patients with HIV encephalopathy, progressive multifocal leukoencephalopathy, and cerebral cryptococcal infection. However, an MRI-based diagnosis is more difficult when single or multiple focal abnormalities with a mass effect are present. The value of localized spin-echo proton MR spectroscopy in differentiating intracranial lymphoma from *Toxoplasma gondii* lesions was tested.

Methods.—Eighteen *T. gondii* lesions and 9 lymphoma lesions were evaluated at 1.5 Tesla. Spectra were obtained from voxels centered on the lesions at an echo time of 135 msec. The metabolite ratios for choline, creatine, N-acetyl, lactate, and lipids were obtained using data from visual analysis and spectral fitting.

Findings.—Three spectral categories were observed: 1 with large lipid peaks with suppression of other metabolites; 1 with an increased choline/creatine ratio with relatively reduced N-acetyl; and 1 with features of the first 2. Each type of spectrum was evident in *T. gondii* lesions and lymphoma lesions; the lesions could not be differentiated by either method of analysis. An overlap of spectra was observed on MR spectroscopy.

Conclusion.—Spin-echo proton MR spectroscopy at an echo time of 135 msec was unable to differentiate between *T. gondii* abscesses and lymphoma of the CNS in patients with AIDS. There was extensive overlap between the 2 types of lesions in the spectra as assessed visually and with a fitting program. Absolute molar quantification of MR spectroscopy may enhance diagnostic specificity.

▶ In patients who are HIV positive, a continuing challenge in differential diagnosis occurs with primary CNS lesions that could be either toxoplasmosis or CNS lymphoma. The authors of this study looked at 27 patients with CNS lesions. A reliable distinction between toxoplasmosis and lymphoma could not be made using MR spectroscopy. In university settings, we are continually bombarded with suggestions that this new technology is going to solve virtually every biological problem. This study indicates that such euphoria is not warranted.

E. Glatstein, M.D.

10 Childhood Leukemia

Chemotherapy in 998 Unselected Childhood Acute Lymphoblastic Leukemia Patients. Results and Conclusions of the Multicenter Trial ALL-BFM 86
Reiter A, Schrappe M, Ludwig W-D, Hiddemann W, Sauter S, Henze G, Zimmermann M, Lampert F, Havers W, Niethammer D, Odenwald E, Ritter J, Mann G, Welte K, Gadner H, Riehm H (Free Univ of Berlin; Georg-August-Univ, Göttingen, Germany; Albert-Ludwigs-Universität, Freiburg, Germany; et al)
Blood 84:3122–3133, 1994   10-1

Background.—The ALL-BFM-86 is the largest multicenter trial of childhood acute lymphoblastic leukemia (ALL) undertaken by the Berlin-Frankfort-Münster (BFM) group. In the previous ALL-BFM 83 trial, in vivo response to initial prednisone treatment was assessed prospectively. Significantly worse prognoses were noted in 10% of patients with peripheral blood blast cell counts of 1,000/μL or more after a 7-day exposure to prednisone and an intrathecal dose of methotrexate (MTX). In the ALL-BFM 86 trial, treatment response was used as an overriding stratification factor for the first time.

Patients and Methods.—A total of 998 evaluable patients were enrolled. Of these, 10.3% with ≥ 1,000/μL blood blasts on day 8 were placed in an experimental group (EG). Those with less than 1,000/μL blood blasts on day 8 were stratified into 2 groups, based on leukemic cell burden. These included a Standard Risk Group (SRG) and a Risk Group (RG), comprising 28.6% and 61.1% of the patients, respectively. The SRG patients were given an 8-drug induction, followed by consolidation protocol M (6-mercaptopurine, high-dose HDF MTX 4 × 5 g/m²) and maintenance. An additional 8-drug reinduction element was used to treat RG patients. Patients in the EG branch received treatment with protocol E (prednisone, HD-MTX, HD-cytarabine, ifosfamide, and mitoxantrone) in place of protocol M. Intrathecal MTX therapy was administered to all patients, and those in the RG and EG branches received cranial irradiation. Patients in the RG branch were randomly assigned to later intensification (prednisone, vindesine, teniposide, ifosfamide, HD-cytarabine) at 13 months. Reinduction therapy was introduced in branch SRG during the trial, because the ALL-BFM 83 follow-up showed that randomized low-risk patients receiving reinduction had significantly better results.

Results.—At a median follow-up of 5 years, the estimated 6-year event-free survival was 72% for the study cohort, 58% in the SRG branch for the first 110 patients without reinduction therapy, and 87% for the next 175 patients with reinduction therapy, 75% in the RG, and 48% in the EG patients. Outcome in RG patients was not significantly affected by late intensification, although only 23% of the eligible patients were randomized. Prednisone poor response remained a negative prognostic indicator, in spite of intensified therapy.

Conclusions.—Intensive reinduction therapy is beneficial, even for low-risk patients. An estimated 75% of unselected patients with childhood ALL may have event-free survival when using an induction, consolidation, and reinduction strategy.

▶ I have included this paper in the section on childhood leukemia for two reasons. First, the results in nearly 1,000 consecutive unselected patients with leukemia are excellent. Second, the article serves as a tribute to the wonderful work carried out by the German leukemia group led by Dr. Riehm. However, this paper illustrates another very important principle that I have long believed to be the case but for which I have had little definitive proof.

Dr. Riehm's group found that if they tried to reduce therapy for so-called "low-risk" patients, the results of treatment seriously deteriorated. It was necessary to maintain a very aggressive and intensive regimen to sustain excellent results.

For years, I have objected to the use of the term "low-risk" leukemia. I do not believe there is such a thing, and I believe it may lead one to the false impression that leukemia is like Wilms' tumor, in which one can simply proportion the amount of treatment based on the stage or extent of the tumor. Although there clearly is a segment of patients with leukemia with more aggressive disease that is less responsive to treatment, we must never forget that leukemia is a disseminated cancer at the time of diagnosis and that the irreducible minimum of therapy consistent with an optimal result remains quite aggressive.

J.V. Simone, M.D.

An Intensive Re-Treatment Protocol for Children With an Isolated CNS Relapse of Acute Lymphoblastic Leukemia
Ribeiro RC, Rivera GK, Hudson M, Mulhern RK, Hancock ML, Kun L, Mahmoud H, Sandlund JT, Crist WM, Pui C-H (St Jude Children's Research Hosp, Memphis, Tenn; Univ of Tennessee, Memphis)
J Clin Oncol 13:333–338, 1995   10–2

Background.—Five percent to 10% of children treated for acute lymphoblastic leukemia (ALL) isolated CNS relapse. The salvage rate and long-term complications of children treated with an intensive chemoirradiation (R-11) protocol after an isolated CNS relapse has developed during first clinical remission were investigated.

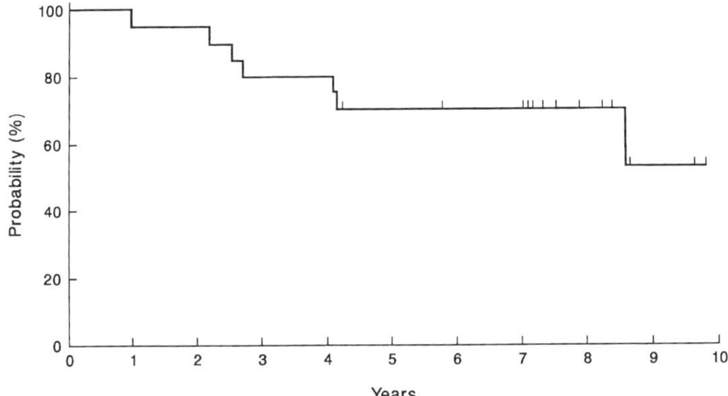

FIGURE 1.—Kaplan-Meier survival estimates for 20 patients treated on the R-11 protocol. (Courtesy of Ribeiro RC, Rivera GK, Hudson M, et al: An intensive re-treatment protocol for children with an isolated CNS relapse of acute lymphoblastic leukemia. *J Clin Oncol* 13:333–338, 1995.)

Methods.—A total of 20 children with ALL who had an isolated CNS relapse as the first adverse event were studied. The 5-drug systemic reinduction treatment involved standard-dose prednisone, vincristine, and asparaginase plus teniposide and cytarabine administered on days 8, 15, and 22. Continuation therapy consisted of 4 rotating drug pairs. Triple-intrathecal therapy was given weekly for 4–5 weeks and then every 6 weeks until craniospinal radiation was delivered.

Results.—The median age at relapse was 7 years. Five of the 20 children had CNS leukemia at presentation, whereas 5 finished treatment before relapse. First complete remission lasted a median of 22.5 months. Ten patients has previously received cranial radiotherapy in conjunction with intrathecal therapy, whereas the others had high-dose intravenous and/or intrathecal methotrexate as CNS-directed treatment. After retrieval therapy, all patients achieved a second complete remission. The 5-year estimate of disease-free survival was 70% (Fig 1). Thirteen children remained in remission at 71–126 months of follow-up, and 10 of 13 patients tested showed normal intelligence quotient scores. Four children had a second relapse (1 CNS and 3 non-CNS relapses), and other malignancies developed in 3. All treatment failures occurred among patients who had previously received cranial irradiation. Only 3 of 10 patients who had previously received irradiation remained in second remission compared with all of the other 10 patients.

Conclusion.—Intensive retrieval therapy is well tolerated and is associated with a high rate of remission in children with ALL in whom an isolated CNS relapse developed during initial complete remission. Apparently, patients who initially receive anti-metabolite-based therapy without CNS irradiation can benefit most from this treatment protocol.

▶ This is a study of children in whom an isolated CNS relapse developed during the course of treatment of ALL. The authors used an intensive regimen of CNS treatment combined with aggressive systemic combination chemotherapy in an attempt to prevent subsequent relapse. They reported good results in a small number of patients. However, a cautionary tale has been pointed out by Dr. Peter Steinherz in an editorial accompanying the original article.[1] He stated that some doubt must be cast on the results, because the standard used by the authors for diagnosing CNS leukemia is not universal. The presence of any leukemic cells in the spinal fluid was sufficient for diagnosing CNS leukemia, whereas other investigators require an elevated CSF cell count as well.

Another point made by both Dr. Steinherz and the authors is that CNS leukemia is probably the tip of the iceberg that reflects an eventual systemic relapse. Central nervous system leukemia, regardless of the standard used to diagnose it, is more evident because of the ability to detect small numbers of cells in an otherwise clear sample. This is not true for leukemia cells in the bone marrow or peripheral blood, or in any internal organ. Therefore, one may simply be detecting the early onset of a general occurrence of leukemia in an easily detectable site. Furthermore, if the treatment were not changed, eventually the patient would relapse systemically. In any case, all agree that systemic and would relapse systemically. In any case, all agree that systemic and CNS treatment is required to give the patient a chance for a cure in spite of a relapse apparently localized in the CNS.

J.V. Simone, M.D.

Reference

1. Steinherz PG: CNS leukemia: Problem of diagnosis, treatment, and outcome. *J Clin Oncol* 13:333–338, 1995.

Low Numbers of CSF Blasts at Diagnosis Do Not Predict for the Development of CNS Leukemia in Children With Intermediate-Risk Acute Lymphoblastic Leukemia: A Childrens Cancer Group Report
Gilchrist GS, Tubergen DG, Sather HN, Coccia PF, O'Brien RT, Waskerwitz MJ, Hammond GD (Mayo Clinic and Found, Rochester, Minn; MD Anderson Cancer Ctr, Houston; Univ of Southern California, Los Angeles; et al)
J Clin Oncol 12:2594–2600, 1994
10–3

Background.—Diagnosing CNS leukemia relies on the confirmation of blast cells in the CSF after cytocentrifugation. The effect on CNS relapse and overall relapse rates of blast cells in the CSF containing 5 cells per µL or fewer at the time of diagnosis of intermediate-risk acute lymphoblastic leukemia (ALL) in children enrolled in a randomized, multicenter, prospective trial was studied.

Methods and Findings.—Outcomes were studied in 1,544 patients who were successfully completing remission-induction treatment. The patients had been randomized to undergo 1 of 4 systemic chemotherapy regimens and to 1 of 2 CNS prophylaxis regimens. A total of 1,450 patients had varying degrees of pleocytosis but no blasts in the CSF at diagnosis, and 94 had blasts in the CSF after cytocentrifugation but a total CSF white blood cell (WBC) count of 5/μL or less. Overall CNS relapse rates and EFS rates did not differ between the 2 groups. No differences were found after analysis of age or WBC count at diagnosis, sex, or type of CNS prophylaxis.

Conclusions.—In this series of patients with intermediate-risk ALL, there were no significant differences in CNS relapse or systemic relapse rates after standard presymptomatic CNS treatment between patients with CSF WBC counts of 5 cells/μL or less and those without detectable blasts in the CSF. Certain treatment approaches may eliminate the need for any further special treatment in patients with CSF blasts.

▶ There has been extensive discussion about the significance of a few leukemia blast cells in the spinal fluid at the time of diagnosis. All the early data suggest that this is a poor prognostic sign. However, that was before routine CNS therapy was given, particularly that which included intrathecal therapy or irradiation. In this study, a large number of patients received routine CNS therapy after the discovery of blast cells in the spinal fluid with a total leukocyte count below 5 cells/μL. The authors found no difference in outcome between that group and the group that had no evidence of blast cells in the spinal fluid.

The caveats in this study are that this is a selected subpopulation of patients, i.e., patients with intermediate-risk ALL, and that this presumes the use of effective and aggressive systemic chemotherapy and "prophylactic" CNS therapy in all patients. We know that virtually all children have some degree of CNS involvement at the time of diagnosis, regardless of whether cells are found in the spinal fluid, because studies in which no CNS therapy is given result in a very high frequency of overt CNS leukemia. Thus, it is not surprising that if all patients received specific CNS therapy and modern multiagent systemic chemotherapy, the presence of a few blasts in the spinal fluid may not portend a bad result. This is a useful study in that it may (in selected patients) allow one to avoid giving additional therapy to the CNS at the end of treatment.

J.V. Simone, M.D.

Case-Control Analysis of Allogeneic Bone Marrow Transplantation Versus Maintenance Chemotherapy for Relapsed ALL in Children
Hoogerbrugge PM, Gerritsen EJA, vd Does-van den Berg A, vd Berg H, Zwinderman AH, Hermans J, Vossen JMJJ (Univ Hosp, Leiden, The Netherlands; Dutch Childhood Leukemia Study Group, The Hague, The Netherlands; State Univ, Leiden, The Netherlands)
Bone Marrow Transplant 15:255–259, 1995   10–4

Introduction.—Current treatment of childhood acute lymphoblastic leukemia (ALL) has resulted in a high remission rate. However, relapse still occurs in 10% to 35% of affected patients. There is substantial disagreement as to the most effective treatment for children with ALL after relapse.

The relative efficacy of allogeneic bone marrow transplant (BMT) vs. maintenance chemotherapy was evaluated in a case-control study of children with relapsed ALL who achieved subsequent remission.

Methods.—The 25 children studied were treated with allogeneic BMT after achieving a second remission (CR2) after relapsed ALL. The 97 control children were treated with high-dose consolidation and maintenance chemotherapy after achieving CR2, and they were matched to the case children for site of relapse, duration of CR1, and leukemia-free interval from onset of CR2. Survival and leukemia-free survival were calculated from the onset of CR2.

Results.—Hazard ratios for the duration of overall survival were 0.81 for the BMT group and 0.76 for the chemotherapy group. Leukemia-free survival tended to be higher in patients with CNS relapse after BMT rather than after chemotherapy, but no differences were significant (Fig 1). Relapse rates were lower, but treatment-related mortality was higher with BMT than with chemotherapy.

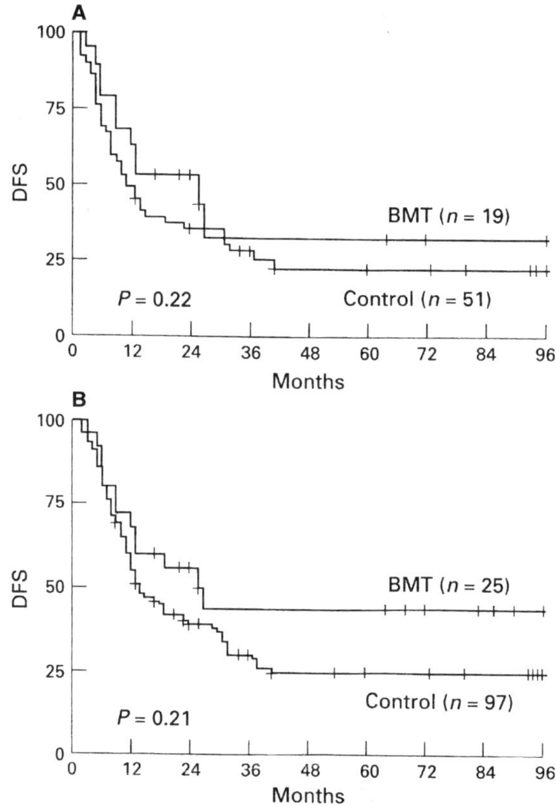

FIGURE 1.—Leukemia-free survival from the second complete remission after allogeneic bone marrow transplantation (*BMT*) or maintenance chemotherapy (controls) for children with relapsed ALL. **A,** only bone marrow relapses. **B,** all relapses. (Courtesy of Hoogerbrugge PM, Gerritsen EJA, vd Does-van den Berg A, et al: Case-control analysis of allogeneic bone marrow transplantation versus maintenance chemotherapy for relapsed ALL in children. *Bone Marrow Transplant* 15:255–259, 1995.)

Discussion.—These data showed a 24% probability of 5-year disease-free survival (26% after CNS relapse and 22% after bone marrow relapse) after chemotherapy and a 44% probability of 5-year disease-free survival (67% after CNS relapse and 42% after bone marrow relapse) after allogeneic BMT. However, these differences did not reach statistical significance with this small group of patients. The lower relapse rate in the patients treated with BMT suggests that myeloablative conditioning and a graft-vs.-leukemia effect have a greater antileukemic effect than does maintenance chemotherapy. However, the higher treatment-related mortality associated with BMT counteracts its antileukemic effect and highlights the need for improved supportive treatment in the early posttransplant period.

▶ For reasons that are not entirely clear, ALL has responded less well to allogeneic BMT than have other forms of leukemia. The authors studied patients who reentered remission after an initial relapse and who were treated either with chemotherapy or BMT. They found the somewhat surprising result that patients who had a bone marrow relapse fared as well with chemotherapy as with transplantation, whereas those who had a CNS relapse did better with transplantation. The authors explain the lack of a difference between the results with chemotherapy and BMT as a result of avoiding the positive selection of patients for transplantation, which may have occurred in other studies. They try to avoid any selection bias in favor of BMT by eliminating patients who relapsed between remission and the planned transplantation. The authors showed once again that transplant patients relapsed less often but had a higher mortality from treatment-related complications, whereas the chemotherapy group had a higher relapse rate but fewer deaths from complications. This article does not settle the issue but, rather, keeps the ball in the air concerning the value of using BMT for ALL in children.

J.V. Simone, M.D.

Intensification of Treatment and Survival in All Children With Lymphoblastic Leukaemia: Results of UK Medical Research Council Trial UKALL X
Chessells JM, for the Med Research Council Working Party on Childhood Leukaemia (Inst of Child Health, London; Paediatric Oncology Day Hosp, Leeds, England; Radcliffe Infirmary, Oxford, England)
Lancet 345:143–148, 1995   10–5

Background.—The United Kingdom Medical Research Council's UKALL X trial was designed to determine the benefit of additional intensification therapy in all children with acute lymphoblastic leukemia, with the exception of those at highest risk for treatment failure. Between 1985 and 1990, more than 90% of eligible patients were enrolled. The principal findings were reported.

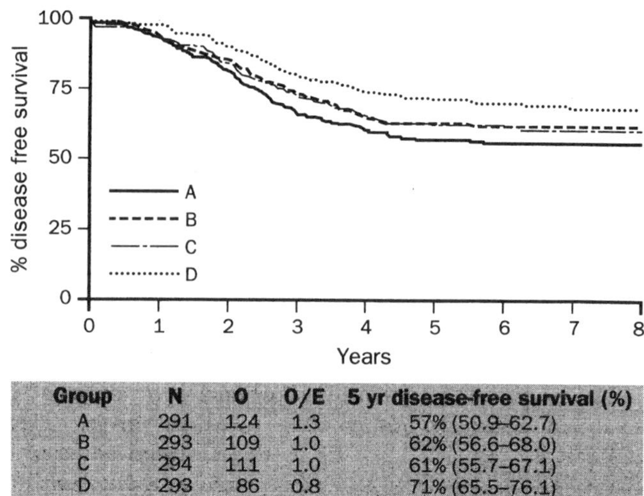

Group	N	O	O/E	5 yr disease-free survival (%)
A	291	124	1.3	57% (50.9–62.7)
B	293	109	1.0	62% (56.6–68.0)
C	294	111	1.0	61% (55.7–67.1)
D	293	86	0.8	71% (65.5–76.1)

FIGURE 4.—Comparison disease-free survival in four randomized treatment arms. (Courtesy of Chessells JM, for the Medical Research Council Working Party on Childhood Leukaemia: Intensification of treatment and survival in all children with lymphoblastic leukaemia: Results of UK Medical Research Council Trial UKALL X. *Lancet* 345:143–148, copyright by The Lancet Ltd., 1995.)

Patients and Methods.—Beginning in 1985, 1,612 children received intensive induction therapy and CNS-directed therapy with cranial irradiation and intrathecal methotrexate. Maintenance chemotherapy was continued for 2 years from the time of remission. Of the 1,612 patients, 1,171 were randomly assigned to receive additional intensification therapy at 5 weeks, 20 weeks, both, or neither. The patients were followed for 3 years or more after termination of the study in 1990.

Results.—At follow-up of at least 3 years, the disease-free survival for all patients was 62% at 5 years. This was a significant improvement over the rate of 56% noted in the preceding MRC UKALL trial. In patients randomized to 2 blocks of intensification, the 5-year disease-free survival was 71%, compared with 62% for patients receiving intensification at 5 weeks, 61% for those receiving intensification at 20 weeks, and 57% for those not receiving intensification (Fig 4). The clinical factors known to influence outcome (age, sex, and initial leukocyte count) had no affect on the benefits of intensification therapy.

Conclusions.—Two courses of intensification therapy led to a 14% improvement in disease-free survival and an 11% improvement in overall survival. All children with acute lymphoblastic leukemia, including those generally considered at lower risk of relapse, will benefit from this additional treatment.

▶ This is an important confirmatory study. It demonstrates that, to a point, children with acute lymphoblastic leukemia must receive an intensive period of chemotherapy at some time in the course of their disease to achieve the best results. This large and careful study done in the United Kingdom clearly shows that two courses of intensive therapy made a significant difference in the outcome. Even more important, it showed that this difference was demonstrable in all risk groups. The results achieved in the best group are equivalent to those now being routinely attained around the world with the more aggressive regimens, e.g., a long-term survival of around 70%.

I may sound like a broken record, but I want to repeat an important point of this study that has been made before: There is no such thing as "low-risk leukemia"; all children with acute lymphoblastic leukemia should receive aggressive multiagent therapy for at least a significant portion of their treatment. Attempts to use relatively simple nontoxic therapy for those patients believed to be in a "super good risk group" will result in failure at a higher rate than would have been attained otherwise.

J.V. Simone, M.D.

Leukemic Cell Growth in SCID Mice as a Predictor of Relapse in High-Risk B-Lineage Acute Lymphoblastic Leukemia

Uckun FM, Sather H, Reaman G, Shuster J, Land V, Trigg M, Gunther R, Chelstrom L, Bleyer A, Gaynon P, Crist W (Univ of Minnesota, Minneapolis; Childrens Cancer Group, Arcadia, Calif; Pediatric Oncology Group, Chicago)
Blood 85:873–878, 1995

10–6

Background.—Mice with severe combined immunodeficiency (SCID) provide a model system for assessing the in vivo homing, engraftment, and growth patterns of normal and malignant human hematopoietic cells. The relationship between leukemic cell growth in this model and treatment outcomes in patients from whom cells were obtained was investigated.

Methods.—Leukemic cells were derived from 42 children with newly diagnosed, high-risk, B-lineage acute lymphoblastic leukemia (ALL) and intravenously inoculated into CB.17 SCID mice. The mice were killed at 12 weeks or when they became moribund from disseminated leukemia. The mice were then examined to determine their burden of human leukemic cells.

Findings.—Twenty-three children whose leukemic cells produced histopathologically detectable leukemia in SCID mice had significantly greater relapse rates than the 19 patients whose leukemic cells did not produce detectable leukemia in the mice. The occurrence of overt leukemia in SCID mice strongly predicted patient relapse.

Conclusion.—Human leukemic cell growth in SCID mice strongly and independently predicts relapse in patients with newly diagnosed, high-risk, B-lineage ALL. The SCID mouse system eliminates some of the problems of other prognostic assessments; appears to complement the prognostic value of conventional risk characteristics, such as age and leukocyte count; and has potential for large-scale assessment of newly diagnosed cases of B-lineage ALL.

▶ This is a fascinating study of the biology of leukemia cells taken from children and implanted in immune-deficient mice. Its purpose was to determine whether the growth characteristics of those cells in the mice revealed anything about the behavior of the leukemia in children. The results are remarkable (see Figure 1 in the original article). Those patients whose cells grew readily, causing leukemia in the SCID mice, had a much poorer prognosis than those whose leukemia cells did not "take" in the mice.

Why would someone like me, who is not a great fan of the profusion of new "prognostic factors," be intrigued by this study? The reason is that this prognostic factor holds the possibility of studying the biological reasons for the difference in outcome. A prognostic factor that identifies an associated condition, such as an increased white blood cell count or an immunologic marker, usually leaves no avenue open for biological investigation as to the reason why. It simply becomes another way of comparing populations of patients that does not offer the possibility of pursuing scientific insights. On the contrary, this study allows one to identify populations of cells that have growth characteristics in an animal model. These cell populations can be studied further for properties that may be instrumental in explaining why the patients from whom the cells were taken do not do as well. Therefore, a whole avenue of investigation to explain treatment failure has been opened.

J.V. Simone, M.D.

A Pilot Study of Isotretinoin in the Treatment of Juvenile Chronic Myelogenous Leukemia

Castleberry RP, Emanuel PD, Zuckerman KS, Cohn S, Strauss L, Byrd RL, Homans A, Chaffee S, Nitschke R, Gualtieri RJ (Univ of Alabama, Birmingham; HL Moffitt Cancer Ctr, Tampa, Fla; Northwestern Univ, Chicago; et al)
N Engl J Med 331:1680–1684, 1994
10–7

Background.—Allogeneic bone marrow transplantation (BMT) is the only effective treatment for juvenile chronic myelogenous leukemia (CML). In vitro studies have shown that isotretinoin attenuates the spontaneous proliferation or leukemic peripheral-blood progenitor cells and their selective hypersensitivity to granulocyte–macrophage colony-stimulating factor (GM-CSF). The clinical efficacy of isotretinoin in juvenile CML was assessed.

Methods.—Eligible patients had newly diagnosed untreated disease, leukocytosis with monocytosis, marrow with less than 25% blasts, hepatosplenomegaly, no chromosomal abnormalities, and negative viral cultures and antibody titers. Ten children with a median age of 10 months were enrolled. Isotretinoin was given in single daily oral doses of 100 mg/m². Patients later underwent BMT when possible.

Findings.—All 10 patients had spontaneous colony formation of leukemic progenitor cells in vitro. The 8 children who were tested had hypersensitivity to GM-CSF. Cheilitis, occurring in 2 patients, was the only toxicity associated with isotretinoin. Disease progressed in 4 children. Two children responded completely, and 3 responded partially. Another child showed a minimal response. The median duration of response was 37

TABLE 3.—Clinical Course of 10 Patients With Juvenile CML Treated With Isotretinoin

Patient No.	Overall Response	Duration of Response*	Outcome
		mo	
1	Complete	83	Continuous complete remission
2	Complete	54	Death from progressive disease
3	Partial	36	Stable with isotretinoin therapy; parents refuse to allow bone marrow transplantation
4	Partial	37	Stable with isotretinoin therapy
5	Partial	6	No evidence of disease >21 mo after bone marrow transplantation
6†	Minimal	7	No evidence of disease >26 mo after bone marrow transplantation
7†	Progressive disease	3	No evidence of disease >42 mo after bone marrow transplantation
8	Progressive disease	NA	Death from juvenile CML
9	Progressive disease	NA	Death from juvenile CML
10†	Progressive disease	NA	Death from juvenile CML

* The values shown for patients 1, 3, and 4 are the durations of response at the time of the most recent follow-up visit.

† The patient had neurofibromatosis.

Abbreviations: CML, chronic myelogenous leukemia; *NA*, not applicable.

(Courtesy of Castleberry RP, Emanuel PD, Zuckerman KS, et al: A pilot study of isotretinoin in the treatment of juvenile chronic myelogenous leukemia. *N Engl J Med* 331:1680–1684, Copyright 1994, Massachusetts Medical Society.)

months. Three of the 4 children who were responding completely or partially and who did not have BMT were alive 36–83 months after juvenile CML was diagnosed. Spontaneous colony formation in vitro was reduced in samples taken from the 5 children reassessed during therapy. In addition, the hypersensitivity of leukemic progenitor cells to GM-CSF was reduced in the 2 patients tested (Table 3).

Conclusions.—Treatment with isotretinoin alone induces durable clinical and laboratory responses in patients with juvenile CML. Further study in a phase II trial of previously untreated patients is now needed to better establish response rates.

▶ This is a very hopeful paper. It demonstrates for the first time the effectiveness of nontraditional chemotherapy for the treatment of a notoriously difficult and rare type of childhood leukemia. The reader is probably aware that all-*trans*retinoic acid is in active use for the treatment of acute promyelocytic leukemia. It is capable of inducing remissions, although it is not curative. In this paper, isotretinoin, or *cis*-retinoic acid, is used for the treatment of juvenile CML. The number of patients is quite small, and only 1 patient achieved a complete response as we would normally define it today. However, 3 other patients achieved control of the leukocyte count with isotretinoin, and several were then successfully treated with BMT. If this were any other chemotherapeutic agent, the results would not be remarkable, because only one patient is in continuous complete remission, having received only isotretinoin. However, the successful use of a biological response modifier, which has a rational scientific basis for its application, gives us hope that this may lead to alternative approaches to the leukemia treatment that we do not currently have in our armamentarium. Even if this and other similar agents simply serve to prepare patients for more aggressive therapies, such as BMT, and thereby increase the likelihood of cure, it would be an advance. It would be preferable, however, if this proves to be an opening to a whole new approach to the treatment of hematopoietic malignancy.

J.V. Simone, M.D.

Clonality in Juvenile Chronic Myelogenous Leukemia

Busque L, Gilliland DG, Prchal JT, Sieff CA, Weinstein HJ, Sokol JM, Belickova M, Wayne AS, Zuckerman KS, Sokol L, Castleberry RP, Emanuel PD (Brigham and Women's Hosp, Boston; Univ of Alabama, Birmingham; All Children's Hosp, St Petersburg, Fla)
Blood 85:21–30, 1995

10–8

Background.—Juvenile chronic myelogenous leukemia (JCML) is a rare myeloproliferative disease of early childhood. The morbidity and mortality of JCML mainly result from nonhematopoietic organ failure caused either by myelomonocytic infiltration or by failure of normal bone marrow. Morphologic evidence of maturation arrest, karyotypic abnormalities, and progression to blast crisis is relatively uncommon. Diagnostic problems can arise when viral infections or other reactive processes mimic the clinical course of JCML. The rarity of JCML and various technical problems have prohibited accurate assessment of clonality in the disease. Multiple assays were used to assess clonality in patients with newly diagnosed JCML.

Methods.—The subjects were 9 untreated girls with newly diagnosed JCML, aged 4–48 months. The diagnosis was made according to clinical criteria and the finding of characteristic "spontaneous" in vitro cell growth, along with negative cultures and titers for various viral agents. Cell separation and RNA and DNA isolation were performed in peripheral blood and bone marrow samples. Three separate, recently developed polymerase chain reaction–based clonality assays were used to evaluate X-chromosome inactivation patterns.

Results.—The assays demonstrated monoclonal derivation of mononuclear cells at the time of diagnosis in all 9 patients. Very few normal hematopoietic elements were present at this time. On cell separation studies, the monoclonal origin of these cells could be traced back to at least the most primitive myeloid progenitor cell. Bone marrow transplantation was followed by reversion to a polyclonal state. In addition, polyclonal reversion occurred in one patient after treatment with 13-*cis*-retinoic acid.

Conclusion.—From the time of diagnosis, JCML is a clonal disorder that evolves from an abnormal myeloid stem cell or perhaps an even earlier level. The finding of clonality distinguishes JCML from the reactive process and establishes a basis for molecular genetic approaches to finding causally associated mutations. The phenomenon of partial reversion to polyclonality with 13-*cis*-retinoic acid therapy is being investigated in a formal phase II protocol.

▶ Juvenile chronic myelogenous leukemia has been an enigma for pediatric oncologists for many years. It has many features that are different from those of traditional leukemias, which makes it difficult to diagnose; these features include an absence of karyotypic abnormalities or morphological evidence of maturation arrest. Furthermore, progression to blast crisis is infrequent. In fact, these patients look a lot like any immunosuppressed patient with chronic debilitating infections and many hematologic features typical of a reaction to such processes. Thus, there has been some dispute as to whether JCML, a very rare form of leukemia, is really leukemia.

The authors studied a group of 9 female patients that fit the criteria for JCML. It was necessary to have female patients because X-chromosome inactivation was used to assess clonality. By sophisticated studies using the polymerase chain reaction method, the authors were able to demonstrate that the disease was clonal in all cases, and they, in fact, traced the origin back to a primitive myeloid cell. These data certainly establish JCML as a monoclonal disease, the usual *sine qua non* of a malignant process. This observation is further evidence, if any was needed, that drastic measures such as bone marrow transplantation may be necessary to treat JCML. However, more recently, some hope has been expressed that retinoic acid may be an affective (and less toxic) adjunct to management of this disease as well.

J.V. Simone, M.D.

Detection of Minimal Residual Disease in Acute Leukemia: Methodologic Advances and Clinical Significance
Campana D, Pui C-H (St Jude Children's Research Hosp, Memphis, Tenn; Univ of Tennessee, Memphis)
Blood 85:1416–1434, 1995   10–9

Introduction.—When patients are given a diagnosis of acute leukemia, they may have approximately 10^{12} malignant cells. Patients with as many as 10^{10} neoplastic cells may be considered to be in complete remission if fewer than 5% of the cells in the bone marrow samples can be morphologically identified as blasts. Patients are treated with the same regimen, regardless of the levels of leukemic cells. Several minimal residual disease (MRD) studies have been undertaken with the assumption that clinical management and, therefore, cure rates could be improved with better estimates of the total body burden of leukemic cells. The methods of assaying MRD, including determining morphologic and cytochemical properties, karyotypic or genetic abnormalities, antigen-receptor gene rearrangements, cell growth requirements in vitro, and immunophenotype, were reviewed.

TABLE 5.—Methodologic Options for Detecting MRD in Patients With Acute Leukemia

Diagnosis	Method	Potentially Suitable Cases (%)	Sensitivity
B-lineage			
ALL	In situ hybridization	25–35	?
	Ploidy determination	5–25	?
	PCR on translocation breakpoints	10–30	10^{-4}–10^{-6}
	Southern blotting for Ig or TCR genes	>90	10^{-2}
	PCR on TCRγ and TCRδ genes	40–60	10^{-3}–10^{-6}
	PCR or IgH genes	>90	10^{-3}–10^{-6}
	Colony assays	?	?
	Immunophenotyping	35	10^{-4}
T-ALL	In situ hybridization	10–20	?
	Ploidy determination	<5	?
	PCR on translocation breakpoints and *TAL-1* deletions	25–35	10^{-4}–10^{-6}
	Southern blotting for TCR genes	90–95	10^{-2}
	PCR on TCRγ and TCRδ genes	40–60	10^{-4}–10^{-6}
	Colony assays	?	?
	Immunophenotyping	90–95	10^{-4}
AML	In situ hybridization	40–60	?
	PCR on translocation breakpoints	20–30	10^{-4}–10^{-6}
	Colony assays	?	?
	Immunophenotyping	35	10^{-4}

Abbreviation: ?, not known; *MRD*, minimal residual disease; *PCR*, polymerase chain reaction; *TCR*, T-cell receptor. (Courtesy of Campana D, Pui C-H: Detection of minimal residual disease in acute leukemia: Methodologic advances and clinical significance. *Blood* 85:1416–1434, 1995.)

Techniques.—Several methods have been developed for measuring MRD in patients with acute leukemia (Table 5). For patients with B-lineage acute lymphocytic leukemia, polymerase chain reaction (PCR) with probes on IgH genes appears to have the most universal suitability and the highest sensitivity. Among patients with T-lineage acute lymphocytic leukemia, Southern blotting for T-cell receptor (TCR) genes has the most universal suitability, whereas PCR with a variety of probes has the highest sensitivity. For patients with acute myelocytic anemia, in situ hybridization has the greatest suitability, whereas PCR on translocation breakpoints has the greatest sensitivity.

Discussion.—Children with leukemia typically have persistent leukemic cells, requiring 2.5–3 years of therapy. The value of early detection and treatment of MRD should be evaluated in controlled clinical studies. Minimal residual disease studies may improve the value of autologous bone marrow transplant by detecting residual leukemic cells in the bone marrow implant. The method of monitoring patients for MRD needs to be carefully chosen, weighing the merits, limitations, and sources of error of each. However, because of the heterogeneous distribution of malignant cells throughout the body, even exceptionally sensitive techniques can miss some residual disease. Clinical studies should focus on relating MRD to prognosis by sampling at all critical points in the course of the disease.

▶ This is a superb review of an emerging and confusing line of research. Clearly, if one could detect and quantitate extremely small numbers of leukemia cells consistently and reproducibly, one might have an advantage during the course of treatment of the disease. These authors do an outstanding job of summarizing all the important work in this area, and Table 5 provides a snapshot of the range of techniques and their suitability and sensitivity. Our summary cannot do justice to the paper, and I would recommend that interested readers obtain a copy for future reference.

J.V. Simone, M.D.

Detection of Minimal Residual Disease in Patients With Childhood Common Acute Lymphoblastic Leukemia After Autologous Bone Marrow Transplantation With *Ex Vivo* Purging and Systemic IL-2 Infusion: Unsuccessful Prediction of Subsequent Relapse

Kiyoi H, Kojima S, Kato K, Matsuyama T, Kodera Y, Ohno R, Naoe T (Nagoya Univ, Japan; Children's Med Ctr; Japanese Red Cross Nagoya First Hosp, Japan; et al)

Bone Marrow Transplant 16:437–442, 1995   10–10

Background.—Some children with common acute lymphoblastic leukemia (ALL) who fail to respond to conventional chemotherapy undergo autologous bone marrow transplantation (ABMT) when no HLA-matched donor is available. There is a good chance that residual leukemic cells will be present in the harvested bone marrow, and the effectiveness of purging with monoclonal antibodies or immunotherapy is uncertain. It is possible to detect minimal residual disease in the bone marrow using the polymerase chain reaction (PCR) technique.

Objective and Methods.—Minimal residual disease was sought in 7 children with common ALL who had undergone ABMT with *ex vivo* purging followed by systemic infusion of interleukin-2. Six of the patients were in second and 1 was in third complete remission at the time marrow was harvested. Marrow engraftment was achieved in all cases. Minimal residual disease was detected using the PCR technique to detect the immunoglobulin heavy-chain third complementary determining region (IgH CDR-III) specific to the leukemic clone.

Findings.—Minimal residual disease was detected in bone marrow harvested from 2 of the 7 patients. Levels of 10^{-5} and 10^{-4} cells, respectively, persisted in the purged bone marrow. One of these patients relapsed 3 months after ABMT, but the other remained in complete remission after 33 months. No minimal residual disease was detected in any bone marrow sample from the other 3 patients who relapsed after ABMT.

Conclusion.—A negative PCR study for minimal residual disease in a patient with common ALL undergoing ABMT does not necessarily indicate that the patient will not have a relapse.

▶ Although this study includes only 7 patients, it points out the difficulty of predicting relapse with modern PCR techniques. The difference between this study and prior studies that alleged that one could determine long-term prognosis by the presence or absence of PCR-based detection of minimal residual disease is that this study includes patients at high risk for treatment failure, i.e., those in second or third remission. The studies with the most promising results for PCR prognostication were those with patients in first remission. These patients are simply more likely to have a good outcome, and the projected number of relapses is likely to be small in any case.

Nonetheless, this study raises a flag of caution that we should not be so confident that modern technology will improve our prognostic ability in childhood leukemia. We still have no reliable technique for accurately identifying those patients who are most likely to relapse with a given treatment.

J.V. Simone, M.D.

Intracellular Metabolites of Mercaptopurine in Children With Lymphoblastic Leukaemia: A Possible Indicator of Non-Compliance?

Lennard L, Welch J, Lilleyman JS (Univ of Sheffield, England)
Br J Cancer 72:1004–1006, 1995

10–11

Introduction.—The thioguanine nucleotides derived from mercaptopurine exert a cytotoxic effect and contribute to an ongoing treatment effect in children with lymphoblastic leukemia (ALL). There is evidence that patients who fail to form adequate amounts of these nucleotides are at increased risk of relapsing.

Objective.—Intracellular concentrations of mercaptopurine metabolites, including thioguanine nucleotides and methylmercaptopurines, were

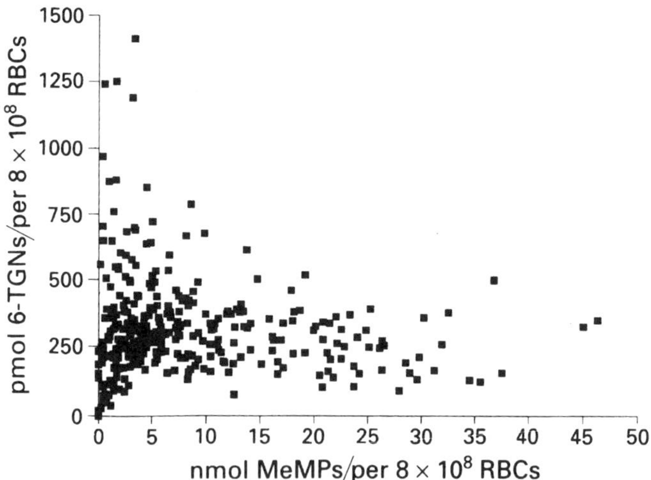

FIGURE 1.—The relationship between red blood cell (*RBC*) thioguanine nucleotides (*6-TGNs*) and methylmercaptopurine metabolites (*MeMPs*) for the 327 children studied. One datum point represents 1 child. (Courtesy of Lennard L, Welch L, Lilleyman JS: Intracellular metabolites of mercaptopurine in children with lymphoblastic leukaemia: A possible indicator of non-compliance? *Br J Cancer* 72:1004–1006, 1995.)

determined in 327 children with ALL from 17 centers in the United Kingdom. All had received mercaptopurine, at least 75 mg/m², for 1 week or longer before the study. The patients were also receiving methotrexate orally in a weekly dose of 10 mg/m².

Findings.—The concentrations of both classes of metabolite varied quite widely. Ten percent of the children had lower quartile levels of both metabolites. In 4 of these patients, only 1 metabolite was detected, and in 6 cases, neither of the metabolites was present. No child had upper quartile concentrations of both metabolites. When the 32 children with low levels of both metabolites were excluded, a significant negative correlation between the levels of thioguanine nucleotides and methylmercaptopurine metabolites was apparent (Fig 1).

Implications.—These findings suggest that some apparent treatment failures in children with ALL might be prevented merely by making sure that patients take all their prescribed medication. The problem of noncompliance is not unique to leukemia.

▶ Mercaptopurine and methotrexate are pillars of treatment of childhood leukemia during remission. Much of the improvement in the outcome of treatment of children with ALL has been the result of therapy with more aggressive regimens using these agents. The authors have studied the metabolites of mercaptopurine in red blood cells. Red blood cells are a convenient source of tissue for study, serving as a surrogate for the bioavailability of the effective antileukemia metabolite.

The authors found an extremely wide variation in the concentration of thioguanine nucleotides and methylmercaptopurine metabolites. They conclude that as many as 10% of patients either are not taking the oral mercaptopurine at all or are taking it only intermittently. Such noncompliance has been reported to be as high as 20% to 40% in other studies, so the 10% figure may actually be low. This failure to comply is generally more common among adolescents and among adolescent boys in particular.

The significance of the study is that it may provide a relatively quick and simple method of measuring effective mercaptopurine metabolite concentrations during the course of treatment so that the dosage may be adjusted or patients may be counseled and encouraged to take all medications. It might also lead to the use of a parenteral form of therapy. Because mercaptopurine is such an important part of effective therapy for this disease and must be administered for an extended period of time, usually 2 years, it is hoped that the authors will extend this study to a large population of patients to determine its utility in controlling effective dosage administration.

J.V. Simone, M.D.

Pediatric Myelodysplasia: A Study of 68 Children and a New Prognostic Scoring System

Passmore SJ, Hann IM, Stiller CA, Ramani P, Swansbury GJ, Gibbons B, Reeves BR, Chessells JM (Inst of Child Health, London; Hosps for Sick Children, London, Childhood Cancer Research Group, Oxford, England; et al)
Blood 85:1742–1750, 1995

10–12

Introduction.—Although the myelodysplastic syndromes (MDS) usually occur in the elderly population, they have also been reported in pediatric patients. The French-American-British (FAB) classification system, based on blood and bone marrow morphological characteristics, has not been very useful with pediatric MDS, which is usually categorized by clinical and cytogenetic features. The cases of pediatric MDS seen during a 21-year period were studied retrospectively for the purpose of developing useful classification and scoring systems for predicting the prognosis.

Methods.—The clinical records, bone marrow aspirates, and blood films of all 68 children given a diagnosis of MDS or chronic myeloproliferative disease between 1971 and 1991 were reviewed to classify the patients using the FAB system. Karyotypic analysis was performed with cultured bone marrow cells, and both the presence or absence of clonal abnormalities and their complexity were scored from 0 to 2.

Results.—With the original FAB classification system, 3 children could not be classified, 35 children were classified as having chronic myelomonocytic leukemia (CMML), 13 with refractory anemia with excess of blasts (RAEB), 11 with refractory anemia, 4 with refractory anemia with excess of blasts in transformation (RAEBT), and 1 with refractory anemia with ringed sideroblasts (RARS).

A modified FAB classification, including fetal hemoglobin levels and cytogenetic findings, allowed reclassification of 31 patients (most originally classified with CMML) as follows: 19 with juvenile chronic myeloid leukemia (JCML) and 12 with infantile monosomy 7 syndrome (IMo7). Transformation to acute myeloid leukemia generally occurred only in patients with refractory anemia, RAEB, RAEBT, or IMo7. Children with JCML had significantly reduced survival compared with those with IMo7 or CMML.

A reduced platelet count and elevated fetal hemoglobin level were predictors of a poor prognosis. In addition, the cytogenetic complexity score revealed significant survival differences between patients with scores of 1 and 2, with all patients with complex abnormalities dying. Therefore, a pediatric scoring system was developed that assigned 1 point for each of the following factors at diagnosis: fewer than 40×10^9/L platelets, a cytogenetic complexity score of 2, and a fetal hemoglobin level higher than 10%.

Discussion.—The FAB classification system and adult scoring systems did not have sufficient discriminative sensitivity for use with pediatric patients with MDS, because many children with MDS have associated abnormalities. Modified classification and scoring systems for children with MDS were developed and need to be assessed in prospective and population-based studies.

▶ Myelodysplasia is rare in children, and the diagnostic challenge is even greater than it is among the adult population. The authors found it difficult to categorize patients by the usual adult classification, so they devised a modified classification—specifically for pediatrics—that was useful in identifying patients with an especially poor prognosis. The main reason for including this paper, however, is to alert the reader that this hemopoietic problem occurs in children as well as in adults. Under the pediatric myelodysplasia rubric, we now include what we have previously called juvenile chronic myelocytic leukemia and infantile monosomy 7 syndrome, as well as myeloproliferative disorders not otherwise specified. In adults, most of these conditions are very difficult to treat successfully. However, children who have only refractory anemia or the features of CMML have a reasonable chance for long-term survival. Nonetheless, patients with this class of diagnosis remain perplexing and challenging, both diagnostically and therapeutically.

J.V. Simone, M.D.

11 Pediatric Solid Tumors

Minimally Invasive Surgery in Children With Cancer
Holcomb GW III, Tomita SS, Haase GM, Dillon PW, Newman KD, Applebaum H, Wiener ES (Children Cancer Group, Arcadia, Calif)
Cancer 76:121–128, 1995   11–1

Background.—The use of minimally invasive surgery in pediatrics is increasing. However, its precise role in the diagnosis and treatment of cancer in children has not been clearly defined.

Methods and Findings.—All 85 patients undergoing a laparoscopic or thoracoscopic procedure at 15 Childrens Cancer Group institutions from 1991 to 1993 were examined. A total of 88 minimally invasive surgery procedures were performed. The mean patient age was 11.6 years. Laparoscopy was performed in 25 patients. Sixty-three thoracoscopic procedures were performed in 60 patients, and tissue biopsy specimens were obtained in 67. In 99% of the biopsies, diagnostic material was obtained. There were 7 complications, all in the thoracoscopic group. Six operations were converted to an open procedure, and atelectasis developed after surgery in 1 patient. None of the patients died.

Conclusion.—Laparoscopy is highly accurate in children with suspected cancer. Morbidity is minimal. Thoracoscopy was almost as efficient, with a slightly higher morbidity. Both procedures are useful for assessing resectability and staging and for evaluating recurrent or metastatic disease.

▶ Use of the endoscope has increased dramatically in adult medicine and surgery over the past several years. It has been slower to develop in pediatrics but, as this paper reports, laparoscopy and thoracoscopy are both very efficient means of obtaining adequate biopsy samples and helping to stage malignant tumors in children. For the moment, the use of these procedures remains intuitively attractive. However, convincing, well-controlled data have yet to emerge to demonstrate whether the procedure reduces the necessity for major surgery or reduces the overall cost of care. Once a critical mass of pediatric surgeons has developed sufficient experience with these procedures, such a study would be indicated.

J.V. Simone, M.D.

Is Neuroblastoma Screening Evaluation Needed and Feasible?

Estève J, Parker L, Roy P, Herrmann F, Duffy S, Frappaz D, Lasset C, Hill C, Sancho-Garnier H, Michaelis J, Philip T (Internatl Agency for Research on Cancer, Lyon, France; Univ of Newcastle upon Tyne, England; Klinik und Poliklinik für Kinderheilkunde, Köln, Germany; et al)
Br J Cancer 71:1125–1131, 1995   11–2

Background.—Neuroblastoma, the most common solid tumor in children, is a lesion of the sympathetic nervous system deriving from embryonic cells of the neural crest. A large screening effort in Japan clearly demonstrated that screening in the first 6 months of life can result in high levels of overdiagnosis. Thus, the efficacy of screening for neuroblastoma is still debated.

The Need for Neuroblastoma Screening.—If neuroblastoma progressed with age from early to late stages, then detecting the disease before it metastasized to bone and marrow would be logical. Most patients with neuroblastoma have excessive amounts of catecholamine metabolites in the urine. Eighty-five percent to 90% of the patients excrete these metabolites. The metabolites are thought to be detectable in the urine of children before symptoms appear. Screening based on the levels of vanillylmandelic acid and homovanillic acid in the urine has been developed using high-performance liquid chromotography.

Screening at 6 months of age has been found to result in overdiagnosis. This is a strong argument against the use of mass screening programs for neuroblastoma. When histologically malignant but clinically benign tumors are detected on screening, heavy treatment with adverse effects may be initiated, leading to unnecessary deaths and long-term morbidity. Even when screenings are done at 12 and 18 months of age, the mortality rate from neuroblastoma may be reduced by only about 25%. Testing the efficacy of this strategy would require a study of half a million children per year during 5–7 years, with follow-up of an equal number of control subjects.

Conclusion.—Screening for neuroblastoma in the first 6 months of life leads to overdiagnosis. However, it is possible that screening at this age confers some protection against neuroblastoma, despite overdiagnosis. This hypothesis can be tested in a case-control study of deaths from neuroblastoma or of patients with stage IV disease.

▶ This paper from European investigators thoughtfully and carefully addresses the issue of the value of screening infants routinely for neuroblastoma. The authors point out the pitfalls in the process, including overdiagnosis or emergence of the tumor between screening tests. It is my opinion that the Japanese, who started this procedure on a large scale, have not yet provided convincing evidence that they are preventing the development of invasive neuroblastoma in a significant proportion of patients. The authors estimate that half a million children would have to be tested annually over a 7-year period, with follow-up of an equal number of controls. This would be a daunting task, to say the least. The authors do present, in a scholarly fashion, the parameters that should be considered if such a major trial is undertaken. They have, therefore, provided a very useful service.

J.V. Simone, M.D.

Localized Resectable Neuroblastoma: Results of the Second Study of the Italian Cooperative Group for Neuroblastoma
De Bernardi B, Conte M, Mancini A, Donfrancesco A, Alvisi P, Tomà P, Casale F, di Montezemolo LC, Cornelli PE, Carli M, Tonini GP, Pession A, Giaretti W, Garaventa A, Marchese N, Magillo P, Nigro M, Kotitsa Z, Tamaro P, Tamburrini A, Rogers D, Bruzzi P (Giannina Gaslini Children's Hosp, Genova, Italy; Natl Inst for Cancer Research, Genova, Italy; Univ of Bologna, Italy; et al)
J Clin Oncol 13:884–893, 1995   11–3

Background.—As many as one fourth of children with newly diagnosed neuroblastoma will have a resectable primary tumor and no metastases. The prognosis is good for these patients; however, a small proportion will relapse, which may prove fatal. Children at risk of relapse cannot be reliably identified by their clinical and biological findings, and the best treatment for reducing the risk of relapse is unclear. In an Italian multicenter study, treatment was optimized for children with localized resectable neuroblastoma.

Methods.—The study included 152 children 0–15 years of age with nondisseminated neuroblastoma. Of those patients, 144 were assessable: 69 had stage 1 disease, defined as complete resection of tumor without tumor rupture (TR); and 75 had stage 2 disease, defined as resection with minimal residual tumor, and/or tumor infiltration of regional lymph nodes (LN$_+$), and/or TR. Forty-nine of the children with stage 2 disease were considered low-risk, i.e., they were younger than 1 year of age or they had negative lymph nodes and no TR. Adjuvant therapy was not used in children with stage 1 and stage 2 LR disease. For the 26 children with stage 2 disease and with high-risk characteristics—i.e., older than 1 year of age with LN$_+$ and/or TR—adjuvant chemotherapy was given for 6 months.

Results.—Three of the 144 children died of treatment-related complications. Another 19 had relapse, and 6 of those patients died of neuroblastoma. The estimated overall survival rate was 93%, and the event-free survival (EFS) rate was 83% at 5 years. One of 69 children with stage 1 disease died postoperatively, and 5 had relapse. There were 1 local and 4 disseminated relapses, with 2 patients dying. The 5-year overall survival rate was 94% and the EFS rate was 90%.

Six of 49 stage 2 low-risk children had relapse, with 4 local and 2 disseminated relapses. Five of 20 children with LN$_+$ and 1 of 4 infants with TR had relapse; the remaining 25 children were relapse-free. One child in this group died of toxicity and another of disease, for an overall survival rate of 96% and an EFS survival rate of 85%.

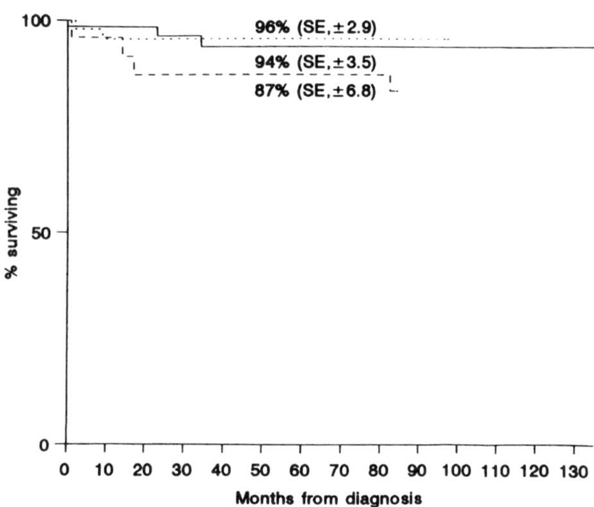

FIGURE 2.—Overall survival curves of patients with stage 1 (*solid line*), stage 2 LR (*dotted line*), and stage 2 HR (*dashed line*) disease. (Courtesy of De Bernardi B, Conte M, Mancini A, et al: Localized resectable neuroblastoma: Results of the second study of the Italian Cooperative Group for Neuroblastoma. *J Clin Oncol* 13:884–893, 1995.)

Eight of 26 stage 2 high-risk children had relapse: 3 of 20 with LN_+, 3 of 4 with TR, and 2 of 2 with LN+ and TR. Three of those children died of disease and 1 of toxicity, for an overall survival rate of 87% and an EFS rate of 61% (Fig 2).

Conclusion.—Children with localized resectable neuroblastoma have an overall good prognosis. Relapse is more likely in patients with LN_+ and TR regardless of age, although the postrelapse course tends to be less aggressive in infants. The overall survival rate is 94% or better in children with stage 1 and stage 2 low-risk disease, supporting a policy of no adjuvant chemotherapy. More intensive chemotherapy may be required for children with stage 2 HR disease.

▶ Neuroblastoma is a devastating disease in children when it is disseminated and occurs after the first year of life. However, as this study reminds us, those with localized disease have an extraordinarily good prognosis. As shown in Figure 2, the overall survival rate for patients with stage 1, stage 2 low-risk, and stage 2 high-risk disease was between 87% and 96%. These results were not caused by any extraordinary therapy given by the authors, which leads one to opine that patients seen with localized disease have a biologically different tumor that will respond favorably to virtually any approach.

One must also keep in mind that roughly half the patients in this study were younger than 1 year of age at the time of diagnosis. This is a critical observation, because it has been well described that children younger than 1 year of age respond well to a variety of relatively simple therapeutic approaches. This reinforces the belief that we should not be patting ourselves on the back too much regarding success in the treatment of this population of patients. We get a lot of help from the inherent biology of the tumor in this case.

J.V. Simone, M.D.

Lack of Correlation of N-*myc* Gene Amplification With Prognosis in Localized Neuroblastoma: A Pediatric Oncology Group Study

Cohn SL, Look AT, Joshi VV, Holbrook T, Salwen H, Chagnovich D, Chesler L, Rowe ST, Valentine MB, Komuro H, Castleberry RP, Bowman LC, Rao PV, Seeger RC, Brodeur GM (Northwestern Univ, Chicago; Univ of Tennessee, Memphis; East Carolina Univ, Greenville, NC)
Cancer Res 55:721–726, 1995   11–4

Introduction.—Neuroblastoma (NB) is a pediatric malignant neoplasm that has a wide prognostic range. Among the biological markers that have been associated with an unfavorable prognosis are N-*myc* amplification, diploid DNA content, chromosome 1p deletion, undifferentiated histology, and high mitotic rate. Amplification of the N-*myc* oncogene is rarely seen in patients with localized NB and is usually associated with a poor prognosis. However, some patients with localized NBs and N-*myc* amplification have had good outcomes without aggressive multimodality therapy. The prognostic significance of N-*myc* amplification in localized NB was investigated in a retrospective study.

Methods.—The data from a study of NB biology were reviewed. Of 850 patients studied, 6 had localized disease with N-*myc* amplification. Outcome neuroblast cellular DNA content, histology, and N-*myc* protein expression were analyzed.

Results.—Of the 6 patients with localized N-*myc*–amplified tumors, 3 had stage A and 3 had stage B NBs. Two of the 3 children with stage A disease were treated with surgical resection only and have remained disease-free for more than 22 and 16 months, respectively. Two of the 3 children with stage B disease have remained disease-free for more than 38 and 20 months, respectively, after treatment with chemotherapy with and without autologous bone marrow transplant and radiotherapy. The other 2 patients were treated with chemotherapy and achieved a complete remission, but they had subsequent recurrences and died. Three patients, including the 2 who died, had unfavorable histology. Only the 2 patients who died had diploid DNA content. Four of the 5 tumors analyzed immunohistochemically had detectable expression of N-*myc* protein, which was not detected in the stromal tumor of 1 patient. The N-*myc* protein expression was at a low level in 1 patient in long remission.

Discussion.—N-*myc* amplification did not clearly correlate with poor clinical outcome in this small group of patients with localized NBs. The findings suggest that the prognostic significance of N-*myc* amplification may vary with different histological features. In addition, N-*myc* amplification may be associated with different genetic composition in localized NBs than in advanced-stage NBs, since tumors in patients with advanced disease usually have diploid DNA content, whereas only 2 of these patients with localized disease had diploid DNA content. The prognostic significance of a low level of N-*myc* protein expression requires further study.

▶ This paper is included simply as a brief wake-up call that biological markers and prognostic factors have a tendency to slip in value or narrow in application as more experience is gained. This study demonstrates that N-*myc* oncogene amplification is uncommon in localized tumors but, when present, does not necessarily portend an adverse outcome. Whether N-*myc* amplification has a role in influencing the aggressiveness of neuroblastoma is open to some question. Is this merely an association, an epiphenomenon, or does it have some biologically important role in determining whether NBs will kill.

J.V. Simone, M.D.

Concordance for Hodgkin's Disease in Identical Twins Suggesting Genetic Susceptibility to the Young-Adult Form of the Disease

Mack TM, Cozen W, Shibata DK, Weiss LM, Nathwani BN, Hernandez AM, Taylor CR, Hamilton AS, Deapen DM, Rappaport EB (Univ of Southern California, Los Angeles; City of Hope Med Ctr, Duarte, Calif)
N Engl J Med 332:413–418, 1995   11–5

Introduction.—Sets of twins concordant for Hodgkin's disease have been reported to be at increased risk for the disease. Between 1980 and 1992, weekly advertisements were placed in large newspapers across the United State and Canada to identify twins with Hodgkin's disease. The genetic susceptibility to the young-adult form of Hodgkin's disease in 432 sets of affected twins was reported.

Methods.—One or both twins were interviewed regarding diagnosis, zygosity, and detailed demographic and medical history. When possible, medical records, pathology reports, and diagnostic slides were obtained. The phenotype of Reed-Sternberg cells and background lymphocytes was determined using standard immunoperoxidase techniques. Specimens for pairs of twins concordant for Hodgkin's disease were evaluated for Epstein-Barr virus (EBV) by polymerase chain reaction. The incidence of Hodgkin's disease before 50 years of age was compared with the national incidence rates in healthy monozygotic and dizygotic twins.

Results.—A total of 179 monozygotic and 187 dizygotic unaffected twins were observed for 14.1 and 14.3 years, respectively, after diagnosis in the affected twin. No pairs of dizygotic twins concordant for Hodgkin's disease were identified. Ten pairs of monozygotic twins were concordant for Hodgkin's disease (Table 2). The mean interval between diagnosis within these pairs was 4.5 years. Monozygotic twins, but not dizygotic

TABLE 2.—Characteristics of 10 Pairs of Monozygotic Twins Concordant for Hodgkin's Disease

| Pair No. | Sex | Year of Birth | Age at Diagnosis (YR) | | Histologic Subtype | | EBV Genome Detection | | | | History of Mononucleosis | | Other 1st-degree relative |
| | | | | | | | PCR | | IN SITU Hybridization | | | | |
			Twin A	Twin B	Twin A	Twin B	Twin A	Twin B	Twin A	Twin B	Twin A	Twin B	
1	M	1936	37	49	NS	NS	−	−	−	−	−	−	−
2	M	1955	16	21	NS	NOS*	−	−	−	−	−	+	+
3	M	1964	18	19	NS	NS	−	−	−	−	−	−	−
4	F	1960	23	26	NS	NS	NA	+	−	+	−	−	−
					(LD)	(LD)							
5	F	1962	16	23	NS	NS	NA	NA	−	−	+	−	−
6	M	1957	20	28	NS	MC	NA	−	−	−	−	−	−
						(LD)							
7†	M	1949	28	29	NOS	MC	NA	NA	+	+	+	+	−
8‡	F	1960	23	30	NS	NS	NA	NA	−	−	−	−	+
9	M	1948	23	24	MC	MC	NA	NA	NA	+	−	−	−
10	M	1953	17	31	NS	NS	−	−	−	−	NA	NA	NA

* There was insufficient tissue for further classification.

† These twins were concordant for eosinophilic infiltrate in tumor specimens; initial reports indicated concordance for mixed-cellularity Hodgkin's disease.

‡ These twins were concordant for minimal-change disease (lipoid nephrosis).

Abbreviations: PCR, polymerase chain reaction, NS, nodular sclerosis, NOS, not otherwise specified; NA, not available, LD, lymphocyte-depleted; MC, mixed cellularity, minus sign, Negative; plus sign, positive.

(Reprinted by permission of *The New England Journal of Medicine*, from Mack TM, Cozen W, Shibata DK, et al: Concordance for Hodgkin's disease in identical twins suggesting genetic susceptibility to the young-adult form of the disease. *N Engl J Med* 332:413–418, Copyright 1995, Massachusetts Medical Society.)

twins, had a greatly increased risk for Hodgkin's disease. However, 90% of monozygotic twins of patients with Hodgkin's disease are expected to remain unaffected. There was a very low incidence of EBV genome in the Reed-Sternberg cells of the tumors of twins concordant for nodular sclerosing Hodgkin's disease.

Conclusion.—An increased incidence of Hodgkin's disease was observed in monozygotic, but not dizygotic, twins. In monozygotic twins, 90% of unaffected twins are expected not to have the disease develop.

▶ Hodgkin's disease has always been a tantalizing subject for those interested in the etiology of cancer. There are well-documented studies of Hodgkin's disease occurring in families, leading to speculation that an infectious agent was responsible. Furthermore, the association of the EBV with this tumor and evidence of its presence in Reed-Sternberg cells certainly draw the circle much tighter. This study strongly suggests that a genetic factor may also play a role. The frequency of Hodgkin's disease occurring in both identical twins was much higher than that observed in fraternal twins. If one needed to conjure up an etiologic sequence that would fit with the state of scientific knowledge today, one could easily suppose that a genetic predisposition or an oncogene was present in certain individuals, which made the development of Hodgkin's disease more likely on exposure to an infectious agent or agents. If that were the case, one would expect the frequency of the disease to be greater in the second of identical twins after Hodgkin's disease had developed in the first twin. A specific gene that might be associated with this observation has not yet been identified.

However, the authors remind us to keep in mind that in spite of the unexpectedly high level of concordance in monozygotic twins, 90% of the monozygotic twins whose twin sibling develops Hodgkin's disease can expect to remain unaffected. Furthermore, no cases of Hodgkin's disease are known to have occurred in other family members of the concordant twins studied. Hodgkin's disease in a twin should alert physicians to the possibility of the disease developing in the other twin, but one should not unduly alarm the family. As shown in Table 2, the time from the development of Hodgkin's disease in the first twin to the time of development in the second twin may be as short as 1 year and as long as 14 years.

J.V. Simone, M.D.

Subsequent Malignancies in Children and Adolescents After Treatment for Hodgkin's Disease
Beaty O III, Hudson MM, Greenwald C, Luo X, Fang L, Wilimas JA, Thompson EI, Kun LE, Pratt CB (St Jude Children's Research Hosp, Memphis, Tenn; Univ of Tennessee, Memphis)
J Clin Oncol 13:603–609, 1995   11–6

Objective.—The risk of subsequent malignancy was estimated in patients treated for Hodgkin's disease in the childhood and adolescent years.

The 499 patients reviewed, who were treated between 1962 and 1993, included 385 who were 10 years of age or older when Hodgkin's disease was diagnosed and 114 preadolescents (younger than 10 years of age).

Treatment.—Both radiotherapy and multiagent chemotherapy were delivered to 346 patients. Thirty received chemotherapy only, and 123 received only radiotherapy. Total radiation doses ranged from 20 to 42 Gy. In the latter years of the review period, patients received either the cyclophosphamide, vincristine, and procarbazine (COP) or the doxorubicin, bleomycin, vinblastine, and dacarbazine (ABVD) regimen. Most recently, patients have received the vinblastine, doxorubicin, methotrexate and prednisone (VAMP) or the vinblastine, etoposide, prednisone, and doxorubicin (VEPA) regimen.

Findings.—The rate of complete response to initial treatment was 92.4%. Nearly half the 68 deaths were the result of recurrent disease. Twenty-five patients had a second malignancy after a median follow-up of 9 years. The 19 solid tumors included 10 carcinomas and 7 sarcomas. Four patients had acute nonlymphoblastic leukemia, and there were single cases of non-Hodgkin's lymphoma and chronic myeloid leukemia. Three patients had a third malignancy. The cumulative risk of a second malignancy increased from 1.5% at 5 years to 7.7% at 15 years. Fourteen of the 25 patients with a second malignancy were free of disease when last seen.

Risk Factors.—Although males predominated in the overall series, 76% of patients with second malignancies were females. Patients initially treated during adolescence were most at risk. The risk also was increased in patients whose Hodgkin's disease recurred. Splenectomy was not a significant risk factor, nor was the type of initial treatment related to the risk of a second malignancy.

Conclusion.—Children and adolescents treated for Hodgkin's disease are at risk of a second, treatment-related malignancy.

▶ The occurrence of second malignancies after treatment for Hodgkin's disease has been a major problem for many years. In this large series of children, the estimated cumulative risk of a second malignancy increased from 1.5% to almost 8% at 15 years. The intriguing observation is that the risk was greater among children who were adolescents at the time of treatment. It is not surprising that the frequency was also greater among those treated a second time for recurrent Hodgkin's disease.

A surprising finding was that there was no difference between patients treated with radiation therapy alone, chemotherapy alone, or radiation plus chemotherapy. In adult studies, it has been demonstrated that patients who received both radiation and multiagent chemotherapy have a significantly higher likelihood of the development of leukemia than those treated with either modality alone. The authors fail to mention one fascinating possibility in this long-term study. This institution has never used nitrogen mustard in the treatment of Hodgkin's disease, a drug that was for years part of the MOPP regimen, and is virtually synonymous with the chemotherapy for Hodgkin's disease. One wonders whether the use of cyclophosphamide instead of nitrogen mustard in these studies resulted in a different likelihood of the development of second malignancies, especially myeloid leukemia.

J.V. Simone, M.D.

Non-Hodgkin's Lymphomas of Childhood and Adolescence: Results of a Treatment Stratified for Biologic Subtypes and Stage. A Report of the Berlin-Frankfurt-Münster Group

Reiter A, Schrappe M, Parwaresch R, Henze G, Müller-Weihrich S, Sauter S, Sykora K-W, Ludwig W-D, Gadner H, Riehm H (Medizinische Hochschule, Hannover, Germany; Christian-Albrechts-Universität, Kiel, Germany; Free Univ of Berlin; et al)

J Clin Oncol 13:359–372, 1995

11–7

Introduction.—The treatment strategy and end results of trial ALL/NHL-BFM 86 for children with untreated non-Hodgkin's lymphoma (NHL) were evaluated. A total of 302 children aged 0.6–17.8 years were followed for a minimum of 3.5 years.

Methods.—Patients were stratified by NHL subtypes into 2 therapy groups; group non-B and group B. Group non-B included patients with lymphoblastic lymphoma and pleomorphic T-cell lymphoma (PTCL). Therapy for this group was an acute lymphoblastic leukemia protocol that included cranial irradiation for advanced disease. Group B included patients with Burkitt's-type lymphoma, acute B-cell leukemia (B-ALL), and most large-cell lymphomas. Therapy for group B was six 5-day therapy

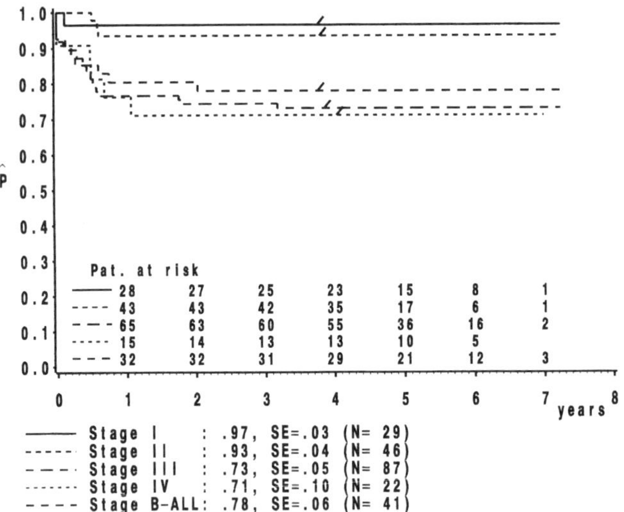

FIGURE 3.—Probability of event-free survival according to stage for patients in therapy group B. *P* values (log-rank test): ≤ .035 for all comparisons between stages I and II vs. stages III, IV, and B-ALL; *P* > .5 for all comparisons between stages III, IV, and B-ALL; *P* > .5 for stage I vs. stage II. (Courtesy of Reiter A, Schrappe M, Parwaresch R, et al: Non-Hodgkin's lymphomas of childhood and adolescence: Results of a treatment stratified for biologic subtypes and stage. A report of the Berlin-Frankfurt-Münster Group. *J Clin Oncol* 13:359–372, 1995.)

courses of dexamethasome, methotrexate, ifosfamide, cytarabine, and etoposide, alternating with cyclophosphamide and doxorubicin. Patients with stages I and II received 3 such courses.

Results.—Distribution of the diagnoses was as follows: 24% lymphoblastic lymphoma; 50% Burkitt's-type lymphomas, including B-ALL; 18% diffuse large-cell lymphomas; and 8% not classified. The probability for event-free survival (pEFS) at 7 years was 80% for the entire group, 78% for the 77 patients in therapy group non-B, and 81% for the 225 patients in therapy group B. At 6 years, pEFS was comparable for patients with stage III and stage IV disease in group non-B. In group B, pEFS at 6 years was significantly higher for patients with stages I and II disease compared with patients with stages III, IV, and B-ALL (Fig 3). Three of 4 patients with large-cell PTCL had a relapse. Otherwise, the rate of adverse events was comparable between patients with varying histologic subsets. The most frequent site of failure was local disease manifestations.

Conclusion.—With the exclusion of patients with PTCL, this treatment strategy provided all patients with a similarly high chance for event-free survival. Local tumor control may become more important with reduced systemic failure.

▶ Although to some extent this paper is confirmatory of results now being obtained around the world, the large group of patients and the overall excellent results, regardless of sub-type, make it important to include this article to underscore the current status of achievable art in the treatment of NHL in children. As shown in Figure 3, the results obtained in this study ranged from a greater-than-70% cure rate to a cure rate of more than 95%. The cure rate for all patients, regardless of histologic subtype or stage, was 80%. This remarkable result offers several lessons to us. First and foremost, this disease is highly curable, provided the patient is in the right hands from the beginning. Any dabbling in the early treatment period could reduce the chance for excellent results. Second, the best results require agressive, modern multiagent therapy. The final lesson is more complex. Randomized trials become much more difficult when the overall results of treatment for any form of cancer are so good. Furthermore, randomized studies may no longer be necessary because, as in this study, one can simply adapt variations in therapy for the particular subtypes of lymphoma and then base one's success on the overall results for the entire group. Randomized trials are more successful when there is likely to be a substantial difference between 2 regimens, either in potential outcome or toxicity (and in this day, cost), and when there is a sufficient number of patients who fail with the conventional approach to allow for differences to be statistically observed. Once the cure rate reaches 70% to 80%, as is true in actue lymphoblastic leukemia, Hodgkin's disease and Wilms' tumor, it is increasingly difficult to accrue enough patients in a study to show a significant difference between treatment regimens.

J.V. Simone, M.D.

The Third Intergroup Rhabdomyosarcoma Study

Crist W, Gehan EA, Ragab AH, Dickman PS, Donaldson SS, Fryer C, Hammond D, Hays DM, Herrmann J, Heyn R, Jones PM, Lawrence W, Newton W, Ortega J, Raney RB, Ruymann FB, Tefft M, Webber B, Wiener E, Wharam M, Vietti TJ, Maurer HM (St Jude Children's Research Hosp, Memphis, Tenn)

J Clin Oncol 13:610–630, 1995   11–8

Introduction.—There has been a dramatic improvement in the cure rate for patients with rhabdomyosarcoma over the past 25 years. Since 1972, the Intergroup Rhabdomyosarcoma Study (IRS) Committee, a cooperative study group, has performed 3 trials. The third trial was designed to devise therapy for the different rhabdomyosarcoma disease categories.

Methods.—A total of 1,062 untreated children with confirmed rhabdomyosarcoma, extraosseous Ewing's sarcoma, or undifferentiated sarcoma were assigned to a clinical group (I–IV) based on the extent of disease or residual disease after resection. They were then randomly assigned to be treated with 1 of several regimens, according to clinical group, tumor site, and histology. Outcome was compared between randomized groups or with results that were obtained in IRS-II.

Results.—Overall, patients in IRS-III had significantly improved therapeutic outcome compared with patients in IRS-II, with 5-year progression-free survival rates of 65% vs. 55% and 5-year survival rates of 71% vs. 63%. Treatment with a 1-year regimen of vincristine and dactinomycin (VA) was as effective as the more intensive regimen of VA plus cyclophosphamide (VAC) in patients in clinical group I with favorable histology. Among patients with clinical group II disease with favorable histology (excluding orbit, head, and paratesticular tumors), adding doxorubicin (ADR) to VA produced a nonsignificant treatment benefit compared with treatment with VA and radiotherapy. Children with clinical group III disease had comparable outcomes, whether treated with pulsed VAC, pulsed VADRC-VAC plus cisplatin, or pulsed VADRC-VAC plus cisplatin plus etoposide. However, the more intensive regimens in each treatment group improved outcomes significantly compared with the results in IRS-II. Patients in clinical group IV (with metastatic disease) did not have improved outcomes with the more intensive regimens compared with comparable patients in IRS-II, and all regimens had similar outcomes. Patients with special pelvic tumors and tumors with unfavorable histology had improved outcomes with the more intensive therapy of IRS-III. The deletion of cyclophosphamide did not reduce the treatment efficacy of regimens in the treatment of orbit and head tumors.

Discussion.—Overall, treatment outcome for children with rhabdomyosarcoma was significantly improved with the treatment regimens used in IRS-III. The data show that cyclophosphamide can be removed from protocols, without compromising outcome and reducing the risk of sterility or secondary cancer. Continued use of sequential VA therapy, along with radiotherapy for patients in clinical groups II and III, is supported.

▶ The lesson from this report is subtle though extremely important because it addresses a fundamental feature in the progress of the treatment of childhood cancer. As Figure 2 in the original article shows, both progression-free survival and survival improved by about 10% between IRS-II and IRS-III. That may not seem like much until one realizes that there are 1,000 patients in each study. That means 100 more patients were saved in the more recent study. The reason for this improvement is more intensive early therapy. That is the hallmark of studies with better outcomes in childhood cancer. The other feature that is characteristic is that the improvement has not come as a giant leap all at once but, rather, has resulted from the series of small improvements over an extended period. One toils in the vineyards and wakes up one day to find out that the results are substantially superior to historical outcomes. These studies are also a reflection of the national cooperation that the vast majority of pediatric oncologists enjoy in carrying out studies on a relatively rare tumor. These are cooperative clinical trials at their best.

J.V. Simone, M.D.

▶ This paper is included simply as a brief wake-up call that biological markers and prognostic factors have a tendency to slip in value or narrow in application as more experience is gained. This study demonstrates that N-*myc* oncogene amplification is uncommon in localized tumors but, when present, does not necessarily portend an adverse outcome. Whether N-*myc* amplification has a role in influencing the aggressiveness of neuroblastoma is open to some question. Is this merely an association, an epiphenomenon, or does it have some biologically important role in determining whether NBs will kill?

J.V. Simone, M.D.

Conservative Surgical Management of Vaginal and Vulvar Pediatric Rhabdomyosarcoma: A Report From the Intergroup Rhabdomyosarcoma Study III
Andrassy RJ, Hays DM, Raney RB, Wiener ES, Lawrence W, Lobe TE, Corpron CA, Smith M, Maurer HM (Houston)
J Pediatr Surg 30:1034–1037, 1995   11–9

Background.—Cytoreductive chemotherapy is currently given before surgery in the treatment of vaginal and vulvar rhabdomyosarcoma (RMS) in children. The Intergroup Rhabdomyosarcoma Study (IRS)-III, conducted between 1984 and 1988, included 27 assessable patients treated according to a preoperative chemotherapy protocol consisting of Adriamycin, cisplatin, vincristine, dactinomycin, and cyclophosphamide.

Patients and Outcomes.—Twenty-four children had primary vaginal tumors, and 3 had vulvar primary tumors. Twenty children with primary vaginal tumors underwent an initial biopsy and had gross residual disease. These children comprised group III. Group IIA consisted of 3 children undergoing resection with positive margins. The 1 patient in group IV had metastatic disease. At surgery, 7 patients had partial or complete vaginectomy. In 6 of those children, no viable tumor was identified in the specimen. One of those 7 patients had a cystectomy, and 5 had a hysterectomy. At 66–108 months after diagnosis, 17 patients had no evidence of disease, 2 died of chemotoxicity, and 1 died of unknown causes after having achieved a complete response. Ten of those 17 children underwent biopsy and chemotherapy only. Radiation therapy was used in the treatment of 4 of these 10 as well. None of the patients in group IIA had evidence of disease, and the 1 patient in group IV died of rapidly progressive disease. Compared with previous experience, the primary chemotherapy protocol resulted in less need for surgical intervention and irradiation. No local recurrences were documented. Twenty of 24 patients continue to be free of relapse, with no evidence of disease. The 3 children with vulvar primary tumors underwent wide local excision and chemotherapy. To date, none of these children have any evidence of disease.

Conclusions.—The preoperative chemotherapy protocol used in the IRS III resulted in excellent local tumor control and less need for surgical resection. The bladder, uterus, and vagina were preserved in most children in this series. Furthermore, there were no local recurrences.

▶ I was a bit surprised to see this paper, because it has long been known in centers that treat this rare tumor that extensive surgical resections were not only permanently disfiguring but unnecessary. However, over a 4-year period, the Intergroup Rhabdomyosarcoma Study Group has collected data from a variety of centers that demonstrate conclusively that either a biopsy alone or a limited resection combined with chemotherapy and/or radiotherapy was sufficient to achieve a cure in a large proportion of these patients. Having spent my entire career in high-volume pediatric oncology institutions, I sometimes forget that this tumor is rare and that a conservative surgical approach, although widely accepted in the major centers, may not be widely recognized as the standard.

J.V. Simone, M.D.

Germline *p53* Mutations Are Frequently Detected in Young Children With Rhabdomyosarcoma
Diller L, Sexsmith E, Gottlieb A, Li FP, Malkin D (Univ of Toronto; Dana-Farber Cancer Inst, Boston)
J Clin Invest 95:1606–1611, 1995

11–10

Introduction.—Alterations in the *p53* gene are common in diverse human malignancies. However, the relationship between constitutional *p53* mutations and malignancy is complex, with germline *p53* mutations occurring in the coding region in most, but not all, patients with cancer who have a family history of cancer and in some patients with cancer with no family history of malignancy. The frequency of constitutional *p53* mutations in 2 groups of pediatric patients with sporadic rhabdomyosarcoma (RMS) was determined, and frequency was correlated with patient and tumor characteristics.

Methods.—Peripheral blood was drawn from 33 children with RMS or a history of RMS and no family history of cancer or Li-Fraumeni syndrome. Genomic DNA was extracted from the blood samples and amplified with primers targeting exons 2–11 of the *p53* gene. Clinical data—including age at diagnosis, sex, tumor histologic type and site, grade, and outcome—were gathered for each patient.

Results.—Of the 33 patients, 3 had genomic DNA samples with heterozygous, specific germline *p53* mutations. The patients with *p53* mutations were younger than those without. The 3 patients received diagnoses of RMS at ages 19 months, 29 months, and 18 months. The *p53* mutations identified were an A-to-G switch at the second position of codon 235 in exon 7, a G-to-C switch at the second position of codon 306 in exon 8, and a T-to-A switch at the first position of codon 227 in exon 7. The 3 patients have been treated and are free of recurrence 2–19 years from diagnosis. There were no correlations between sex, tumor histologic type, site, or grade and *p53* mutations.

Discussion.—Although constitutional *p53* mutations are common in patients with a family history of cancer, an uncommonly high proportion of these patients with RMS and no family history of cancer harbored *p53* mutations predicting amino acid substitutions. Three of 13 children younger than 3 years of age but none of the 20 children with diagnosis after the age of 3 years carried *p53* mutations, suggesting an association between young age at diagnosis and genetic predisposition. Genetic testing for constitutional *p53* mutations has a potential predictive role in relatives of patients with RMS.

▶ This study of *p53* mutations has a more subtle message than the simple association with the mutation and the development of cancer in children. The authors found that 3 of 13 children younger than 3 years of age at diagnosis carried the mutations, whereas none of 20 children older than 3 years of age had a detectable constitutional *p53* mutation. The authors, therefore, add weight to the evidence that suggests that *p53* mutations may predispose individuals to malignancy at an early age, leading one to the conclusion that it might be fruitful to study the parents and close relatives of these patients. This is especially true because RMS was one of the tumors found with some frequency in the Li-Fraumeni syndrome, in which there is a germline mutation of *p53*. Thus, the role of *p53* may differ, depending on the circumstances under which the mutation occurs. It will not be long before every tumor will have a genetic profile performed along with histologic examination.

J.V. Simone, M.D.

B-Cell Lineage Confers a Favorable Outcome Among Children and Adolescents With Large-Cell Lymphoma: A Pediatric Oncology Group Study
Hutchison RE, Berard CW, Shuster JJ, Link MP, Pick TE, Murphy SB (State Univ of New York, Syracuse; St Jude Children's Research Hosp, Memphis, Tenn; Univ of Florida, Gainesville; et al)
J Clin Oncol 13:2023–2032, 1995   11–11

Background.—Recent research suggests that a high proportion of childhood large-cell lymphomas (LCLs) are of T-cell type as well as B-cell type and that many T-cell LCLs in children express antigens associated with anaplastic large-cell lymphoma (ALCL). The immunophenotype of children treated uniformly for large-cell non-Hodgkin's lymphoma (NHL) was investigated to determine the prognostic importance of B-cell and T-cell lineages and of CD30 positivity.

Methods.—Sixty-nine patients underwent immunochemical analysis, histologic classification, and uniform staging. Treatment was delivered according to 1 of 2 protocols for stage I or II NHL or for stage III or IV large-cell NHL.

Findings.—An immunophenotypic analysis identified 25 B-cell, 23 T-cell, and 21 indeterminate lineages. In 27 patients, CD30 was expressed. Twenty-two of those patients had ALCL histology. Patients with B-cell lineages were older and had better survival rates than those with T-cell or indeterminate lineages, with 3-year event-free survivals of 96%, 67%, and 74%, respectively (Fig 2). Patients with limited-stage disease more commonly had B-cell lineage, but this lineage was still associated with favorable survival when stratified for stage. Survival was not significantly associated with CD30 expression or ALCL histologic type.

Conclusions.—Proportionately, B-cell lineage is less frequent in pediatric LCLs than in adults. The CD30 antigen-expressing lymphomas are common among patients with T-cell and indeterminate lineages. The B-cell phenotype, which tends to occur in older children, is associated with improved survival rates.

▶ I include this study from the Pediatric Oncology Group, which has a relatively straightforward message, because it is not widely appreciated that LCL occurs in children. This type of lymphoma was thought for many years to be limited to adults, but more sophisticated histologic analysis and the use of immunochemistry have enabled identification and the study of pediatric NHLs in great detail. Because lymphomas are relatively uncommon in children compared with adults, and because the large-cell type represents a minority of those found in children, gathering these data required the resources of a large cooperative group.

The primary conclusion of this study is that patients with B-cell lineage lymphomas have a better outcome than those with T-cell or indeterminant markers; the striking difference is shown in Figure 2. This difference holds up even when the tumors and patients are stratified for other known risk factors. Although the outcome for the T-cell and indeterminant types is not

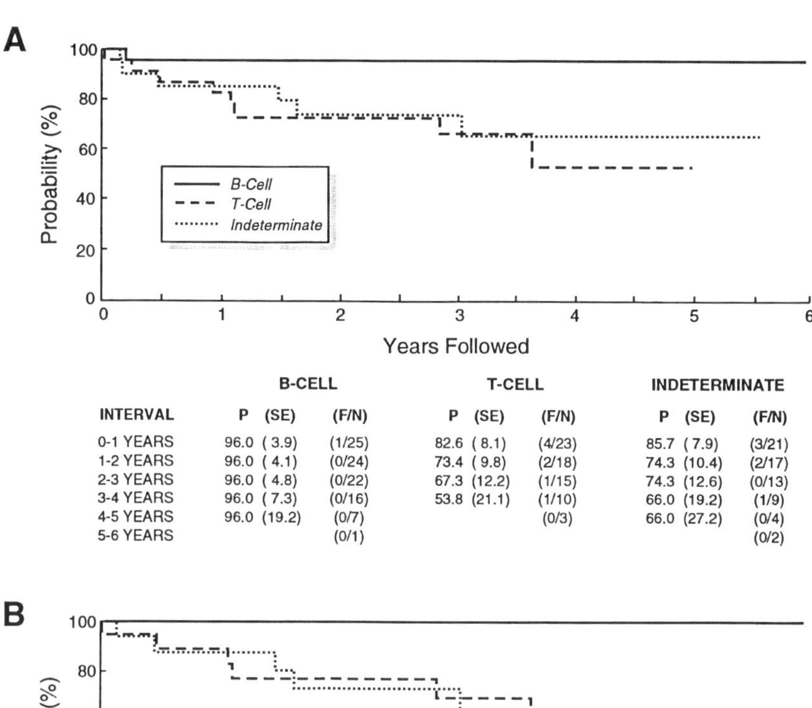

A

	B-CELL			T-CELL			INDETERMINATE		
INTERVAL	P	(SE)	(F/N)	P	(SE)	(F/N)	P	(SE)	(F/N)
0-1 YEARS	96.0	(3.9)	(1/25)	82.6	(8.1)	(4/23)	85.7	(7.9)	(3/21)
1-2 YEARS	96.0	(4.1)	(0/24)	73.4	(9.8)	(2/18)	74.3	(10.4)	(2/17)
2-3 YEARS	96.0	(4.8)	(0/22)	67.3	(12.2)	(1/15)	74.3	(12.6)	(0/13)
3-4 YEARS	96.0	(7.3)	(0/16)	53.8	(21.1)	(1/10)	66.0	(19.2)	(1/9)
4-5 YEARS	96.0	(19.2)	(0/7)			(0/3)	66.0	(27.2)	(0/4)
5-6 YEARS			(0/1)						(0/2)

B

	B-CELL			T-CELL			INDETERMINATE		
INTERVAL	P	(SE)	(F/N)	P	(SE)	(F/N)	P	(SE)	(F/N)
0-1 YEARS				88.9	(7.7)	(2/18)	87.5	(8.6)	(2/16)
1-2 YEARS	100.0	( )	(0/14)	77.0	(10.7)	(2/15)	72.9	(12.0)	(2/13)
2-3 YEARS	100.0	( )	(0/13)	69.3	(13.6)	(1/12)	72.9	(14.3)	(0/10)
3-4 YEARS	100.0	( )	(0/10)	46.2	(24.0)	(1/8)	62.5	(22.1)	(1/7)
4-5 YEARS	100.0	( )	(0/6)			(0/2)	62.5	(27.1)	(0/3)
5-6 YEARS			(0/1)						(0/2)

FIGURE 2.—A, event-free survival of B-cell cases ($n = 25$) showed superior survival vs. T-cell ($n = 23$) or indeterminate cases ($n = 21$) ($P = .027$). **B,** advanced-stage B-cell cases ($n = 14$) also showed superior survival vs. advanced T-cell ($n = 18$) and advanced indeterminate cases ($n = 16$) ($P = .036$). *Abbreviations: P,* estimated percent failure-free through end of interval; *F,* number of failures in interval; *N,* number at risk at start of interval. (Courtesy of Hutchison RE, Berard CW, Shuster JJ, et al: B-cell lineage confers a favorable outcome among children and adolescents with large-cell lymphoma: A Pediatric Oncology Group study. *J Clin Oncol* 13:2033–2032, 1995.)

terrible (an approximate 50% survival at 4 years), the lines do not show the same tendency to plateau as they do for the B-cell type. Thus, late relapses are likely to occur in T-cell and indeterminant types of LCL but not in B-cell lymphoma. The behavior of the B-cell type resembles that of Burkitt's lymphoma, i.e., if one can get past the first 6 months safely, the patient is usually cured.

J.V. Simone, M.D.

Our 10-Year Experience With Embolized Wilms' Tumor
Županić B, Bradić I, Batinica S, Radanović B, Šimunić S, Županić V, Popović L, Belina D (Univ of Zagreb, Croatia)
Eur J Pediatr Surg 5:88–91, 1995
11–12

Background.—Wilms' tumor is the most common genitourinary malignancy in children. Although there appears to be a hereditary component in some patients, the tumor is usually diagnosed in 2- or 3-year-old children. In most patients, the initial finding is an abdominal tumor. Other symptoms are abdominal pain, hematuria, hypertension, and varicocele. Intravenous urography, CT, ultrasound, and angiography are used to establish the diagnosis. Surgery alone is effective in the treatment of the disease in infants. At later stages, surgery must be combined with other modalities, such as preoperative embolization, radiation therapy, and chemotherapy. One 10-year experience with Wilms' tumor was reported.

Patients and Findings.—The cases of 33 children were reviewed. Age at diagnosis ranged from 2 to 16 years. The most common finding was a palpable mass. Complete clinical, laboratory, and radiologic examinations were performed, the latter including a plain radiograph of the abdomen, IV urography, ultrasonography, CT, aortorenovasography, and selective renal angiography. A new invasive diagnostic and therapeutic procedure—preoperative percutaneous transcatheter intra-arterial embolization (PTIE) of the renal artery—was introduced. The goal of this method was to decrease vascularization, to reduce the mass of the kidney affected by the tumor, to separate it from the surrounding tissue, and to decrease intraoperative spillage of malignant cells into the blood stream and their spread. This procedure made nephrectomy easier to perform. Nephrectomy was best performed 48 hours after embolization.

Conclusion.—With the procedure used in this series, locally inoperable tumors may be resectable. This procedure carries no risk of intraoperative malignant cell-shedding because of complete occlusion of intrarenal arterial blood flow. Typically, the renal vein is empty except for a malignant or nonmalignant thrombus arising from local tumor pressure or impaired renal blood flow. In addition, capsular veins are thrombotic. Within a day after PTIE, a loose capsule forms around the aseptic tumor necrosis. By the fourth day, the capsule is more solid and slightly vascularized. The risk of intraoperative transvenous malignant cell spillage from intraoperative tumor manipulation is minimized by tumor sequestration. In the patients reviewed, the amount of blood transfused during surgery was less than 300 mL.

▶ I include this paper for its novelty, because I do not know of a single institution in this country where embolization of Wilms' tumors is a normal part of therapy. These investigators report the use of tumor embolization followed 2 days later by nephrectomy. However, except for the claim that an inoperable Wilms' tumor may become operable, it is hard to accept that this process has a role in the treatment of this disease.

Although I am trying to keep an open mind, the tools of modern-day therapy for Wilms' tumor make it impossible to recommend, or even condone, the use of this practice. Inoperable Wilms' tumor can often be controlled with preoperative chemotherapy, because they are such a chemosensitive type of tumor. That approach has the additional advantage of having a cytocidal effect on any tumor cells that may have escaped the primary Wilms' tumor. At this point, a commentator usually suggests that a controlled trial be performed to determine whether this procedure is of value. However, it is not clear that a controlled trial would pass muster at an institutional review board or scientific review today.

J.V. Simone, M.D.

Improved Outcome for Children With Hepatoblastoma
Stringer MD, Hennayake S, Howard ER, Spitz L, Shafford EA, Mieli-Vergani G, Saxena R, Malone M, Dicks-Mireaux C, Karani J, Mowat AP, Pritchard J
(King's College Hosp, London; Hosp for Sick Children, London)
Br J Surg 82:386–391, 1995   11–13

Background.—Hepatoblastoma is the most common primary malignant liver tumor in infants and children. Improved management of these tumors has primarily resulted from the use of better cytotoxic agents and treat-

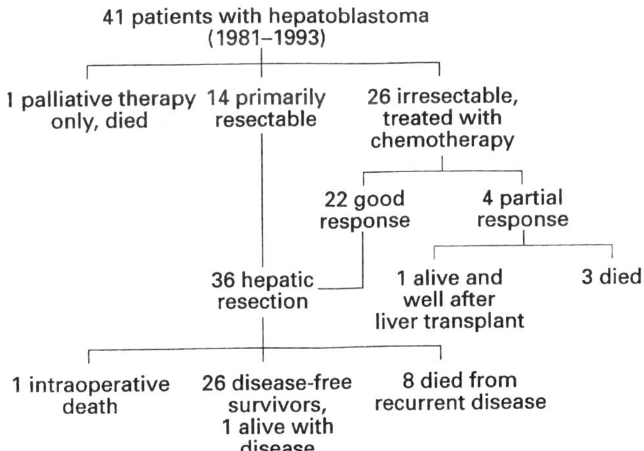

FIGURE 2.—Outcome of 41 patients with hepatoblastoma. (Courtesy of Stringer MD, Hennayake S, Howard ER, et al: Improved outcome for children with hepatoblastoma. *Br J Surg* 82:386–391, 1995, Blackwell Science Ltd.)

ment regimens. Surgical techniques and outcome were reviewed in a relatively large series of patients treated with modern chemotherapy.

Methods and Findings.—Forty-one children treated for hepatoblastoma between 1981 and 1993 were studied. The clinical, radiologic, and pathologic findings were reviewed. Primary resection of the hepatic tumor was performed in 14 children. Palliative treatment only was given to 1 infant with severe congenital anomalies. Among the 26 children with irresectable disease, pulsed cytotoxic chemotherapy with cisplatin and doxorubicin enabled subsequent surgical excision in 22. One child with irresectable and persistent extensive intrahepatic disease was successfully treated by liver transplantation. With a policy of selective preoperative chemotherapy, 90% of hepatoblastomas were resectable. No perioperative deaths resulted from hemorrhage, but 1 child died of an intraoperative tumor embolus. The 28 survivors were followed for a median of 5 years. Twenty-seven were free of disease (Fig 2). Patients treated with intent to cure had a cumulative survival probability of 67%. Survival data analysis suggested that the outcome was favorable for patients with a pure fetal histologic tumor subtype.

Conclusion.—In this patient series, the combination of improved chemotherapy and technical advances in hepatic resection and transplantation contributed to an actuarial long-term survival rate of 67%. This represents significant progress in the treatment of hepatoblastoma.

▶ Primary hepatic tumors have generally been resistant to all forms of therapy, with the exception of surgical resection. If the tumors were unresectable, historically there was little hope for cure. A major change began in the early 1980s, when investigators around the world began to use preoperative chemotherapy as a means of reducing the size of unresectable tumors to make them potentially resectable.

This paper illustrates such an approach, and the results are diagrammed in Figure 2. The intriguing thing about this study is that there was no significant difference in the overall survival rates between patients who underwent primary resection (11 of 14 were alive at a median of 84 months) and those treated by delayed resection after chemotherapy (16 of 22 were alive at a median of 60 months). This indicates that preoperative chemotherapy followed by resection can cure a significant proportion of patients with hepatoblastoma who previously were not curable.

J.V. Simone, M.D.

12 Brain Tumors

Metastatic Medulloblastoma: The Experience of the French Cooperative M7 Group
Bouffet E, Gentet JC, Doz F, Tron P, Roche H, Plantaz D, Thyss A, Stephan J-L, Lasset C, Carrie C, Alapetite C, Choux M, Mottolese C, Visot A, Zücker JM, Brunat-Mentigny M, Bernard JL (Centre Leon Berard, Lyon, France; Hôpital de la Timone, Marseille, France; Institut Curie, Paris; et al)
Eur J Cancer 30A:1478–1483, 1994   12–1

Introduction.—In recent series, the overall disease-free survival of patients with medulloblastoma ranged from 50% to 60% at 10 years to 30% to 40% for patients with metastases at diagnosis. With the lack of relevant prognostic data for patients with metastatic medulloblastoma, the optimal treatment is not well established. The outcomes of children with metastatic medulloblastoma treated according to the French M7 protocol were reported.

Methods.—Sixty-eight newly diagnosed, previously untreated patients with medulloblastoma entered the M7 study between 1985 and 1988. Twenty-three patients had metastatic disease, as detected by conventional staging procedures, CSF examination, myelogram and/or spinal axis MRI, and cranial CT or MRI. This high-risk group was treated uniformly with

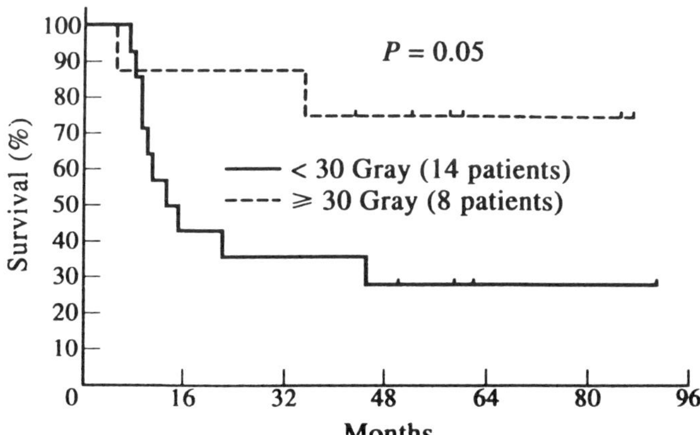

FIGURE 1.—Event-free survival as a function of radiation dose to the brain. (Courtesy of Boffet E, Gentet JC, Doz F, et al: Metastatic medulloblastoma: The experience of the French Cooperative M7 Group. *Eur J Cancer* 30A:1478–1483, 1994, with kind permission from Elsevier Science Ltd, The Boulevard, Langford Lane, Kidlington 0X5 1GB, UK.)

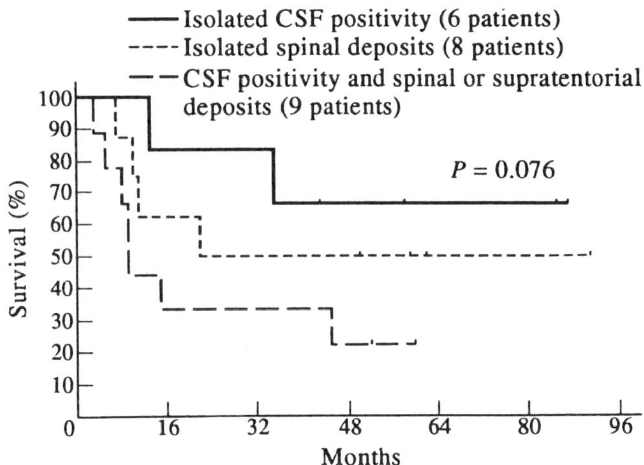

FIGURE 2.—Event-free survival as a function of metastatic disease. (Courtesy of Bouffet E, Gentet JC, Doz F, et al: Metastatic medulloblastoma: The experience of the French Cooperative M7 Group. *Eur J Cancer* 30A:1478–1483, 1994, with kind permission from Elsevier Science Ltd, The Boulevard, Langford Lane, Kidlington 0X5 1GB, UK.)

surgery, 2 courses of the 8-in-1 chemotherapy regimen, and craniospinal radiotherapy. The patients were followed up for at least 3.5 years or until death. Various factors were examined for prognostic significance.

Results.—Complete or subtotal resection of the primary tumor was achieved in 17 patients, whereas the other 6 had macroscopic residual disease. Recurrent disease occurred in 54% of 22 evaluable patients. There was a correlation between survival and the dose to the cranial field, with a threshold dose of 30 Gy (Fig 1). Event-free survival was better for patients with isolated CSF positivity and worse for those with both CSF positivity and spinal or supratentorial deposits (Fig 2). The patients with metastatic disease had a 7-year relapse-free survival of 43% compared

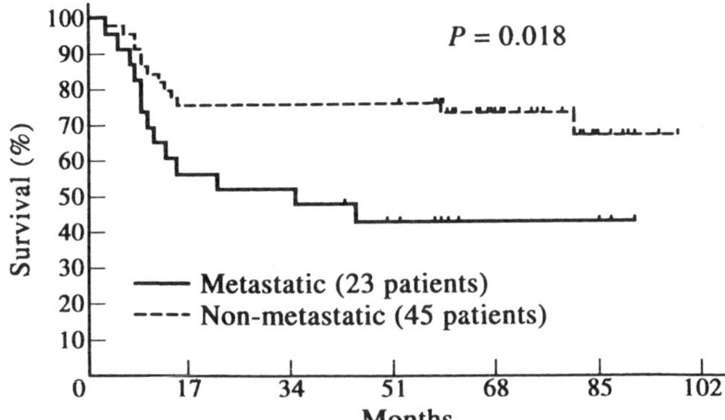

FIGURE 3.—Event-free survival for patients who were seen with metastatic disease compared with patients without detectable metastasis treated with the M7 protocol. (Courtesy of Bouffet E, Gentet JC, Doz F, et al: Metastatic medulloblastoma: The experience of the French Cooperative M7 Group. *Eur J Cancer* 30A:1478–1483, 1994, with kind permission from Elsevier Science Ltd, The Boulevard, Langford Lane, Kidlington 0X5 1GB, UK.)

with 68% for patients with localized disease (Fig 3). Survival was unrelated to age, sex, location of metastases, extent of initial surgery, and radiation dose to the posterior fossa.

Conclusions.—Because of their worse prognosis, patients with metastatic medulloblastoma require more aggressive treatment at the time of diagnosis. A 30-Gy radiation dose to the whole brain appears to be appropriate for these high-risk patients. Further evaluation of the different sites of metastatic disease in cooperative studies is needed.

▶ It is important to remind ourselves periodically that some brain tumors are curable. This long-term study by the French group in Lyon shows in its figures that it is certainly possible to cure some of these patients, depending on the extent of metastases at the time of diagnosis. Furthermore, outcome depends on whether the patients receive at least 30 Gy of radiotherapy. Thus, for all children who are seen with medulloblastoma, including those with metastatic disease, one is justified to expect a 60% long-term disease-free survival. More important yet, because this disease is responsive to therapy, it is reasonable to expect that refinements of that therapy might further push up the cure rate.

J.V. Simone, M.D.

Preliminary Experience With MR-Guided Thermal Ablation of Brain Tumors

Anzai Y, Lufkin R, DeSalles A, Hamilton DR, Farahani K, Black KL (Univ of California, Los Angeles)
AJNR 16:39–48, 1995

12–2

Introduction.—Magnetic resonance–guided stereotactic radiofrequency ablation of brain tumors is possible using stereotactic neurosurgery for accurate placement of devices, radiofrequency energy for establishing focal thermal coagulation, and MRI for pinpointing the tumor and monitoring the therapeutic effect. Twelve patients with 14 primary or metastatic tumors underwent this procedure to evaluate its feasibility and to determine MR features and sequential evolution of radiofrequency lesions created within the tumors.

Methods.—Neurologic status was monitored throughout because patients remained awake. Stereotactic coordinates of the tumor were determined for placement of the biopsy needle using MRI. Histopathologic diagnosis was confirmed by frozen section, and then an MR-compatible radiofrequency probe was introduced through the same opening. A radiofrequency lesion was generated by increasing the temperature to 80°C for 1 minute. This procedure was repeated at varying locations throughout the tumor until the entire tumor volume was treated. The treatment goal was to cover the entire tumor seen on pretreatment, plus a small rim of normal surrounding tissue. Magnetic resonance imaging was performed before, during, immediately after, and 1 day, 1 week, 1 month, 3 months and 6 months after radiofrequency ablation.

Results.—Well-defined radiofrequency lesions were detected on MRI. These were helpful for follow-up treatment. Contrast-enhanced T1-weighted images showed ring enhancement. The T2-weighted images showed the lesion boundary as a well-defined dark signal rim. Disease progression was not detected in any lesion treated with radiofrequency ablation.

Conclusion.—Stereotactic MR-guided radiofrequency brain tumor ablation is a very possible brain tumor treatment alternative. With MRI, accurate tumor location and visualization of feedback of thermal tissue changes are possible for determining therapeutic effect.

▶ I have included this article because I am always on the outlook for new approaches to the treatment of brain tumors. Two features that make this approach interesting are that it is noninvasive and that, by generating a radiofrequency lesion, it is possible to provide real-time feedback for treatment. Because the radiofrequency creates focal tissue coagulation, the technique can be used in previously irradiated patients and can be used repeatedly. The entire procedure takes about 3 hours, including pre- and post-treatment MR examinations. Another advantage is that this procedure is done with the patient under local anesthesia, so the patient is responsive and his or her neurologic symptoms can be monitored during the entire procedure.

If this sounds too good to be true, it almost is. The most serious shortcoming of these treatments for a malignant brain tumor is the lack of precise target definition by MR energy. Tumors are often spatially disseminated and spread undetected beyond the reach of surgery or this focal approach. Nonetheless, a noninvasive procedure is certainly preferable, even if it is effective for palliation only.

J.V. Simone, M.D.

Stereotactic Radiosurgery for the Definitive, Noninvasive Treatment of Brain Metastases
Alexander E III, Moriarty TM, Davis RB, Wen PY, Fine HA, Black PM, Kooy HM, Loeffler JS (Brigham and Women's Hosp, Boston; Beth Israel Hosp, Boston)
J Natl Cancer Inst 87:34–40, 1995   12–3

Introduction.—Patients with cancer commonly experience brain metastasis. Untreated, these metastases are typically fatal within one month. Surgical resection or whole brain radiotherapy can significantly increase survival. Stereotactic radiosurgery is a minimally invasive treatment option that delivers a high-energy, focal dose of radiation. Its effectiveness in treating brain metastasis was evaluated retrospectively.

Methods.—The records of all patients with brain metastasis treated with radiosurgery over a 7-year period were reviewed. All patients had a Kar-

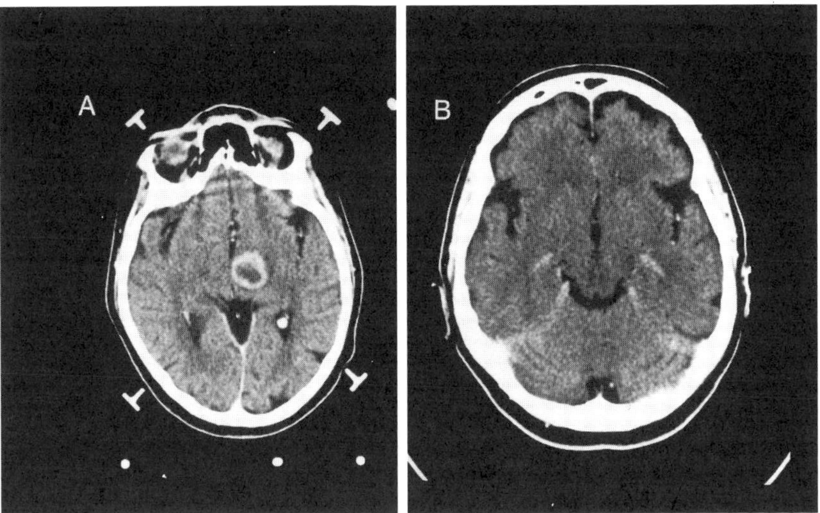

FIGURE 1.—Woman, 62, with metastatic ovarian carcinoma **A.** contrast-enhanced CT scan at the time of radiosurgery showing a 2- x 2.5-cm mass in the left thalamus and midbrain. **B.** contrast-enhanced CT scan at the same level 3 months after radiosurgery. (Courtesy of Alexander E. III, Montary TM, Davis RB, et al: Stereotactic radiosurgery for the definitive, noninvasive treatment of brain metastases. *J Natl Cancer Inst* 87:34-40, 1995.)

nofsky performance score above 70, no clinical evidence of emergent neurologic deterioration, and had previously been treated with whole brain radiotherapy. Follow-up consisted of neurologic examination and contrast-enhanced CT or MRI 6–10 weeks after treatment and then every 3 months. Contrast-enhanced CT scans of metastatic ovarian carcinoma at radiosurgery and 3 months later are seen in Figure 1. Survival and local tumor control were analyzed. Patient and treatment characteristics were analyzed to determine an association with survival or local tumor control.

Results.—Survival ranged from 0.5 to 88 months, with a median of 9.4 months. There was local failure in 11% of the tumors at a median time of 8.4 months after treatment. Reduced survival was associated with systemic disease at the time of radiosurgery, age greater than 60 years, male sex, and 3 or more brain lesions, with age and systemic disease contributing independently. Local tumor control failure was associated with infratentorial tumors, tumors larger than 3 cm^3 in volume, and previously treated lesions, with infratentorial and recurrent lesions contributing independently (Fig 4). Karnofsky performance scores changed by a median of 15% at 6 months and 10% at 1 year. There was low perioperative morbidity and mortality, with a 2% 30-day mortality.

Discussion.—These data suggest that radiosurgery may be a treatment option with outcomes comparable to those for craniotomy in patients with brain metastasis. Radiosurgery may be particularly suitable for patients with inoperable lesions or multiple metastases, but it is unsuitable for

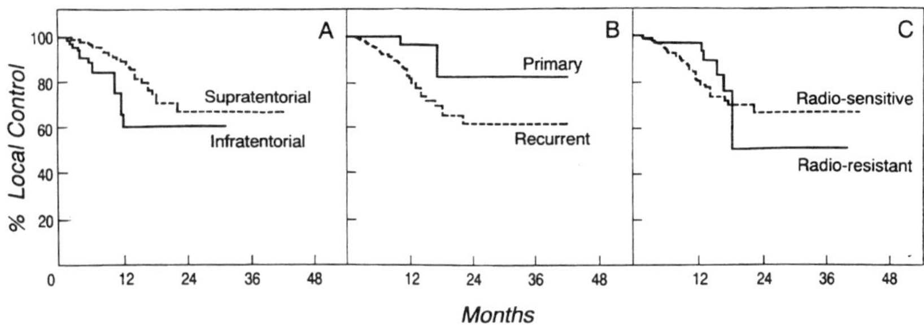

FIGURE 4.—Factors associated with failure of local control. Kaplan-Meier curves showing the time from treatment to local failure: **A.** for lesions above (dashed line) or below (solid line) the tentorium: **B.** for lesions that had failed previous therapies (recurrent: dashed line) compared with those being treated for the first time (primary: solid line); and **C.** for metastatic lesions believed to be responsive to conventional radiotherapy, including lung, breast, colon, and germ cell cancers (radiosensitive: dashed line), compared with lesions that are usually unresponsive to conventional radiotherapy, including melanoma, sarcoma, and renal cell cancer (radioresistant: solid line) (Courtesy of Alexander E III, Moriarty TM, Davis RB, et al: Stereotactic radiosurgery for the definitive, noninvasive treatment of brain metastases. *J Natl Cancer Inst* 87:34-40, 1995.)

treating large tumors causing acute neurologic deterioration, especially when they are located infratentorially.

▶ Stereotactic radiosurgery, as practiced in this country, typically represents a single shot of treatment, and in this series from Boston, it is used for brain metastases. The data that the authors present are impressive, although obviously there are not many patients who are alive 24 months later. Local control in that group of patients is of unclear meaning, largely because so many patients have died and autopsies are seldom obtained. Some of these patients are still dying of metastatic disease, although if one selects patients whose metastases are confined to the CNS and who are far enough from the initial treatment, there potentially is some curability in this group, as has been reported to be the case for surgical resection. In this series, all patients received fractionated whole brain radiotherapy before the stereotactic boost. That type of treatment seems fairly reasonable to me, in sharp distinction to the single-dose boost delivered by stereotactic technique only.

Exactly what the role of stereotactic treatment will be is still unclear, as it has yet to be compared with other forms of treatment in a randomized approach. The costs are significant, although in this particular series, the morbidities are described as being associated with "very few acute or long-term complications." The expenditures were said to be 20% to 35% less than the charges for surgery, which mostly revolve around the multiday hospitalization. It is still unclear how much better this is than conventional treatment with a conventional fractionated boost for those patients who only have 1 or 2 lesions. The ideal study still needs to be carried out soon.

E. Glatstein, M.D.

Linac Radiosurgery for High-Grade Gliomas: The University of Florida Experience
Buatti JM, Friedman WA, Bova FJ, Mendenhall WM (Univ of Florida, Gainesville)
Int J Radiat Oncol Biol Phys 32:205–210, 1995   12–4

Introduction.—Even with aggressive surgery, radiotherapy, and chemotherapy, most patients with high-grade gliomas die rapidly of their disease. Stereotactic radiosurgery offers a noninvasive way to deliver a large focal boost to radioresistant tumors, and it has given promising results in selected patients with high-grade gliomas. Eleven patients treated with linac radiosurgery for high-grade gliomas were studied.

Methods.—The patients were carefully selected for radiosurgery from a referral base of 85 patients. All were believed to have a lesion located in an area that could tolerate a 10-Gy or greater boost dose. Six patients had glioblastoma multiforme and 5 had anaplastic astrocytoma. The median age was 42.1 years, and all patients had a Karnofsky performance status of at least 90. The median dose of external beam radiotherapy was 60 Gy. Stereotactic radiosurgery was generally administered 2–3 weeks later, and it was delivered to the enhancing tumor volume without margin. The median treatment volume was 14 cm^3, with a maximum of 22.5 cm^3. The median radiosurgical boost dose was 12.5 Gy, and the median prescription sphere was the 80% isodose shell.

Results.—The median actuarial survival was only 17 months. Intracranial disease progressed within 1 year after radiosurgery. At a median follow-up of 13 months, only 3 patients were still alive. Only patients with reoperation after recurrence had a significant survival advantage.

Conclusion.—Compared with previously reported series and despite careful patient selection and aggressive treatment, poor results were obtained with linac radiosurgery for high-grade gliomas. Tumor volume may be an important prognostic factor when selecting patients to receive radiosurgical boost treatment. Given these inconsistent results, performing stereotactic radiosurgery for malignant glioma outside of a study setting is of uncertain benefit.

▶ This series comes from the University of Florida, which has traditionally been a major center for innovative techniques in cancer treatment. In this study, the authors are looking at stereotactic radiosurgery used as a boost for selected patients with high-grade glioma. The authors make the point that they carefully selected patients who had small lesions and conditions thought to be very favorable. The benefits of the stereotactic boost are somewhat obscure in this series, but it is a small series that should not be overinterpreted.

Nonetheless, the authors raise excellent questions about the selection process regarding patients who are receiving stereotactic radiosurgery in various other reports. This, together with the process of a single-shot treatment for the stereotactic boost, makes it difficult for anyone thinking objectively to believe that this treatment has established value. Its value obviously is not established as yet, and it must be considered as research. This must be done because the experience regarding tumors with these large doses is essentially nil on this side of the Atlantic. Moreover, on the opposite side of the Atlantic, the experience is predominantly for arteriovenous malformations, not neoplasms. At the moment, I believe radiosurgery must be described as a treatment in search of a disease.

E. Glatstein, M.D.

Bystander Tumoricidal Effect in the Treatment of Experimental Brain Tumors

Wu JK, Cano WG, Meylaerts SAG, Qi P, Vrionis F, Cherington V (Tufts Univ, Boston; New England Med Ctr, Boston; Univ of Amsterdam)
Neurosurgery 35:1094–1103, 1994   12–5

Background.—The retrovirus-mediated transfer of the herpes simplex virus–thymidine kinase (HSV-tk) gene into tumor cells sensitizes them to the cytocidal effect of ganciclovir, an antiviral agent. This technique has yielded promising results in experimental studies of brain tumors. The bystander tumoricidal effect may be a major mechanism for the efficacy of HSV-tk retroviral gene therapy. Given that the efficacy of in vivo gene transfer to tumor cells is less than 100%, the bystander effect was hypothesized to explain tumor eradication.

Methods and Findings.—The bystander tumoricidal effect was found to be a major contributor to the tumoricidal effect of ganciclovir in cell culture experiments using the mouse K1735 C19 cerebral melanoma line. The bystander effect was assessed in vitro by co-culturing wild-type C19 melanoma cells with HSV-tk–expressing C19 cells. The maximal tumoricidal effect occurred when only 1 in 10 tumor cells expressed the HSV-tk gene, suggesting that 1 tumor cell with the HSV-tk gene, when given ganciclovir, will destroy 10 neighboring or bystander cells. The destruction of bystander cells was apparently unmediated by a soluble factor released into the media. Rather, it required close cell proximity or cell contact. Also, HSV-tk–expressing C19 cells exerted an antitumoral effect on a variety of different tumor cell lines along with wild-type C19 cells, including a human glioblastoma multiforme cell line. The bystander tumoricidal effect could be harnessed directly without retrovirus-producing cells to increase survival in the mouse C19 brain tumor model.

Conclusions.—The bystander tumoricidal effect is an important contributor to the tumoricidal effect of ganciclovir in cell culture experiments in the mouse K1735 C19 cerebral melanoma line. This expands the observation of the bystander phenomenon to a wider range of tumor types. With further study and refinement, the use of HSV-tk–containing tumor cell lines may possibly be added to the current armamentarium of human brain tumor treatment.

▶ There is a flurry of activity aimed at trying to treat brain tumors by inserting genetic material that renders the cells vulnerable to antiviral agents. This study in animals demonstrates that the effect on the brain tumor is not simply mediated by direct action on each infected cell, but also through a "bystander" effect, i.e., cells that are touching the targeted tumor cell but which are themselves uninfected may be destroyed indirectly by the antiviral agent. This so-called bystander effect is an extremely important principle because it may be virtually impossible to infect every tumor cell with a retrovirus to make it sensitive to the antiviral agents. Because we have few effective tools in the treatment of brain tumors, it is important to keep tracking the progress in experimental models to spot hopeful trends that may lead to more effective treatment of our patients.

J.V. Simone, M.D.

The Increasing Incidence of Malignant Gliomas and Primary Central Nervous System Lymphoma in the Elderly
Werner MH, Phuphanich S, Lyman GH (Univ of South Florida, Tampa)
Cancer 76:1634–1642, 1995   12–6

Introduction.—Cancer, in general, is more prevalent in the elderly population, and in particular, there is evidence that primary malignant brain tumors are becoming more frequent. This may, however, be an artifact resulting from more widespread CT scanning.

Objective.—The incidence of various histologic types of primary malignant brain tumor was examined by analyzing data from the Florida Cancer Data System covering 1981–1984 and 1986–1989. A total of 6,353 cases were available. Malignant meningiomas, chordomas, choroid plexus papillomas, teratomas, and germinomas were excluded.

Findings.—The average annual incidence rates increased gradually with advancing age, peaking at 18.3 cases per 100,000 at ages 70–74 years and subsequently decreasing (Fig 1). The incidence of tumors in individuals who were 20–64 years of age did not change appreciably between the 2 review periods, but it increased by 36% in those aged 80–84 years and more than fivefold in those aged 85 and older. Astrocytomas actually became less frequent in older individuals in the later review, but anaplastic astrocytomas, glioblastomas, and lymphomas were all more frequent. The incidence of all cancers in those older than age 65 years increased by 7.6%, which is not a significant change. The incidence of pancreatic cancer, which also is diagnosed by CT, did not increase significantly from the earlier to the later period.

Conclusion.—Primary brain tumors are being detected more frequently in older patients, peaking at 70–74 years of age. The increase involves

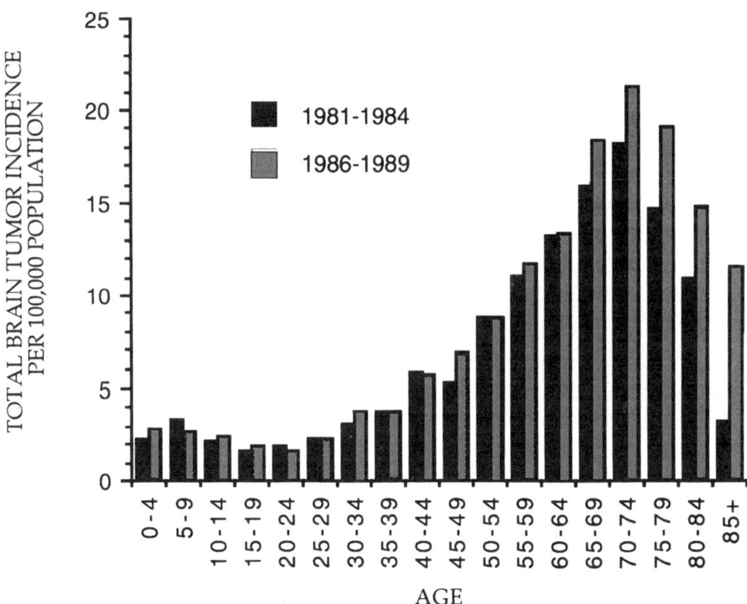

FIGURE 1.—Age-specific average annual incidence rates of primary brain tumors in Florida for the years 1981–1984 and 1986–1989. (Courtesy of Werner MH, Phuphanich S, Lyman GH: The increasing evidence of malignant gliomas and primary central nervous system lymphoma in the elderly. *Cancer* 76:1634–1642, 1995. Reprinted by permission of Wiley-Liss, Inc., a division of John Wiley & Sons, Inc.)

specific histologic types and cannot be ascribed to increased case ascertainment.

▶ This study demonstrates a clear-cut and substantial increase in the incidence of certain primary brain tumors in Florida during the 1980s. The increased incidence is mainly in the elderly population and is largely caused by the increase in gliomas and primary lymphomas. The authors do not believe that this increase in incidence is the result of better diagnostic tools such as CT scans or some other technical artifact. Others have reported an increasing incidence in brain tumors as well, particularly primary brain lymphomas. Part of that increase is caused by the very high incidence among patients with AIDS, but even if this is taken into account, the overall incidence appears to be increasing.

Unfortunately, this study offers no clues as to the reason for the alarming increase in brain tumors. This is doubly disappointing because (1) our therapeutic methods, particularly for gliomas, are not very effective, and (2) there are no new exciting therapeutic tools that will be ready in the near future.

J.V. Simone, M.D.

Intraarterial Administration of Melphalan for Treatment of Intracranial Human Glioma Xenografts in Athymic Rats
Kurpad SN, Friedman HS, Archer GE, McLendon RE, Petros WM, Fuchs HE, Guaspari A, Bigner DD (Duke Univ, Durham, NC; Burroughs Wellcome Co, Research Triangle Park, NC)
Cancer Res 55:3803–3809, 1995   12–7

Background.—Sixty-five percent of all primary brain tumors are malignant gliomas, which carry a dismal prognosis. Adjuvant chemotherapy is hindered by insufficient drug delivery, systemic toxicity, and a highly variable biological sensitivity. By improving tumor drug delivery and decreasing systemic toxicity, selectivity may be enhanced by intra-arterial (IA) treatment. A series of experiments was conducted to test the efficacy of IA melphalan in human glioma xenografts implanted intracerebrally in athymic rats.

Methods and Findings.—Male athymic nude rats with a mean weight of 300 g were inoculated intracerebrally with D-54 MG and D-456 MG. On days 6 and 7 and days 9 and 10, respectively, rats that were randomized by body weight and treated with single-dose melphalan given IA at 0.5 or 0.75 mg had a significantly greater median survival than did those given IA saline or IV melphalan at 0.75 and 0.9 mg or at 0.5 and 0.75 mg. Although there was a dose-dependent increase in median survival associated with IA melphalan, no signficant difference was found between 0.5 and 0.75 mg in either tumor model (Fig 5). In toxicity studies of non–tumor-bearing

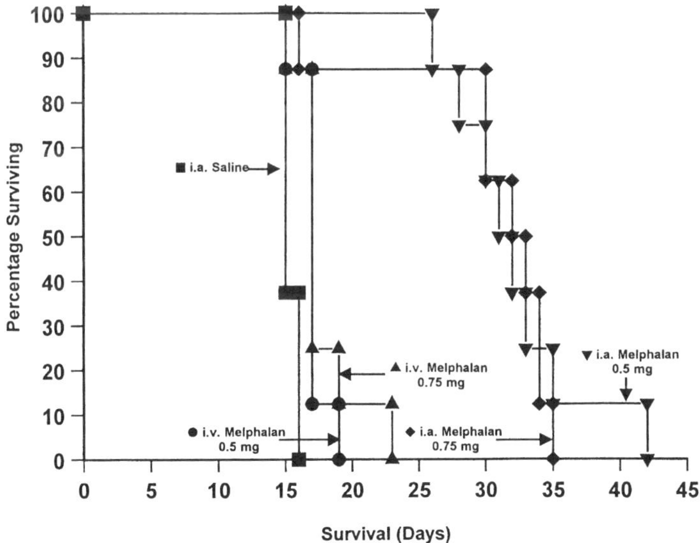

FIGURE 5.—The response rate of intracerebral D-54 MG in athymic rats (*n* = 8 in all groups) to treatment with equivalent doses of melphalan given intra-arterially and IV. (Courtesy of Kurpad SN, Friedman HS, Archer GE, et al: Intraarterial administration of melphalan for treatment of intracranial human glioma xenografts in athymic rats. *Cancer Res* 55:3803–3809, 1995.)

athymic rats, the maximum tolerated dose for IA melphalan was 0.8 mg. This dosage was best despite differences in xenograft permeabilities. In the pharmacokinetic experiments, IA melphalan showed a significant first pass advantage vs. IV melphalan administration.

Conclusions.—Intra-arterially delivered melphalan yields significantly better results than IV melphalan in athymic rats with intracerebral human glioma xenografts. Tumor drug uptake is also significantly increased with IA delivery. Its high antiglioma activity, short half-life, and low lipophilicity suggest that IA melphalan may have significant clinical potential for patients with malignant brain tumors.

▶ Both surgery and radiotherapy for brain tumors face the same problem: How far into normal tissue must one go to achieve the desired effect and control? Gliomas are notoriously invasive beyond the apparent borders of the tumor, making them extremely difficult to cure. Systemic chemotherapy has been comparatively ineffective for a variety of reasons, including failure to penetrate the tumor properly and systemic side effects of the large doses that might be necessary. Kurpad and colleagues describe an attempt to overcome this problem by the IA administration of melphalan, which has 2 virtues. First, an extremely high dose can be delivered on first pass to the tumor without dilution. Second, chemotherapy penetration does not stop at the apparent borders of the tumor but, rather, enters normal tissues in substantial concentrations as well, presumably attacking microscopic extension into what appears to be normal tissue.

As shown in Figure 5, IA melphalan prolonged the survival of the animals twofold or more. Comparatively speaking, this is a relatively simple method of treatment that might be a more effective adjuvant to radiation and surgery than systemic therapy. However, all of us have been chastened by the resilience of gliomas in our patients. One notes that the survival graph shows no cures with any of the treatments given to these animals. That may be an unfair standard for this particular experiment, but it does keep us from unwarranted exuberance rather than a more appropriate cautious optimism.

J.V. Simone, M.D.

Radiation Therapy and Bromodeoxyuridine Chemotherapy Followed by Procarbazine, Lomustine, and Vincristine for the Treatment of Anaplastic Gliomas
Levin VA, Prados MR, Wara WM, Davis RL, Gutin PH, Phillips TL, Lamborn K, Wilson CB (Northern California Cancer Ctr, Union City; Univ of California, San Francisco; MD Anderson Cancer Ctr, Houston)
Int J Radiat Oncol Biol Phys 32:75–83, 1995   12–8

Background.—5-Bromo-2'-deoxyuridine (BrdU) and other halogenated pyrimidine analogues are preferentially incorporated into dividing cells, substituting for thymidine. Therefore, it makes tumor cells more sensitive to the effects of irradiation. A phase II study of BrdU combined with radiotherapy for patients with anaplastic glioma was undertaken.

Methods.—The analysis included 138 patients with nonglioblastoma multiforme anaplastic glioma. The median patient age was 43 years; 116 patients had anaplastic astrocytoma (AA), and 22 had astrocytoma stratum. The patients received a total radiation dose of 60 Gy, given in daily fractions of 1.7–1.8 Gy on Monday through Friday. On the Thursday before the start of radiotherapy and for the subsequent 5 weeks, the patients received BrdU in a continuous 96-hour IV infusion at 0.8 g/m²/24 hr. After radiotherapy, chemotherapy with procarbazine, lomustine, and vincristine (PCV) was started. Chemotherapy continued for 1 year or until tumor progression.

Results.—The estimated survival rate was 46% for the patients with AA at 4 years and 79% for the patients with astrocytoma stratum at 6 years. The estimated 4-year progression-free survival rates were 42% and 68%, respectively. Seventy-seven percent of the patients received limited-field irradiation and 23% received whole-brain irradiation; survival was better in the former group. Fifteen percent of the patients had total tumor resection, 53% had partial resection, and 32% had biopsy only. Forty-two percent of the patients with recurrences received at least 1 additional treatment. On Cox proportional hazards regression, several covariates were individually predictive of survival in patients with AA: younger age, Karnofsky performance score, and extent of surgery, but not limited-field irradiation. Fourteen percent of the patients had a rash during radiotherapy that required dose modification, 18% had grade III or greater leukopenia, and 9% had grade III or greater thrombocytopenia.

Conclusion.—In patients with anaplastic gliomas, BrdU plus radiotherapy followed by PCV chemotherapy can yield a better progression-free survival than other reported therapies. With aggressive treatment, patients with astrocytoma stratum can achieve significant increases in survival. Confirmatory studies of this treatment approach are needed.

▶ The University of California in San Francisco has long led the country in innovative approaches to tumors of the CNS. In this paper, these authors present their experience with so-called anaplastic astrocytomas: grade III gliomas. Using their approach of definitive radiation therapy along with BrdU sensitization followed by PCV, the authors have an enviable 4-year survival rate of 46%. The median age of their patients (43 years) is a little younger than that of some other series, but there can be little doubt that their median survival figures are excellent, even though the authors used limited-field radiation ports, in today's world of CT and MRI. The authors have looked carefully at their age factor, and they believe they have distinguished it.

If these authors' results are confirmed by others, this would appear to be a new standard of treatment. Of course, exactly what the contribution of the postradiation chemotherapy is remains unclear; and exactly how much is derived from the BrdU radiosensitizer is also unclear without the definitive study. Hopefully, those definitive studies can be done soon, because if this is confirmed, it is the best evidence I know of that BrdU is an effective radiosensitizer of selected lesions in the CNS. It is worth noting one of their comments: For grade IV glioma (glioblastoma), the halogenated pyrimidines have shown little effect.

E. Glatstein, M.D.

Large Effect of Age on the Survival of Patients With Glioblastoma Treated With Radiotherapy and Brachytherapy Boost
Sneed PK, Prados MD, McDermott MW, Larson DA, Malec MK, Lamborn KR, Davis RL, Weaver KA, Wara WM, Phillips TL, Gutin PH (Univ of California, San Francisco)
Neurosurgery 36:898–904, 1995   12–9

Objective.—The use of brachytherapy boosts after external-beam radiotherapy for patients with primary glioblastoma multiforme was studied. Age significantly affects survival; however, the survival results were not analyzed by various age strata. The effects of age and other potential prognostic factors on survival in patients undergoing brachytherapy boost for glioblastoma multiforme were assessed.

Methods.—One hundred fifty-nine adult patients with primary glioblastoma multiforme were examined. Ninety-eight were men and 61 were women. The median age was 52 years, and the median Karnofsky performance score was 90. All patients underwent a high-activity iodine-125 brain implant boost after external-beam radiotherapy. Before radiotherapy, 7% of the patients underwent biopsy only, 66% had subtotal resection, and 27% had gross total resection. The dose of external beam radiotherapy ranged from 39.6 to 76.8 Gy; 91% of the patients received a dose in the range of 59.4–61.2 Gy. The median brachytherapy dose was 55 Gy, and the median dose rate was 0.43 Gy/hr. Fifty-one percent of the patients underwent reoperation.

Findings.—Fourteen patients were alive at 3 years, and information on the quality of life was available for all but 1. Ten patients were steroid independent. The mean Karnofsky performance score decreased from 92 when brachytherapy was given to 75 at last follow-up. On univariate and multivariate analyses, age was the most important variable affecting survival. For 9 patients aged 18–29.9 years, the 3-year survival probability was 78%. The median survival had not yet been reached at a median follow-up of 322 weeks in survivors. The median survival rate was 109 weeks for the 19 patients aged 30–39.9 years, 96 weeks for the 45 patients aged 40–49.9 years, 77 weeks for the 46 patients aged 50–59.9 years of age, and 76 weeks for the 40 patients aged 60 years or older (Fig 1).

Conclusion.—For patients with glioblastoma mulitforme treated with radiotherapy and brachytherapy boosts, age is an important prognostic indicator. The probability of survival is surprisingly good for adult patients

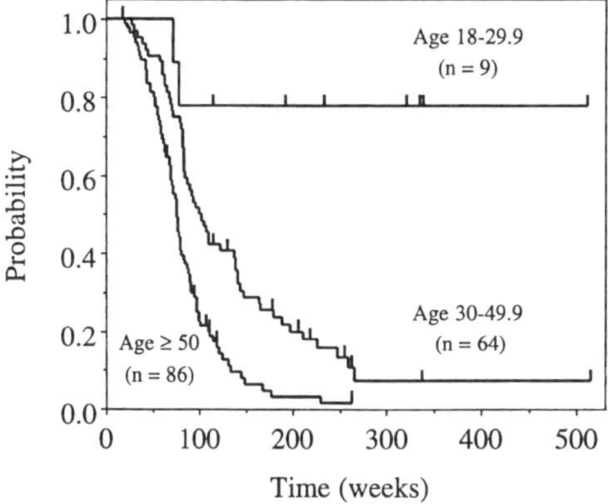

FIGURE 1.—Kaplan-Meier actuarial survival curves were significantly different among patients aged 18–29.9 years (*n* = 9; median survival, not reached; 3-year survival, 78 ± 14%), patients aged 30–49.9 years (*n* = 64; median survival, 102 weeks; 3-year survival, 29 ± 6%), and patients aged ≥ 50 years (*n* = 86; median survival, 76 weeks; 3-year survival, 6 ± 3%). (Courtesy of Sneed PK, Prados MD, McDermott MW, et al: Large effect of age on the survival of patients with glioblastoma treated with radiotherapy and brachytherapy boost. *Neurosurgery* 36:898–904, 1995.)

up to 29.9 years of age, justifying the use of aggressive treatment in young patients. New approaches are needed to improve survival for older patients.

▶ It has long been known that age is an important prognostic factor in the management of patients with glioblastoma. This paper comes from the University of California at San Francisco and looks retrospectively at the authors' experience with radiotherapy plus brachytherapy boost. Again, age is demonstrated to be an important factor that must be accounted for in any long-term interpretation, especially when there are no true controls. The results for patients aged 18–30 years appear surprisingly good, but that group represents only 9 patients.

E. Glatstein, M.D.

The Treatment of Brain Stem and Thalamic Gliomas With 78 Gy of Hyperfractionated Radiation Therapy

Prados MD, Wara WM, Edwards MSB, Larson DA, Lamborn K, Levin VA (Univ of California, San Francisco; MD Anderson Cancer Ctr, Houston)
Int J Radiat Oncol Biol Phys 32:85–91, 1995   12–10

Background.—Outcomes are poor for patients with intrinsic brain stem tumors. With standard radiotherapy doses of 50–60 Gy, the median survival is about 1 year. Several clinical trials have tried strategies to permit higher radiation doses. The survival effects of increasing the dose of

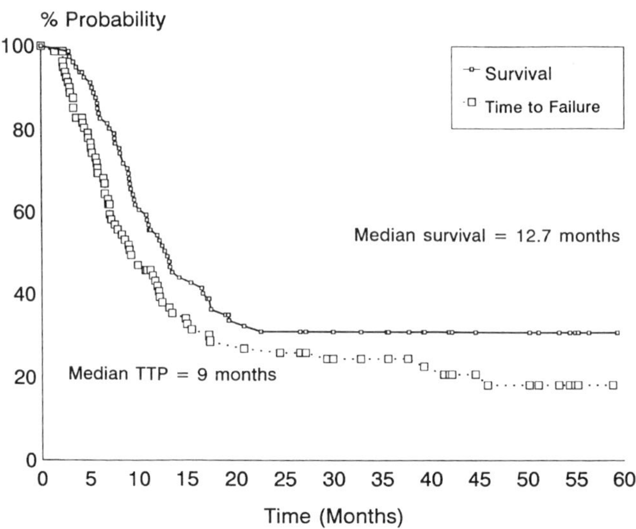

FIGURE 1.—Kaplan-Meier survival and tumor progression curves for the 81 evaluable patients enrolled to receive 78 Gy of hyperfractionated radiation therapy. *Abbreviation: TTP,* time to tumor progression. (Courtesy of Prados MD, Wara WM, Edwards MSB, et al: The treatment of brain stem and thalamic gliomas with 78 Gy of hyperfractionated radiation therapy. *Int J Radiat Oncol Biol Phys* 32:85–91, 1995, with kind permission from Elsevier Science Ltd, The Boulevard, Langford Lane, Kidlington 0X5 1GB, UK.)

hyperfractionated radiotherapy from 72 to 78 Gy in patients with gliomas were assessed, with an emphasis on patients with brain stem or thalamic tumors.

Methods.—The study included 78 patients with a clinical and radiographic diagnosis of brain stem or thalamic glioma, as well as 6 patients with disease in other sites. Thirty-nine patients were aged 17 years or younger. All patients received 78 Gy of radiation, given in 1-Gy fractions twice a day. The initial and subsequent responses to therapy were assessed by comparing pretreatment and posttreatment MRI scans and neurologic examinations. The effects of different variables on survival were estimated by Cox proportional hazards analysis.

Results.—Eighty-one patients were evaluable. Of these, 68 received 76 Gy or more, 10 received 70–75 Gy, and 3 received 60–68 Gy. The overall rate of stabilization or response was 70.4%. Thirty-one percent of the patients had a decrease in tumor size, 39.5% had stabilization of disease, and 29.6% had immediate progression. The median survival time—measured from the start of radiation therapy until death—was 12.7 months: 16.1 months for adults and 10.8 months for children. The median time to tumor progression—measured from the start of radiation therapy until documented radiographic or clinical progression—was 9 months: 11.4 months for adults and 8.4 months for children (Fig 1). Survival and time to progression were shorter for patients who had had symptoms for 2 months or less and for those with a diffuse lesion (Table 2). Some patients had evidence of radiation necrosis.

TABLE 2.—Survival and Tumor Progression in Evaluable Patients Enrolled to Receive 78 Gy*

Group	Number	Median survival (months)	Median time to tumor progression (months)
Overall	81	12.7	9.0
Children < 18 years	39	10.8	8.4
Adults	42	16.1	11.4
Symptoms ≤ 2 months	31†	9.8	6.3
Symptoms > 2 months	45†	16.1	11.4
Radiation dose ≥ 76 Gy	68	12.7	10.4
Radiation dose < 76 Gy	13	9.3	6.0
Brain stem location	58	12.2	8.8
Thalamic location	17	12.7	6.8

* Patients with 2 months or less of symptoms had significantly shorter survival ($P = .008$) and tumor progression ($P = .033$) rates than did those with more than 2-month histories.

† Information is missing for 5 patients.

(Courtesy of Prados MD, Wara WM, Edwards MSB, et al: The treatment of brain stem and thalamic gliomas with 78 Gy of hyperfractionated radiation therapy. *Int J Radiat Oncol Biol Phys* 32:85–91, 1995 with kind permission from Elsevier Science Ltd, The Boulevard, Langford Lane, Kidlington 0X5 1GB, UK.)

Conclusion.—Increasing the radiotherapy dose from 72 to 78 Gy does not appear to improve survival for patients with brain stem or thalamic gliomas. A 78-Gy dose may be the limit beyond which unacceptable risks of radiation injury occur. There is a clear need for different treatment approaches to these tumors.

▶ These authors have used hyperfractionated radiation therapy with doses up to 78 Gy, to treat a series of patients with brain stem gliomas and thalamic gliomas. So far, the only scheme they have published uses 1 Gy twice daily. Most of us would try to distinguish the brain stem tumors from the thalamic lesions, because most of us do not have data that suggest similarity in outcome. It would have been interesting to see what would have happened had the authors chosen numbers such as 125–150 rad twice a day, but they did not. Therefore, the conclusions from this study are very limited. There is no suggestion of an improvement in survival, although it is possible that improvement is being obscured by the inclusion of the thalamic lesions with the rest of the brain stem. It would be of some help to separate them.

E. Glatstein, M.D.

In-111 DTPA Ommayagrams in Leptomeningeal Carcinomatosis

Korkmaz M, Kim EE, Wong FC-L, Podoloff DA, Haynie TP, Yung A (Univ of Texas MD Anderson Cancer Ctr, Houston; Univ of Ankara, Turkey)
Clin Nucl Med 20:610–612, 1995   12–11

Objective.—In patients with metastatic solid tumors or leukemias, it is not uncommon to find circulating blast cells in the leptomeningeal and subarachnoid spaces. Chemotherapy delivered to the ventricular system via an Ommaya shunt device results in better distribution and less discomfort. Radionuclide Ommayagrams were used to evaluate CSF-Ommaya shunt communication, CSF flow patterns, blockage of the CSF pathway, and prediction of distribution of chemotherapeutics in patients with leptomeningeal carcinomatoses.

Methods.—Ommayagrams, using 500 mCi of indium-111 diethylenetriaminepentaacetic acid (DTPA) injected into the reservoir of the shunt device, were performed in 25 patients (8 males; age, 1–61 years): for lymphoma in 8 patients, melanoma in 7, breast cancer in 6, leukemia in 2, lung cancer in 2, ovarian cancer in 1, and undifferentiated rhabdomyosarcoma in 1. Gamma camera images were obtained at 5 minutes and at 2, 4, and 24 hours after injection, and they were correlated with MRI findings. Activity that did not reach basal cisterns within 2 hours was termed abnormal. Any distortion of the CSF space was noted.

Results.—Six of 9 patients with a spinal fluid space abnormality had complete obstruction of the CSF space according to MRI findings. Ommayagrams confirmed 3 of the 6 complete obstructions. Magnetic resonance imaging showed spinal and cerebral fluid space abnormalities in 11 patients, and Ommayagrams confirmed 8 of those. Omayagrams were 73% sensitive, 100% specific, and 88% accurate for any CSF space abnormality, and they were 100% sensitive, specific, and accurate for CSF space obstruction. Magnetic resonance imaging was 100% sensitive, 86% specific, and 88% accurate for CSF space obstruction. There were no side effects of treatment.

Conclusion.—Ommayagrams were less sensitive than MRI but were more specific for complete obstruction. Evaluation of CSF patterns in these patients is important, because patients with MRIs showing complete obstruction may not be completely obstructed and may be able to benefit from intrathecal chemotherapy.

▶ Among patients who have metastatic solid tumors or leukemias, it is not uncommon these days to find spread to the leptomeningeal space and dissemination throughout the subarachnoid space and ventricular systems. This particular study looks at radioactive ^{111}In DTPA injected into Ommaya shunt reservoirs to assess CSF shunt communication in patients with a variety of solid tumors or leukemia. The authors looked at 25 patients with leptomeningeal carcinomatosis and were able to show that the Ommaya reservoirs were frequently obstructed by CSF space abnormalities. In 3 patients, they were able to show total obstruction of the CSF. This technology is sufficiently simple to perform, and I am confident we will see many more reports in the future evaluating CSF formation by this kind of technology.

E. Glatstein, M.D.

Surgical Treatment of Spinal Cord Compression From Epidural Metastasis

Sundaresan N, Sachdev VP, Holland JF, Moore F, Sung M, Paciucci PA, Wu L-T, Kelligher K, Hough L (Mount Sinai Hosp and Med School, New York)
J Clin Oncol 13:2330–2335, 1995   12–12

Objective.—Although treatment of patients with cancer with spinal cord compression is mainly palliative, survival times can be doubled if the condition is treated aggressively with surgery. To determine the quality of life and potential morbidity in patients with spinal metastases treated surgically, a retrospective 5-year analysis was performed.

Methods.—Surgical complications and postsurgical morbidity were recorded in 110 patients (age, 28–85 years) who were treated for neoplastic spinal cord compression. The primary tumor sites included breast, chordoma, sarcoma, lung, kidney, plasmacytoma, and colorectum. There were 55 patients who had undergone prior treatment, and 47 of those had failed to respond to radiation therapy.

Results.—Before surgery, 48 patients could not walk, and 21 of those had severe paraparesis. Staged anterior-posterior resection and instrumentation was performed in 53 patients, anterior resection with instrumentation in 33, resection in 18, and posterior resection and instrumentation in 6. Ninety patients improved after surgery, and 20 did not improve. Thirty-two of the 48 nonambulatory patients were able to walk after surgery, and 11 of 21 patients with severe paraparesis were able to walk. In 18 of 20 patients with severe pain, there was improvement in pain relief after surgery. After surgery, radiation was administered to 20 of 51 patients who had not been treated previously with radiation. The rate of complications after surgery was 48% and included wound breakdown in 18 patients, stabilization failure in 11, infection in 13, hemorrhage in 10, respiratory failure in 4, intraoperative vascular/visceral injury in 6, and CSF leak in 4. The complication rate was higher in patients older than 65 years (71%), those having prior treatment (67%), and those with paraparesis (64%). Overall survival was 16 months, with 46% alive at 2 years. The 44 patients with paraparesis had an average survival of 6 months and a 2-year survival rate of 19%, whereas ambulatory patients had an average survival time of 36 months and a 2-year survival rate of 54%.

Conclusion.—Aggressive surgical treatment of patients with neoplastic cord compression, involving anterior-posterior resection with instrumentation, provides good long-term survival in selected patients.

▶ Until recently, the primary strategy in management of spinal cord compression resulting from tumor had been the combination of irradiation and steroids. Chemotherapy was also used in those patients who had chemotherapy-sensitive tumors such as lymphoma. In many centers, surgical intervention has been reserved for those patients in whom steroids and radiation failed to halt the neurologic progression or when neurologic deterioration was rapid. Recently, 2 factors have led to reassessment of the standard approach. Magnetic resonance imaging studies and more effective surgical techniques that allow for reconstruction of the spine will permit, in many cases, a complete resection of all gross tumor as defined in the radiologic studies. Furthermore, the current treatment of spinal cord compression has been palliative. Early diagnosis has repeatedly been emphasized, because patients with minimal neurologic dysfunction had the best results when treated with radiation and steroids.

Because survival was still in the range of only 3–6 months, the primary goal of treatment was to improve quality of life and to permit ambulation during the terminal phases of the patient's illness. However, the data in this study indicate that there may be a subset of patients in whom more aggressive surgery can actually lead to a significant prolongation of life in addition to impacting upon the quality of life. The authors report a 2-year survival rate of 46% with a postoperative complication rate of 48%. Postoperative radiation therapy to the spine was administered to 20 of the 51 patients who had not received prior radiation.

This report emphasizes the aggressive nature of the surgery, with staged anterior-posterior resections being done in almost one half of the patients and with all patients requiring spinal instrumentation for reconstruction. Nevertheless, the impact of this surgery upon quality of life and, particularly, preservation of motor function, ambulation, and relief of pain indicates that this approach should more frequently be considered in select patients with spinal cord metastases.

R.F. Ozols, M.D., Ph.D.

13 Lung Cancer

Liposarcoma of the Anterior Mediastinum and Thymus: A Clinicopathologic Study of 28 Cases
Klimstra DS, Moran CA, Perino G, Koss MN, Rosai J (Mem Sloan-Kettering Cancer Ctr, New York; Armed Forces Inst of Pathology, Washington, DC)
Am J Surg Pathol 19:782–791, 1995   13–1

Objective.—The clinical and histologic findings were reviewed in 28 patients with anterior mediastinal liposarcoma. The patients were 16 males and 12 females, 14–72 years of age.

Clinical Findings.—Most patients had no symptoms, and many of them received the diagnosis when routine chest radiographs revealed a mass. Four patients had pain, 4 were short of breath, and 1 had a cough. One patient had a superior vena cava syndrome and 1 had a collapsed lung. Two patients had had other lipomatous tumors.

Pathology.—The tumors averaged 16 cm in size, with an average weight of 1,500 g. Most of them were lobulated and circumscribed. Twenty-five of the 28 tumors were low-grade neoplasms. Sixty percent were well-differentiated lipoma-like or sclerosing lesions, 28% were myxoid tumors, and 12% had mixed features. There were 3 high-grade pleomorphic neoplasms. There were no pure round-cell liposarcomas. Most of the well-differentiated tumors contained at least focal areas of sclerosis. In 7 cases, residual thymic tissue was seen within or adjacent to the tumor.

Outcome.—Twenty-three patients were followed for up to 6 years. Complete resection was attempted in all cases. Seven of the 22 patients who survived surgery (32%) had recurrences after an average of 3 years. Three of these patients and 4 others died of their tumors. Only 4 of the 15 surviving patients have been followed for 3 years or longer. Patients with myxoid tumors had the highest mortality rate (44%), and they died sooner than those with well-differentiated neoplasms. No patient had metastatic disease.

► This is a surprisingly large series of patients with anterior mediastinal liposarcoma. Although I have seen a few of these patients in my career, I have not seen many, and the size of this series is really quite remarkable. The experience is of note precisely because the series is so large. For most of us, liposarcoma of the anterior mediastinum remains an interesting entity that is rarely seen. The patients have done fairly well as a group, reflecting what is apparently a fairly low-grade level of neoplasm in the majority of the patients.

E. Glatstein, M.D.

Malignancies in the Lung and Pleura Mimicking Benign Processes
Colby TV (Mayo Clinic Scottsdale, Arizona)
Semin Diagn Pathol 12:30–44, 1995   13–2

Objective.—Although it is not uncommon for benign lung lesions to be mistaken for malignant lesions, it is rare for malignant lesions to be misinterpreted as benign. Five such cases representing well-differentiated adenocarcinoma, spindle-cell carcinoma, intravascular lymphomatosis, sarcomatous mesothelioma, and metastatic angiosarcoma were seen.

Histologic Pitfalls in Diagnosing Well-Differentiated Adenocarcinoma of the Lung.—Well-differentiated carcinomas do not look malignant, and significant inflammatory changes in the lung tissue resemble honeycombing. The key to identifying this tumor as malignant is the observance of uniform mucinous cells growing in the alveolar spaces.

Histologic Pitfalls in Diagnosing Spindle-Cell Carcinoma of the Lung.—This type of carcinoma is difficult to distinguish from sarcomas and products of fibroblastic proliferation. It can be identified by locating the nodules or fascicles of spindled or polygonal cells, which are the foci of the atypical cells. Vessel invasion and the epithelial nature of the tumor are also characteristic findings.

Histological Pitfalls in Diagnosing Intravascular Lymphomatosis of the Lung.—This type of carcinoma looks like an inflammatory interstitial pneumonia with numerous alveolar macrophages, hyaline membranes, prominent endothelial cell nuclei, and lack of mass lesions. The diagnostic key is recognition of the intravascular neoplastic cells and confirmation of their lymphoid nature by staining and phenotyping.

Histologic Pitfalls in Diagnosing Sarcomatous Mesothelioma.—This carcinoma resembles reactive fibrous tissue with cellular foci that may not be very apparent. Malignant cytologic factors are usually absent. Clues to the malignant nature of the disease are the thickness of the proliferation; the lack of zonation; the proliferative nodules; a storiform pattern of spindle cells; a waxy hyalinized stroma; and invasion of the chest wall.

Histological Pitfalls in Diagnosing Metastatic Angiosarcoma.—This carcinoma can be misinterpreted as an infarct, hemorrhagic pneumonia, or diffuse alveolar hemorrhage. The key to diagnosis is the presence of multiple nodules, microscopic hemorrhagic and sometimes necrotic nodules on the pulmonary artery, and invasive spindle cells.

Conclusion.—Particular attention should be paid to those lung malignancies that can mimic benign processes.

▶ In my opinion, this paper is very interesting reading. It discusses 5 specific entities that pathologists apparently have trouble with in the lung and pleura. The problem is that well-differentiated lesions are sometimes hard to distinguish from benign processes. The lesions that Colby describes are well-differentiated adenocarcinomas (especially bronchioloalveolar carcinoma, spindle-cell carcinoma of the lung, intravascular lymphomatosis, sarcoma of the mesothelioma, and angiosarcoma). Although most of these diagnoses are relatively infrequent, I think this article would be very helpful to the nonsurgical pathologist who sees a case that has been referred as belonging to one of these categories. To be aware of these different diagnoses is important, in the sense that these particular problems probably mandate a second pathologic opinion. For that reason, I think this is an important paper.

E. Glatstein, M.D.

Telomerase Activity in Small-Cell and Non–Small-Cell Lung Cancers

Hiyama K, Hiyama E, Ishioka S, Yamakido M, Inai K, Gazdar AF, Piatyszek MA, Shay JW (Univ of Texas, Dallas; Hiroshima Univ, Japan)
J Natl Cancer Inst 87:895–902, 1995   13–3

Hypothesis.—The enzyme telomerase adds hexameric nucleotide repeats onto the ends of vertebrate chromosomal DNA to make up for losses that take place during DNA replication. Normal somatic cells lack telomerase activity and cease dividing after the telomeric ends of at least some

---

TABLE 1.—Telomerase Activity in Lung Cancer Tissues Surgically Resected from 136 Patients

Histology	No. (%) of telomerase-negative samples	No. (%) of telomerase-positive samples	No. (%) of telomerase-positive tumors after serial dilutions*	
			10×	100×
Small-cell lung cancer†	0	11 (100)	11 (100)	9‡ (81.8)
Non-small-cell lung cancer§	27	98 (78.4)	72 (57.6)	36 (28.8)
Adenocarcinoma	20	45 (69.2)	34 (52.3)	19 (29.2)
Squamous	6	46 (88.5)	33 (63.5)	15 (28.8)
Other‖	1	7 (87.5)	5 (62.5)	2 (25.0)
Total	27 (19.9)	109 (80.1)	83 (61.0)	45 (33.1)

* Positive samples (n = 109) using tumor tissue extracts containing 6 μg of protein were subjected to sequential dilutions, and the numbers of positive samples were listed: 10× = positive using 0.6 μg of protein; 100× = positive using 0.06 μg of protein.
† n = 11.
‡ One of 2 negative tumors at 100× dilution was not a typical small-cell lung cancer but a poorly differentiated large-cell neuroendocrine carcinoma.
§ n = 125.
‖ Includes 5 adenosquamous carcinomas (1×, 1×, 10×, 10×, and 100×), 2 large-cell carcinomas (negative and 100×), and 1 carcinoid tumor (10×).
(Courtesy of Hiyama K, Hiyama E, Ishioka S, et al: Telomerase activity in small-cell and non–small-cell lung cancers. *J Natl Cancer Inst* 87:895–902, 1995.)

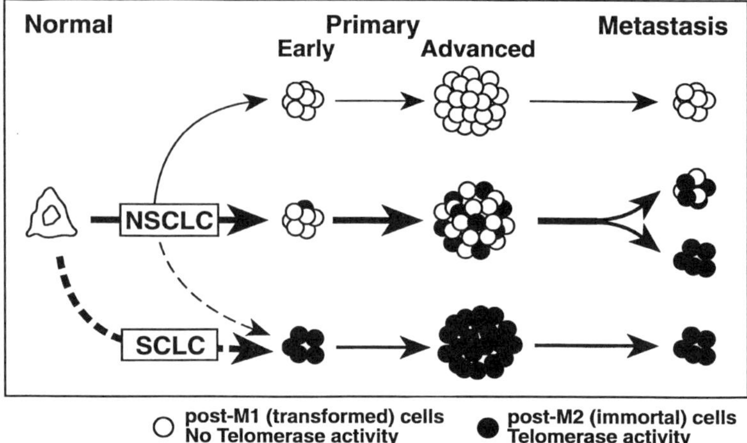

FIGURE 3.—A model of lung cancer progression. Whereas some early, late, and metastatic lung tumors consist of only mortal cells, this is likely (based on the present study) to be the exception rather than the rule. Most small-cell lung cancers (*SCLC*), when clinically diagnosed, have already experienced many cell divisions (i.e., have overcome both stages of cellular senescence [M1 and M2]) and have stabilized telomere repeat lengths and high telomerase activity. However, whereas most non-small-cell lung cancer (*NSCLC*) cells have overcome M1, they still contain many mortal cells in which telomeres continue to shorten and, in general, express low telomerase activity. In the course of tumor progression (after many additional cell divisions), a rare cell overcomes the M2 mechanism and acquires telomerase activity (immortality). Whereas the early and, perhaps, advanced stage primary NSCLC tumors contain a large fraction of mortal (post-M1, telomerase negative) cells, only immortal (post-M2) cells would be able to survive and would represent the majority of the metastatic tumors. The relative size of the arrows indicates the suggested frequency of cells in the hypothesized pathway to lung cancer. (Courtesy of Hiyama K, Hiyama E, Ishioka S, et al: Telomerase activity in small-cell and non–small-cell lung cancers. *J Natl Cancer Inst* 87:895-902, 1995.)

of the chromosomes have decreased to a critical length. It is conceivable that immortalized cells—including some cancer cells—continue proliferating because they express telomerase.

Objective and Methods.—The role of telomerase in carcinogenesis was examined by assaying telomerase activity in 136 operative samples of primary lung cancer and 68 samples of noncancerous lung tissue from the same patients. Four other primary and 23 metastatic lesions were sampled at autopsy or biopsy. Pleural fluid from 3 patients with lung adenocarcinoma was also examined. A polymerase chain reaction–based assay—the telomeric repeat amplification protocol (TRAP)—was used.

Findings.—Telomerase activity was present in 80% of the surgical samples of lung cancer (Table 1). All small-cell lung cancers were positive. Only 4% of the samples of adjacent, noncancerous lung tissue were positive for telomerase. Most squamous cell lung cancers were strongly positive. High enzyme levels generally were found in metastatic lesions and in tumors whose telomeric length was altered. All 3 pleural fluid samples were telomerase-positive.

Interpretation.—It is conceivable that tumors with high telomerase activity consist chiefly of immortal cells, whereas those with low or absent activity may contain mortal cancer cells (Fig 3). It might prove feasible to use telomerase inhibitors therapeutically.

▶ Telomerase is an enzyme that is generally not found in somatic cells. It appears that immortalized cancer cells proliferate indefinitely, and this proliferation appears to correlate with the expression of telomerase. This particular series of a large number of patients with primary lung cancer included 11 with small-cell lung cancer; all showed high levels of telomerase activity. In patients who had primary non–small-cell lung cancer, there was quite a range from undetectable to high levels, but typically high levels of telomerase activity were seen. The authors seem to think that telomerase may be useful as a diagnostic marker in lung cancer as well as a potential target for therapeutic intervention. The telomerase story is just beginning, but it appears to be an important factor in a large number of cancers, and we may well be hearing much more about this one in the future.

E. Glatstein, M.D.

Aberrant Expression of *p53* or the Epidermal Growth Factor Receptor is Frequent in Early Bronchial Neoplasia, and Coexpression Precedes Squamous Cell Carcinoma Development
Rusch V, Klimstra D, Linkov I, Dmitrovsky E (Sloan-Kettering Inst, New York; Mem Sloan-Kettering Cancer Ctr, New York)
Cancer Res 55:1365–1372, 1995   13–4

Background.—New strategies for detecting and treating lung cancer must be based on a better understanding of lung carcinogenesis. Although molecular genetic abnormalities are frequent in non–small-cell lung cancer (NSCLC), little is known about which of these precede an invasive carcinoma. The expression of *p53*, epidermal growth factor receptor (EGFR), and transforming growth factor-α, the most common molecular genetic abnormalities in NSCLC, was examined in preneoplastic bronchial lesions.

Methods.—In a retrospective review of resected tumors at one center, primary NSCLC and associated bronchial lesions were identified. Immunohistochemistry was used to compare expression in the invasive carcinomas, the associated bronchial lesions, and normal lung. The study included 34 NSCLC associated with 62 bronchial lesions. The invasive tumors were 15 squamous cell carcinomas (SCCs) and 19 non-SCCs. Bronchial lesions include areas of squamous metaplasia in 14 cases, inflammatory atypia in 19, dysplasia in 17, and carcinoma in situ in 12.

Findings.—Fifty-six percent of the NSCLCs and 16% of the bronchial lesions demonstrated aberrant *p53* immunostaining. Fifty-three percent of the NSCLCs and 48% of the bronchial lesions showed abnormal EGFR immunostaining. Positive staining for transforming growth factor-α occurred in 47% of the NSCLCs but was inconsistent in the bronchial lesions and normal bronchial epithelium. Only bronchial lesions associated with SCCs showed *p53* staining. Aberrant EGFR expression was not correlated with a specific type of invasive carcinoma or with specific preneoplastic lesions. However, there was a trend toward increased expression in dys-

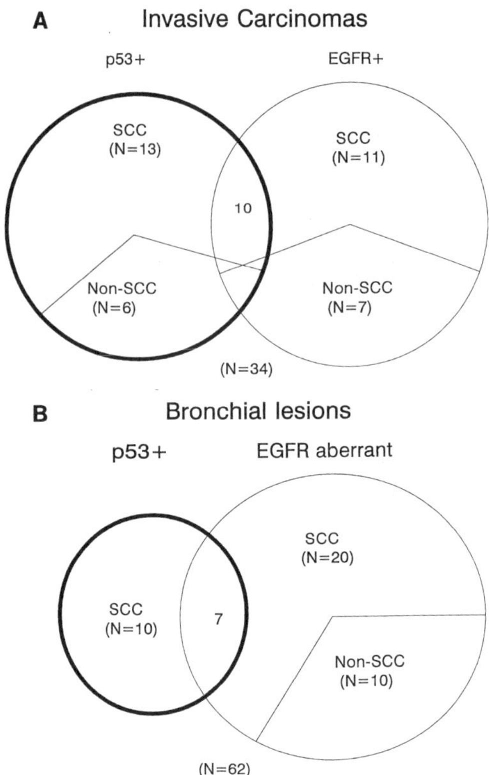

FIGURE 5.—Number of invasive carcinomas (**A**) and bronchial lesions (**B**) that exhibited staining for either *p53* or epidermal growth factor receptor (*EGFR*) simultaneously. The notations regarding cell type on the diagram for the bronchial lesions refer to the histology of the associated invasive carcinoma. Only one of the invasive tumors of nonsquamous histology exhibited positive staining for both *p53* and EGFR. All 7 of the bronchial lesions that showed positive *p53* and aberrant EGFR staining were associated with squamous cell carcinoma (*SCC*). (Courtesy of Rusch V, Klimstra D, Linkov I, et al: Aberrant expression of *p53* or the epidermal growth factor receptor is frequent in early bronchial neoplasia, and coexpression precedes squamous cell carcinoma development. *Cancer Res* 55:1365–1372, 1995.)

plasia and carcinoma in situ relative to metaplasia and atypia. All but one NCSLC demonstrating aberrant *p53* and EGFR staining simultaneously were SCC (Fig 5).

Conclusions.—Transforming growth factor-α is variably expressed in normal respiratory epithelium and reactive and preneoplastic bronchial lesions. The expression of *p53* occurs in preneoplastic bronchial lesions but not in reactive or metaplastic epithelium. Aberrant EGFR expression is seen in both reactive and preinvasive bronchial lesions and may be an early marker of neoplastic transformation. The simultaneous aberrant expression of EGFR and *p53* occurs mostly in SCC and associated bronchial lesions.

▶ Slowly, the story of *p53* and its relationship to lung cancer is starting to emerge. This paper from the Memorial Sloan-Kettering Cancer Center looks at the expression of *p53,* EGFR, and the transforming growth factor-α, and examines their relationships to preneoplastic NSCLC. In the case of *p53,* only bronchial lesions associated with SCC stained positively for that material. The data from this paper appear to reach the conclusion that the transforming growth factor-α is variably expressed in normal respiratory epithelium as well as preneoplastic bronchial lesions. By contrast, *p53* expression is seen in preneoplastic bronchial lesions but is not present in reactive or metaplastic epithelia. The aberrant EGFR occurs in both reactive and preinvasive bronchial lesions. Finally, when both the aberrant EGFR and *p53* occur, they are most likely to occur in SCC and their associated bronchial lesions. This information may make it easier to define patients at high risk for later lung cancers than has been possible in the past.

E. Glatstein, M.D.

Phase II Study of All-*trans*-Retinoic Acid and α-Interferon in Patients With Advanced Non-Small Cell Lung Cancer

Athanasiadis I, Kies MS, Miller M, Ganzenko N, Joob A, Marymont MA, Rademaker A, Gradishar WJ (Northwestern Univ, Chicago)
Clin Cancer Res 1:973–979, 1995   13–5

Background.—Non–small-cell lung cancer (NSCLC) is a major public health problem for which surgery offers the only chance of cure. Unfortunately, only a small proportion of patients can be cured. Innovative systemic strategies are urgently needed for patients with NSCLC.

Methods.—Twenty-nine patients with unresectable, locally advanced, or metastatic NSCLC received *trans*-retinoic acid (TRA), 150 mg/m²/day, orally in 3 divided doses plus interferon-alpha (IFN-α), 3×10^6 units/day, subcutaneously. The patients ranged in age from 41 to 80 years. Twenty-four patients had an Eastern Cooperative Oncology Group performance status of 0–1, and 5 patients had a status of 2. In all patients, disease was advanced and refractory to conventional treatment. The histologic types were adenocarcinoma in 21 patients, squamous cell carcinoma in 6, and large-cell carcinoma in 2.

Findings.—Only 3 patients completed 8 weeks of therapy without interruption or dose modifications. Eighty-eight percent of the patients had fatigue. Sixty-four percent of the patients had a syndrome characterized by dry oral and nasal mucosa, recurrent sinus infections, and epistaxis. Fifty-two percent of the patients had grade 2 or 3 dermatitis. Seven patients, or nearly half the men in the study, had severe scrotal dermatitis. Eleven patients had moderate-to-severe hypertriglyceridemia. Three patients needed gemfibrozil for levels up to 1,660 mg/dL. None of the patients had hematologic toxicity or leukocytosis. One patient died of complications of myocardial infarction during TRA/IFN-α treatment. Twenty-five patients undergoing more than 2 weeks of therapy were assessable. Another 2 patients died early of complications of cancer, and the remaining 2 wished to stop treatment after only 3 and 5 days. Of the assessable patients, responses were complete in 2 patients at 17 months and after 18 months, and were partial in 2 patients at 7 and 14 months. Responses occurred in all histologic types.

Conclusions.—Combined differentiation therapy with TRA/IFN-α has modest, objective activity but considerable toxicity in patients with NSCLC. Further research is needed to determine the biological basis of TRA/IFN-α and the prognostic parameters that predict response.

▶ For more than 70 years, it has been known that retinoids are important in maintaining the integrity of epithelial tissue and play a role in both differentiation and proliferation. *cis*-Retinoic acid has proved useful in preventing the development of second primary epithelial malignancies in patients with resected primary head and neck cancer. Most importantly, all-*trans*-retinoic acid (ATRA) induces complete remission in the majority of patients with acute promyelocytic leukemia (APL) through differentiation of the leukemic cells. The leukemic cells contain a translocation between chromosomes 15 and 17. The retinoic acid receptor α gene is located on chromosome 17 and is translocated to chromosome 15. Whether retinoids will play a major therapeutic role in patients with other hematologic malignancies or solid tumors has not been determined. However, the approach of differentiation therapy is an attractive alternative to intensive cytotoxic chemotherapy.

The results reported in this study are of some interest, because they suggest that retinoids—and potentially differentiating therapy in general—may play a therapeutic role in diseases other than APL. This study suggests that there is synergism between retinoids and interferon in this setting. Preclinical data also suggest that this may be the case. The study is provocative enough to suggest that further investigations in this direction are worth pursuing.

M.S. Tallman, M.D.

Phase III Trial of Thoracic Irradiation With or Without Cisplatin for Locally Advanced Unresectable Non–Small-Cell Lung Cancer: A Hoosier Oncology Group Protocol
Blanke C, Ansari R, Mantravadi R, Gonin R, Tokars R, Fisher W, Pennington K, O'Connor T, Rynard S, Miller M, Einhorn L (Hoosier Oncology Group, Indianapolis, Ind; Walther Cancer Inst, Indianapolis, Ind; Indiana Univ, Indianapolis)
J Clin Oncol 13:1425–1429, 1995   13–6

Background.—As many as 30% of patients with non–small-cell lung cancer (NSCLC), by far the most common primary malignant lung tumor, have locally advanced neoplasms that are not resectable and, consequently, have a poor prognosis. The best approach to stage III NSCLC remains uncertain, but combined-modality treatment has been proposed.

Study Plan.—Whether it is worthwhile to add cisplatin therapy to irradiation was studied in a series of 240 patients who either had biopsy-

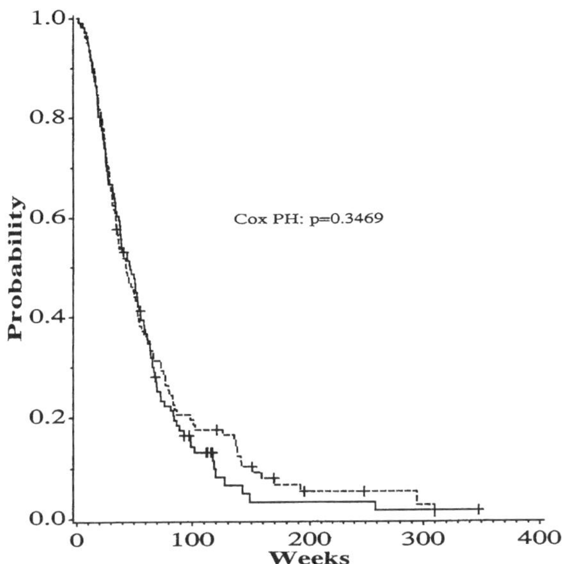

FIGURE 2.—Survival. The solid line indicates administration of thoracic radiation therapy (*XRT*): censored, 10; death, 101; total, 111; median (weeks), 46. *Dashed line* indicates administration of XRT and cisplatin; censored, 6; death, 98, total, 104; median (weeks), 43. (Courtesy of Blanke C, Ansari R, Mantravadi R, et al: Phase III trial of thoracic irradiation with or without cisplatin for locally advanced unresectable non–small-cell lung cancer: A Hoosier Oncology Group protocol. *J Clin Oncol* 13:1425–1429, 1995.)

proven disease that was unresectable or stage I/II disease that was inoperable for medical reasons. The patients were randomized to receive either thoracic irradiation alone in a total tumor dose of 60–65 Gy or radiotherapy combined with cisplatin. Three cycles of chemotherapy were given at 3-week intervals, starting on the first day of radiotherapy. The dose was 70 mg/m². The 215 evaluable patients were followed for a median of 52 months. The 2 treatment groups were well matched.

Results.—Half the patients given combined treatment and 38% of those given radiotherapy only had an objective response. Another 35% and 40% of patients, respectively, remained stable. Overall survival curves did not differ substantially (Fig 2). Patients with nonsquamous tumors did better with combination treatment.

Toxicity.—Patients who received cisplatin had more nausea and vomiting than those given radiotherapy alone. Hematologic toxicity was moderate. Renal insufficiency developed in 1 patient in the combined treatment group, but none had significant neuropathy. Both treatment-related deaths—1 caused by radiation pneumonitis and 1 by heart, respiratory, and renal failure—were in the combined treatment group.

Conclusion.—There is no clear advantage to adding cisplatin chemotherapy to radiotherapy for patients with locally advanced NSCLC.

▶ There has been a great deal of interest in adding cisplatin to radiation therapy for locally advanced, unresectable NSCLC. Exactly what the cisplatin has contributed is not clear. This randomized study was designed to assess the cisplatin as a pure adjuvant. The chemotherapy actually began on the first day of radiation, but it was not exploited specifically as a radiation-sensitizing compound. In terms of response, progression-free survival, or overall survival, there is no suggestion that the cisplatin significantly added to the effects of radiation alone. This is disappointing in light of the typical approach to using cisplatin these days, but I think we all have to acknowledge that NSCLC is extraordinarily difficult for all of us to treat, regardless of modality. We really need better weapons.

E. Glatstein, M.D.

Radical Radiotherapy for Early Nonsmall Cell Lung Cancer

Graham PH, Gebski VJ, Langlands AO (Westmead Hosp, NSW, Australia)
Int J Radiat Oncol Biol Phys 31:261–266, 1995   13–7

Introduction.—Survival rates have varied widely in reports of the results of radical radiotherapy for early-stage non–small-cell lung cancer, in part because of methodological problems and/or small populations in the studies. A large group of patients with long-term follow-up were retrospectively reviewed to determine the impact of radical radiotherapy.

Methods.—The records of 150 patients treated between 1979 and 1985 for stage I and II non–small-cell lung cancer were reviewed. The patients were divided into 4 groups for analysis: those who were not treated (18 patients) and those who were treated with palliative radiotherapy (21), radical radiotherapy (103), or surgery (8). The patients treated with radical radiotherapy had a median age of 67 years and were more likely to be male. The median primary radiotherapy dose was 60 Gy in 30 fractions. All patients were assessed for comorbidity and were followed until death or for at least 5 years.

Results.—Patients who were untreated or treated with palliative radiotherapy had a similar survival rate. Survival was not calculated for the 8 surgical patients. Survival was significantly improved in the group treated with radical radiotherapy. The overall 5-year survival rate in this group was 13%. However, patients without weight loss and significant comorbidity had a 25% 5-year survival rate, and patients with T1 tumors, stable weight, and age younger than 70 years had a 50% 5-year survival rate. There were no treatment-related deaths or instances of rare late toxicity or mild acute toxicity.

Discussion.—Although the overall prognosis for patients with non–small-cell lung cancer remains very poor, radiotherapy can be a potentially curative strategy in a small subset of patients, particularly in patients with small tumors, stable weight, and no comorbidity.

▶ There are many people who seem to question the role of radiation therapy in the management of non–small-cell lung cancer. Most of us believe that for early-stage cancer, a patient should undergo a resection if possible. On the other hand, if the patient is not a suitable candidate, for whatever reasons, definitive radiation therapy has a reasonable chance of benefiting the patient long-term; the outcome we think is reasonably comparable to surgery, although we still believe surgery to be preferred. This series from Australia looks at the experience with non–small-cell lung cancer between 1979 and 1985. The authors identified 150 patients with stage I and II disease, 103 of whom were treated by radical radiotherapy. The overall 5-year survival rate of patients treated with radical intent was 13%, although in a small subset of patients (those younger than 70 years with T1 lesions not associated with weight loss), the 5-year survival rate was a respectable 50%.

I think the point is that when one tries to compare radiation therapy and surgery, one has to take into account that there are certain patients who are usually treated by one modality or the other. Definitive radiation therapy for lung cancer is usually restricted to an elderly subset of patients or one that is medically compromised in some way. Simple survival alone may be misleading in attempts to compare the modalities. This article certainly confirms the observations of many others in that there is a group of patients that can be cured with radiation therapy. Unfortunately, it is a modest proportion of the total population.

E. Glatstein, M.D.

Hypofractionated Irradiation for Inoperable Non-Small Cell Lung Cancer
Stevens MJ, Begbie SD (Royal North Shore Hosp, Sydney, Australia)
Australas Radiol 39:265–270, 1995   13–8

Background.—Inoperable non–small cell lung cancer (NSCLC) is associated with a very high mortality rate. These patients are generally treated with radiation therapy, although the optimal radiation dose and fractionation schedule are controversial. Conventional radiotherapy schedules, which deliver a high dose in small fractions over 6–8 weeks, are both toxic and cost-ineffective and deliver a higher radiation dose than is needed to achieve symptom control. Therefore, hypofractionation has been suggested. Experience with a hypofractionation schedule allowing only 2 high-dose fractions was reported.

Methods.—Over 21 months, 38 patients with inoperable NSCLC and predominantly chest symptomatology were treated with a total mid-plane dose of 1,700 cGy given in 2 fractions of 850 cGy separated by an interval of 1 week. The majority of the patients had good performance status and minimal preradiation weight loss. Patients were assessed for acute toxicity, symptomatic response, duration of response, and time to disease progression at 6 weeks, 12 weeks, and then every 3 months.

Results.—The patients were followed for a median of 25 weeks (range, 0.2–83 weeks). The overall survival was closely related to freedom from systemic disease (Fig 1). Local disease-free survival was closely related to freedom from symptoms (Fig 2). Complete symptom relief was achieved in 70% of the patients. Only 2 patients had local failure after irradiation.

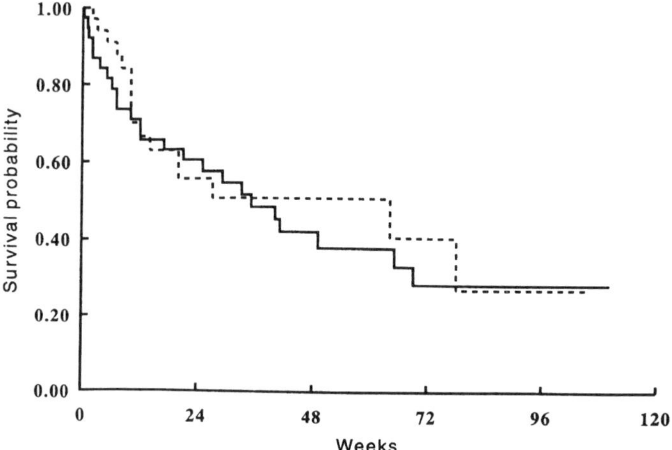

FIGURE 1.—Relationship between overall survival (*solid line*) and systemic (extra-thoracic) failure-free survival (*broken line*) after irradiation. (Courtesy of Stevens MJ, Begbie SD: Hypofractionated irradiation for inoperable non-small cell lung cancer. *Australas Radiol* 39:265–270, 1995.)

Acute toxicity—most commonly somatic pain lasting 2–7 days or mild esophagitis—occurred in 42%. Only 1 patient had serious late toxicity with the probable development of radiation myelopathy.

Conclusion.—The course of radiation therapy can be shortened without compromising symptomatic relief in patients with inoperable NSCLC. The median survival in this series was comparable with that in other international studies. A high proportion of the patients were symptom-free until death, with hemoptysis, cough, and chest pain more controllable than

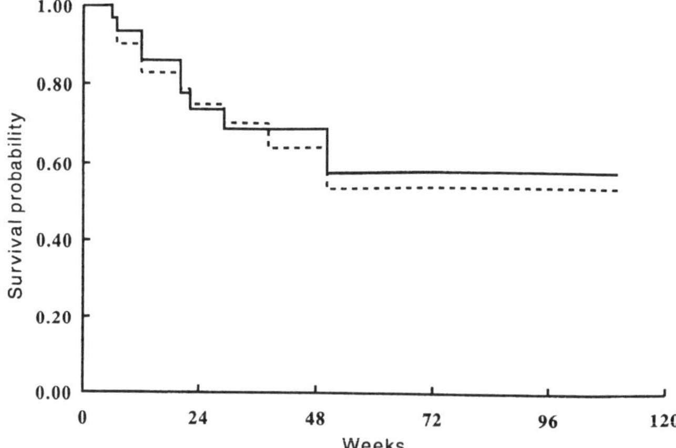

FIGURE 2.—Relationship between symptom-free survival (*solid line*) and local disease-free survival (*broken line*) after irradiation. (Courtesy of Stevens MJ, Begbie SD: Hypofractionated irradiation for inoperable non-small cell lung cancer. *Australas Radiol* 39:265–270, 1995.)

dyspnea. There was a relatively low rate of mild toxicity, with late radiation injury of the spinal cord the most serious potential risk.

▶ In today's world of cost containment, palliative thoracic irradiation is under considerable scrutiny. This paper from Australia looked at 2 fractions of 850 cGy, each given 1 week apart. My only concern with this kind of treatment is that one must be sure that the patient is, in fact, a candidate for palliative measures, i.e., he or she has either metastasis or other serious medical conditions or compromise of performance status that essentially obviates any effort for cure.

An incredible self-fulfilling prophecy exists among physicians who deal with lung cancer. Obviously, it is a difficult problem, but for patients who are in good shape—even those who have nodal involvement—there is still a reasonable chance of survival, even when the disease cannot be resected. We would like those results to be better, and this approach obviously will not do that. On the other hand, in cases that are clearly palliative, it will save a lot of time and money.

E. Glatstein, M.D.

Effects of Postoperative Mediastinal Radiation on Completely Resected Stage II and Stage III Epidermoid Cancer of the Lung

Weisenburger TH (Univ of California, Los Angeles)
Chest 106:297S–301S, 1994   13–9

Introduction.—Approximately 44% of patients with lung cancer have disease that apparently is limited to the chest at the time of presentation. With early detection and surgical treatment, survival ranges from 60% to 70% and decreases significantly for patients with more advanced primary disease or nodal involvement. Retrospective studies have suggested that postoperative radiotherapy can improve survival for patients with hilar or mediastinal lymph node metastases from epidermoid carcinoma. This hypothesis was tested in a randomized trial.

Methods.—Two hundred thirty patients with stage II or III epidermoid carcinoma and complete surgical resection were stratified and randomly assigned to radiotherapy and control groups. Complete resection was defined as negative resection margins, with the most proximal or cephalad of the mediastinal lymph nodes being free of tumor. Patients in the radiation group were scheduled to receive a total dose of 50 Gy to the chest delivered by megavoltage equipment. A third arm, which was to have consisted of radiotherapy plus levamisole, was dropped for accrual reasons. The final analysis included 210 eligible patients, including 13 who did not receive their assigned treatment. The mean time from randomization to analysis was 3.5 years.

Results.—Toxicity was increased in the radiation group, but the pulmonary toxic reactions did not significantly differ. Recurrent disease developed in 94 patients, with no significant differences between groups. There was a significant difference in local recurrence—21 patients in the control groups had local failure at the first site compared with just 1 patient in the radiation group. Survival or disease-free survival did not significantly differ. The 44 patients with N2 disease showed a significant reduction in the overall recurrence rate, regardless of group assignment.

Conclusions.—In patients with stage II or III epidermoid carcinoma of the lung, postoperative mediastinal irradiation appears to significantly reduce local recurrence rates; however, the large number of other recurrences prevents any benefit in terms of survival. The early metastatic behavior of lung cancer makes it unlikely that local treatment will be sufficient; effective systemic therapy is needed.

▶ This brief paper represents the long-term follow-up of the prospectively randomized study done by the Lung Cancer Study Group, initially published in *The New England Journal of Medicine* in 1986. There are no substantive changes, but there are a few comments about this study that are worth making. First of all, when the paper was initially published, the focus of interest was patients who had positive mediastinal nodes. It is important to note that only 20% of the patients in this study fell into that N2 category. The second point to emphasize is that most people have concluded from this study that postoperative radiation to the mediastinum is not indicated for patients who have stage II or III carcinoma of the lung. This is incorrect.

This study is unusual from the standpoint of surgery. The surgery that was carried out was essentially a clean-out procedure of the mediastinum. This is not generally done at the community level or even at most university centers (most likely, this is a reflection of the fact that most of the thoracic surgery being done in this country is not being done by thoracic surgical oncologists). Be that as it may, the typical resection done in this country presently does *not* include a full dissection of the mediastinum.

A third factor to remember about this study is that it is restricted only to epidermoid carcinoma and to patients in whom the complete mediastinal dissection showed that the most proximal mediastinal nodes were negative. This is a very special subset of patients who undergo surgery. One can come to this conclusion simply by noting that for this group of patients, surgery alone has a 5-year survival rate of approximately 40%. This clearly is not representative, because it reflects an extraordinarily highly selective group. Unfortunately, the exclusion of patients whose nodes were positive at the northernmost line of resection makes it virtually impossible to compare this particular study with anything else that has been in the literature.

If the surgery performed on a patient with lung cancer includes this kind of extensive mediastinal node resection, then the author's conclusion about omitting postoperative radiation therapy can be rationalized because there is no improvement in survival. The gains in local control are not statistically significant, although it is important to note that this is a relatively small study, with only 230 patients randomized over 7 years at several institutions. To me, if the extensive surgery done in the study is not performed in a given patient, I would certainly recommend supplementing the limited type of surgery that is generally done with postoperative radiation therapy when the mediastinal nodes are positive. For stage II disease where the hilum is positive, it once again comes down to exactly how much surgery occurs. The more limited the mediastinal resection is, the less confident one can be about whether postoperative radiation therapy should be withheld for stage II disease. If a reasonable number of mediastinal nodes (most likely 10 or 12, or some such number) are all negative, then I would be willing to withhold radiation therapy. On the other hand, if there are only 2 nodes taken from the mediastinum at the time of surgery, I cannot be confident about the absence of mediastinal nodal disease. These kinds of decisions need to be made by experienced physicians who understand the devil and all his disguises.

The Lung Cancer Study Group should be complimented for publishing these long-term data. How many studies are published prematurely, when the results are provocative, but fail to be updated in the long term because the data do not hold up? One only has to try to find 5-year figures (with *every* patient having at least 5 years of follow-up, as opposed to actuarial projections with one patient out 5 years) in lymphoma and in ovarian cancer!

E. Glatstein, M.D.

A Prospective Randomized Trial to Determine the Benefit of Surgical Resection of Residual Disease Following Response of Small Cell Lung Cancer to Combination Chemotherapy
Lad T, Piantadosi S, Thomas P, Payne D, Ruckdeschel J, Giaccone G (The Lung Cancer Study Group; Eastern Cooperative Oncology Group; European Organization for Research and Treatment of Cancer)
Chest 106:320S–323S, 1994   13–10

Background.—Small-cell lung cancer is almost always a systemic disease, prompting controversy as to the role of surgery in its management. Although patients who have advanced disease have high response rates to chemotherapy, relapse is common and long-term survival is poor. Several lines of evidence suggest that surgical resection after a response to chemotherapy induction may be a rational approach. A phase 3 study of surgery's role in the treatment of small-cell lung cancer was launched in 1983. The main goal of the study was to compare mortality for patients who did and did not undergo surgery. The results were recently reported.

Methods.—The study sample comprised 328 patients who had limited-stage small-cell lung cancer. Sixty-five percent were men, and the median patient age was 59 years. All patients received 5 cycles of cyclophosphamide, doxorubicin, and vincristine chemotherapy, which was administered every 21 days. Those who had a partial or complete objective response, who had confirmation of pure small-cell histologic features, and who had resectable tumors were randomized to undergo or not to undergo pulmonary resection. Radiotherapy to the chest and brain was administered to all randomized patients, with 50 Gy given in 25 fractions to the chest and 30 Gy given in 15 fractions to the brain. The patients were followed up every 3 months.

Results.—There were 90 complete and 127 partial responses to chemotherapy, for an objective response rate of 66%. The total number of patients randomized was 146, including 66% of the responders and 44% of the patients overall. The 70 patients who had surgery had a resection rate of 83% and a 91% rate of pathologic complete remission; 9% were left with residual non–small-cell histologic features only. Therefore, a total of 28% of patients had complete eradication of small-cell lung cancer. The median survival was 12 months for the overall group of 328 patients and 16 months for those who were randomized. The patients who underwent surgery had a median survival of 15 months, compared with 19 months for those who did not undergo surgery. The actuarial survival at 2 years was 20%. No patient subsets that appeared to benefit from the addition of surgery were identified.

Conclusions.—Pulmonary resection does not appear to be a useful addition to the multimodality treatment of small-cell lung cancer. It does not improve survival for patients whose disease responds to chemotherapy, nor does it affect the pattern of relapse. In contrast to one previous report, "salvage" surgery for non–small-cell residual disease was not successful.

▶ This is another study of the role of surgery in lung cancer, this time following the response of small-cell lung cancer to combination chemotherapy. The role of surgery in small-cell lung cancer has seen a resurgence of interest, and this abstract represents a controlled clinical trial done to assess its value. The authors are to be commended for attempting randomized study on surgery. Such studies are very difficult to perform. Their results, however, fail to show any benefit of surgery used on a routine basis.

There probably is a role for surgery in highly selected patients who are in good shape. Unfortunately, the typical patient with small-cell cancer has already suffered significant pulmonary injury from the decades of cigarette consumption responsible for the genesis of the problem in the first place.

In my own career, I can think of one patient in whom I honestly wish I had performed surgery first. This patient had a huge mass that was barely touching the mediastinum but was overlying a large amount of lung parenchyma. In retrospect, I think it would have been smart to resect that mass and then give postoperative radiation to the mediastinum, where there was presumably some involvement, and to leave the lung parenchyma to the chemotherapy. The role of surgery in these highly selected patients needs to be *extremely* tailored to meet the needs of patients who have relatively unusual problems. The decision must be made by the nonsurgeons that it will help. This particular study substantiates not using surgery on a routine basis, even for "limited-stage" patients.

E. Glatstein, M.D.

Randomized Trial of Lobectomy Versus Limited Resection for T1 N0 Non-Small Cell Lung Cancer

Lung Cancer Study Group, Ginsberg RJ, Rubinstein LV (Mem Sloan-Kettering Cancer Ctr, New York)
Ann Thorac Surg 60:615–623, 1995   13–11

Background.—Lobectomy is the standard treatment for early-stage lung cancer. Recently, however, lesser resections have been advocated as treatment for patients with T1 N0 non–small-cell lung cancer (NSCLC). This strategy has the theoretical advantages of preserving pulmonary function, decreasing perioperative mortality and morbidity, and allowing further resections if a second primary lung cancer develops. The efficacy of lobectomy was compared with that of limited resection for the treatment of T1 N0 NSCLC in a prospective, randomized trial.

Methods.—A total of 276 patients with a clinical T1 N0 peripheral NSCLC tumor were stratified according to age and pulmonary function and were randomly assigned to surgical treatment with either lobectomy or limited resection (segmentectomy or adequate wedge resection). Of those 276 patients, 247 were assessable. The patients were assessed at 3-month intervals for 2 years, at 6-month intervals for the next 3 years, and annually thereafter.

Results.—There were no significant differences between the 2 treatment groups for the stratification variables and selected prognostic variables. The 2 groups had similar types and numbers of postoperative complications, except that 6 patients in the lobectomy group and no patients in the limited resection group had respiratory failure requiring ventilatory assis-

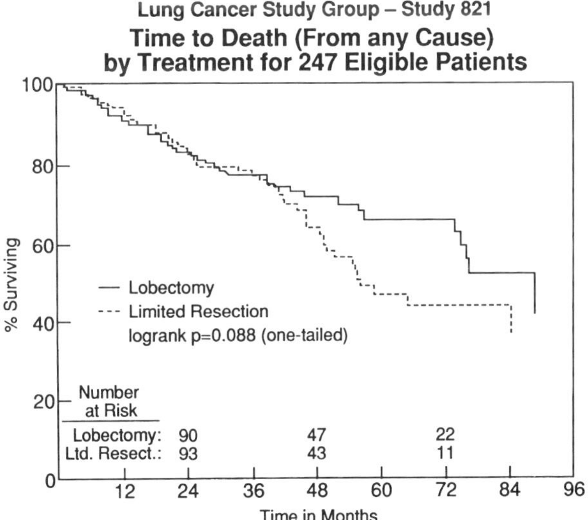

FIGURE 1.—Time to death (from any cause) by treatment for 247 eligible patients. (Courtesy of Lung Study Group, Ginsberg RJ, Rubinstein LV: Randomized trial of lobectomy versus limited resection for T1 N0 non-small cell lung cancer. *Ann Thorac Surg* 60:615–623, 1995. Reprinted with permission from the Society of Thoracic Surgeons.)

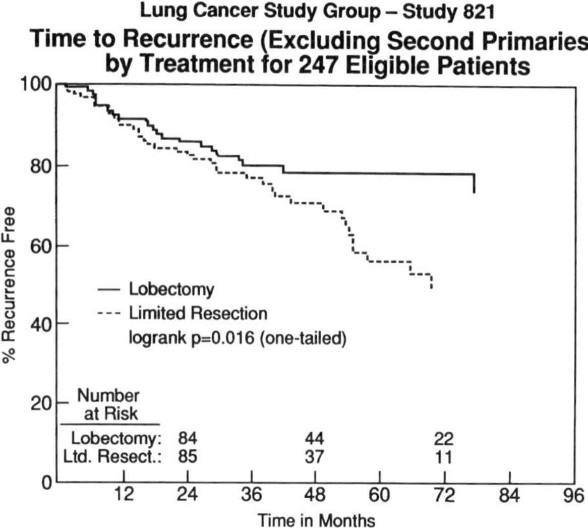

FIGURE 2.—Time to recurrence (excluding second primaries) by treatment for 247 eligible patients. (Courtesy of Lung Cancer Study Group, Ginsberg RJ, Rubinstein LV: Randomized trial of lobectomy versus limited resection for T1 N0 non-small cell lung cancer. *Ann Thorac Surg* 60:615–623, 1995. Reprinted with permission from the Society of Thoracic Surgeons.)

tance. Compared with the lobectomy group, the limited resection group had a 30% increase in the mortality rate from all causes (Fig 1) and a 50% increase in the rate of death from cancer. In addition, the limited resection group demonstrated a 75% increase in the rate of recurrence (Fig 2), which was attributable to a tripled locoregional recurrence rate.

Conclusions.—Patients treated with limited resection have a significantly increased risk of local recurrence and a lesser chance of overall and disease-free survival than do patients treated with lobectomy. Therefore, lobectomy with systematic hilar and mediastinal lymph node sampling or dissection is recommended as the continued standard surgical treatment for patients with T1 N0 NSCLC tumors.

▶ In managing patients who have lung cancer, the most important factor in decision-making is the patient's overall performance status, which is critical in this study's population of largely heavy cigarette smokers. The point is that whatever amount of lung is removed, the remaining lung usually is not normal but, rather, is compromised to some degree by smoking. How much compromise is present is frequently difficult to assess, even with modern pulmonary function studies. Therefore these authors addressed the problem of limited lung cancer (clinically T1 N0 NSCLC) that could be managed by either a lobectomy or a limited wedge resection all the way up to a segmentectomy. This study is randomized in that the patients had only peripheral lesions that were amenable to either procedure. The limited resection, ranging from wedge resection to segmentectomy, resulted in a moderate increase both in recurrence rates and the overall death rate.

Optimal decisions for favorable patients are hard to define. Although one knows the clinical stage, one does not really know the pathologic stage, which is important in making a decision regarding what needs to be done. For patients who want and mandate relatively conservative treatment options, one frequently can deliver such options. On the other hand, some of these things are easier said than done.

E. Glatstein, M.D.

Videothoracoscopy and Video-Assisted Small Thoracotomy for the Treatment of Pulmonary Malignancies

Casadio C, Giobbe R, Cianci R, Molinatti M, Oliaro A, Maggi G (Univ of Turin, Italy)
J Cardiovasc Surg 35:445–448, 1994 13–12

Background.—Video-assisted thoracic surgery is done with increasing frequency; however, its role in the treatment of pulmonary malignancies or metastatic mediastinal adenopathies has not yet been defined. The use of a video-assisted minimally invasive approach for the treatment of pulmonary malignancies and mediastinal lymph node sampling was reported.

Methods and Findings.—One hundred consecutive video-assisted thoracic operations were analyzed. Twenty-two patients were affected by a malignancy in the lung or in the subcarinal lymph nodes. Six of these patients had a primary lung cancer and underwent surgery with a video-assisted small thoracotomy of 5 cm because of a very poor respiratory reserve. Nine patients underwent a video-assisted wedge resection of a nodule that, at frozen section analysis, yielded metastasis. An 8-cm thoracotomy was made, and the entire lung was palpated carefully through the thoracic cage. Five patients had enlarged lymph nodes in the posterior and inferior mediastinum only, which were inaccessible by cervical mediastinoscopy or anterior mediastinotomy.

Conclusions.—Video-assisted thoracic surgery can be used for resection or assessment of thoracic malignancies in selected patients. With thoracoscopic exploration, a useful mediastinal nodal sampling can be obtained for these adenopathies.

▶ I think this is a very interesting paper dealing with a series of patients who have undergone video-assisted thoracic operations. Twenty-two of them had a malignancy in the lung or subcarinal nodes. The reason I think this study is interesting is that it suggests that it would be *possible* to do conservative excisional surgery (i.e., a sleeve resection), sampling and removing selected nodes as well as the primary tumor mass, but leaving the lung in place. The big problem in doing radical surgery, as we traditionally know it in these patients, is that a huge proportion of them have chronic obstructive lung disease resulting from the excessive consumption of cigarettes. Cigarette use in this group of patients puts major limitations on what the surgeon can do. If the lung parenchyma were left intact, without removal of a whole lobe or a whole lung, I think it could be possible for radiation to be superimposed after such "conservative" surgery and still allow us to achieve the same degree of success that we do at the moment, and possibly more. If the tumor mass could be effectively removed with only microscopic residual disease, radiation should be very effective.

Obviously, the metastatic potential is a major issue among patients with lung cancer, because so many of them have nodal involvement and/or overt metastases at the time of their diagnosis. Even so, new techniques evolving from this type of surgery could permit this kind of sleeve resection with a very tight margin of the primary tumor and, also, selected nodal removal. If radiation or chemotherapy could be shown to be effective after resection, these patients might be much better off in terms of their pulmonary function. It will take a somewhat adventuresome surgeon to try doing this kind of work, but I believe this is the way that thoracic surgery for cancer will be performed in the next century.

E. Glatstein, M.D.

Striking Changes in Smoking Behaviour and Lung Cancer Incidence by Histological Type in Southeast Netherlands, 1960-1991
Janssen-Heijnen MLG, Nab HW, van Reek J, van der Heijden LH, Schipper R, Coebergh JWW (Comprehensive Cancer Centre South, Eindhoven, The Netherlands; Erasmus Univ, Rotterdam, The Netherlands; Univ of Limburg, Maastricht, The Netherlands; et al)
Eur J Cancer 31A:949–952, 1995   13–13

Background.—Previous studies of Dutch men have indicated that the mortality rates for lung cancer have decreased after a dramatic increase since World War II. Conversely, steady increases in the lung cancer mortality rate in females have been noted. Temporal trends in the incidence of lung cancer in the southeast Netherlands between 1960 and 1991 were examined.

Methods and Findings.—Data from the Eindhoven Cancer Registry were used. Changing trends were analyzed according to the period of diagnosis and the 10-year birth cohort and histologic type. Regional patterns in smoking habits were also analyzed using data from national surveys conducted since 1958. A total of 10,223 patients with lung cancer were registered between 1960 and 1991, including 9,412 men and 811 women. In men, lung cancer incidence rates increased dramatically from birth cohorts 1890–1899 to 1910–1919, after which a decrease was noted. The peak incidence for both squamous cell and small-cell carcinomas was reached in 1978; for adenocarcinoma, the peak was reached in 1985. In females, an increasing trend in lung cancer incidence was observed up to 1988 for each consecutive birth cohort and for each histologic category. The changes in lung cancer incidence rates were, in all likelihood, associated with the pattern of past smoking behaviors. The percentage of male adult smokers in the southern part of The Netherlands decreased from

95% in 1960 to 40% in 1981. Conversely, the percentage of female adult smokers increased from 27% in 1960 to 40% in 1967, with slight reductions occurring only after 1979.

Conclusion.—The observed trends in smoking habits suggest that incidence rates for male lung cancer will decrease even further in the near future. In contrast, the incidence of lung cancer in females will not be expected to decrease until after the year 2000.

▶ This epidemiologic study is from The Netherlands, where the population is considerably less mobile than in this country. In this paper, the authors emphasize that when they look at the incidence of smoking, they see a reliable relationship between smoking habits and the incidence of lung cancer. I think the evidence is very strong. If anyone is really serious about preventing cancer, they should begin by making cigarettes illegal. Although that is not a political reality at this time, all efforts to prevent cancer pale in comparison with that action. Any environmental movement to prevent pollution of other agents will be relatively small in its ability to prevent cancer compared with what could be achieved by eliminating cigarettes.

When one considers the amount of money that we spend on cigarette-related diseases, the indifference of our society is staggering. The tragedy of both lung and head and neck cancers, in particular, is that they are largely preventable. The lag time between the cessation of smoking and the decrease in lung cancer appears to be approximately 20–25 years. I truly hope that someday someone will be able to effect some political solution to this problem, but I doubt very much whether that will occur. In the meantime, the sad truth is that there will continue to be business (and disgraceful profits) as usual.

E. Glatstein, M.D.

14 Head and Neck Cancer

The Head and Neck Manifestations of Mycosis Fungoides
Brennan JA (Johns Hopkins Hospital, Baltimore, Md)
Laryngoscope 105:478–480, 1995

14–1

Introduction.—Mycosis fungoides (MF), a common T-cell lymphoma, is typically seen cutaneously, but it may spread to the lymph nodes and viscera. The prognosis depends on the extent of dissemination. Mycosis fungoides can be seen with varying head and neck manifestations. Because early detection is crucial, these manifestations were studied retrospectively.

Methods.—The records of all 45 patients receiving a diagnosis of MF between 1983 and 1992 were reviewed, with attention to demographic data, clinical presentations, diagnostic methods, treatment, and relapses.

Results.—The patients had a mean age of 56.8 years (range, 16–85 years); there were 20 men and 25 women; 29 were white and 16 were black. The diagnosis was made an average of 6 years after the onset of cutaneous symptoms (range, 2 months to 36 years). Cutaneous or extra-cutaneous involvement was found in 70% of the patients. The cutaneous head and neck lesions included skin patches in 7%, skin plaques in 37%, skin tumors in 21%, and erythroderma in 5%. The most common extra-cutaneous manifestation, by far, was cervical lymphadenopathy. Others included alopecia, facial nerve paralysis, leonine facies, hypopigmentation, serous otitis media, tongue ulcerations, trismus with masseter tumor, and accessory nerve paralysis (Table 2). Biopsy specimens usually revealed atypical lymphoid cells with hyperchromatic, convoluted nuclei and scant cytoplasm infiltrating the epidermis and dermis.

Patients were treated most commonly with radiation therapy, particularly total body electron-beam therapy with or without spot orthovoltage treatment. Other common treatments included photochemotherapy (47% of patients), topical chemotherapy (44%), and systemic chemotherapy (31%). Relapses requiring further treatment occurred in 76% of the patients.

Conclusion.—The majority of these patients with MF had head and neck cutaneous and extracutaneous manifestations. Because biopsies of

---

TABLE 2.—Extracutaneous Head and Neck Manifestations of Mycosis Fungoides

Manifestation	No. of Patients ($N = 43$)
Cervical lymphadenopathy	17 (40%)
Alopecia	2 (5%)
Facial nerve paralysis	2 (5%)
Leonine facies	1 (2%)
Hypopigmentation	1 (2%)
Serous otitis media	1 (2%)
Tongue ulcerations	1 (2%)
Trismus with masseter tumor	1 (2%)
Accessory nerve paralysis	1 (2%)

Note: Two of the 45 patients in whom mycosis fungoides was evaluated had no documented physical examination on chart review.

(Courtesy of Brennan JA: The head and neck manifestations of mycosis fungoides. *Laryngoscope* 105:478–480, 1995.)

---

both cutaneous lesions and lymph nodes should be performed for staging the disease, head and neck specialists should be familiar with the diagnosis and treatment of MF.

▶ To me, MF is different from a cutaneous T-cell lymphoma. Mycosis fungoides is an extraordinarily relentless disease that appears to be of lymphoid origin. Nonetheless, the major organ affected is the skin, with secondary involvement of other organs. This report documents an experience with MF in 45 patients at Johns Hopkins Hospital, approximately 70% of whom had cutaneous or extracutaneous involvement of the head and neck areas.

Once there is extensive involvement of the skin, the long-term prognosis is extraordinarily poor for patients with this disease. I find MF to have its own clinical course that is much different from that of lymphomas involving the skin, which may or may not be of T-cell origin. They are both indolent, but in the case of MF, the patient appears to die by a micron each day. Patients may live a long time, during which their existence can be quite miserable because of the relatively ineffective methods of treatment and the impact that visible neoplasm has on the patient's psyche. Over time, I have become more impressed with the results of psoralen plus ultraviolet light. These days, I prefer to reserve total skin treatment for patients who have skin involvement that needs palliation. I do believe that a significant proportion (approximately 50%) of patients who have stage IA disease (with less than 10% of the skin involved, without other disease) can be cured with electron-beam therapy. However, beyond that, I am not convinced about most patients.

The manifestations listed in Table 2 leave out 1 manifestation that I have seen in 2 patients who lost hearing on at least 1 side as a result of their entire external auditory canal becoming occluded with skin involvement, making it impossible for sound waves to ever get to the tympanic membrane. These patients were benefited by local radiation therapy when nothing else seemed to affect their disease. I may add that this disease is highly responsive to treatment but very difficult to eradicate. When it finally does become "resistant," this disease is as resistant as anything I know of to the various interventions that we have.

E. Glatstein, M.D.

Papillary Hürthle Cell Carcinoma With Lymphocytic Stroma: "Warthin-Like Tumor" of the Thyroid
Apel RL, Asa SI, LiVolsi VA (Univ of Toronto; Univ of Pennsylvania, Philadelphia)
Am J Surg Pathol 19:810–814, 1995

14–2

Introduction.—As many as 11% of papillary carcinomas of the thyroid are oxyphilic, or Hürthle cell, neoplasms that exhibit a papillary structure but consist predominantly—or totally—of Hürthle cells. A subtype of papillary Hürthle cell carcinoma characterized by a lymphocytic stroma was described for the first time.

Clinical Aspects.—Twelve women and 1 man 26–66 years of age were affected; the average age was 44. The tumors were located randomly within the thyroid gland. All patients but 2 had a palpable thyroid nodule. The patients were all free of disease when followed for 3 months to 9 years.

Histology.—The tumors had a definite papillary structure, and the infiltrate consisted primarily of lymphocytes. Some tumor cell nuclei were pleomorphic and resembled typical Hürthle cells, but features of papillary carcinoma were apparent in most cases. In all but 3 cases, the surrounding thyroid parenchyma exhibited chronic lymphocytic inflammation. The infiltrate consisted of T lymphocytes, B lymphocytes, and plasma cells that were immunohistochemically reactive for kappa and lambda light chains. Three patients had an associated follicular-variant papillary carcinoma. Perithyroidal or cervical node metastases were present in 3 cases, and 1 tumor extended into skeletal muscle.

Conclusion.—This tumor, which closely resembles Warthin's salivary gland tumor (papillary cystadenoma lymphomatosum), may be described as a "Warthin-like tumor of the thyroid."

▶ This is an unusual series of 13 cases from 2 different institutions. The lesion apparently is an unusual thyroid cancer with a papillary appearance with oxyphilic or Hürthle cell characteristics. A lymphocytic stroma contributes to an appearance under the microscope that is very similar to the so-called Warthin's tumor of the salivary gland, a papillary cystadenoma lymphomatosum. This is a very unusual tumor, and to have a series of 13 cases makes the study a potentially useful reference. Twelve of the 13 patients were women. The clinical behavior is fairly indolent, consistent with papillary carcinoma of the thyroid gland. The lymphocytic infiltrate, as well as what appears to be an association with chronic lymphocytic thyroiditis, suggests immunologic interactions that are as yet uncharacterized and that presumably play some role in the pathogenesis of this lesion.

E. Glatstein, M.D.

Follicular Lesions of the Thyroid: Does Frozen Section Evaluation Alter Operative Management?
Chen H, Nicol TL, Udelsman R (Johns Hopkins Univ, Baltimore, Md; Johns Hopkins Thyroid Tumor Center, Baltimore, Md)
Ann Surg 222:101–106, 1995   14–3

Background.—The criteria for malignancy in patients with follicular lesions of the thyroid, namely, capsular or vascular invasion, cannot be reliably determined by fine-needle aspiration. Frozen section (FS) evaluation is therefore widely used to guide the intraoperative management of these lesions. The accuracy and clinical value of FS evaluation in the operative management of follicular lesions of the thyroid were assessed.

Methods.—Of 210 consecutive patients with follicular thyroid lesions diagnosed by FNA or FS evaluation, 125 underwent surgical resection at the study hospital. Seventy-six percent of the patients were women, and the median patient age was 43 years. The clinical and histologic findings were reviewed. One hundred eighteen patients underwent preoperative FNAs, and 120 had intraoperative FS evaluations. The definitive pathologic diagnosis was made from permanent sections.

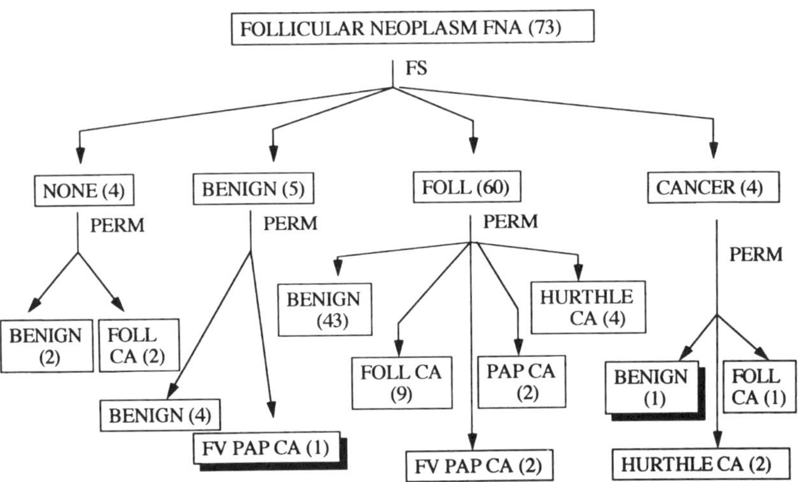

FIGURE 2.—Patients with a fine-needle aspiration *(FNA)* diagnosis of "follicular neoplasm" and their subsequent frozen section *(FS)* evaluation and permanent histologic diagnosis *(PERM)*. The bold background indicates a misguided surgical intervention. Abbreviations: *FOLL,* follicular lesion, defer to permanent histology: *FOLL CA,* follicular cancer; *FV PAP CA,* follicular variant of papillary cancer; *PAP CA,* papillary cancer; *HURTHLE CA,* Hurthle cell carcinoma. (Courtesy of Chen H, Nicol TL, Udelsman R: Follicular lesions of the thyroid: Does frozen section evaluation alter operative management? *Ann Surg* 222:101–106, 1995.)

Results.—In 87% of the FS evaluations performed, the categorization was "follicular lesion, defer to permanent section." Thus, these evaluations yielded no useful clinical information. The results of FS evaluation correctly modified the operative procedure in just 3% of patients. In another 5%, the surgeon was misled by an incorrect FS evaluation, which resulted in 4 misguided operations (Fig 2).

Conclusions.—For patients with follicular thyroid lesions, FS evaluation offers minimal useful diagnostic information. It is an expensive procedure that leads to longer and sometimes misguided operations. Pending the development of some more definitive diagnostic tool for follicular thyroid lesions, the recommendation is to omit FS, resect the lobe with the nodules, and perform the definitive operative management according to the final permanent histologic findings.

▶ Fine-needle aspiration of thyroid nodules in the presence of follicular lesions is frequently indeterminant. Pathologic diagnosis will frequently indicate "follicular neoplasms," with a subset of these being follicular cancer. Hence, many patients undergo surgical resection. The general strategy is to ultimately use the intraoperative frozen section to determine the extent of operation. This report from an experienced thyroid, surgical, and pathology group indicates the inadequacy of this strategy. As shown in Figure 2, in most cases frozen section evaluation was also indeterminant. Even in expert hands, definitive diagnosis of cancer was rarely provided. Twenty-eight percent of indeterminant lesions that required the permanent sections proved to be malignant. The authors suggest that routine frozen section evaluation be omitted in the operative management of follicular thyroid lesions.

The data support their argument that resection of the thyroid lobe containing the follicular nodule be performed, and that in the absence of gross determinance of definitive diagnosis, management be based on the final permanent sections. The major exceptions are the clinical indicators of malignancy with tumor extending into contiguous structures. This is another in a series of very important articles concerning the determinants of local recurrence after surgery for rectal cancer. The data suggest that distal intramural spread is generally less than 1 cm[1] and that the lateral or tangential margin is pivotal.[2]

A.M. Cohen, M.D.

References

1. Williams NS, Dixon MF, Johnston D: Reappraisal of the 5 centimetre rule of distal excision for carcinoma of the rectum. *Br J Surg* 70:150–154, 1983.
2. Quirke P, Durdy P, Dixon MF, et al: Local recurrence of rectal adenocarcinoma due to inadequate surgical resection. *Lancet* 2:996–999, 1986.

Distant Metastases in Papillary Thyroid Carcinoma: 100 Cases Observed at One Institution During 5 Decades

Dinneen SF, Valimaki MJ, Bergstralh EJ, Goellner JR, Gorman CA, Hay ID
(Mayo Clinic, Rochester, Minn)
J Clin Endocrinol Metab 80:2041–2045, 1995   14–4

Background.—Although the long-term cause-specific survival of patients with papillary thyroid carcinoma is favorable, patients in whom distant metastases (DM) develop have a worse prognosis. The factors predicting survival in patients with DM from papillary thyroid carcinoma were sought.

Methods.—The medical records of 100 consecutive patients who had DM after primary treatment at one institution between 1940 and 1989 were analyzed retrospectively. The patients were 55 males and 45 females aged 8–91 years. The 20 survivors had a median follow-up of 21 years.

Findings.—Cause-specific survival was 40% at 5 years, 27% at 10 years, and 24% at 15 years. These rates did not differ significantly among the early, middle, and late eras. In a univariate analysis, age at diagnosis of DM best predicted survival (Fig 3). Survival was better in younger patients. Tumor-related factors associated with improved survival were complete resection of the primary tumor, histologic grade 1, diploid nuclear DNA, and lung as first site of DM. Radioiodine treatment was associated with improved survival in a univariate analysis. However, according to multivariate analysis, the only significant predictors of survival were age, DM site, and degree of extrathyroidal invasion of the primary tumor. None of

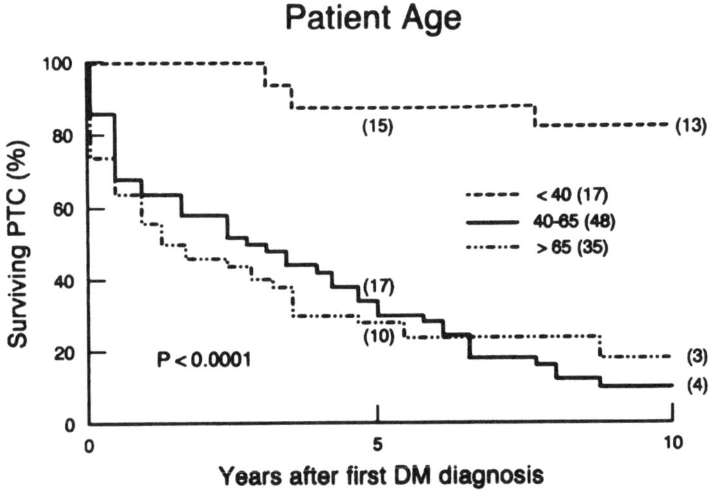

FIGURE 3.—Influence of age on the cause-specific survival of 100 patients with distant metastases from papillary thyroid carcinoma. *Numbers in parentheses* refer to the number of patients remaining in the analysis at each time point. (Courtesy of Dinneen SF, Valimaki M, Bergstralh EJ, et al: Distant metastases in papillary thyroid carcinoma: 100 cases observed at one institution during 5 decades. *J Clin Endocrinol Metab* 80:2041–2045, 1995, Copyright The Endocrine Society.)

the 4 treatment variables (external radiation, surgery, chemotherapy, or radioiodine) significantly predicted survival in the Cox model.

Conclusion.—In the past 5 decades, outcome has changed little for patients with DM from papillary thyroid carcinoma. Current treatments apparently do not affect survival.

▶ In general, papillary thyroid carcinoma is associated with long-term survival, even in the presence of extensive regional disease. In a small subset of patients, metastatic disease will develop. As with primary disease, the major determinant of long-term survival is the age at diagnosis. These data support the dramatic dichotomy in this disease based on age.

A.M. Cohen, M.D.

Definitive Radiotherapy for T1 and T2 Squamous Cell Carcinoma of the Tonsil

Moose BD, Kelly MD, Levine PA, Constable WC, Cantrell RW, Larner JM (Univ of Virginia, Charlottesville)
Head Neck 17:334–338, 1995

14–5

Background.—Most studies of radiotherapy for early-stage squamous cell carcinoma of the tonsillar region have claimed local control rates similar to those achieved operatively using average tumor doses of 65–70 Gy. It has been suggested that lower doses may be equally effective.

Series.—The efficacy of moderate-dose radiotherapy was examined in 185 patients with tonsillar carcinoma. Of 99 patients who had T1 or T2 tumors arising from the tonsillar fossa or faucial pillars, 36 had their lesions resected or received palliative radiotherapy. Fifty-three of the 63 patients given definitive radiotherapy were available for follow-up 2 years later. These patients, who had a mean age of 57 years, were observed for a median of 5 years.

Therapy.—Patients with T1 tumors received an average tumor dose of 63 Gy from either a cobalt-60 unit or a 6-MV linear accelerator. The average dose for T2 cases was also 63 Gy. More than 90% of patients were treated at a rate exceeding 200 cGy per fraction. Twenty-one of 30 patients with palpable lymph nodes underwent planned neck dissection 4–6 weeks after radiotherapy.

Results.—Determinate 3-year survival rates were 75% for patients with T1 cancers and 80% for those with T2 lesions. Patients with lesions of the

TABLE 3.—Local Control by T-Stage at 2 Years

	Local control	Number salvaged	Ultimate control
T1	25/30 (83%)	1/5	26/30 (87%)
T2	18/23 (78%)	2/5	20/23 (87%)

(Courtesy of Moose BD, Kelly MD, Levine PA, et al: Definitive radiotherapy for T1 and T2 squamous cell carcinoma of the tonsil. *Head Neck* 17:334–338, 1995. Reprinted by permission of John Wiley & Sons, Inc.)

TABLE 5.—Summary of Series Reporting Results of Definitive Radiotherapy for Squamous Cell Carcinomas of the Tonsillar Region

Series	No. of patients (T1/T2)	Dose (Gy)	Local Control (T1/T2) (%)
Dubois	49/84	>70	69/46
Amornmarn	23/50	60–80	94/80
Lusinchi	48/145	>71	88/79
Bataini	36/93	64.9	89/84
*Wang	11/72	60–65	82/60
*Remmler	14/35	65–75	100/94
*Wong	17/59	64.3/67.8	94/79
*Perez	55/0	60–70	64/0
*Lee	9/36	66/76.8 (b.i.d.)	100/94
†Wang	7/46	60–65	71/46
†Lo	0/93	63.8/66.34	71/70
†Lee	14/51	66/76.8 (b.i.d.)	79/69

* Fossa lesions.
† Pillar lesions (Wang and Lo series also included retromolar trigone lesions).
(Courtesy of Moose BD, Kelly MD, Levine PA, et al: Definitive radiotherapy for T1 and T2 squamous cell carcinoma of the tonsil. *Head Neck* 17:334–338, 1995. Reprinted by permission of John Wiley & Sons, Inc.)

faucial pillars had a 3-year survival rate of 54% compared with 86% for those with tumors of the tonsillar fossa, despite comparable average doses. Local control was achieved in 87% of all patients (Table 3). Six of 8 patients whose treatment failed in the neck had concurrent failure at the primary tumor site. Three patients had serious complications.

Discussion.—The results of previous trials of radiotherapy for tonsillar cancer are given in Table 5. The findings in this study indicate that T1 and T2 lesions, particularly those arising from the tonsillar fossa, are adequately treated by doses of 63 Gy or less.

▶ This paper from the University of Virginia shows the excellent results of using definitive radiation alone, without surgical resection, for patients with T1 and T2 squamous cell carcinoma of the tonsil. The local control and survival figures were really excellent. It is interesting that these authors used a slightly lower dose than most people would generally recommend, without paying any price in terms of local control. I must say that I would have preferred to have seen actuarial curves rather than determinate survival figures, because the determinate figures virtually always look better than other analyses; however, that does not change the fact that the local control is excellent, and the authors have included a nice tabulation regarding references dealing with the effectiveness of using radiation therapy alone for stage T1 and T2 lesions.

E. Glatstein, M.D.

Local Control of Oropharyngeal Carcinoma by Irradiation Alone

Wang CC, Montgomery W, Efird J (Massachusetts Gen Hosp, Boston; Harvard Med School, Boston)
Laryngoscope 105:529–533, 1995   14–6

Introduction.—Squamous cell carcinomas of the oropharynx occur fairly commonly, especially in the faucial tonsil and at the base of the tongue. They tend to be asymptomatic in the early stages and exhibit aggressive and deeply infiltrative characteristics involving the tongue musculature and lymph nodes. Management of squamous cell carcinomas of the oropharynx with radiation therapy alone was reviewed.

Methods.—The review involved the records of 402 patients with squamous cell carcinomas of the faucial tonsil and the base of the tongue treated with irradiation between 1970 and 1993. Early in the study, the patients were typically given 1.8–2 Gy per fraction once daily, for a total dose of 65–70 Gy in 7–8 weeks. However, after 1979, the typical protocol was twice daily 1.6-Gy fractions given 5 days each week for 12 days, followed by a 10-day to 2-week rest period and resumption of the twice-daily 1.6-Gy fractions for a total of 64–67.2 Gy in 6 weeks.

Results.—Of the 402 patients, 210 received the once-daily radiation protocol and 192 received the twice-daily protocol. The 5-year local control rates for T1 and T2 disease of the faucial tonsil were 91% with the twice-daily protocol and 75% with the once-daily protocol (Fig 1); for T3 disease of the faucial tonsil, local control rates were 80% with twice-daily irradiation and 45% with once-daily treatment (Fig 2). Among patients

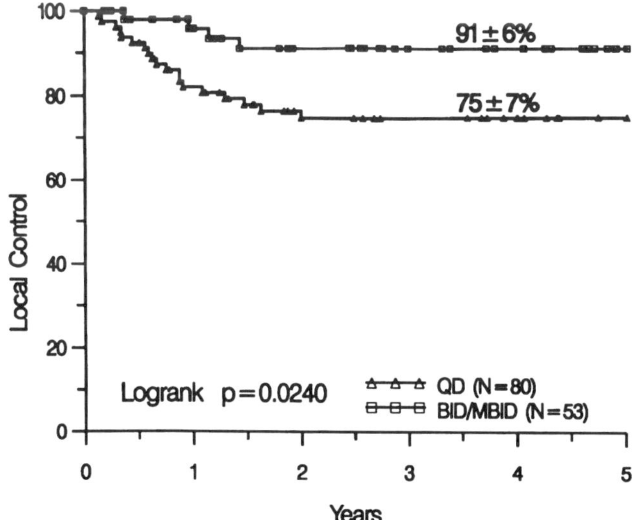

FIGURE 1.—Five-year actuarial local tumor control rates for T1 and T2 squamous cell carcinomas of the faucial tonsil after once-daily (*QD*) and twice-daily (*BID/MBID*) radiation therapy. (Courtesy of Wang CC, Montgomery W, Efird J: Local control of oropharyngeal carcinoma by irradiation alone. *Laryngoscope* 105:529–533, 1995.)

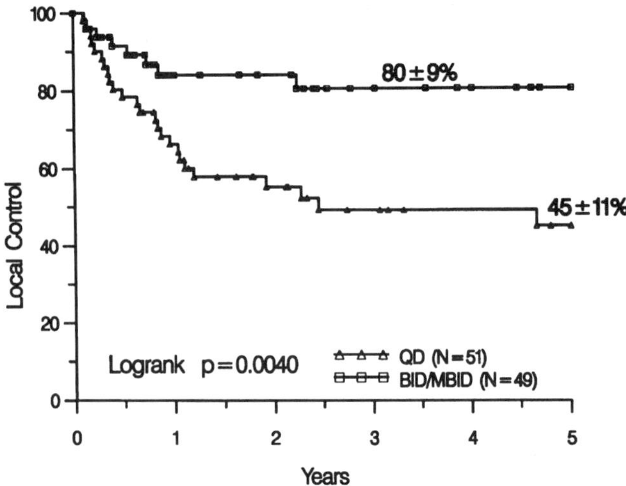

FIGURE 2.—Five-year actuarial local tumor control rates for T3 squamous cell carcinomas of the faucial tonsil after once-daily (*QD*) and twice-daily (*BID/MBID*) irradiation. (Courtesy of Wang CC, Montgomery W, Efird J: Local control of oropharyngeal carcinoma by irradiation alone. *Laryngoscope* 105:529–533, 1995.)

with squamous cell carcinomas of the base of the tongue, the 5-year local tumor control rates for T1 and T2 disease were 85% with twice-daily treatment and 79% with once-daily treatment (Fig 3); for T3 disease, the rates were 54% with twice-daily irradiation and 26% with once-daily irradiation (Fig 4). Twice-daily irradiation was also associated with higher

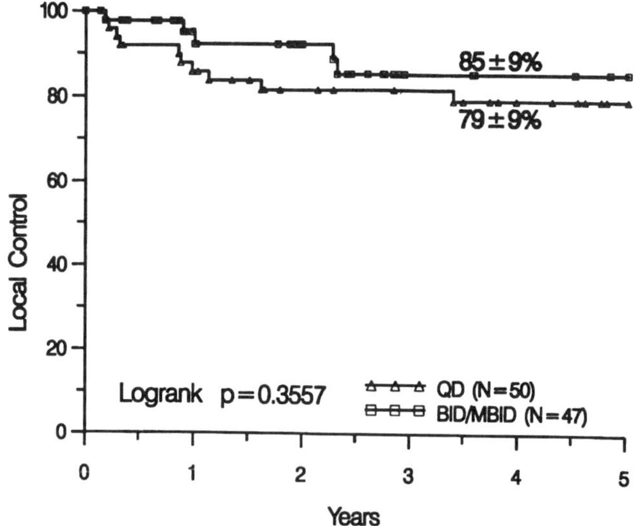

FIGURE 3.—Five-year actuarial local tumor control rates for T1 and T2 squamous cell carcinomas of the base of the tongue after once-daily (*QD*) and twice daily (*BID/MBID*) irradiation. (Courtesy of Wang CC, Montgomery W, Efird J: Local control of oropharyngeal carcinoma by irradiation alone. *Laryngoscope* 105:529–533, 1995.)

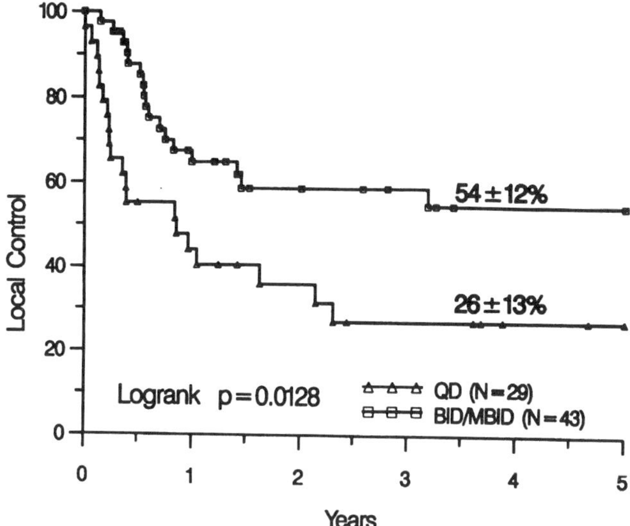

FIGURE 4.—Five-year actuarial local tumor control rates for T3 squamous cell carcinomas of the base of the tongue after once-daily (*QD*) and twice-daily (*BID/MBID*) irradiation. (Courtesy of Wang CC, Montgomery W, Efird J: Local control of oropharyngeal carcinoma by irradiation alone. *Laryngoscope* 105:529–533, 1995.)

5-year disease-specific survival rates compared with once-daily treatment: 77% vs. 67% with T1 and T2 faucial tonsil tumors, 68% vs. 33% with T3 faucial tonsil tumors, 76% vs. 65% with T1 and T2 tumors of the base of the tongue, and 53% vs. 14% with T3 tumors of the base of the tongue.

Conclusion.—These data indicate significant improvements in local tumor control and in disease-free survival for patients with squamous cell carcinomas of the faucial tonsil and base of the tongue treated with accelerated irradiation schedules. The improvements are particularly marked in patients with T3 lesions.

▶ This excellent paper reviews a large number of patients with squamous carcinoma of the faucial tonsil and base of the tongue. Their management was with radiation therapy alone after biopsy. This includes the experience at Massachusetts General Hospital with accelerated hyperfractionated radiation therapy twice daily. These are retrospective data, rather than prospectively randomized data, but the point is that the treatment results obtained using radiation therapy alone are excellent until they get to the T4 category. These results for T1, T2, and T3 disease certainly raise questions about the need for combined-modality treatment on a routine basis, as is being done throughout much of the country today.

Quite frankly, the only problem I have with twice-a-day treatment is that many patients are unwilling to come in twice a day because they believe they cannot do this and hold down a job effectively. There is great concern about losing one's job, and unfortunately, in today's world, there are not a lot of jobs out there to choose from if one *does* lose one's position.

The tonsillar data are particularly outstanding, as are the T1 and T2 base-of-tongue data. The T3 base-of-tongue data are not quite as impressive as the data on the T3 tonsil; however, even so, the majority of the T3 base-of-tongue lesions are controlled by twice-a-day treatment alone. The numbers in this experience are excellent, and that seriously suggests to me that we are not performing enough definitive treatments involving radiation alone.

E. Glatstein, M.D.

Decreased Acute Toxicity by Using Midline Mucosa-Sparing Blocks During Radiation Therapy for Carcinoma of the Oral Cavity, Oropharynx, and Nasopharynx

Perch SJ, Machtay M, Markiewicz DA, Kligerman MM (Univ of Pennsylvania, Philadelphia)
Radiology 197:863–866, 1995   14–7

Background.—Acute toxicity from mucositis during head and neck irradiation may be minimized by decreasing the volume of mucosal surface exposed to unnecessary irradiation. Narrow midline blocks in the lower neck can be used to protect the mucosa of the aerodigestive tract. However, some clinicians believe that such blocks may shield cervical lymph nodes at risk for occult disease and that inhomogeneity from the higher match lines may result in underdosing of the upper neck nodes. It was determined whether midline mucosa-sparing blocks (MSBs) can significantly decrease acute toxicity during radiation therapy for head and neck cancer without compromising tumor control.

Methods and Findings.—The radiation records and simulation films of 125 patients were reviewed. All had carcinoma of the oral cavity, oropharynx, or nasopharynx. Acute toxicity was measured by weight loss, hospitalization for nutritional support, and unplanned treatment interruptions. Weight loss occurred in 26 of 50 patients with MSBs, compared with 37 of 47 patients without MSBs. Hospitalization for nutritional support was needed in 1 of 61 patients with MSBs and in 7 of 64 without MSBs. These differences were significant (Table 4). In patients with MSBs, there was

TABLE 4.—Acute Toxicity as a Function of Midline Blocks

Parameter	MSB	No MSB	*P* Value
Weight loss ≥ 5%	26/50 (52)	37/47 (79)	.006
Hospitalized for nutritional support	1/61 (2)	7/64 (11)	.04
Missed ≥ 5d	10/61 (16)	19/64 (30)	.07

Note: Numbers in parentheses are percentages.
Abbreviation: MSB, mucosa-sparing block.
(Courtesy of Perch SJ, Machtay M, Merkiewicz DA, et al: Decreased acute toxicity by using midline mucosa-sparing blocks during radiation therapy for carcinoma of the oral cavity, oropharynx, and nasopharynx. *Radiology* 197:863–866, 1995. Radiological Society of North America.)

TABLE 5.—Neck Failure Rates With and Without MSBs When Controlling for N Stage and Neck Dissection

Parameter	MSB (*n* = 61)	No MSB (*n* = 64)	*P* Value
N0			
Crude	18% (6/33)	15% (2/13)	NS
3-yr Actuarial	19%	16%	
N1			
Crude	25% (2/8)	11% (1/9)	NS
3-year Actuarial	30%	25%	
N2			
Crude	18% (3/17)	21% (7/34)	NS
3-yr Actuarial	27%	26%	
N3			
Crude	33% (1/3)	50% (4/8)	NS
3-yr Actuarial	33%	38%	
Neck dissection			
Crude	19% (6/32)	36% (8/22)	NS
3-yr Actuarial	21%	35%	
No neck dissection			
Crude	21% (6/29)	14% (6/42)	NS
3-yr Actuarial	28%	18%	

Abbreviations: NS, not significant; *MSB*, mucosa-sparing block.
(Courtesy of Perch SJ, Machtay M, Merkiewicz DA, et al: Decreased acute toxicity by using midline mucosa-sparing blocks during radiation therapy for carcinoma of the oral cavity, oropharynx, and nasopharynx. *Radiology* 197:863–866, 1995. Radiological Society of North America.)

also a trend toward fewer treatment interruptions than in those without MSBs. The 2 groups had similar 3-year actuarial tumor control rates (Table 5).

Conclusion.—In this series, the use of midline blocks decreased acute toxicity during radiation treatment for head and neck carcinoma without adversely affecting tumor control. Midline blocks and higher match lines should be used when possible.

▶ This simple but important study looks at the question of whether a midline block over the lower neck in the treatment of patients with head and neck cancer can significantly reduce acute toxicity without compromising tumor control. The study involved 2 groups of patients who were reasonably similar in terms of their diagnosis and disease stage, roughly half of whom received these midline MSBs and roughly half of whom did not. Those who underwent that kind of blockage had less weight loss, fewer hospitalizations for nutritional support, and a smaller likelihood of requiring an interruption of treatment than did those patients who did not receive that kind of blockage.

This nice retrospective study makes the point that as long as there is no midline disease in the lower neck, this kind of block can be very helpful in minimizing morbidities without exacting a major price for that advantage. The authors make the very important point that to maximize the benefit of this block, they need a high match in the neck compared with a lower neck match. Obviously, this depends to some degree on the location of the primary tumor itself, as one must try to avoid matching across the tumor volume to the maximum degree possible. This study is worthwhile reading for those who are trying to maximize the tolerance of their treatments.

E. Glatstein, M.D.

The Influence of Positive Margins and Nerve Invasion in Adenoid Cystic Carcinoma of the Head and Neck Treated With Surgery and Radiation
Garden AS, Weber RS, Morrison WH, Ang KK, Peters LJ (MD Anderson Cancer Ctr, Houston)
Int J Radiat Oncol Biol Phys 32:619–626, 1995   14–8

Background.—Adenoid cystic carcinomas arising from the major and minor salivary glands are usually treated surgically. However, the infiltrative growth pattern and perineural spread of these head and neck tumors make local recurrence common. Since 1962, postoperative radiotherapy has been used at a university cancer center to reduce the risk of local recurrence and to avoid the need for radical surgery in patients with adenoid cystic carcinomas of the head and neck. The results of this combined approach were examined in a 30-year review.

Methods.—One hundred ninety-eight patients with adenoid cystic carcinoma of the head and neck were included in the review. The patients, treated from 1962 to 1991, ranged from 13 to 82 years of age. All received postoperative radiotherapy for known or suspected microscopic residual disease. The primary tumor site was parotid in 30 patients, submandibu-

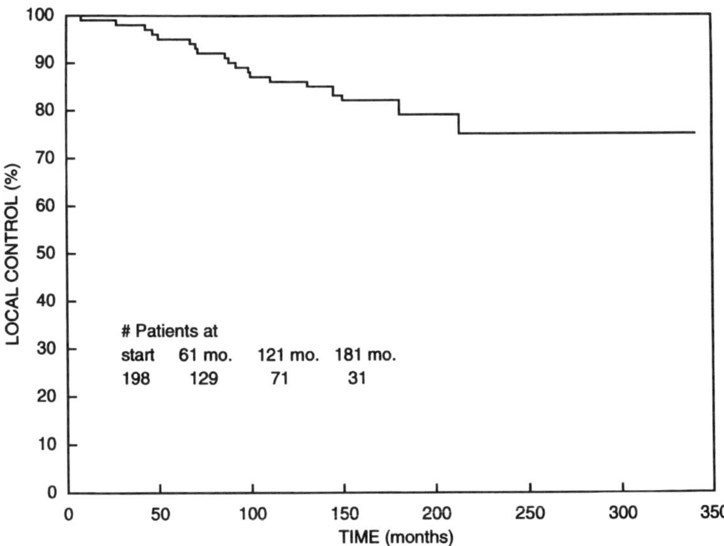

FIGURE 1.—Actuarial local control in 198 patients with adenoid cystic carcinoma treated with surgery and postoperative radiotherapy. (Courtesy of Garden AS, Weber RS, Morrison WH, et al: The influence of positive margins and nerve invasion in adenoid cystic carcinoma of the head and neck treated with surgery and radiation. *Int J Radiat Oncol Biol Phys* 32:619–626, 1995, with kind permission from Elsevier Science Ltd, The Boulevard, Langford Lane, Kidlington 0X5 1GB, UK.)

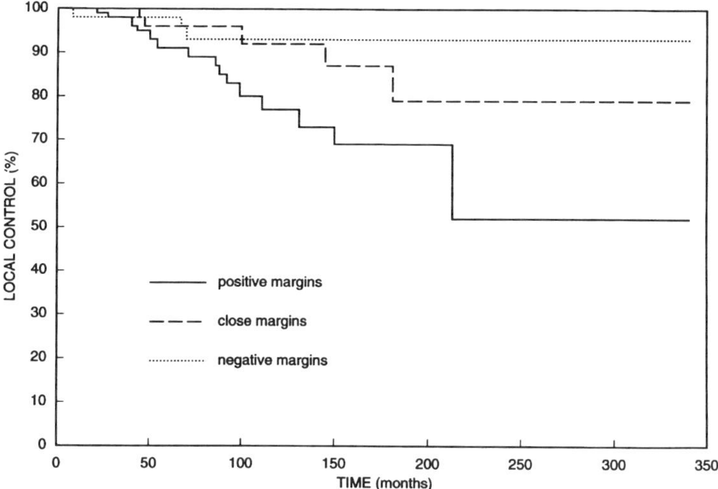

FIGURE 2.—Actuarial local control in 198 patients with adenoid cystic carcinoma treated with surgery and postoperative radiotherapy. Patients are grouped by margin status. (Courtesy of Garden AS, Weber RS, Morrison WH, et al: The influence of positive margins and nerve invasion in adenoid cystic carcinoma of the head and neck treated with surgery and radiation. *Int J Radiat Oncol Biol Phys* 32:619–626, 1995, with kind permission from Elsevier Science Ltd, The Boulevard, Langford Lane, Kidlington 0X5 1GB, UK.)

lar/sublingual in 41, lacrimal in 5, and minor salivary glands in 122. The margins were microscopically positive in 42% of patients and close or uncertain in 28%. Sixty-nine percent of the patients had perineural spread, and 28% had invasion of a major, i.e., named, nerve. The median radiation dose to the tumor bed was 60 Gy. The patients were followed for a median of 93 months, with at least 2 years' follow-up for all survivors.

Results.—The local recurrence rate was 12%, and the actuarial local control rate was 95% at 5 years, 86% at 10 years, and 79% at 15 years (Fig 1). The local recurrence rate was 18% in patients with positive margins, 9% in those with close or uncertain margins, and 5% in those

TABLE 2.—Local Failure by Site Stratified by Positive Margins and Named Nerve Involvement

Site	No. of failures (%)	Failures with positive margins (%)	Failures with named nerve involvement (%)
Minor salivary gland	16 (13)	10 (19)	5 (16)
Submandibular/sublingual gland	1 (2)	1 (9)	1 (7)
Parotid gland	4 (13)	3 (20)	4 (40)
Lacrimal gland	2 (25)	1 (33)	0 (0)
Total	23 (12)	15 (18)	10 (18)

(Courtesy of Garden AS, Weber RS, Morrison WH, et al: The influence of positive margins and nerve invasion in adenoid cystic carcinoma of the head and neck treated with surgery and radiation. *Int J Radiat Oncol Biol Phys* 32:619–626, 1995, with kind permission from Elsevier Science Ltd, The Boulevard, Langford Lane, Kidlington 0X5 1GB, UK.)

with negative margins (Fig 2). The crude treatment failure rate was 18% for patients with involvement of a major nerve and 9% for those without (Table 2).

Local control tended to improve with increasing radiation dose, significantly so for patients with positive margins. In this group, the crude control rate was 40% for doses of less than 56 Gy vs. 88% for doses of 56 Gy or greater. The actuarial rate of freedom from relapse was 68% at 5 years, 52% at 10 years, and 45% at 15 years. Failures occurred at the base of the skull and neck in just 2% of patients with and 3% of those without elective treatment. Distant metastases developed in 37% of patients, including 31% of those who were disease-free at the primary tumor site—this was the most frequent type of disease recurrence.

Conclusion.—For patients with adenoid cystic carcinomas of the head and neck, surgery followed by radiotherapy yields excellent local control. Involvement of a major nerve is an adverse prognostic factor, as is the presence of microscopically positive margins, but the local control rate can still exceed 80%. A 60-Gy radiation dose to the tumor bed (66 Gy for patients with positive margins) is effective. However, distant metastases still occur in about one third of patients, and there is no good treatment for this problem.

▶ Adenoid cystic carcinoma of the head and neck (also called cylindroma by some) remains a major therapeutic dilemma. It has an enormous propensity to recur locally, as well as to metastasize. It has an extraordinarily long fuse, with many patients having recurrence after 10-year intervals or longer. This is a large series from the M.D. Anderson Cancer Center showing surprisingly good local control achieved by postsurgical radiation therapy, but the point is clearly made that local treatments are fairly effective at present. However, one third of the patients fail systemically, and good systemic treatment is one of our major needs in treating this neoplasm.

E. Glatstein, M.D.

Voice Evaluation Before and After Laser Excision vs. Radiotherapy of T1A Glottic Carcinoma

Rydell R, Schalén L, Fex S, Elner Å (Univ Hosp of Lund, Sweden)
Acta Otolaryngol (Stockh) 115:560–565, 1995   14–9

Background.—Although both radiation and carbon dioxide laser therapy are believed to be equally effective in eliminating glottic carcinoma, their respective effects on voice quality remain controversial. Voice quality after laser treatment was, therefore, compared with that after radiotherapy in patients with T1A glottic squamous cell carcinoma.

Patient and Methods.—Thirty-six men with T1A glottic squamous cell carcinoma (mean age, 65 years) were studied. Of these, 18 patients had undergone CO_2 laser cordectomy and 18 had been treated with full-dose radiotherapy. Fifteen men without laryngeal disorders (mean age, 64 years) served as controls. Voice recordings were obtained before and at 3 months and 2 years after treatment. The Soundscope program was used to evaluate acoustic measures of shimmer, jitter, breathiness, harmonic-to-noise ratio, and fundamental frequency. Both the time required to read a running speech voice sample and the number of breaths were also analyzed. Perceptual voice analysis was performed in a blinded fashion by 4 experienced listeners (group A) and 4 naive listeners (group B). Group A evaluated quality of voice based on a modified grade, roughness, breathiness, asthenia, and strain score. Group B evaluated grade only.

Results.—Patients undergoing radiotherapy were found to have significantly better voice quality at both 3 months and 2 years after treatment, compared with the laser treatment group, as determined by the acoustic measures of breathiness, jitter, fundamental frequency average, running speech voice sample readings, and number of breaths. The perceptual measures of grade, breathiness, asthenia, and strain were also significantly better after radiotherapy. Significant differences in roughness were noted between the radiotherapy and laser groups and controls, but no differences were observed between the 2 treatment groups.

Conclusion.—When deciding on treatment for T1A glottic cancer, patients should be advised regarding the possible effects of both radiation and laser therapy on quality of voice.

▶ I have never understood why there was a big controversy about how to treat patients with early-stage carcinoma of the vocal cord. Nonetheless, a number of different treatments for this lesion have evolved, with the most recent being cordectomy done by laser. As best as I can tell, the cure rates are comparable by all these different means and, thus, the real issue comes down to just how good the voice is.

This very good study from Sweden focuses on evaluation of the voice before and after treatment. The authors studied 36 patients who had treatment for vocal cord cancer, and they also listened to 15 controls who had no problem with their larynx. Studies were done before treatment, at 3 months, and at 2 years after treatment. To summarize briefly, this objective study found that voice quality at both 3 months and 2 years after treatment was significantly better after radiation therapy than after laser treatment.

I must admit that I am not surprised by this, but I am not sure what the complications of this will be with respect to the HMOs, which seem to look only at cost as the basis for decision-making. I do hope I live long enough to see issues other than cost enter into the equation.

E. Glatstein, M.D.

Rehabilitation Outcomes of Long-Term Survivors Treated for Head and Neck Cancer
de Boer MF, Pruyn JFA, van den Borne B, Knegt PP, Ryckman RM, Verwoerd CDA (Univ Hosp, Rotterdam, The Netherlands; Inst for Health and Environmental Issues, Willemstad, The Netherlands; Univ of Limburg, Maastricht, The Netherlands; et al)
Head Neck 17:503–515, 1995   14–10

Introduction.—Although T1 glottic larynx carcinoma is the most common head and neck cancer, there have been no studies on the physical and psychosocial rehabilitation outcomes of patients with this disease. In addition, there are few studies of the psychosocial outcomes of cancer in long-term survivors of cancer of the larynx, oral cavity, or oropharynx. Therefore, new instruments were developed to assess the physical and psychosocial outcomes in patients in 3 treatment groups; factors associated with these outcomes were analyzed.

Methods.—The study population consisted of patients who had survived 2–6 years after treatment for head and neck cancer in 3 groups: patients with T1 larynx carcinoma treated with radiotherapy; patients who underwent total laryngectomy and radiotherapy for laryngeal carcinoma; and patients who underwent a commando procedure (resection of the primary site, partial mandibulectomy, a radical neck dissection, reconstruction of the bone and soft-tissue defect, and tracheotomy) for carcinoma in the oral cavity and/or oropharynx. A questionnaire addressing physical and psychosocial outcomes (uncertainty, negative feelings, loss of control, and threatened self-esteem) was mailed to 177 patients; 110 returned completed questionnaires.

Results.—Physical problems with speech production were reported by 78% of the laryngectomy patients and 58% of the commando procedure patients. More than half (58%) of the T1 larynx patients still had hoarseness. Problems with eating and drinking were reported by half of the commando procedure patients and 22% of the laryngectomy patients. The majority of patients in each group experienced phlegm in the mouth or throat, with the highest proportion of complaints in the commando procedure group. Other common complaints were dry mouth and difficulty with chewing. Substantially damaged appearance was reported by 56% of the laryngectomy patients and 55% of the commando procedure patients (Fig 1). Respiratory complaints and difficulties in breathing were most common in laryngectomy patients, but T1 larynx patients also commonly complained of frequent colds and coughing. Uncertainty regarding the disease and treatment was reported in more than half of all the patients and was particularly common in laryngectomy patients.

Laryngectomy and commando procedure patients often reported diminished self-esteem and negative feelings. Laryngectomy patients were also most likely to feel a loss of control (Fig 2). Patients also reported significant changes in their social and everyday functioning, including alterations in

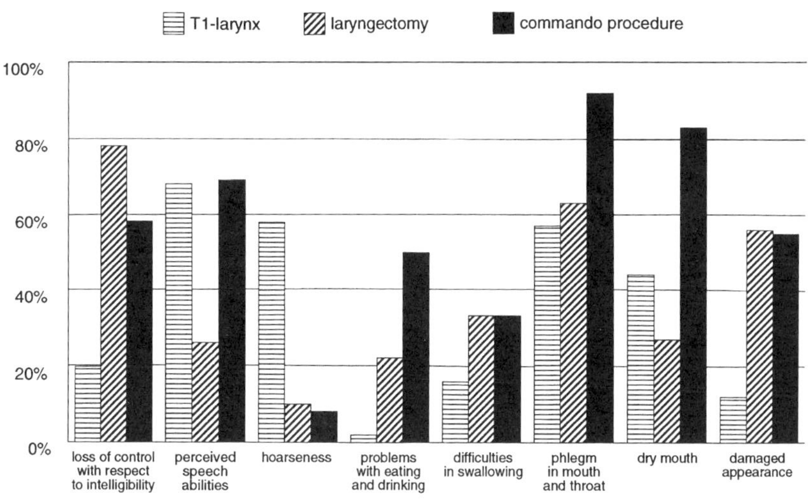

FIGURE 1.—Physical problems experienced by 3 treatment groups. Percentages of high scores are given. (Courtesy of de Boer MF, Pruyn JFA, van den Borne B, et al: Rehabilitation outcomes of long-term survivors treated for head and neck cancer. *Head Neck* 17:503–515, 1995. Reprinted by permission of John Wiley & Sons, Inc.)

personal contact, family tensions, reduced sexual contact, and loss of employment (Fig 3). Factors significantly associated with rehabilitation outcome included open discussion with family members, social contact, thorough information from the physician, and time passed since treatment.

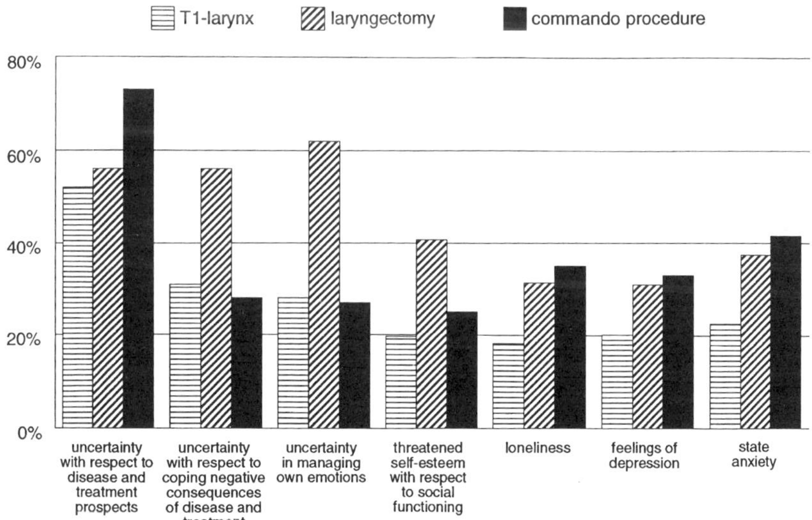

FIGURE 2. —Psychosocial problems experienced by the 3 treatment groups. Percentages of high scores are given. (Courtesy of de Boer MF, Pruyn JFA, van den Borne B, et al: Rehabilitation outcomes of long-term survivors treated for head and neck cancer. *Head Neck* 17:503–515, 1995. Reprinted by permission of John Wiley & Sons, Inc.)

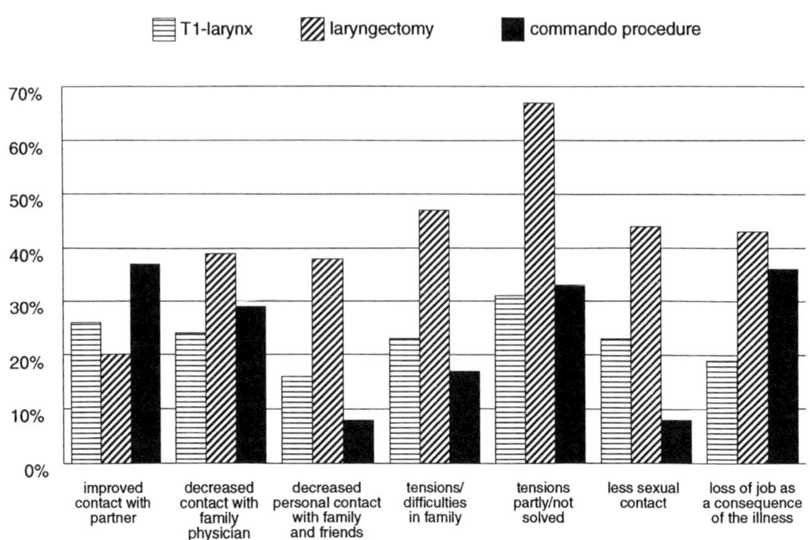

FIGURE 3.—Social/everyday functioning of the 3 treatment groups. Percentages of high scores are given. (Courtesy of de Boer MF, Pruyn JFA, van den Borne B, et al: Rehabilitation outcomes of long-term survivors treated for head and neck cancer. *Head Neck* 17:503–515, 1995. Reprinted by permission of John Wiley & Sons, Inc.)

Negative psychosocial outcomes were associated with swallowing difficulty.

Conclusion.—Patients treated for laryngeal, oral, or oropharyngeal carcinoma with radiotherapy or surgery experience substantial physical and psychosocial complaints, even up to 6 years after treatment. The psychosocial distress is related to hampered communication abilities in laryngectomy patients and to eating problems and disfigurement in patients who have undergone the commando procedure. Open discussion of the disease in the family, social support, and adequate medical information can predict positive rehabilitation outcomes.

▶ This paper from The Netherlands looks at the rehabilitation of long-term survivors of head and neck cancer. The authors comment that there are few studies on the rehabilitation outcome of such patients, despite the fact that they are the majority of the long-term survivors. From this study, the reason for that is fairly clear. The data indicate that there is a high percentage of patients treated with laryngectomy or commando procedures who experience major psychosocial distress years after their treatment. This is a significantly higher risk than among patients treated with radiotherapy alone. Psychosocial and physical complaints reported by laryngectomy patients result from major problems related to ineffective communication. Patients who have undergone commando procedures with reconstruction of the pharynx frequently have major problems not only with disfigurement but, also, with aspiration of food.

The real questions are whether the patients who survive would undergo the treatment again if they knew what they were getting into and how the outcomes differ according to treatment. Unfortunately, these issues are not commented upon; however, even so, this article should be required reading for those who deal with patients who have head and neck cancer.

E. Glatstein, M.D.

15 Skin Cancer

The Orderly Progression of Melanoma Nodal Metastases
Reintgen D, Cruse CW, Wells K, Berman C, Fenske N, Glass F, Schroer K, Heller R, Ross M, Lyman G, Cox C, Rappaport D, Seigler HF, Balch C (Univ of South Florida, Tampa; MD Anderson Cancer Ctr, Houston; Duke Univ Med Ctr, Durham, NC)
Ann Surg 220:759–767, 1994　　　　　　　　　　　　　　　　15–1

Purpose.—The pattern of nodal metastases is generally thought to be random in most solid tumors. Because of the occurrence of skip nodal metastases, pathologic staging cannot be adequately done by sampling of first-station nodal basins. However, in malignant melanoma, the cutaneous lymphatic flow is better defined than in other malignancies and can be accurately mapped. If the sentinel node is negative in patients with malignant melanoma, "higher" nodes are unlikely to contain micrometastases. Preoperative and intraoperative mapping was performed in patients with malignant melanoma who were candidates for elective lymph node dissection (ELND) to assess the pattern of nodal metastases.

Methods.—The subjects were 42 patients with malignant melanoma and a primary tumor thickness of more than 0.76 mm. All were candidates for ELND, based on the preoperative lymphoscintigraphic findings of drainage to a single basin. The axilla was dissected in 27 patients, the groin in 12, and the posterior cervical triangle in 3. Mapping of the lymphatics from the primary melanoma was performed preoperatively and intraoperatively in an attempt to identify the sentinel lymph node in the regional basin, which was defined as the first node in the basin from which the primary site drained. After this node was submitted separately for pathologic evaluation, complete node dissection was performed. The analysis sought to determine the degree of skip metastases and to evaluate the likelihood of metastatic disease in the sentinel nodes vs. other nodes in the basin.

Results.—Sentinel nodes were histologically negative in 34 patients. The rest of the nodes in the basin were negative as well; therefore, these patients had no skip metastases. Sentinel nodes were positive in the other 8 patients, and in all but one patient, the sentinel node was the only site of disease. Thus, the frequency of sentinel nodal metastases in this group was 92%, with none of the higher nodes having metastatic disease. Binomial distribution was used to compare nodal involvement between the sentinel and nonsentinel nodal groups. On testing of the null hypothesis that nodal metastases would occur in equal proportions among sentinel and nonsentinel nodes, the probability that all 7 unpaired observations would consist of involvement of the sentinel nodes was only 0.008.

Conclusions.—Nodal metastases from cutaneous melanomas are not random events. Mapping and identification of the sentinel lymph nodes in the lymphatic basins show that these nodes contain the first evidence of metastases. The histologic findings in the sentinel node accurately reflect the findings in the rest of the lymphatic basin. With this information, complete node dissection can be reserved only for those patients with evidence of nodal metastatic disease. Information from sentinel node biopsy can also be used as a prognostic factor. This approach can achieve effective pathologic staging with no decrement in the standard of care and with reduced morbidity.

▶ The data in this multicenter trial confirm the report from Morton et al.,[1] which demonstrates the efficacy of identifying melanoma nodal metastases by excision of the "sentinel" node. This paper confirms the very low risk of "skip" metastases in regional lymph nodes in patients with cutaneous melanoma. The use of a vital dye allows the sentinel node(s) to be excised. If this lymph node is negative, it is highly unlikely that there are any other metastases. This is an ideal strategy when the surgeon believes an elective or prophylactic regional lymphadenectomy is indicated in a patient with a melanoma of median thickness.

It is possible to perform a minimally morbid procedure and limit a full lymphadenectomy to only those patients who have a positive sentinel node. As pointed out in this manuscript, it is more appropriate to perform a sentinel lymph node excision as a staged preliminary procedure. This will allow the pathologist to use immunohistochemical staining to detect micrometastatic foci. Because the benefit of prophylactic or elective lymph node dissection for cutaneous melanoma appears to be marginal at best, the use of sentinel node excision before a formal regional lymphadenectomy would now appear to be the standard of care.

A.M. Cohen, M.D.

Reference

1. Morton DL, Wen DR, Wong JH, et al: Technical details of intraoperative lymphatic mapping for early stage melanoma. *Arch Surg* 127:392–399, 1992.

Prognostic Parameters in Localised Melanoma: Gender Versus Anatomical Location
Karakousis CP, Driscoll DL (Roswell Park Cancer Inst, Buffalo, NY)
Eur J Cancer 31A:320–324, 1995   15–2

Background.—Two favorable prognostic factors in primary melanoma are location in an extremity and female sex. However, because these

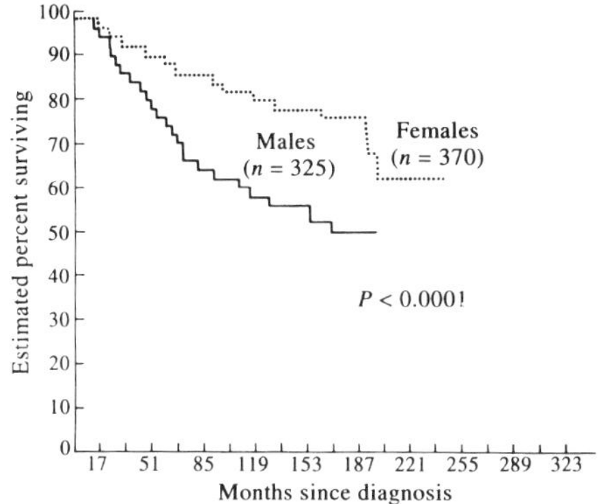

FIGURE 5.—Survival curves of patients with malignant melanoma, according to sex. (Courtesy of Karakousis CP, Driscoll DL: Prognostic parameters in localised melanoma: Gender versus anatomical location. *Eur J Cancer* 31A:320–324, 1995, with kind permission from Elsevier Science Ltd, The Boulevard, Langford Lane, Kidlington 0X5 1GB, UK.)

factors cluster in the same group of patients, it is not known whether they are independent variables.

Methods.—Six hundred ninety-five patients with localized melanoma referred between 1976 and 1988 were studied. Several prognostic parameters were analyzed. The effects of sex and anatomical location were compared directly in a multivariate analysis by sequentially controlling 1 factor while the other was free.

Findings.—Significant prognostic factors associated with survival were primary lesion thickness, the age of the patient at diagnosis, sex, and anatomical location of the primary lesion (Fig 5). Poorer prognoses were associated with thicker lesions; patients older than age 50 years; male sex; and location in the trunk, head, and neck. Survival differed significantly according to sex within each location (extremity or trunk, head, and neck). However, survival did not differ according to anatomical location within each sex.

Conclusion.—Primary lesion thickness, patient age at diagnosis, gender, and anatomical location of the melanoma are all significant prognostic indicators in localized melanoma. Sex seems to have a greater effect on survival than does anatomical location.

▶ Patients with malignant melanoma frequently perceive their disease as lethal. However, patients with relatively thin extremity melanoma—particularly women with thin extremity melanoma—have an excellent prognosis, with a 5-year survival rate of 90%. Multiple studies indicate that sex is an important prognostic factor, but it has not been clear as to whether the female sex is more highly associated with extremity melanoma, hence the more favorable prognosis. In this series of almost 700 patients at the Roswell Park Cancer Institute, multivariate analysis of all the major prognostic factors indicated that female sex is an important independent prognostic factor. The thickness of the primary lesion, the age of the patient at diagnosis, the sex, and the anatomical location are all important prognostic factors. At every anatomical location, women had an improved prognosis. The biological basis for this remains unknown.

A.M. Cohen, M.D.

Prognostic Factors in 1,521 Melanoma Patients With Distant Metastases

Barth A, Wanek LA, Morton DL (St John's Hosp and Health Ctr, Santa Monica, Calif)

J Am Coll Surg 181:193–201, 1995   15–3

Purpose.—The incidence of malignant melanoma of the skin is rapidly increasing, with 7,200 deaths from metastatic melanoma expected in 1995. However, little prognostic information for patients with metastatic melanoma is available. Variables predicting outcome in patients with melanoma who had distant metastases were assessed retrospectively.

Methods.—The analysis included 1,521 patients with American Joint Committee on Cancer (AJCC) stage IV melanoma who were treated at 1 cancer center from 1971 to 1993. The median patient age was 51 years, and 61% of patients were male. The patients received a wide range of treatments. Ten clinical and pathologic variables were evaluated as potential predictors of outcome by Cox proportional hazard regression analysis. The review also sought to determine whether survival for this patient group had changed over the years.

Results.—Just 2% of the patients had stage IV disease when first seen. The patients had a median survival of 7.5 months and an estimated 5-year survival rate of 6%. Independent predictors of survival were initial site of metastasis, disease-free interval before distant metastasis occurred, and disease stage before distant metastasis occurred. The site of the initial metastasis could be used to divide the patients into 3 prognostic groups. Those with cutaneous, nodal, or gastrointestinal metastasis had a median survival of 12.5 months and an estimated 5-year survival rate of 14%; those with pulmonary metastasis had a survival time of 8.3 months and a 5-year survival rate of 4%; and those with liver, brain, or bone metastasis had a survival time of 4.4 months and a 5-year survival rate of 3%. Survival was significantly longer for patients with a disease-free interval before distant metastasis of 72 months or longer. Across the 22-year experience, the survival rate did not improve significantly.

Conclusion.—The initial site of metastasis, disease-free interval before distant metastasis, and stage of disease before distant metastasis are independent prognostic factors for survival in patients with malignant melanoma. These variables should be taken into account in planning future treatment trials. The past 2 decades have seen no significant improvement in survival for patients with AJCC stage IV melanoma, despite advances in diagnostic imaging and the development of new treatment techniques.

▶ This study from a surgical oncology unit with a long-standing interest in this disease is a multivariate analysis of prognostic factors in patients with metastatic melanoma. The study base was over 22 years, and 10 clinical and pathologic variables were studied. Despite innovative new treatment options, the survival rate of patients with metastatic melanoma has not changed significantly. The independent variables that predicted survival included the initial site of metastasis, the disease-free interval, and the initial tumor stage. These data provide important background for ongoing clinical trials of new treatment strategies in the treatment of patients with metastatic melanoma. It is imperative that such studies use the major predictors of survival in comparing their results.

A.M. Cohen, M.D.

Primary Cutaneous Melanoma: Optimized Cutoff Points of Tumor Thickness and Importance of Clark's Level for Prognostic Classification
Büttner P, Garbe C, Bertz J, Burg G, d'Hoedt B, Drepper H, Guggenmoos-Holzmann I, Lechner W, Lippold A, Orfanos CE, Peters A, Rassner G, Stadler R, Stroebel W (Steglitz Med Center, Berlin; Federal Health Office, Berlin; German Univ, Würzburg, Germany; et al)
Cancer 75:2499–2506, 1995   15–4

Background.—The principal established prognostic factors for patients with primary cutaneous melanoma are maximum tumor thickness and the level of invasion. However, there is considerable disagreement regarding the classification of tumor thickness. A large number of patients with primary cutaneous melanoma were studied retrospectively to determine the best cutoff points of tumor thickness in relation to survival probability and to ascertain whether the combined data on tumor thickness and level of invasion improve prognostic classification compared with tumor thickness data alone.

Methods.—The records of 5,093 patients with primary cutaneous melanoma followed every 3–6 months for up to 10 years were reviewed. The histologic slide preparations were also reviewed to determine tumor thickness, level of invasion, and histologic subtype. Survival probabilities were calculated for 17 separate tumor thicknesses, ranging from 0.40 to 45 mm. Multivariate Cox proportional hazard analysis was performed, including data on age, sex, anatomical tumor location, tumor thickness, level of invasion, histologic subtype, and treatment center.

Results.—Univariate analysis of 10-year survival showed an almost linear decrease in survival from 100% to 50% in relation to tumor thickness from 0.1 to 6 mm, with no further significant survival decreases with tumor thickness greater than 6 mm (Fig 1). This relationship was also found by multivariate analysis. The best fit of classification cutoffs to survival curves was found with cutoff points at 1, 2, and 4 mm. Multivariate analysis revealed a significant independent influence of level of

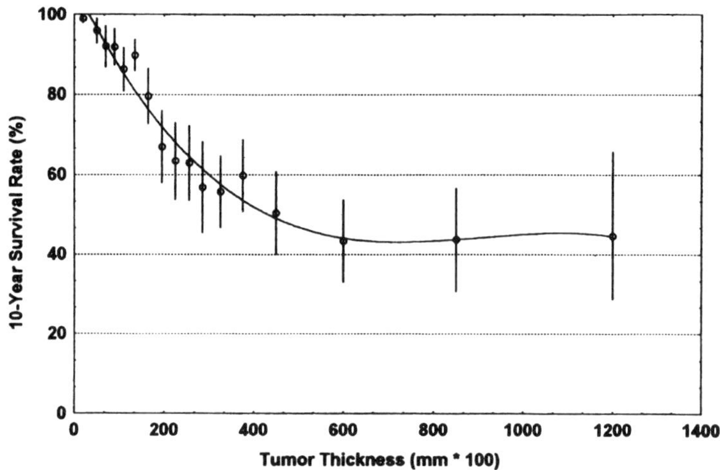

FIGURE 1.—Relationship between tumor thickness and 10-year survival rates in primary cutaneous melanoma. *Solid curve* represents an estimation of the observed relationship. *Vertical lines* indicate the 95% confidence intervals. (Courtesy of Büttner P, Garbe C, Bertz J, et al: Primary cutaneous melanoma: Optimized cutoff points of tumor thickness and importance of Clark's level for prognostic classification. *Cancer* 75:2499–2506, copyright ©1995. Reprinted by permission of Wiley-Liss, Inc., a division of John Wiley & Sons, Inc.)

invasion on survival only when the tumor thickness was ≤1 mm, whereas sex and anatomical site of tumor were important prognostic factors.

Conclusion.—Prognostic classification of patients with primary cutaneous melanoma should be based predominantly on tumor thickness, using cutoff points of 1, 2, and 4 mm, with secondary consideration of level of invasion in patients with relatively thin tumors.

Primary Cutaneous Melanoma: Prognostic Classification of Anatomic Location

Garbe C, Büttner P, Bertz J, Burg G, d'Hoedt B, Drepper H, Guggenmoos-Holzmann I, Lechner W, Lippold A, Orfanos CE, Peters A, Rassner G, Stadler R, Stroebel W (Steglitz Med Center, Berlin; Federal Health Office, Berlin; German Univ, Würzburg, Germany; et al)
Cancer 75:2492–2498, 1995   15–5

Background.—Although anatomical location has been identified as a significant prognostic factor in patients with primary cutaneous melanoma, the specific sites associated with high and lower risk have not been established. The prognostic impact of anatomical cutaneous melanoma sites was evaluated with multivariate analysis.

Methods.—A total of 5,093 patients with invasive primary cutaneous melanoma were examined every 3–6 months for up to 10 years. The anatomical location was classified into 13 sites. Survival probabilities were calculated. Cox proportional hazard analysis was used to determine the prognostic significance of various factors for predicting the increased risk of death from cutaneous melanoma.

Results.—Mean tumor thickness varied by anatomical site, from 1.83 mm at the lower arm and lower leg to greater than 2.50 mm at the scalp, foot, buttocks, and hand. The 10-year survival rates were related to tumor thickness of a particular anatomical location, but not consistently. The univariate 10-year survival rates varied from 63.4% with tumors of the scalp to 87.7% with tumors of the lower arm. In women, the most favorable site-specific survival rates occurred with tumors in the lower arm, followed by the thigh, the buttocks, and the lower leg. In men, the most favorable site-specific survival rates occurred with tumors in the abdomen, followed by the lower leg, the face, and the hand. Using the survival outcome associated with tumors of the lower leg as the baseline, the risk associated with the other anatomical sites was analyzed, controlling for tumor thickness, level of invasion, and sex. The back and breast, upper arm, neck, and scalp (TANS regions) were identified as high-risk sites, whereas the thigh, lower leg, foot, lower arms, hand, abdomen, buttocks, and face were identified as low-risk sites.

Conclusion.—The prognostic significance of anatomical location of primary cutaneous melanoma was confirmed, with tumors in the TANS regions identified as the areas of greatest risk. The locations of the low- and high-risk sites suggest that lymphatic drainage may be important factors in determining survival.

Primary Cutaneous Melanoma: Identification of Prognostic Groups and Estimation of Individual Prognosis for 5093 Patients
Garbe C, Büttner P, Bertz J, Burg G, d'Hoedt B, Drepper H, Guggenmoos-Holzmann I, Lechner W, Lippold A, Orfanos CE, Peters A, Rassner G, Stadler R, Stroebel W (Steglitz Med Ctr, Berlin; Federal Health Office, Berlin; German Univ, Würzburg, Germany; et al)
Cancer 75:2484–2491, 1995   15–6

Introduction.—Various prognostic indicators for patients with primary cutaneous melanoma have been identified, yet little research has focused on the definition of prognostic groups. The records of more than 5,000 patients with primary cutaneous melanoma were examined in an attempt to determine the relative importance of the different prognostic factors and to define prognostic categories based on combinations of prognostic factors, establishing a model for individual prognosis estimation.

Methods and Results.—Patient follow-up spanned 18 years, and the records of 5,093 of the 5,264 patients enrolled were analyzed via the multivariate Cox model. A classification and regression tree analysis was used to further analyze the records of 4,371 patients. Independent highly significant effects were revealed for tumor thickness, level of invasion, patient sex, and anatomical location of the tumor. Histologic subtype and patient age were less significant. The classification and regression tree analysis disclosed 12 well-defined subgroups of patients with primary cutaneous melanoma. Those groups were defined primarily by tumor thickness, patient sex, and tumor anatomical location. Through further analysis incorporating data from Kaplan-Meier survival curves, 5 groups were established that showed prognoses significantly different from other groups and between pairs of groups. That prognostic stratification was superior to that of the standard TNM model. Individual survival probabilities were calculated, based on the significant factors identified with the Cox model, and correlation with the observed Kaplan-Meier survival curve was good.

Discussion.—The prognostic factors identified were consistent with those recognized in other large studies. Although tumor thickness was a major factor, consideration of several additional factors significantly contributed to a better estimation of patient outcome. The final 5 groups identified provide the basis for a suggested clinical classification of patients with cutaneous melanoma. Ten-year survival rates among those 5 groups differed significantly, whereas survival rates among groups defined by tumor thickness alone or by tumor thickness and level of invasion (TNM) were less diverse. Hence, substantial improvement in prognosis estimation is possible with application of the suggested prognostic classification system.

▶ I will comment on Abstracts 15–4 through 15–6 as a group, as they represent multivariate analyses of the same group of more than 5,000 patients analyzed for prognosis. There are many patient and tumor determinants of prognosis. These result in a wide variation of long-term survival after potentially curative surgery, with a range of 14% to 97% at 10 years. Such data are important, not only for stratification in prospective clinical trials but also for advising patients as to their likely long-term survival. Many patients (as well as physicians) believe that melanoma is a highly lethal disease in almost all patients. However, as demonstrated in this series of papers, there is a large subset of patients who undergo treatment with a highly favorable outcome.

Many previous studies have suggested that anatomical location is an important prognostic factor. However, univariate analyses of site do not take into account many other known prognostic variables. The initial description of the BANS site grouping as representing the upper back, posterior arm, posterior neck, and posterior scalp as high-risk sites was not confirmed. In Abstract 15–5, comparable high-risk areas defined by Cox proportional hazards suggested the TANS regions as representing the back, breast, upper arm, neck, and scalp.

Depth of penetration, as determined by either the Clark's level by micrometer-determined tumor thickness (Breslow), was analyzed for the optimal categorization as a prognostic determinant (Abstract 15–4). Figure 1 demonstrates in a compelling fashion the relationship between tumor thickness and survival, particularly over the common range of 1–4 mm. Tumor thickness alone appears to be highly accurate in providing tumor-related prognostic information, and the stratification of 1, 2, and 4 mm was recommended by the authors. However, as shown in Figure 1, thickness appears to be a continuous variable in the large majority of patients.

Abstract 15–6 contains an exhaustive utilization of the proportional hazards model not only to identify broad prognostic groups, but to provide a mathematical model for estimating long-term prognosis in a single individual. Such categorization allows use of the major independent determinants of prognosis, which include tumor thickness, sex, anatomical location, histologic subtype, and the age of the patient.

Of particular interest in all these studies is the lack of impact of surgical treatment on overall survival. Prospective, randomized trials have evaluated prophylactic vs. therapeutic regional lymphadenectomy as well as margins in the local excisions. These studies have indicated that, in general, 2-cm margins are adequate for most patients and that a clear-cut survival benefit from prophylactic lymphadenectomy remains unproven. Ongoing studies of selective lymphadenectomy based on "sentinel node" excision are of particular interest because such strategies avoid unnecessary morbidity associated with a full lymphadenectomy when the nodes are negative.

A.M. Cohen, M.D.

Evidence That a Low-Fat Diet Reduces the Occurrence of Non-Melanoma Skin Cancer

Black HS, Thornby JI, Wolf JE Jr, Goldberg LH, Herd JA, Rosen T, Bruce S, Tschen JA, Scott LW, Jaax S, Foreyt JP, Reusser B (Baylor College of Medicine, Houston; Veterans Affairs Med Ctr, Houston)
Int J Cancer 62:165–169, 1995   15–7

Objective.—Solar ultraviolet (UV) radiation, the main cause of skin cancer, is a difficult environmental factor to avoid. Various extrinsic factors, including dietary fat, may also affect the expression of this disease. Dietary lipid affects UV-induced skin cancer in experimental animals, and a low-fat diet can ameliorate the expression of UV-induced skin cancer. A low-fat diet was studied for its preventive effects against nonmelanoma skin cancer.

Methods.—The 2-year dietary intervention trial included 101 patients with skin cancer. They were randomly allocated into 2 groups: a control group who consumed an average of 38% of calories as fat and made no change in their dietary habits and an intervention group who were instructed to limit their fat intake to 20% of total calories. Every 4 months, the patients were examined by a dermatologist who was unaware of their group assignment. Nutrient analyses were performed at the end of each follow-up visit.

Results.—The patients in the intervention group were consuming 21% of calories as fat at the 4-month follow-up visit, and they continued to follow a low-fat diet throughout the 2-year study. The 2 groups were similar in total calories and mean body weight, with no differences in the polyunsaturated/saturated fat ratio until the end of the study. For the control group, there was no change in the number of skin cancer occurrences from baseline. In contrast, patients in the low-fat diet group showed

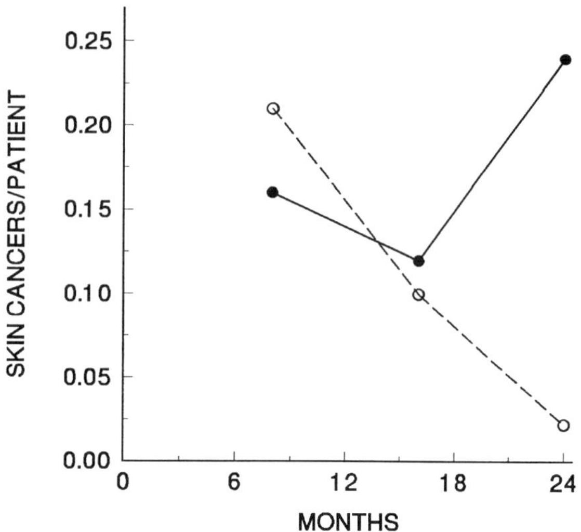

FIGURE 4.—Effect of a low-fat diet on the occurrence of skin cancer. *Filled circles,* control group; *open circles,* low-fat dietary-intervention group. *Data points* reflect number of tumors per patient for each 8-month period. (Courtesy of Black HS, Thornby JI, Wolf JE Jr, et al: Evidence that a low-fat diet reduces the occurrence of non-melanoma skin cancer. *Int J Cancer* 62:165–169, 1995. Copyright 1995, Wiley-Liss, Inc. Reprinted by permission of Wiley-Liss, Inc., a subsidiary of John Wiley & Sons, Inc.)

a decline in cancer occurrence starting at 8 months. By the end of the study, this difference had become significant. The intervention group had significantly fewer cancers in the last 8 months of the study than the control group (Fig 4). Within the intervention group, significantly fewer patients had skin cancer during the last 8 months of the study than during the first 8 months.

Conclusions.—A low-fat diet appears to reduce the occurrence of non-melanoma skin cancers. The rates of skin cancer occurrence begin to fall after as little as 1 year of following a low-fat diet. These findings are supported by previous studies showing that a reduced fat intake decreases the incidence of premalignant actinic keratosis.

▶ People in westernized societies generally obtain approximately 40% of their dietary calories from fat. It has been suggested that reducing that fat intake in half, in association with a high-fiber diet, is useful in terms of cancer prevention as well as cardiovascular disease. In this very important, prospective, randomized, 2-year dietary intervention trial, a considerable reduction in numbers of new basal or squamous cell skin cancers was noted at 2 years. This is remarkable considering the relatively short duration of this trial. These data should encourage other groups looking at prevention of breast, colorectal, and prostate cancer with dietary fat reduction. Current recommendations are to reduce dietary fat calories from 40% to 30%. However, patients who are committed to disease prevention should be encouraged to reduce their dietary fat to 20% of total calories.

A.M. Cohen, M.D.

Multiple Courses of High-Dose Total Skin Electron Beam Therapy in the Management of Mycosis Fungoides
Becker M, Hoppe RT, Knox SJ (Stanford Univ, Calif)
Int J Radiat Oncol Biol Phys 32:1445–1449, 1995   15–8

Introduction.—Many therapeutic strategies have been developed for the treatment of cutaneous mycosis fungoides (MF). The most effective single treatment method is radiation therapy either to localized lesions or to the total skin. The results of multiple courses of high-dose total skin electron beam therapy have not been published previously. The efficacy and sequelae of 2 courses of high-dose total skin electron beam therapy in 15 patients were reviewed to determine the indications, outcome, and complications of this management strategy.

Methods.—The records were reviewed of 15 patients with MF who had received 2 courses of high-dose total skin electron beam therapy between 1968 and 1990. The 9 men and 6 women had a mean age of 52 years when treated with the first course of total skin electron beam therapy. Staging before the first course revealed 3 patients with stage I, 9 with stage II, 1 with stage III, and 2 with stage IV disease. Restaging before the second course of therapy revealed 2 with stage I, 5 with stage II, 1 with stage III, and 7 with stage IV disease. The total dose to the skin was 25–36 Gy for the first course and 10–36 Gy for the second course of total skin electron beam therapy. Patient data were analyzed to determine indications for a second course of high-dose total skin electron beam therapy and to assess the response and complications in the selected patients.

Results.—Of the 15 patients, 11 had a complete response (with a mean duration of 11.6 months) and 4 had a partial response to the initial course of total skin electron beam therapy. The first and second courses of total skin therapy were separated by 6–96 months, with average intervals of 39.4 months in those with a complete response and 46.8 months in those with a partial response to the first course. Between the 2 courses, all patients received therapy with other local modalities for control of either persistent disease or relapse. Response to the second course of total skin therapy was complete in 6 patients and partial in 9. Complete responses generally had a shorter duration after the second than after the first course of therapy. Acute side effects were the same after both courses, with the most common being erythema, edema, alopecia, and dry skin. Twelve of the 15 patients have died (with death directly attributable to MF in 9), 2 are living, and 1 was lost to follow-up. Death occurred 2–66 months after the second course of total skin therapy. The 2 survivors have stable disease with topical nitrogen mustard therapy at 33 and 54 months after the second course of total skin therapy. Their long-term sequelae include scattered telangiectasias, hyperpigmentation, hypopigmentation, partial alopecia, and diffuse xerosis.

Conclusions.—The use of 2 courses of total skin electron beam therapy is effective and tolerable in appropriately selected patients. The selection criteria include initial response to total skin electron therapy followed by a long disease-free interval, exhaustion of other treatment options, diffuse recurrence, and a long interval between the 2 courses.

▶ The subject of re-treatment is very rarely discussed in the literature. This particular paper looks at re-treatment of the whole skin for mycosis fungoides, delivering high-dose electron beam therapy to the skin for 2 separate courses. The reader must understand that the point of the second course is clearly to deliver palliation. The decision to use a second course of total skin electron beam therapy virtually always is predicated upon exhaustion of all other options. If the patient genuinely got some reasonable mileage out of the first course (i.e., complete regression), has exhausted all other options, and at the same time does not show any stigmata of cutaneous morbidities from the first course, then it is reasonable to consider this type of treatment. I have done it myself on several occasions. I do think it is important to emphasize that the goal is palliative and that the patient has to be selected on the basis of not only a good response to the first course, but also no major cutaneous side effects of treatment. Telangiectasias, edema, or thin skin representing a chronic effect of the initial course of treatment are in my opinion contraindications. In addition, the long-term morbidities of the occasional patient who may survive another 15 years or so after the second course may ultimately prove excessive. Only time and good investigators will tell.

E. Glatstein, M.D.

Radiotherapy for Merkel Cell Carcinoma of the Skin of the Head and Neck
Sauntharalingam M, Rudoltz MS, Mendenhall WM, Parsons JT, Stringer SP, Million RR (Univ of Florida Health Science Ctr, Gainesville)
Head Neck 17:96–101, 1995   15–9

Background.—Merkel cell carcinoma, a relatively rare neuroendocrine carcinoma of the skin, arises in the head and neck region in approximately half of all cases. It is an aggressive tumor, predispoing patients to locoregional recurrence and distant metastases after surgical excision alone. Radiotherapy had been used in the management of this disease. An experience with Merkel cell carcinoma of the head and neck and an evaluation of the role of radiotherapy in the treatment of primary and recurrent disease were reported.

Methods.—Twelve of 18 patients with Merkel cell carcinoma treated at one center were reported. All had primary tumors in the head and neck region. Eight patients, comprising group A, were treated at initial diagnosis, and 4 patients, comprising group B, were treated at the time of locoregional recurrence.

Findings.—Locoregional control was achieved in 7 group A patients and in all group B patients. Distant metastases developed in 1 group A patient and in all group B patients, all of whom eventually died of disease. One patient had bone exposure, which required surgical débridement and hyperbaric oxygen treatment.

Conclusions.—Aggressive treatment is needed in patients with Merkel cell carcinoma of the head and neck. Locoregional recurrence appears to be a harbinger of distant metastases. Patients with such recurrence should receive treatment to both the primary site and draining lymphatics at initial presentation. The role of chemotherapy is still not clear.

▶ For whatever reasons, we are now seeing a fairly large number of patients with Merkel cell carcinoma, and it is hard to find out what the natural history is. This experience from the University of Florida consists of 12 patients with primary tumors in the head and neck region, 8 of whom were treated initially (group A) and 4 of whom were treated at time of locoregional recurrence (group B). The data show that this very radiosensitive problem frequently can be controlled locally but has a high risk of dissemination, similar to that of small cell carcinoma. In light of our lack of information on the natural history of this particular entity, this paper is important.

E. Glatstein, M.D.

The Importance of Postoperative Radiation Therapy in the Treatment of Merkel Cell Carcinoma
Meeuwissen JA, Bourne RG, Kearsley JH (Royal Brisbane and Mater Misericordiae Hosp, Queensland, Australia)
Int J Radiat Oncol Biol Phys 31:325–331, 1995   15–10

Introduction.—Merkel cell carcinoma (MCC) is a rare skin malignancy that tends to be locally aggressive and develops locoregional and distant metastases. Optimal treatment strategies are still being studied. The importance of radiotherapy was investigated, using retrospective data from a large cohort of patients.

Methods.—Over 10 years, 80 patients with histologically proven MCC were treated. Of these 80 patients, 51 were referred for initial treatment and 29 were referred for treatment of recurrent disease. Treatment strategies included surgery alone in 38 patients, surgery and postoperative radiotherapy in 34 patients, incomplete surgery and postoperative radiotherapy in 7 patients, and chemotherapy and radiotherapy in 1 patient. The patients were followed for 4–140 months (median, 20 months).

Results.—At 3 years, the disease-free survival rate was 29%, and the overall survival rate was 68%. Relapse after primary treatment occurred in 55 of the 80 patients. All 38 patients treated with surgery alone (either local excision or local plus regional lymph node excision) experienced recurrence at a median of 5.5 months. At 3 years, overall survival in this group was 65%, with a 0% disease-free survival rate. Ten of the 34 patients treated with surgery and postoperative radiotherapy had disease recurrence at a median of 16.5 months. Overall survival in this group at 3 years was 86%, with a 68% disease-free survival rate. Six of the 7 patients treated with radiotherapy after incomplete surgery relapsed. The patient treated with chemotherapy and radiotherapy has been disease-free for 21 months.

Discussion.—These data indicate that both complete surgical excision and adjuvant radiotherapy are important in treating this very aggressive malignancy.

▶ The diagnosis of MCC has become much more common in the past decade and a half. I truly do not remember seeing one case of MCC during residency or the first few years of my postresidency career. These days, I seem to bump into a case every few months or so. I do not know what they used to be called, but today they are being called Merkel cell carcinoma.

Obviously, it is not easy to find information on this entity, because most of the series represent 6 to 12 cases. This paper from Australia represents a series of 80 patients. They were reviewed retrospectively, but an indication for postoperative radiation therapy seems reasonably clear. The natural history of the disease appears to be one of high propensity for local recurrence as well as metastatic spread. It appears to be a tumor that requires both aggressive local treatment and systemic treatment, and is, in many ways, analogous to small cell cancer.

E. Glatstein, M.D.

Randomised Trial of Hyperthermia as Adjuvant to Radiotherapy for Recurrent or Metastatic Malignant Melanoma

Overgaard J, Gonzalez DG, Hulshof MCCM (Aarhus Univ Hosp, Denmark; Academisch Medisch Centrum, Amsterdam, The Netherlands; Haukeland Hosp, Bergen, Norway)
Lancet 345:540–543, 1995   15–11

Background.—Recurrent or metastatic malignant melanoma responds well to radiotherapy delivered in large doses per fraction. Uncontrolled studies suggest that adjuvant hyperthermia may improve this response.

TABLE 4.—Proportional Hazard Analysis With 2-Year Local Control as End Point

	p	Relative risk (95% CI)
Hyperthermia	0·023	1·73 (1·07–2·78)
Tumor size (largest diameter in cm)	0·050	0·91 (0·85–0·99)
Radiation dose (27 vs 24 Gy)	0·049	1·17 (1·01–1·36)
Sex (female)	0·15	..
Time to recurrence (months)	0·24	..
Tumor site (node vs cutaneous)	0·79	..
Number of tumors (multiple vs single)	0·63	..

(Courtesy of Overgaard J, Gonzalez DG, Hulshof MCCM: Randomised trial of hyperthermia as adjuvant to radiotherapy for recurrent or metastatic malignant melanoma. *Lancet* 345:540–543, copyright by The Lancet Ltd., 1995.)

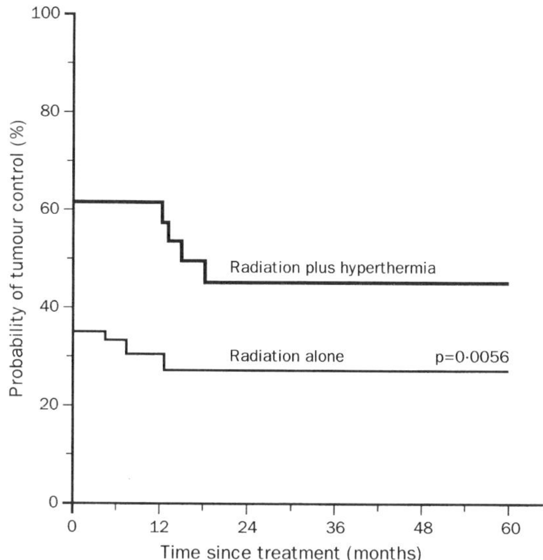

FIGURE.—Probability of tumor control after treatment with radiation alone or radiation plus hyperthermia. (Courtesy of Overgaard J, Gonzalez DG, Hulshof MCCM: Randomised trial of hyperthermia as adjuvant to radiotherapy for recurrent or metastatic malignant melanoma. *Lancet* 345:540–543, copyright by The Lancet Ltd., 1995.)

Therefore, this tumor type may provide a suitable clinical model for investigating the interaction between radiotherapy and hyperthermia. In a European multicenter trial, the value of hyperthermia as an adjuvant to radiotherapy in patients with malignant melanoma was assessed.

Methods.—Seventy patients with a total of 134 metastatic or recurrent lesions of malignant melanoma were studied. By random assignment, lesions were treated with radiotherapy alone, at a dosage of 3 fractions of 8 or 9 Gy in 8 days, or with hyperthermia, 43°C for 60 minutes.

Findings.—The overall 2-year actuarial local tumor control was 37%. In a univariate analysis, a beneficial effect of hyperthermia and radiation dose was noted, but tumor size had no effect. According to a Cox multivariate regression analysis, the most important prognostic variables were hyperthermia, tumor size, and radiation dose (Table 4). Adding hyperthermia did not significantly increase acute or late radiation reactions. Although hyperthermia was well tolerated, only 145 of the treatments achieved the protocol objective because of problems with the equipment. The overall 5-year survival rate was 19%. However, 38% of the patients for whom all known disease was controlled survived for 5 years (Figure).

Conclusions.—When given with radiation therapy, adjuvant hyperthermia significantly improved local tumor control in patients with malignant melanoma. The curative potential of successful local treatment of patients with one or a few metastatic malignant melanoma lesions was significant.

▶ Melanoma continues to be a major problem for radiation oncologists. There has been some interest, largely based on the work of Dr. Overgaard, that has led to the use of a few fractions of large size. The idea of 2,400 or 2,700 rad frankly does not seem enough, in my mind, to be able to control a melanoma, and it is interesting that this amount can control melanoma in approximately one third of the patients. On the other hand, similar radiation followed by a single exposure of 43°C of hyperthermia for 60 minutes is associated with almost half the patients having local control. This is an important study in terms of its execution. There was no increase in tissue reactions resulting from the addition of hyperthermia, and it may well be that hyperthermia truly is indicated for these patients. Certainly, based on this study, one would conclude that. Obviously, this study needs to be confirmed, but it is interesting nonetheless to see that the benefit of hyperthermia can be demonstrated in this way.

It is still surprising to me to be able to detect local control with only 3 fractions of radiation therapy, in large-size fractions. It is not clear to me why melanoma should be dramatically different from other neoplasms, virtually all of which show less morbidity and more local control (paradoxically) associated with increasing the number of fractions. This paper is provocative in terms of its demonstration of the efficacy of pauci-fraction treatment with radiation in melanoma and also in its demonstration of a benefit resulting from the administration of hyperthermia.

E. Glatstein, M.D.

16 Sarcomas

Molecular Assays for Chromosomal Translocations in the Diagnosis of Pediatric Soft Tissue Sarcomas
Barr FG, Chatten J, D'Cruz CM, Wilson AE, Nauta LE, Nycum LM, Biegel JA, Womer RB (Univ of Pennsylvania, Philadelphia; Children's Hosp of Philadelphia)
JAMA 273:553–557, 1995   16–1

Background.—Soft-tissue tumors in children commonly pose diagnostic problems. Several small round-cell tumors have been associated with consistent chromosomal translocations, and molecular assays have been developed for the detection of these translocations in clinical specimens. The value of these molecular assays for differential diagnosis was assessed in comparison with standard histopathologic and cytogenetic analysis.

Methods.—The study included frozen tumor tissue and histopathologic slides from 79 patients with soft-tissue sarcoma. The reverse transcriptase–polymerase chain reaction (RT-PCR) was used to assay tumor RNA. The chromosomal translocations detected by these assays include PAX3-FKHR and PAX7-FKHR chimeric transcripts in alveolar rhabdomyosarcoma, EWS-FLI1 and EWS-ERG chimeric transcripts in Ewing's sarcoma, and EWS-WT1 chimeric transcripts in desmoplastic small round-cell tumor (Table 1). The RT-PCR results were compared in blinded fashion with the cytogenetic and histopathologic results.

Results.—The RT-PCR assays detected chimeric transcripts in all tumors shown to have translocations by standard cytogenetic study. Chimeric transcripts were also found in additional cases without cytogenetically detectable translocations. Eighteen of 21 alveolar rhabdomyosarcomas

TABLE 1.—Consistent Chromosomal Translocations in Small Round-Cell
Tumors of Childhood

Tumor	Translocation	Chimeric Product
Alveolar rhabdomyosarcoma	t(2:13)(q35:q14)	PAX3-FKHR
	t(1:13)(p36:q14)	PAX7-FKHR
Ewing's sarcoma	t(11:22)(q24:q12)	EWS-FLI1
	t(21:22)(q22:q12)	EWS-ERG
Desmoplastic small round-cell tumor	t(11:22)(p13:q12)	EWS-WT1

TABLE 5.—Comparison of Reverse Transcriptase-Polymerase Chain Reaction (RT-PCR) and Histopathologic Results

| | Histopathologic Results | | | | | | |
RT-PCR Results	ARMS	ERMS	Ewing	DSRCT	USRCT	Other	Total
PAX3-FKHR	16	1	0	0	1	0	18
PAX7-FKHR	2	1	0	0	0	1*	4
EWS-FLI1	0	0	4	0	1	0	5
EWS-ERG	0	0	2	0	0	0	2
EWS-WT1	0	0	0	3	0	0	3
Negative	3	28	2	0	5	9	47
Total	21	30	8	3	7	10	79

* This PAX7-FKHR fusion occurred in a rhabdomyosarcoma that could not be further classified because of treatment effect.

Abbreviations: ARMS, alveolar rhabdomyosarcoma; *ERMS*, embryonal rhabdomyosarcoma; *Ewing*, Ewing's sarcoma, including peripheral primitive neuroectodermal tumors; *DSRCT*, desmoplastic small round-cell tumor; *USRCT*, undifferentiated small round-cell tumor.

(Courtesy of Barr FG, Chatten J, D'Cruz CM, et al: Molecular assays for chromosomal translocations in the diagnosis of pediatric soft tissue sarcomas. *JAMA* 273:553–557, Copyright 1995, American Medical Association.)

showed PAX3-FKHR or PAX7-FKHR fusions, as did 2 of 30 embryonal rhabdomyosarcomas and 1 of 7 undifferentiated sarcomas. Six of 8 Ewing's sarcomas and 1 of 7 undifferentiated sarcomas showed EWS-FLI1 or EWS-ERG fusions. All 3 desmoplastic small round-cell tumors in the series showed the EWS-WT1 fusion (Table 5).

Conclusion.—A genetic approach to the differential diagnosis of soft-tissue sarcomas in children is possible with molecular assays for specific gene fusions. There is close correlation between the genetic findings and the standard histopathologic categories. The assays used in this study are useful tools for routine application in the rapid and objective assessment of pediatric soft-tissue sarcomas.

▶ Genetic methods are well established in the treatment decision-making process of patients with hematologic malignancies. For example, a 9;22 translocation can be found in chronic myelogenous leukemia and in variants of acute myelogenous leukemia, and it has important diagnostic and therapeutic implications. The presence of this marker chromosome can be detected by cytogenetic and molecular genetic assays for the translocation, as well as by methods that can detect the fusion protein. The use of such methods in the management of patients with solid tumors is not well established. Among the sarcomas arising in children, distinct chromosomal markers have been described in alveolar rhabdomyosarcoma, Ewing's sarcoma, and desmoplastic small round-cell tumors (see Table 1).

"Small round-cell tumors" are a diverse group of morphologically similar tumors including the rhabdomyosarcomas, osseous and extraosseous Ewing's sarcoma, neuroblastoma, and lymphoma. Therapy differs for these tumors and, therefore, a precise diagnosis is necessary to choose proper treatment. The authors compared the results of molecular assays for the chromosomal translocation with standard histopathologic and cytogenetic analysis. The molecular assay used was the PCR. Informative tumor karyotypes were obtained in only 29 of 74 evaluable tumors (39%), and a characteristic translocation was identified in 11. The PCR technique identified the fusion transcript in all 11 cases in which cytogenetic analysis was successful, plus an additional 4 cases that did not demonstrate the characteristic translocation. This suggests that the PCR technique is more sensitive than cytogenetic analysis.

The 79 cases chosen for analysis included both embryonal and alveolar rhabdomyosarcoma, Ewing's sarcoma, desmoplastic small round-cell tumors, undifferentiated small round-cell tumors, and other tumors of similar morphology (Table 5). The histopathologic classification corresponded to the PCR result in 18 of 21 (86%) alveolar rhabdomyosarcomas, 28 of 30 (93%) embryonal rhabdomyosarcomas, 6 of 8 (75%) Ewing's sarcomas, 3 of 3 (100%) desmoplastic small round-cell tumors, 5 of 7 (71%) undifferentiated small round-cell tumors, and 9 of 10 (90%) other small round-cell tumors. Therefore, the concordance was good. However, 4 additional cases of alveolar rhabdomyosarcoma and 1 additional case of Ewing's sarcoma were identified by the use of PCR among tumors that had been classified differently. In addition, 3 tumors morphologically characterized as alveolar rhabdomyosarcoma and 2 classified as Ewing's sarcoma did not contain characteristic transcripts. Therefore, on the basis of molecular analysis, 10 of 79 (13%) would have been classified differently on the basis of molecular analysis and, perhaps, would have undergone different therapy.

These data suggest that routine histopathology can be enhanced by molecular diagnostics. The era of molecular diagnosis for solid tumors has arrived, and as additional characteristic lesions are identified among the more common solid tumors, one can expect that these techniques will become routinely available in general pathology laboratories and that the results will have important clinical decision-making implications.

G.J. Bosl, M.D.

Doxorubicin Versus CYVADIC Versus Doxorubicin Plus Ifosfamide in First-Line Treatment of Advanced Soft Tissue Sarcomas: A Randomized Study of the European Organization for Research and Treatment of Cancer Soft Tissue and Bone Sarcoma Group
Santoro A, Tursz T, Mouridsen H, Verweij J, Steward W, Somers R, Buesa J, Casali P, Spooner D, Rankin E, Kirkpatrick A, Van Glabbeke M, van Oosterom A (Istituto Nazionale Tumori, Milan, Italy; Hosp General de Asturias, Oviedo, Italy; Institut Gustave Roussy, Paris; et al)
J Clin Oncol 13:1537–1545, 1995   16–2

Background.—More active chemotherapy regimens are needed to improve the final outcomes of patients with soft-tissue sarcomas. In a European Organization for Research and Treatment of Cancer (EORTC) Soft Tissue and Bone Sarcoma Group phase II trial, begun in 1984, doxorubicin, 50 mg/m², plus ifosfamide, 5,000 mg/m², given in a 24-hour continuous infusion with mesna as a uroprotector produced a 35% response rate in evaluable patients with advanced disease. Toxicity was acceptable. A phase III trial was, therefore, initiated to compare this combination of doxorubicin and ifosfamide with single-agent doxorubicin as well as a multidrug regimen without ifosfamide—cyclophosphamide, vincristine, doxorubicin, and dacarbazine (CYVADIC).

Methods.—Thirty-five centers associated with the EORTC participated in a prospective, randomized trial. Six hundred sixty-three eligible patients were randomly assigned to receive doxorubicin, 75 mg/m^2, on treatment arm A; CYVADIC on arm B; or ifosfamide, 5 g/m^2, plus doxorubicin, 50 mg/m^2, on arm C.

Findings.—The overall response rate among eligible patients was 24%, and among evaluable patients it was 26%. The response rates among the 3 treatment arms did not differ significantly. They were 23.3% in arm A, 28.4% in arm B, and 28.1% in arm C. The duration of remission in arms A, B, and C was 46 weeks, 48 weeks, and 44 weeks, respectively, which also was not significantly different. The median overall survival rates among the 3 arms were comparable, at 52, 51, and 55 weeks, respectively. The degree of myelosuppression was significantly greater for ifosfamide plus doxorubicin than for the other 2 regimens. Cardiotoxicity was also more common in arm C, although other toxicities were similar.

Conclusion.—Single-agent doxorubicin remains the standard against which more intensive or new drug chemotherapies should be compared in adults with advanced soft-tissue sarcomas. Combination chemotherapy is not recommended outside of a controlled clinical trial from which patients requiring significant tumor volume reduction are excluded.

▶ It has been 20 years since the value of doxorubicin chemotherapy was demonstrated in the treatment of metastatic adult soft-tissue sarcoma. The initial reports indicated a response rate of 20% to 25%. As with other diseases, with the demonstration that responses were obtained with a number of other drugs, the use of combination chemotherapy in this disease was recommended.

This article reports a decade of experience from 35 cancer centers representing the EORTC Soft Tissue and Bone Sarcoma Group. More than 600 patients were treated, and as reported in the abstract, neither the response rate nor survival in the combination chemotherapy arms showed any measurable difference from the relatively less toxic arm receiving doxorubicin alone. This article points out the importance of progressing from phase II trials to randomized protocols if advances in chemotherapy for advanced disease are to be elucidated.

A.M. Cohen, M.D.

Liposomal Doxorubicin: Antitumor Activity and Unique Toxicities During Two Complementary Phase I Studies
Uziely B, Jeffers S, Isacson R, Kutsch K, Wei-Tsao D, Yehoshua Z, Libson E, Muggia FM, Gabizon A (Univ of Southern California, Los Angeles; Hadassah Hebrew Univ, Jerusalem)
J Clin Oncol 13:1777–1785, 1995   16–3

Introduction.—Liposomal doxorubicin preparations have been suggested as an alternative to prolonged infusions of doxorubicin, as they may increase efficacy, decrease toxicity, or overcome resistance. A liposomal doxorubicin preparation with a polyethylene glycol coating, DOX-SL, has been formulated. Preclinical studies of DOX-SL showed enhanced accumulation in tumors and substantial antitumor activity in murine models. In addition, DOX-SL has demonstrated a significantly different pharmacokinetic profile, compared with free doxorubicin. The maximal tolerated dose of DOX-SL and the toxicities associated with its administration were studied in 2 phase I trials.

Methods.—The study populations included patients with a variety of assessable solid tumors that had not responded to therapy. In 1 trial, the dose of DOX-SL was begun at 20 mg/m^2 every 3 weeks, with the dose escalating in increments of 20 mg/m^2. In the other trial, patients were initially given DOX-SL doses of 60 mg/m^2 every 3 weeks, which was changed to the same dose every 4 weeks because of skin toxicity with the initial dosing schedule. The patients were assessed for antitumor response and for toxicity.

Results.—Six patients exhibited an acute reaction to the infusion at the first exposure, characterized by flushing, choking sensation, back pain, or hypotension, which resolved after the infusion was discontinued. Two of these patients were successfully re-treated with slower infusions and premedication with hydrocortisone, cimetidine, and diphenhydramine. The major dose-limiting toxic reactions were mucositis (stomatitis-pharyngitis) and skin toxicity (hand-foot syndrome). Other toxicities were generally mild and reversible and included alopecia, pigmentation, conjunctivitis, and nausea and vomiting.

Doses of 20 and 40 mg/m^2 were well tolerated, but higher doses resulted in increasing need for dose reduction. The dosing schedule was also important; dose reduction was required more frequently at higher doses with 3-week intervals than with 4-week intervals. Of the 45 assessable patients, 8 (18%) had a partial antitumor response, 7 (16%) showed improvement, and 4 had stable disease. There were no antitumor responses with the dose of 20 mg/m^2. Responsive tumors included breast, prostate, non–small-cell lung, renal cell, mesothelioma, head and neck, and ovary cancers.

Discussion.—The enhanced antitumor activity and reduced toxicity profile with DOX-SL compared with free doxorubicin may be the result of the effects of slow-release and prolonged systemic exposure or of preferential extravasation of liposomal drug in the tumor. Phase II testing of DOX-SL in patients with solid tumors is warranted.

▶ Liposomal delivery of drugs may have a role in cancer treatment because of alterations in the pharmacokinetic properties of the cytotoxic moiety as well as in improved drug-tissue distribution. Preclinical studies with polyethylene glycol-n-coated long-circulating liposomes have shown enhanced accumulation of DOX-SL in both ascitic and solid tumors. Liposome extravasation through microvascular beds leads to deposition of the liposomal contents in the extracellular fluid compartment, thereby improving drug delivery.

This is one of the most comprehensive clinical studies examining the toxicity and antitumor activity of liposomal doxorubicin. The toxicity profile that was observed resembles that associated with a prolonged continuous infusion of doxorubicin. The 18% overall response rate in this phase I trial is encouraging, as is the demonstration that there were some responses to the liposomal doxorubicin in patients who had received prior therapy with doxorubicin. Whether the liposomal formulation can overcome resistance to doxorubicin, however, remains to be established.

R.F. Ozols, M.D., Ph.D.

Aggressive Fibromatosis: Optimisation of Local Management With a Retrospective Failure Analysis
Catton CN, O'Sullivan B, Bell R, Cummings B, Fornasier V, Panzarella T (Univ of Toronto, Ont, Canada; Princess Margaret Hosp, Toronto, Ont, Canada; Wellesley Hosp, Toronto, Canada)
Radiother Oncol 34:17–22, 1995
16–4

Background.—Aggressive fibromatosis, a cellular tumor composed of well-differentiated fibroblasts, is an uncommon, benign soft-tissue neoplasm. Decision-making about treatment is difficult because of the variable natural history of the disease. A retrospective review of the outcomes in 40 consecutive patients treated for aggressive fibromatosis at one center was performed.

Patients and Findings.—The patients were 27 females and 13 males, aged 11 to 78 years at diagnosis, treated between 1979 and 1988. The median follow-up was 86 months. Excision was attempted in 36 patients, and biopsy was performed in 4. Thirty-one patients had no overt disease after surgery, 26 of whom received adjuvant irradiation. Eight patients underwent radiotherapy alone. Another patient was treated with azathioprine and prednisone. Sixty percent of the patients had recurrent disease at presentation. The overall relapse-free rate at 5 and 10 years was 63% (Fig 2). Combined surgery and irradiation was associated with a 46% relapse rate compared with 25% for irradiation alone. Thirty-six percent of the failures in the combined group were marginal. The relapse rate after surgery alone was 20%, and after chemotherapy, 0. Relapse could be

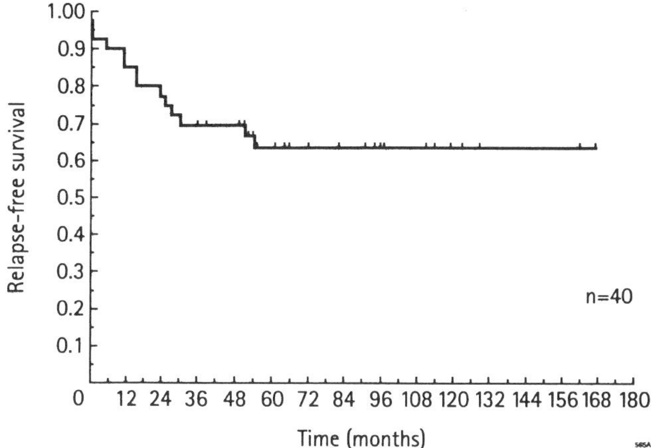

FIGURE 2.—Forty patients treated for aggressive fibromatosis. Relapse-free survival estimated by the Kaplan-Meier method. (Courtesy of Catton CN, O'Sullivan B, Bell R, et al: Aggressive fibromatosis: Optimisation of local management with a retrospective failure analysis. *Radiother Oncol* 34:17–22, 1995, with kind permission of Elsevier Science—NL, Sara Burgerhartstraat 25, 1055 KV Amsterdam, The Netherlands.)

predicted by tumor size greater than 8 cm but not by tumor site, status of surgical margins, and the presence or absence of a history of relapse. Twelve patients with subsequent treatment failure underwent successful salvage surgery. Ninety-two percent were free of disease at the last follow-up. A functional assessment showed that 46% of patients had poor functional outcomes after all treatment compared with 25% at referral. Ninety-one percent of the patients with a grade of 2 or less had a history of recurrence. Amputations were performed because of painful recurrence in 4 of 5 patients.

Conclusions.—In this series, treatment planning was hindered by insufficient information on tumor location. Few patients had clinically apparent disease when seen by the radiation oncologist, and even fewer patients had preoperative cross-sectional imaging available. Relapse and poor functional outcome were related. A thorough pretreatment assessment of local disease and optimal selection, integration, and delivery of available treatment modalities is needed to attain high rates of local control with good functional outcomes. Combined treatment with surgery and irradiation should be considered and planned jointly for patients at risk for relapse or those with disease in sites where relapse would subsequently compromise function.

▶ Aggressive fibromatosis represents a particular type of sarcoma that basically has no predilection for dissemination but has a tremendous predisposition toward local recurrence. These lesions can also be categorized as desmoids. There are not many large series of patients with aggressive fibromatosis, and this article represents one of the better studies, assessing 40 patients treated between 1979 and 1988. It takes a long time to feel comfortable about the adequacy of treatment for such lesions; fortunately, this series has a long follow-up (median, 86 months). One of the interesting features of this series is that the local relapse rate was worse for patients who had surgery and radiation combined (46%) than it was for patients treated with radiation therapy alone (25%). Many of the failures in the combined group represented failures at the edge of the field rather than in the middle, suggesting that the radiation oncologist put too much emphasis on the adequacy of the surgery and did not use a big enough target volume.

I have had the experience of treating many of these patients myself, and if there is one thing I have learned over the years, it is that you need a large volume for aggressive fibromatosis. It does come up at the edge of the field, and you have to make allowance for extremely generous margins. These margins, by definition, must be greater than what one would ordinarily use, even if there has been "a complete surgical resection." Histologically, these lesions are sufficiently bland that the description of the adequacy of the margins is not terribly helpful. This is one reason why one has to use generous fields.

This series form the Princess Margaret Hospital, one of the great institutions in cancer treatment in the world, is less than ideal because of problems associated with tumor imaging. Twelve percent of the patients did not have pretreatment cross-sectional imaging in the form of CT or MRI. Many patients required an amputation for recurrence; this is not unusual in the management of what is a local disease. If one is going to perform surgery, one has to do an extensive surgical procedure for this diagnosis. Over the years, the most common mistake that I have seen associated with this diagnosis is inadequate surgery and/or inadequate radiation in terms of volume. It is incredibly easy to underestimate the extent of the problem, either surgically or radiotherapeutically, and one has to allow for this in the management strategy. This series represents a useful and valuable experience for the reader.

E. Glatstein, M.D.

Supraomohyoid Neck Dissection as a Staging Procedure for Squamous Cell Carcinomas of the Oral Cavity and Oropharynx
Henick DH, Silver CE, Heller KS, Shaha AR, El GH, Wolk DP (Montefiore Med Ctr, Bronx, NY)
Head Neck 17:119–123, 1995   16–5

Background.—In patients with squamous cell carcinoma of the oral cavity and orophayrnx, the presence or absence of cervical metastasis is an important indicator of survival. Many surgeons perform supraomohyoid neck dissection (SOHND) to detect clinically occult cervical metastatic disease. The efficacy of this practice was investigated.

Methods.—Seventy-five previously untreated patients with clinically negative necks were assessed in a multi-institutional retrospective study. Twenty-three percent of the neck specimens showed occult metastatic disease, and 77% were negative histologically. Ninety-four percent of the patients with positive specimens and 22% of those with negative specimens underwent postoperative irradiation. Patients were followed for 2 years or longer, until neck disease recurred.

Findings.—Cervical metastasis subsequently developed in one fourth of the treated patients with positive specimens. Metastasis developed in none of the untreated patients with positive specimens, in 8% of the treated patients with negative specimens, and in 11% of the untreated patients with negative specimens. Supraomohyoid neck dissection had a sensitivity of 82% for cervical metastasis, a negative predictive value of 91%, and an accuracy of 94%.

Conclusions.—Supraomohyoid neck dissection in patients with primary squamous cell carcinoma of the oral cavity and oropharynx effectively predicts occult metastasis because of its high sensitivity, negative predictive value, and overall accuracy. The pathologic findings in SOHND apparently influence the choice of further treatment. That patients with positive and negative specimens had identical 2-year survival rates may reflect the effect of more aggressive treatment, as influenced by positive SOHND findings. Extensive lymph node dissection seems to offer no diagnostic advantage over a more limited neck dissection in the assessment of occult cervical metastasis.

▶ This study represents a multi-institutional retrospective analysis evaluating the efficacy of SOHND for the detection of occult cervical metastases in squamous cell carcinoma of the oral cavity and oropharynx. A total of 75 previously untreated patients with clinical negative necks were studied. Seventeen patients (23%) revealed occult metastatic disease, whereas 58 patients (77%) were histologically negative. Postoperative irradiation was received by 94% of the patients who had positive specimens and by only 22% of those with negative specimens. Of those that received postoperative radiation therapy for a positive neck, only 4 patients had local recurrence in the neck, and a total of 6 patients had recurrence in the primary site. Of those who received postoperative radiation for negative neck specimens, only 1 had recurrence in the neck nodes, and 2 had recurrence in the primary site.

The authors claim they could not demonstrate a significant difference in the recurrence rate among the postoperatively irradiated and nonirradiated patients in this small sample. This is not surprising because they are two totally separate groups that cannot be compared because the patients who were irradiated basically represented a group of positively explored patients who had a high risk of recurrent disease, whereas the nonirradiated patients represented those who had a low risk of recurrent disease, i.e., most of them were patients who were pathologically negative. That the recurrence rates were similar statistically confirms the benefit of radiation therapy in the high-risk (i.e., node-positive) group.

The authors concluded that the SOHND is a valuable procedure for staging patients with squamous cell carcinoma of the oral cavity and oropharynx. That may be true, but how much value is it really? In patients who have no known disease in the neck, what would happen if they were simply irradiated? How many of them would, in fact, have recurrence without any dissection? I suspect that most of them would not have recurrence, even without a staging procedure. Somehow, it seems to me that the need for the dissection to help stage the disease is really excessive frosting on the cake.

E. Glatstein, M.D.

Management of Extremity Soft Tissue Sarcomas With Limb-Sparing Surgery and Postoperative Irradiation: Do Total Dose, Overall Treatment Time, and the Surgery-Radiotherapy Interval Impact on Local Control?

Fein DA, Lee WR, Lanciano RM, Corn BW, Herbert SH, Hanlon AL, Hoffman JP, Eisenberg BL, Coia LR (Fox Chase Cancer Ctr, Philadelphia, Pa)
Int J Radiat Oncol Biol Phys 32:969–976, 1995
16–6

Objective.—Adjuvant radiotherapy has become a routine part of management for patients with extremity soft-tissue sarcomas. However, the effects of various radiation treatment factors on local control—total dose, surgery-radiotherapy interval, and overall treatment time—remain unclear. These and other potential prognostic factors were evaluated for their effects on local control, distant metastases, and overall survival in patients with extremity soft-tissue sarcomas.

Methods.—The analysis included 67 patients with extremity soft-tissue sarcomas who underwent limb-sparing surgery and postoperative radiation therapy over 21 years. All patients were treated with curative intent. The median dose of external beam radiation was 60.4 Gy, and 13 patients received interstitial brachytherapy as a part of treatment. The patients were followed for a median of 31 months. Clinical and treatment variables were examined for their effects on local control, survival, and distant metastasis.

Results.—The 5-year local control rate was 87% overall, 95% for those who received more than 62.5 Gy of radiation, and 78% for those who received a lower dose (Fig 2). The patients in the higher radiation dose group had significantly larger tumors, a higher percentage of grade 3 tumors, and a higher percentage of positive surgical margins. Patients with negative or close surgical margins had a 5-year local control rate of 100% compared with 56% for those with positive margins. The covariates in Cox proportional hazards regression analysis were tumor dose, overall treatment time, time from surgery to the start of radiation therapy, margin status, grade, and tumor size. Of those, only total dose and marginal status had a significant impact on local control. The only factor that significantly influenced distant metastasis or survival was tumor size.

Conclusions.—For patients with extremity soft-tissue sarcomas, a postoperative radiation therapy dose of greater than 62.5 Gy is needed to make a significant improvement in local control. This is the first study to show that total dose has an independent effect on local control of extremity

By Total Dose Groups

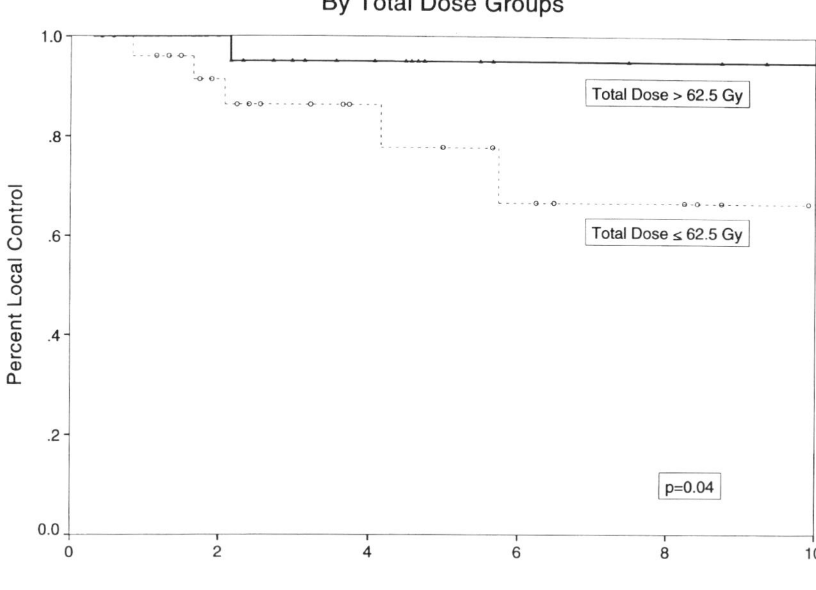

FIGURE 2.—Local control by total dose group of extremity soft tissue sarcomas after postoperative irradiation. (Courtesy of Fein DA, Lee WR, Lanciano RM, et al: Management of extremity soft tissue sarcomas with limb-sparing surgery and postoperative irradiation: Do total dose, overall treatment time, and the surgery-radiotherapy interval impact on local control? *Int J Radiat Oncol Biol Phys* 32:969–976, 1995. Copyright 1995 with kind permission from Elsevier Science Ltd, The Boulevard, Langford Lane, Kidlington OX5 1GB, UK.)

soft-tissue sarcomas. Although the higher dose brings an improvement in local control, there may be an associated increase in the rate of complications.

▶ The treatment of soft-tissue sarcoma frequently involves combined surgical resection and adjuvant radiation therapy. Radiation therapy may be given preoperatively, postoperatively, or by iridium-192 brachytherapy. In this Cox proportional hazards regression analysis of covariants associated with local control, surgical resection margin status and radiation therapy dose were the important predictors of local control. The data suggest that at a dichotomy of 62.5 Gy with negative margins, local control can be expected in 95% of patients. Once again, we have data demonstrating the importance of careful surgical/radiation oncology interaction to maximize functional and cancer eradication results in the multimodality treatment of cancer.

A.M. Cohen, M.D.

17 Bone Marrow Transplantation and Stem Cell Support

Autologous Bone Marrow Transplantation for Acute Myeloid Leukemia in First Remission: Identification of Modifiable Prognostic Factors
Mehta J, Powles R, Singhal S, Horton C, Tait D, Milan S, Meller S, Pinkerton CR, Treleaven J (Royal Marsden Hosp, Sutton, England)
Bone Marrow Transplant 16:499–506, 1995

17–1

Introduction.—Despite complete remission rates as high as 80%, no more than 30% of adult patients with acute myeloid leukemia (AML) achieve long-term disease-free survival when given conventional chemotherapy. Intensive consolidation therapy improves the outcome somewhat. Allogeneic marrow transplantation is indicated for young patients when a sibling donor is available, but only a minority of patients are candidates.

Objective.—Modifiable treatment-related and transplant-related factors were sought in 74 consecutive patients in first remission of AML who received unpurged autologous bone marrow after conditioning with melphalan and total-body irradiation.

Results.—Four patients died of transplant-related causes before neutrophil recovery. Ultimately, 14 patients died of this cause. There was no unusual toxicity. Thirty patients (40.5%) relapsed a median of 7.5 months after marrow transplantation. The same number of patients were alive and well in continued remission when last followed for a median of 37.5 months after transplantation.

Prognostic Factors.—The factor most closely associated with a decreased risk of relapse and improved disease-free survival was the administration of 2 or more courses of consolidation chemotherapy before marrow transplantation. Patients given more than 2×10^8 nucleated cells/kg had more than a twofold better chance of surviving without disease because of a decreased risk of transplant-related death.

Conclusion.—The single most effective way of limiting the risk of relapse of AML is to administer adequate consolidation chemotherapy before bone marrow transplantation. In addition, providing an adequate number of nucleated cells will lessen the risk of transplant-related death.

▶ For patients who are candidates for allogeneic bone marrow transplantation but cannot undergo the procedure because of the lack of an available suitable donor, autologous bone marrow transplantation is an alternative strategy that is receiving a great deal of attention. Although this procedure is associated with less risk of morbidity and mortality, relapse after transplantation is common. This study identifies prognostic variables for patients with AML who are undergoing autologous bone marrow transplantation.

A multivariant analysis was done, the important finding of which was that the administration of 2 or more courses of consolidation chemotherapy before the harvest and transplant was found to be the most significant factor associated with a decreased risk of relapse and an improved disease-free survival. A nucleated cell dose greater than 2×10^8/kg resulted in an improved disease-free survival by decreasing the transplant-related mortality. Although this study suggests that 2 or more cycles of consolidation chemotherapy significantly improved disease-free survival and diminished the relapse rate, the consolidation chemotherapy administered was unconventional.

Most other studies have suggested that high-dose cytarabine may provide the optimal consolidation chemotherapy regimen, but this study included patients who received 6-thioguanine and cytarabine, the latter administered at a dose of 60 mg/m² every 12 hours in 3 blocks of 3, 4, and 5 days, respectively, at 5-day intervals. Other patients received the regimen just described, followed by a cycle of amsacrine and cytarabine at a dose of 200 mg/m² on days 1 through 5 and etoposide at 100 mg/m² on days 1 through 5. Therefore, although the consolidation chemotherapy regimen was not completely uniform and was not what is often administered as high-dose cytarabine, the observations that were made do suggest that multiple cycles of postremission chemotherapy may benefit patients who subsequently undergo autologous bone marrow transplantation.

M.S. Tallman, M.D.

Allogeneic Sibling Umbilical-Cord-Blood Transplantation in Children With Malignant and Non-Malignant Disease
Wagner JE, Kernan NA, Steinbuch M, Broxmeyer HE, Gluckman E (Univ of Minnesota, Minneapolis; Mem Sloan Kettering Cancer Ctr, New York; Indiana Univ, Indianapolis; et al)
Lancet 346:214–219, 1995   17–2

Background.—Since the first successful umbilical cord blood transplant procedure was performed in 1988, many patients with malignant and nonmalignant disorders undergoing high-dose chemotherapy and radiotherapy have been treated with the infusion of umbilical cord blood from

HLA-identical and HLA-disparate donors. The first 44 consecutive cases reported to the International Cord Blood Transplant Registry were reviewed to determine outcomes.

Methods.—The children included in the analysis had acquired or congenital lymphohematopoietic disorders, neuroblastoma, or metabolic diseases. The first of their procedures was done in September 1994. Umbilical cord blood from sibling donors was used to reconstitute hematopoiesis in all cases.

Findings.—Engraftment probability at 50 days after transplantation was 85% in patients with HLA-identical and HLA-1 antigen disparate grafts. There was no instance of late graft failure. The 100-day probability of grade II–IV graft-vs.-host disease (GVHD) was 3%. At 1 year, this probability was 6%. The recipients of HLA-identical or HLA-1 antigen disparate grafts had a 72% probability of survival with a median 1.6-year follow-up.

Conclusions.—In this series, GVHD was uncommon. Grade II acute GVHD developed in only 1 of 30 patients with HLA-identical or HLA-1 antigen disparate sibling donors. The rest of the patients had no GVHD or only limited cutaneous rashes. Grade I GVHD developed in 2 of the 4 patients with HLA-2 and HLA-3 mismatches, grade II developed in a third patient, and grade III in the last. The 2 patients with grade II and III acute GVHD had donors disparate at the noninherited paternal allele, whereas the 2 patients who did not have significant acute GVHD had donors disparate at the noninherited maternal allele, supporting earlier observations that partial tolerance to the noninherited maternal allele may develop during gestation.

▶ This is a fascinating compilation by the International Cord Blood Transplant Registry of patients treated with high-dose chemotherapy and radiotherapy with the infusion of umbilical cord blood. Why cord blood? There are 2 main reasons: first, it is available with ease when a newborn sibling presents itself at the appropriate time; and second, there is experimental and clinical evidence that stem cells from cord blood are less likely to cause GVHD. Those hypotheses were essentially confirmed in this report.

Bone marrow transplanters are continuously exploring ways to overcome several problems with the use of this technology. The first problem is the unavailability of matched donors for allogeneic transplants. The ability to use cord blood from a newborn infant, although a relatively rare occasion, provides a useful additional source of stem cells. Second, stem cells obtained from cord blood have the unusual property of causing less GVHD, particularly if there are mismatch sites on the maternal side, because partial tolerance apparently develops during gestation. Transplanters are also pushing the frontiers by doing more allogeneic transplants with greater mismatches and are beginning to find ways to overcome the consequences, i.e., severe GVHD, which would also enlarge the pool of marrow or stem cell donors.

The day may come when the effects of giving mismatched transplants can be sufficiently mitigated so that the availability of donors is more akin to that of blood transfusion donors.

J.V. Simone, M.D.

Unrelated Bone Marrow Donor Transplants for Children With Leukemia or Myelodysplasia
Casper J, Camitta B, Truitt R, Baxter-Lowe LA, Bunin N, Lawton C, Murray K, Hunter J, Pietryga D, Garbrecht F, Taylor CK, Drobyski W, Horowitz M, Flomenberg N, Ash R (Med College of Wisconsin, Milwaukee; Blood Ctr of Southeastern Wisconsin, Milwaukee; Children's Hosp of Wisconsin, Milwaukee)
Blood 85:2354–2363, 1995

17–3

Introduction.—Many types of childhood leukemia are treated by allogeneic bone marrow transplantation (BMT). The best donor in this situation is an HLA-matched sibling; however, a matched related donor is available for only about 30% of the patients. The chances of finding an unrelated donor have increased with the creation of the National Marrow Donor Program and other registries. The results of unrelated donor BMT for 50 children with leukemia or myelodysplasia were studied.

Methods.—The patients were 31 boys and 19 girls (median age, 9 years). Twenty-five had acute lymphoblastic leukemia, 3 had acute myeloid leukemia, 3 had juvenile chronic myelogenous leukemia, 10 had chronic myeloid leukemia, and 9 had myelodysplastic syndrome. All received BMT from an unrelated donor between 1986 and 1991. Thirteen patient-donor pairs were serologically matched at HLA-A, B, DR, and DQ; 6 of these were reactive in mixed lymphocyte culture. Thirty-six patients were mismatched for 1 HLA antigen, and 1 patient was mismatched for more than 1 antigen. The conditioning regimens included cytosine arabinoside, cyclophosphamide, fractionated total body irradiation, and methylprednisolone. Busulfan was given to high-risk patients. T-cell depletion with IgM monoclonal antibody T10B9 plus complement and posttransplant cyclosporine A were used for prophylaxis against graft-vs.-host disease (GVHD).

Results.—The engraftment rate was 98%. The recipients took a median of 18 days to reach a polymorphonuclear leukocyte count of greater than 500/µL and 20 days to reach a platelet count of more than 25,000/µL. Thirty-three percent of the patients had grade II or greater GVHD, and 81% of these died. Although 30 of 40 patients at risk had chronic GVHD, it was extensive in only 5. At a median follow-up of 49 months, the event-free survival rate was 44%, and the overall survival rate was 50%. The event-free survival rate was 60% for patients with low-risk disease—i.e., acute lymphoblastic leukemia or acute myeloid leukemia in first or second remission or chronic myelogenous leukemia in chronic phase—compared with 34% for patients with high-risk disease. The event-free

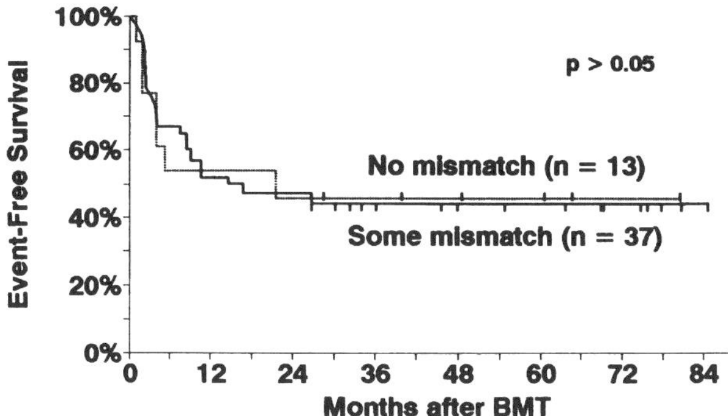

FIGURE 3.—Probability of event-free survival for patients who received matched or mismatched marrow from an unrelated donor. Patients currently disease free are represented by tick marks. (Courtesy of Casper J, Camitta B, Truitt R, et al: Unrelated bone marrow donor transplants for children with leukemia or myelodysplasia. *Blood* 85:2354–2363, 1995.)

survival rate was 46% for patients who were serologically matched with their donors and 43% for those who were partially mismatched (Fig 3).

Conclusion.—Unrelated donor BMT can be successful in children with leukemia or myelodysplasia, even with a major HLA mismatch. These transplants offer a chance for long-term disease-free survival and cure for patients who would otherwise die of their disease. The results compare favorably with previous reports of HLA-matched sibling donor transplants and suggest that unrelated donor transplants should be considered earlier rather than later in the course of disease.

▶ When I read this paper I had a "good news, bad news" reaction. First, the good news. One of the limitations of BMT as a treatment for leukemia is that only one fourth to one third of patients will have matched donors available. The national data bank for finding unrelated matched donors is expensive and cumbersome to use. An alternative is to offer transplants from donors who are partially HLA-mismatched. As these and other authors report, techniques have been developed to mitigate the anticipated worsening GVHD so that surprisingly good results can be obtained. This requires carefully controlled conditions that include T-cell depletion in the donor marrow and a more aggressive approach to controlling GVHD.

What is the bad news? At the risk of being considered an Ebenezer Scrooge, it is important to point out that 13 of the patients were largely HLA-matched, with 6 of these reactive in mixed lymphocyte culture. Furthermore, 36 of the 37 remaining patients were mismatched for only 1 HLA antigen; only 1 patient was mismatched for more than 1 antigen. The point I am making is that although the patients were not precisely matched, they were not randomly mismatched either. Therefore, one should not gain from this article the impression that the donors were selected from a random population. Rather, the difference between the traditional HLA-matched donor and the donors in this paper was incremental. This is an important distinction, because the workup for such donors remains as extensive (if not more so) as it would be for identifying an HLA-matched donor. Furthermore, although the circle is larger, the number of potential donors is still restricted with this approach.

Nonetheless, it is promising that the universe of potential donors for any given patient is becoming larger. Now all we have to do in the changing world of managed care is to make sure that the increased transplant capability is not a technique in search of a patient and that the indications for this very expensive procedure are carefully constructed.

J.V. Simone, M.D.

Treatment of Steroid-Resistant Acute Graft-Versus-Host Disease With an Anti-IL-2-Receptor Monoclonal Antibody (BT 563) in Children Who Received T Cell-Depleted, Partially Matched, Related Bone Marrow Transplants

Herbelin C, Stephan J-L, Donadieu J, Le Deist F, Racadot E, Wijdenes J, Fischer A (Hôpital des Enfants Malades, Paris; Centre Régional de Transfusion Sanguine, Besançon, France)
Bone Marrow Transplant 13:563–569, 1995   17–4

Background.—Recent studies have found that murine antihuman IL-2R moAb is effective in patients with steroid-resistant acute graft-vs.-host disease (GVHD). A pilot study of BT 563, an anti-p55 moAb, was initiated to test its safety and efficacy in children with inherited diseases who had received T-cell–depleted partially matched relative marrow.

Methods.—Fifteen children with steroid-resistant acute GVHD, grades II–IV, were enrolled in the study. Patient ages ranged from 1 month to 5 years. All had inherited bone marrow diseases and had received T-cell–depleted marrow from a partially matched related donor. Murine monoclonal antibody treatment consisted of BT 563 antibody, 0.2 mg/kg, daily. Therapy was continued until GVHD was controlled, and methylprednisolone administration was tapered to 2 mg/kg/day or less.

Findings.—Eleven children had complete remission, and 2 had partial remission. There were no adverse treatment effects. Compared with previously published data on the use of BT 563 antibody, good response rates were correlated with early therapy, initiated a mean 7.7 days after GVHD onset, and prolonged therapy, given for a mean 25.9 days. Six of the 13 responders had relapses, but the same treatment induced further remission. Chronic GVHD developed in 6 children, 1 of whom died of an associated infection. Ten patients are currently long-term survivors free of chronic GVHD.

Conclusions.—Early, prolonged therapy with anti-IL-2R monoclonal antibody is safe and effective in young children with steroid-resistant GVHD. Additional studies of anti-IL-2R antibody use as a first-line treatment for acute GVHD are needed.

▶ Treatment of steroid refractory GVHD is currently complicated by a high infectious mortality rate caused by an inability to wean patients from steroids. Other therapies are needed. Promising new approaches involve infusion of monoclonal anticytokine or anti–T-cell-antibodies. Although this approach results in an initial good response rate, most patients have relapse shortly after stopping antibody infusion.

This paper is important because it suggests that early and lengthy infusion of antibody may result in more durable remissions.

R. Burt, M.D.

Thalidomide in the Management of Chronic Graft-Versus-Host Disease in Children Following Bone Marrow Transplantation

Cole CH, Rogers PCJ, Pritchard S, Phillips G, Chan KW (British Columbia Children's Hosp, Vancouver, Canada; Vancouver Gen Hosp, BC, Canada)
Bone Marrow Transplant 14:937–942, 1994   17–5

Background.—Chronic graft-vs.-host disease (GVHD) is a major long-term complication of allogeneic bone marrow transplantation in children, with a reported incidence of 25% to 30%. Although corticosteroids and other immunosuppressive agents are used to treat GVHD in children, long-term treatment may lead to growth retardation, an increased risk for infection, and other adverse effects. Thalidomide, initially used as a sedative but discontinued because of its teratogenic side effects, has demonstrated immunosuppressive properties. This agent, therefore, has been investigated as a possible alternative to other immunosuppressive medications, and recently was shown to be safe and effective in patients with high-risk or refractory chronic GVHD. The outcomes of 5 children treated with thalidomide for severe chronic GVHD were assessed.

Patients and Methods.—The children, aged 6 months and 2, 4, 10, and 12 years, had severe corticosteroid-dependent chronic GVHD. They were treated with 12–25 mg of thalidomide per kg per day and clinically evaluated on a monthly basis. Response to treatment was based on symptom resolution and withdrawal of other immunosuppressive agents.

Results.—Clinical response to thalidomide was observed in all children. Improved Lansky play-performance scores were noted, and termination or reduction in other immunosuppressive medications was achieved. Thalidomide-induced peripheral neuropathy did not occur in any patient, and treatment-related side effects were minimal. All children have survived 48–65 months after transplantation.

Conclusion.—Children with chronic GVHD can be safely and effectively treated with thalidomide. Use of this agent also may help avoid the need for long-term corticosteroid therapy.

▶ I could not resist including this article in the Year Book of Oncology. If there ever was an example of a drug behaving like a phoenix rising from the ashes, this is it. The immunosuppressive effects of thalidomide were discovered serendipitously after it had fallen into disuse as a sedative because of its profound teratogenic effects. It now appears to be a safe and effective alternative to corticosteroids and other immunosuppressive agents. More likely, it will be another of the several agents that may be tried alone or in combination to control this terrible side effect of bone marrow transplantation.

J.V. Simone, M.D.

Reconstitution of Cellular Immunity Against Cytomegalovirus in Recipients of Allogeneic Bone Marrow by Transfer of T-Cell Clones From the Donor
Walter EA, Greenberg PD, Gilbert MJ, Finch RJ, Watanabe KS, Thomas ED, Riddell SR (Fred Hutchinson Cancer Research Ctr, Seattle; Univ of Washington, Seattle)
N Engl J Med 333:1038–1044, 1995   17–6

Introduction.—For immunocompromised patients, reactivation of latent cytomegalovirus (CMV) infection can result in substantial morbidity and mortality. The occurrence of CMV disease in immunocompromised allogeneic bone marrow recipients is associated with a deficiency of CMV-specific CD8+ cytotoxic T lymphocytes. Clones of these lymphocytes were evaluated for safety and immunologic efficacy for immunotherapy in recipients of allogeneic bone marrow transplants.

Methods.—Donor bone marrow was obtained, and clones of CMV-specific CD8+ cytotoxic T cells were isolated. Starting 30 to 40 days after bone marrow transplantation, 14 patients each received 4 IV infusions of the T-cell clones isolated from their donors. The recipients were monitored for up to 12 weeks after the last infusion for reconstitution of their cellular immunity against CMV. The persistence of the transferred T cells was evaluated by assessment of the rearranged genes encoding the T-cell receptor.

Results.—The T-cell clone infusions had no observable toxic effects. All patients demonstrated reconstitution of cytotoxic T cells specific for CMV. Eleven patients who had deficient cytotoxic activity against CMV before the infusions showed a significant increase afterward, similar to those measured in the donors. Studies of rearranged T-cell–receptor genes in 2 recipients suggested that the transferred clones persisted for at least 12 weeks. Patients with a deficiency of CMV-specific CD4+ T-helper cells had a decrease in cytotoxic T-cell activity. None of the recipients had CMV viremia or other forms of CMV disease.

Conclusion.—The T-cell transfer technique appears to offer a safe and effective means of reconstituting cellular immunity against CMV in bone marrow recipients; further research is needed to establish its efficacy as prophylaxis against CMV infection. Persistence of the transferred CD8+ T cells appears to require T-helper cell function.

▶ Cytomegalovirus is a major cause of morbidity and mortality after allogeneic bone marrow transplantation. In approximately 50% of allogeneic recipients, CMV viremia develops between days 30 and 100 after allogeneic bone marrow transplantation. Cytomegalovirus pneumonitis will develop in approximately one half of these patients unless preemptive therapy is initiated with ganciclovir. Ganciclovir therapy is complicated by myelosuppression and late recurrence of CMV. The ultimate ability to prevent recurrence of this latent organism depends on the redevelopment of natural immunity to CMV.

Dr. Riddell et al. showed the feasibility of adoptive transfer of immunity to CMV by infusion of CMV-specific CD8+ donor lymphocytes in an earlier publication.[1] In this article based on their phase I study, they show that adoptive infusion of CMV-specific donor lymphocytes is a safe method of reconstituting immunity against CMV after allogeneic bone marrow transplantation. Specifically, no patient had an exasperation of graft-vs.-host disease, despite infusion of between 33 million and 1 billion cells per square meter of body surface area given 1 week apart for 4 weeks. The absence of graft-vs.-host disease was probably caused by the infusion of lymphocytes that were clones expanded ex vivo for their specificity against CMV. The authors also demonstrate that immunity after adoptive immunotherapy to CMV was lost over time unless CD4+ T-helper cells specific for CMV developed in the host.

These results suggest that transfer of immunity to specific viruses may be safely performed after allogeneic bone marrow transplantation.

R. Burt, M.D.

Reference

1. Riddell SR, Watanabe KS, Goodrich JM, et al: Restoration of viral immunity in immunodeficient humans by the adoptive transfer of T cell clones. *Science* 257:238–241, 1992.

Phase I–II Study of Interleukin-2 After High-Dose Chemotherapy and Autologous Bone Marrow Transplantation in Poorly Responding Neuroblastoma
Valteau-Couanet D, Rubie H, Meresse V, Farace F, Brandely M, Hartmann O (Institut Gustave Roussy, Villejuif, France; Hôpital Purpan, Toulouse, France; Roussel-Uclaf, Romainville, France)
Bone Marrow Transplant 16:515–520, 1995   17–7

Rationale.—Despite the use of high-dose chemotherapy and autologous bone marrow transplantation (ABMT), patients with treatment-resistant metastatic neuroblastoma continue to have a poor outlook. The use of recombinant interleukin-2 (rIL-2) after ABMT has been considered with the goal of enhancing the immune response against the tumor.

Objective.—Twelve children with poorly responding neuroblastoma received 5 courses of rIL-2 treatment after ABMT. The patients had metastases that had failed to remit completely after first-line chemotherapy.

Treatment.—Patients received rIL-2 by infusion at 2-week intervals. The initial course lasted 5 days, and the remaining 4 courses lasted 2 days each. The plan was to begin rIL-2 therapy within 4 months after ABMT. Treatment began in a dose of 12×10^6 units/m^2 of body surface, with increments of 4×10^6 units/m^2 daily.

Efficacy.—Of 7 patients who had measurable disease at the time of ABMT, 2 had complete and 2 had partial responses to rIL-2 treatment. Two others had stable disease, whereas 1 progressed. Four patients remained alive in complete remission 36–54 months after ABMT. The other 8 patients died of progressive disease.

Safety.—Patients received 90% of the planned dose of rIL-2 on average, but dose escalation was not feasible. All patients became febrile and anorexic. Half the patients vomited but not severely. Only 9 of 56 treatment courses were complicated by hypotension. Eight courses were associated with neuropsychiatric disorder, which in 2 instances was severe. Five treatment courses were ended because of thrombocytopenia, but there were no hemorrhagic complications. Anemia was made worse by rIL-2 treatment. Twelve courses were attended by liver dysfunction.

Conclusion.—It is feasible to administer rIL-2 shortly after ABMT to children with treatment-resistant metastatic neuroblastoma.

▶ The outcome of patients with high-risk neuroblastoma—who are either those children older than 1 year of age who have stage IV disease or patients with stage II or III disease who have n-*myc* amplification—remains very poor, in spite of intensive chemotherapy followed by high-dose chemotherapy with stem-cell rescue. The authors of this paper attempted to find other avenues for improving survival in patients with this high-risk disease.

This study was a feasibility study and demonstrated that the clinical toxicity of rIL-2 given to these patients was similar to that observed in adult patients and was worse when given immediately after ABMT. It also has to be noted that half of the patients did not receive the planned rIL-2 therapy after ABMT; only 6 of 12 patients received 100% of the planned dose. Previous reports of stem-cell transplantation for this disease have shown that these patients remain very susceptible to toxic agents, primarily because of the intensity of the therapy with nephrotoxic agents, such as cisplatinum, carboplatinum, and ifosfamide, and that most of these patients have second-look operations in which at least 1 of the kidneys is sacrificed. Nevertheless, the effects of rIL-2 in neuroblastoma have not been proven, and this paper failed to do so.

M. Kletzel, M.D.

Phase III Randomized, Double-Blind Placebo-Controlled Trial of rhGM-CSF Following Allogeneic Bone Marrow Transplantation

Nemunaitis J, Rosenfeld CS, Ash R, Freedman MH, Deeg HJ, Appelbaum F, Singer JW, Flomenberg N, Dalton W, Elfenbein GJ, Rifkin R, Rubin A, Agosti J, Hayes FA, Holcenberg J, Shadduck RK (Texas Oncology, PA/Sammons Baylor, Dallas; Med College of Wisconsin, Milwaukee; Hosp for Sick Children, Toronto; et al)

Bone Marrow Transplant 15:949–954, 1995   17–8

Background.—Studies have shown that morbidity caused by allogeneic bone marrow transplantation (BMT) may be reduced by administration of yeast-derived recombinant human granulocytic-macrophage colony-stimulating factor (rhGM-CSF). In a prospective, randomized, placebo-controlled study of patients undergoing sibling BMT, the efficacy of the procedure and the toxicity associated with administration of rhGM-CSF were compared between subjects and controls administered a placebo.

Methods.—Patients undergoing sibling BMT were identified as high or low risk for morbidity and mortality according to specific criteria. Patients were treated with a preparative regimen of IV cyclosporine, 3–5 mg/kg/day, followed by oral cyclosporine, 12.5 mg/kg/day, combined with methylprednisolone, 0.5 mg/kg/day. On the day of the bone marrow transplant, 53 patients were treated with rhGM-CSF, 250 µg/m²/day; infusion was continued to day 20. Control patients (56) were treated with an infusion of placebo in the same manner. Neutrophil recovery was defined as the number of days required to reach 2 consecutive absolute neutrophil count readings of 0.1, 0.5, or 1.0×10^9 cells/L; a platelet count $\geq 20 \times 10^9$ cells/L was defined as platelet recovery. Mucositis was graded objectively. Grades of toxicity were identified and recorded. Data were interpreted using the Cochran-Mantel-Haenzel row means test, chi-square tests, and Kaplan-Meier plots.

Results.—Most patients receiving rhGM-CSF treatment tolerated it well. In the placebo group, 3 patients who had achieved the absolute neutrophil count and 3 others withdrew because of toxic complications; 11 in the rhGM-CSF group withdrew because of toxicity. The subjects treated with rhGM-CSF took less time (13 days) to reach neutrophil recovery than did patients who received placebo (17 days) and experienced less mucositis and infection. No differences in platelet or lymphocyte recovery, graft-vs.-host disease, or survival occurred between groups. Patients receiving rhGM-CSF treatment spent less time in the hospital after transplantation.

Discussion.—Patients undergoing HLA-matched BMT can be safely treated with an infusion of rhGM-CSF when the infusion has been preceded by cyclosporine and prednisone prophylaxis for graft-vs.-host disease. They are likely to experience a more rapid recovery and fewer complications than untreated patients.

▶ Although the administration of hematopoietic growth factors in patients undergoing autologous BMT has diminished the morbidity of this intensive approach by reducing the duration of neutropenia, less information is available regarding the potential benefits and hazards in the setting of allogeneic BMT. This report reviews the results of a phase III prospective, multicenter, randomized, double-blind, placebo-controlled trial of yeast-derived rhGM-CSF or placebo, given by 4-hour IV infusion starting on the day of marrow infusion to day 20 and continued among a cohort of patients with a variety of hematopoietic malignancies receiving histocompatibly matched sibling BMT.

The time to neutrophil recovery to >500/µL was less in patients receiving rhGM-CSF compared with patients receiving placebo (day 13 vs. day 17; PE was 0.0001). Moreover, the incidence of grade III–IV mucositis and infection was significantly reduced in patients receiving rhGM-CSF. Not surprisingly, no differences in platelet recovery or lymphocyte recovery were seen. Furthermore, the instances of renal occlusive disease and graft-vs.-host disease were not different between the 2 groups. In addition, there was no apparent impact on the rate of relapse or overall survival.

This study is important because it suggests that there are considerable benefits and few hazards associated with the administration of rhGM-CSF to patients undergoing histocompatibly matched sibling BMT with cyclosporine and prednisone for graft-vs.-host disease prophylaxis. Although in this study more patients receiving rhGM-CSF relapsed or died than did those receiving placebo, the difference was not statistically significant. This report provides support for a practice that is already beginning to be widely applied. The long-term impact, if any, of hematopoietic growth factors in this setting will require longer-term follow-up.

M.S. Tallman, M.D.

Ex vivo Expansion and Subsequent Infusion of Human Bone Marrow-Derived Stromal Progenitor Cells (Mesenchymal Progenitor Cells): Implications for Therapeutic Use

Lazarus HM, Haynesworth SE, Gerson SL, Rosenthal NS, Caplan AI (Univ Hosps of Cleveland, Ohio; Case Western Reserve Univ, Cleveland, Ohio)
Bone Marrow Transplant 16:557–564, 1995   17–9

Objective.—A phase I trial was planned to determine whether it is feasible to collect human bone marrow–derived progenitor stromal cells (mesenchymal progenitor cells [MPCs]) from patients with hematologic malignancy in complete remission, expanding them in ex vivo culture, and infusing them intravenously.

Methods.—Twenty-three patients who were 18–68 years of age were enrolled in the study. Twelve had undergone autologous or syngeneic bone marrow transplantation 4–52 months previously. Marrow mononuclear cells obtained from the posterior iliac crest were separated, and adherent cells were culture-expanded in vitro in Complete Medium for 4–7 weeks before being reinfused. The cells were examined by phase microscopy whenever the culture medium was changed to gauge mitotic expansion and confirm normal cell morphology.

Results.—A median of 364 × 10⁶ nucleated marrow cells were used for expansion. The median number of MPCs obtained after expansion was 59 × 10⁶, representing a median of 13 cell doublings. Mesenchymal progenitor cells were infused into 15 patients from 28 to 49 days after collection. Groups of 5 patients received 1, 10, or 50 × 10⁶ cells. There were no apparent adverse reactions. In no case did marrow cellularity change by more than 20% within 2 weeks after infusion of MPCs.

Conclusion.—It seems feasible to expand MPCs and use them for various therapeutic purposes in both the hematologic and orthopedic settings.

▶ Stromal cells derived from pluripotent MPCs constitute a distinct cell population within the human bone marrow, which provides both the microenvironment and cellular regulators for hematopoiesis. Many groups are focusing research efforts on the ex vivo expansion of hematopoietic progenitors, with the goal of supplementing or replacing the conventional autograft and reducing the period of aplasia that follows high-dose chemotherapy. Lazarus and colleagues have, instead, isolated and expanded the supporting stroma that facilitates engraftment. They hypothesize that the infusion of sufficient numbers of MPCs at the time of autotransplant will enhance recovery of peripheral blood cells.

Beginning with a single 10- to 15-mL bone marrow aspirate from 23 patients with hematologic malignancies in remission, the investigators inoculated cultures designed to promote the growth of MPCs preferentially. Expansion occurred in 21 of 23 cultured specimens, including cases in which the patient had undergone prior bone marrow transplantation. After 2–3 passages, a median of 59 × 10⁶ MPCs—identified by their reactivity with monoclonal antibodies that react with stromal cells but not bone marrow–derived hematopoietic cells—were harvested. Based on the rarity of this cell type within normal bone marrow aspirates, 16,000-fold expansion was calculated. Infusion of as many as 50 million MPCs was not associated with toxicity and provides a basis for further clinical investigation involving larger numbers of MPCs in the setting of autotransplantation. Such an approach may accelerate engraftment. Ex vivo expanded MPCs also provide attractive targets for gene transfer protocols and provide a model system for novel therapeutic applications.

J.N. Winter, M.D.

18 Pharmacology

Docetaxel: An Active New Drug for Treatment of Advanced Epithelial Ovarian Cancer
Piccart MJ, Gore M, Ten Bokkel Huinink W, Van Oosterom A, Verweij J, Wanders J, Franklin H, Bayssas M, Kaye S (Jules Bordet Inst, Brussels, Belgium; Royal Marsden Hosp, London; Netherlands Cancer Inst, Amsterdam; et al)
J Natl Cancer Inst 87:676–681, 1995

18–1

Background.—Natural paclitaxel, or Taxol, has recently been recognized as a highly cytotoxic agent for use in platinum-refractory ovarian cancer. Because of its relative scarcity, synthetic and semisynthetic substitutes have been pursued. The new semisynthetic taxoid, docetaxel, has consistently produced antitumor responses in patients with ovarian cancer in phase I trials. Therefore, a phase II trial was conducted to assess the efficacy and toxic effects of docetaxel.

Methods.—Ninety-seven patients with advanced epithelial ovarian cancer were enrolled in the study. Eligible patients had disease relapse or progression within 12 months of the last administration of a first-line or second-line platinum-based regimen with at least 1 bidimensionally measurable target lesion. Docetaxel was given in a dose of 100 mg/m² as a 1-hour infusion every 3 weeks without premedication to minimize potential hypersensitivity.

Findings.—The 76 assessable patients had an overall response rate of 23.6%. When all 90 eligible patients were included in the comparison, that rate was 20%. The response rate was 23.5% in the 34 eligible patients whose tumor progressed on the most recent platinum treatment. For all eligible patients, the median progression-free survival was 3.9 months, and the median overall survival was 8.4 months. Docetaxel-related toxicity consisted of short-lived neutropenia in 81 patients, or 90%; this was complicated by fever and hospitalization in 8%. Hypersensitivity reactions occurred in 31% of patients, with 8% having significant reactions. Neurotoxicity occurred in 48%, with grade 3 or greater toxicity in 3%. Sixty-four percent of the patients had skin reactions, but only 4% had grade 3 reactions. Twelve percent of the patients had pleural effusions—the adverse effect of greatest concern. Peripheral edema was noted in 44% of the patients, and weight gain from fluid retention was seen in 19%.

Conclusion.—Docetaxel appears to be active against platinum-resistant tumors. Because of its toxic effects, however, it is unlikely that docetaxel will have a better therapeutic index than paclitaxel for palliative treatment in patients with advanced ovarian cancer. The toxic effect of greatest concern is fluid retention, which is related to the cumulative dose administered. Therefore, a trial exploring the contribution of 3–4 courses of docetaxel to the classic management of advanced ovarian cancer with platinum compounds may be considered.

▶ This study demonstrates that docetaxel, the first semisynthetic taxane to be evaluated in clinical trials, has a similar degree of activity (23.5% response rate) as paclitaxel in patients with platinum-resistant advanced ovarian cancer. Although the activity profile is similar, there is a different pattern of toxicity compared with that of paclitaxel. Fluid retention, manifested as weight gain, and pleural effusions were observed in 44% and 12% of patients, respectively, in this study. The authors conclude that until this toxicity is successfully circumvented, docetaxel is unlikely to have a better therapeutic index than paclitaxel in patients with advanced ovarian cancer.

It is important to emphasize that premedication was not administered in this trial. More recent clinical studies with docetaxel have used varying regimens of steroids and diuretics, although it remains to be determined how effective they are as a prophylactic measure against fluid retention. As with paclitaxel, the duration of administration may also have a marked effect on the pattern of toxicity, and different schedules of docetaxel may also have different effects on fluid retention. The current optimum management for patients with advanced ovarian cancer, at least in the United States, is a combination of paclitaxel and a platinum compound. If the fluid retention toxicity can be circumvented, docetaxel will have to be evaluated together with a platinum compound, because most studies in ovarian cancer suggest that the combination chemotherapy is superior to treatment with single agents.

R.F. Ozols, M.D., Ph.D.

Paclitaxel: A Radiation Sensitizer of Human Cervical Cancer Cells
Rodriguez M, Sevin B-U, Perras J, Nguyen HN, Pham C, Steren AJ, Koechli OR, Averette HE (Univ of Miami, Fla)
Gynecol Oncol 57:165–169, 1995   18–2

Introduction.—Radiotherapy is an important treatment modality in the management of cervical carcinoma, particularly with advanced disease. Various radiosensitizing agents have been investigated in attempts to enhance radiation cytotoxicity. Paclitaxel is a relatively new and promising cytotoxic agent that has demonstrated activity in several types of cancer. The radiation sensitizing effects of paclitaxel were evaluated in cervical cancer cell lines.

Methods.—Three cervical cell lines were irradiated with 1 of 6 radiation doses (0, 2, 4, 6, 8, or 10 Gy), with some cells pretreated with 1 of 5 doses of paclitaxel 48 hours before irradiation. The combination doses of paclitaxel and radiation were kept at fixed ratios. On the seventh day after irradiation, the adenosine triphosphate cell viability assay was performed to measure cellular response.

Results.—Combination treatment with both paclitaxel and radiation increased cytotoxicity in all 3 cell lines, with mean inactivation D values decreasing from 6.70 to 4.33, 6.08 to 4.54, and 7.03 to 5.97 in the 3 cell lines, respectively. The interaction between paclitaxel and radiation therapy was supra-additive in the ME-180 and SiHa cell lines, but subadditive in the MS-751 cell line.

Conclusion.—Paclitaxel administered at therapeutic concentrations has a modest radiosensitizing effect on cervical cancer cells. These findings warrant further clinical study to determine the radiosensitizing effect of paclitaxel on cervical cancer cells in vivo and the potential impact on prognosis.

▶ Paclitaxel, or Taxol, is an interesting compound. This study from Miami demonstrates that it is capable of sensitizing cervical carcinoma cells from humans. The data look interesting and, hopefully, will have clinical relevance down the road. This particular paper by Rodriguez et al. uses an assay documenting the percentage of adenosine triphosphate that remains in culture after exposure to both radiation and drug. I would have preferred to see this evaluated by a classic cell survival approach, but the authors' data are not inconsistent with those of Liebmann et al.[1] The interesting thing about this particular drug is that low doses of Taxol have radiosensitizing properties as well as cytotoxic properties. In the paper by Liebmann et al., Taxol was shown to have most of its cytotoxicity at relatively low doses, with a very steep decrease in cell survival of 2 to 2½ logs resulting from exposure before the curve broke.

If this is true in vivo, then it may well be that Taxol doses do not have to be pushed to the level of maximum toxicity to obtain the benefits of the compound, especially in combination with other agents. It may also be that Taxol is best administered in a continuous low-dose infusion, both from a sensitizing point of view and from a cytotoxic one. Time will tell regarding these issues, but this kind of study seems to be very important and may be very valuable in the future in helping us to use Taxol in the most beneficial way possible.

E. Glatstein, M.D.

Reference

1. Liebmann J, Cook J, Teague D, et al: Taxol mediated radiosensitization in human tumor cell lines. Presented at the Second National Cancer Institute Workshop on Taxol and Taxus, 1992.

Phase I Study of Paclitaxel and Topotecan in Patients With Advanced Tumors: A Cancer and Leukemia Group B Study
Lilenbaum RC, Ratain MJ, Miller AA, Hargis JB, Hollis DR, Rosner GL, O'Brien SM, Brewster L, Green MR, Schilsky RL (Univ of California, San Diego; Univ of Chicago Med Ctr; Univ of Tennessee, Memphis; et al)
J Clin Oncol 13:2230–2237, 1995   18–3

Introduction.—Paclitaxel and topotecan are 2 promising newer chemotherapeutic agents that have distinct mechanisms of action. Paclitaxel's cytotoxic actions occur by its promotion of microtubule assembly and the stabilization of the assembled microtubules, which prevents the depolymerization and reorganization of the mitotic spindle. Topotecan achieves its effects by inhibiting the nuclear enzyme topoisomerase I. The dose-limiting toxicities of the combination of paclitaxel and topotecan were investigated in a phase I trial in patients with advanced solid tumors.

Methods.—Over 1 year, 46 patients with assessable solid tumors were given paclitaxel as a 3-hour IV infusion on day 1 and topotecan as a 30-minute infusion on days 1 through 5 of each 21-day cycle. The dose of topotecan was fixed at 1 mg/m^2/day, and the dose of paclitaxel was escalated until the maximum tolerated dose, with the starting dose at 50 mg/m^2 and cohorts of 3–8 patients treated at each dose level. Once the maximum tolerated dose with the 2 agents was defined, filgrastim, 5 µg/kg/day, was added to the regimen, administered on days 6–14 to control neutropenia. All patients were monitored for toxic effects at least weekly, and tumor response was evaluated every 2 cycles.

Results.—Without filgrastim, the maximum tolerated dose of paclitaxel was 80 mg/m^2, with hematologic toxicity being the dose-limiting complication. With filgrastim added to the regimen, the maximum tolerated dose of paclitaxel was 230 mg/m^2. This dose level induced hematologic dose-limiting toxicity in 1 patient (febrile neutropenia) and dose-limiting myalgias and arthralgias in another patient. Two patients died of treatment-related toxicity. Of the remaining 44 patients, 3 had a partial response (1 patient each with head and neck carcinoma, non–small-cell lung cancer, and metastatic colon cancer), 16 had stable disease after 2 cycles, and 25 had progressive disease.

Conclusions.—The recommended doses for phase II studies are paclitaxel, 80 mg/m^2, on day 1 and topotecan, 1 mg/m^2, on days 1–5 when filgrastim is not used. When filgrastim is added to the regimen, the recommended dose of paclitaxel is increased to 230 mg/m^2 on day 1, with the same schedule for topotecan with 21- to 28-day intervals between cycles.

▶ Paclitaxel has been demonstrated to be a highly active agent in a wide variety of malignancies, particularly ovarian cancer, breast cancer, and lung cancer. Not only is the drug active as a single agent, but paclitaxel combinations also appear to have at least additive, if not synergistic, activity. Topotecan, an inhibitor of topoisomerase I, also appears to be a promising agent in its own right for lung cancer and ovarian cancer. This study demonstrates the feasibility of combining paclitaxel and topotecan. The dose-limiting neutropenia can be managed with filgrastim.

An unusual but interesting observation from this study is that the dose of paclitaxel used in combination with topotecan is higher than what one would have expected from single-agent trials of paclitaxel. This observation is similar to what has been reported for the use of paclitaxel and carboplatin, for which there appears to be significantly less thrombocytopenia than one would have expected with the doses of carboplatin that can be administered. Whether this is attributable to the pharmacokinetic or pharmacodynamic interactions between paclitaxel and other drugs needs to be explored in more detail.

R.F. Ozols, M.D., Ph.D.

Pharmacokinetics of All-*trans*-Retinoic Acid Administered on an Intermittent Schedule

Adamson PC, Bailey J, Pluda J, Poplack DG, Bauza S, Murphy RF, Yarchoan R, Balis FM (Natl Cancer Inst, Bethesda, Md)
J Clin Oncol 13:1238–1241, 1995   18–4

Introduction.—Treatment with all-*trans*-retinoic acid (ATRA) induces, but does not maintain, remission in many patients with acute promyelocytic leukemia (APL). Pharmacokinetic studies have found that the plasma concentration of ATRA is decreased substantially during continuous therapy, thereby reducing systemic exposure. It was hypothesized that an intermittent administration schedule would result in repetitive periods of high plasma concentrations of drug and systemic exposure. The pharmacokinetics of this administration strategy were studied.

Methods.—Ten HIV-infected patients with Kaposi's sarcoma who were enrolled in a phase II trial of ATRA served as the study population. The participants were given ATRA (40 mg/m²/day) for 7 consecutive days every other week. Pharmacokinetic monitoring was performed after an overnight fast on days 1 and 7 of the first week and on the first day of the third and eleventh weeks of treatment. On those days, the plasma concentration of ATRA was measured, using high-performance liquid chromatography, with heparinized blood samples obtained every 30 minutes for 8 hours.

Results.—During the first week, plasma concentrations of ATRA decreased significantly. The mean area under the plasma concentration–time curve (AUC) was 145 µmol/L on day 1, but only 18 µmol/L on day 7. Plasma concentrations of ATRA had a mean AUC of 177 µmol/L on the first day of week 3 and of 128 µmol/L on the first day of week 11, which were comparable to the levels on the first day of week 1.

Conclusion.—An intermittent schedule of ATRA administration appears to overcome the low systemic drug exposure resulting from continuous daily administration. However, because daily administration of ATRA is highly effective in inducing remission, an intermittent schedule is not recommended during induction therapy. The role of intermittent administration for maintaining remission in patients with APL will be further studied.

▶ The vitamin A derivative ATRA promotes terminal differentiation of leukemic promyelocytes in the majority of patients with APL. Since the initial observations by Huang and colleagues appeared in 1988,[1] investigators in both France[2] and the United States[3] have confirmed that ATRA induces the malignant clone to differentiate into mature neutrophils, with rapid improvement in the characteristic life-threatening coagulopathy. However, several limitations to differentiation therapy have been identified. One complication is that although the percentage of patients achieving complete morphological remission is high, the duration of these remissions is not long unless conventional cytotoxic chemotherapy is subsequently administered.

It has been suggested that one reason for retinoic resistance is that the plasma levels of ATRA decrease after a number of months, despite continued administration of the same dose. The reason for this reduction is not clear, but it may be related to the induction of cytoplasmic binding proteins with continued administration of the retinoid. Adamson and colleagues have performed a pharmacokinetic study in which they show that an intermittent schedule of ATRA, whereby the drug is administered in repetitive cycles of 7 consecutive days of drug followed by 7 days without the drug, results in periods of exposure to concentrations of ATRA that are normally only observed on the first day of treatment. Although the plasma exposure to ATRA, as measured by the AUC, decreases significantly during the first week of drug administration, plasma ATRA concentrations at the start of weeks 3 and 11 during this every-other-week schedule were equivalent to those achieved on day 1 of treatment.

The information reported in this article is important because it suggests that an intermittent schedule of ATRA may circumvent the decreased plasma AUC normally observed with a continuous administration and may have an impact on the relapse rate after only ATRA administration. One problem has to do with interpatient variability in the plasma AUC after oral administration of the drug. This has been seen in other pharmacokinetic studies and was observed in the study abstracted here. Although this study demonstrates that an intermittent schedule of administration may result in potentially more favorable plasma concentrations of ATRA, it is not clear whether such a schedule of administration will translate into longer remission durations for patients. Future trials will be needed to address this issue. In addition, other strategies for maintaining higher plasma ATRA concentrations, such as the administration of p-450 inhibitors (e.g., ketoconazole), which may block the rate-limiting step in a catabolism of ATRA, may be productive.

M.S. Tallman, M.D.

References

1. Huang ME, Ye YC, Chen SR, et al: Use of all-*trans*-retinoic acid in the treatment of acute promyelocytic leukemia. *Blood* 72:567–577, 1988.

2. Castaigne S, Chomienne C, Daniet MT, et al: All-*trans*-retinoic acid as differentiation therapy for acute promyelocytic leukemia: I. Clinical results. *Blood* 76:1704–1709, 1990.
3. Warrell RP, Frankel SR, Miller WH, et al: Differentiation therapy of acute promyelocytic leukemia with tretinoin (all-*trans*-retinoic acid). *N Engl J Med* 374:1385–1393, 1991.

Decreased Mutation Rate for Cellular Resistance to Doxorubicin and Suppression of mdr 1 Gene Activation by the Cyclosporin PSC 833

Beketic-Oreskovic L, Durán GE, Chen G, Dumontet C, Sikic BI (Stanford Univ, Calif)
J Natl Cancer Inst 87:1593–1602, 1995   18–5

Background.—Overexpression of the multidrug transporter P-glycoprotein by the mdr 1 gene is the predominant mechanism involved in cellular resistance to doxorubicin, a commonly used anticancer drug. Other less common mechanisms have been identified, including decreased expression and/or activity of topoisomerase II (Topo II), altered glutathione levels, overexpression of multidrug resistance–associated protein, and increased expression of the p110 protein called the major vault protein. The mutation rate and mechanisms of drug resistance were investigated in tumor cells exposed to doxorubicin in the presence of the cyclosporin PSC 833, an effective multidrug resistance modulator.

Methods.—Populations of the human MES-SA sarcoma cell line were incubated with both doxorubicin and PSC 833 after expansion of the populations in the experimental group and without population expansion in the control group, and the surviving colonies were analyzed for the mutation rate with fluctuation analysis. Resistance to various other anticancer agents was tested in the surviving clones. The reverse transcriptase polymerase chain reaction was used to determine the presence of mdr 1 transcripts, MRP gene expression, and Topo II transcripts. Topoisomerase II-DNA cleavable complex formation with 3 concentrations of etoposide was measured with the K-SDS precipitation assay, and Topo II catalytic activity was evaluated with decatenation of kinetoplast DNA. Topoisomerase IIα protein, glutathione, and p110 major vault protein expression were measured using the appropriate monoclonal antibodies.

Results.—There were surviving colonies in 8 of the 10 populations exposed to both doxorubicin and PSC 833 after population expansion, whereas none of the control populations survived, suggesting that drug resistance resulted from spontaneous mutations, rather than from cellular function changes induced by drug exposure. Of the 16 surviving isolated clones, 6 did not have drug resistance. The surviving clones had cross-resistance to etoposide (a Topo II–related agent) but not to vinblastine, paclitaxel, cisplatin, camptothecin, or mitomycin C. The surviving clones expressed no detectable mdr 1 transcripts. There were no differences between surviving clones and parental cells in expression of the MRP gene, cellular glutathione content, or expression of the p110 major vault protein. Although the clones and parental cells had similar levels of Topo IIβ transcripts, the clones had significantly decreased levels of Topo IIα transcripts and Topo IIα protein. There was also decreased complex formation with all concentrations of etoposide in the selected clones, and Topo II activity was reduced to 8% to 56% of the catalytic activity level in the parental MES-SA cells.

Conclusion.—Treatment of tumor cells with both doxorubicin and PSC 833 resulted in a decreased mutation rate for resistance to doxorubicin and inhibited mdr 1 gene activation. Therefore, multidrug resistance modulation therapy may prevent clinical drug resistance in some patients. The cross-resistance seen in some of the clones indicates an unmasked prominence of alterations in Topo IIα expression in the development of drug resistance; the nature of this mechanism requires further study.

▶ Clinical trials evaluating the potential for reversing multidrug resistance have been disappointing. Although numerous agents have been identified in preclinical models to be capable of reversing multidrug resistance associated with efflux pumps, clinical trials have identified a series of problems that appear to markedly limit this therapeutic strategy. The intrinsic toxicity of many resistance-reversing agents has not permitted the achievement of plasma levels that may be necessary to reverse drug resistance in preclinical models of cancer. In addition, the reversing agents frequently alter the pharmacokinetics of the anticancer drug being tested. Furthermore, in those studies in which it appears that there may have been some evidence of reversal of drug resistance, the duration of these remissions has been disappointingly short.

This study suggests that a more appropriate strategy may be to use modulators of drug resistance as part of initial treatment approaches, because it may be possible to delay or suppress the emergence of mdr 1 mutants. Not only was the overall mutation rate decreased when tumor cells were treated with doxorubicin and the resistance modulator PSC 833, there was also decreased activation of the mdr 1 gene. Such a potential strategy would be limited to those patients in whom there is no intrinsic expression of the mdr 1 gene in tumor cells.

R.F. Ozols, M.D., Ph.D.

Prediction of Carboplatin Clearance From Standard Morphological and Biological Patient Characteristics

Chatelut E, Canal P, Brunner V, Chevreau C, Pujol A, Boneu A, Roché H, Houin G, Bugat R (Université Paul Sabatier, Toulouse, France)
J Natl Cancer Inst 87:573–580, 1995

18–6

Background.—The hematologic toxicity of the antineoplastic drug carboplatin depends mainly on the drug's pharmacokinetics. Its treatment efficacy may be associated with plasma drug exposure. Some authorities have proposed dosage adjustment based on isotopic determination of glomerular filtration rate. Dosage adjustment based on creatinine clearance depends on accurate measurement of urine volume per unit time. The relationship between carboplatin clearance and patient characteristics was investigated in a population pharmacokinetics study.

Methods.—Seventy patients (age, 23–84 years) were studied. They were treated with different combination regimens with carboplatin at doses ranging from 184 to 950 mg for various types of tumors. Plasma carboplatin pharmacokinetics were determined as ultrafilterable platinum, and data were analyzed in the nonlinear mixed effects model. Data on 46 cycles in 34 patients were used to derive the most predictive formula, and data on another 43 cycles in the 36 remaining patients were analyzed to assess the reliability of the formula.

Findings.—Carboplatin clearance was best predicted by the formula, $0.134 \times$ weight $+ [218 \times$ weight $\times (1 - 0.00457 \times$ age$) \times (1 - 0.314 \times$ sex$)]$/creatinine expressed in micromolar concentration. The formula prospectively predicted the carboplatin clearance with precision and minimal bias. This predictive method was as accurate as the method derived from measures of glomerular filtration rate after [51]chromium–ethylenediamine tetra-acetic acid injection.

Conclusion.—This formula for assessing carboplatin clearance permits clinicians to determine individualized dosages in adults in a simple manner. The calculated carboplatin clearance is multiplied by the area under the curve to yield the desired dosage.

▶ Carboplatin is rapidly cleared from the kidneys, and the area under the curve (AUC) in the plasma depends on the glomerular filtration rate (GFR). The GFR, for which the creatinine clearance can be substituted, is markedly dependent on numerous physiologic factors, in particular, the patient's age. Dosing of carboplatin based on body surface area fails to take into account, for example, that a 40-year-old patient with ovarian cancer and a serum creatinine value of 0.6 has at least a 2-times-greater GFR than a 70-year-old patient with ovarian cancer and a serum creatinine level of 1.2.

Several methods have been proposed for individualizing carboplatin dosing based on individual differences in GFR. The investigators in this study reported a formula for determining an individual patient's carboplatin clearance based on the patient's age, weight, and serum creatinine value. Regardless of the formula used, individualized dosing of carboplatin will lead to predictable AUCs and protect patients from excessive toxicity.

R.F. Ozols, M.D., Ph.D.

Ketoconazole in the Management of Paraneoplastic Cushing's Syndrome Secondary to Ectopic Adrenocorticotropin Production

Winquist EW, Laskey J, Crump M, Khamsi F, Shepherd FA (Toronto Hosp; Univ of Toronto)

J Clin Oncol 13:157–1614, 1995

18–7

Introduction.—Fifteen to twenty percent of cases of Cushing's syndrome (CS) result from ectopic production of pro-opiomelanocortin–derived peptides, such as adrenocorticotropin. Most patients with such ectopic Cushing's syndrome (ECS) have neuroendocrine tumors; half of the cases are associated with small-cell lung cancer (SCLC). Ketoconazole is a potent, rapid, and reversible inhibitor of testicular and adrenal steroidogenesis that has been successfully used for the treatment of patients with CS with tumors arising in the adrenal and pituitary glands. An experience with ketoconazole in the treatment of ECS was reported.

Patients.—The 12-year experience included 15 consecutive patients with ECS who were treated with ketoconazole. Eleven were men and 4 were women; the median age was 59 years. The tumor diagnosis was SCLC in 9 patients, mixed SCLC/non-SCLC in 1, and non-SCLC lung cancer in 1; bronchial and pancreatic carcinoid in 1 each; and medullary carcinoma of the thyroid in 1. The diagnosis of ECS was made at the same time as the tumor diagnosis in 8 patients. The most common clinical findings were proximal muscle weakness in 10 patients; peripheral edema in 8 patients; and hypertension in 8 patients. On biochemical evaluation, 14 patients had hypokalemia, 13 had metabolic acidosis, and 10 had new or worsened diabetes mellitus.

Treatment and Outcomes.—All patients were treated with ketoconazole; 9 received anticancer chemotherapy also. The dosages ranged from 400 to 1,200 mg/day, adjusted according to urinary free-cortisol levels. Ketoconazole treatment continued for a median of 26 days. Strict criteria were applied to define the clinical, biochemical, and hormonal responses to ketoconazole.

Most patients showed improvement in hypokalemia, metabolic alkalosis, diabetes mellitus, and hypertension. A hormonal response was observed in 10 patients, including 7 complete responses that lasted a median of 25 days. The longest of these lasted 989 days. Three patients had definite symptomatic hypoadrenalism develop, and another probably had this complication. Progression of cancer led to death in most patients, accompanied by escape from hormonal control by ketoconazole. The overall median survival was 19 weeks.

Conclusions.—For most patients with ECS, ketoconazole treatment yields a reduction in cortisol excess. Even without a complete hormonal response, clinical improvement in hypokalemia, metabolic alkalosis, diabetes mellitus, and hypertension may occur. Ketoconazole is therefore a safe and effective treatment for ECS; however, successful treatment of the underlying cancer is the key to control of ECS.

▶ Ketoconazole has been used infrequently for the treatment of SC secondary to ectopic production of adrenocorticotropic hormone (ACTH) by tumors. The drug previously had been established to be useful in the management of CS secondary to primary adrenal and pituitary causes. The efficacy relates to its potent, rapid, and reversible effect as an inhibitor of steroidogenesis. The majority of the patients in this study had small-cell lung cancer, which accounts for almost half of all cases of ECS. Other tumors associated with this syndrome include carcinoid tumors, islet cell tumors, medullary carcinoma of the thyroid, and pheochromocytoma. An occasional patient with adenocarcinoma of the lung, breast, prostate, or pancreas will also exhibit ECS. All patients in this study demonstrated a biochemical and/or hormonal response to ketoconazole.

A response to chemotherapy alone often is associated with decreased production of ACTH and control of the syndrome. However, in this study ketoconazole was effective even in those patients who had tumor progression while receiving chemotherapy. There were a few adverse side effects from this agent, and clinical improvement in hypokalemia, metabolic alkalosis, diabetes mellitus, and hypertension were significant. This study demonstrated that ketoconazole is an effective and safe treatment for ECS and appears to be particularly useful in those patients in whom there is no effective treatment for the underlying malignancy.

R.F. Ozols, M.D., Ph.D.

Effects of Tamoxifen on Cardiovascular Risk Factors in Postmenopausal Women After 5 Years of Treatment
Love RR, Wiebe DA, Feyzi JM, Newcomb PA, Chappell RJ (Univ of Wisconsin Comprehensive Cancer Ctr, Madison)
J Natl Cancer Inst 86:1534–1539, 1994   18–8

Introduction.—Cardiovascular disease is seen in about two thirds of postmenopausal women, nearly one third of whom will die of heart diseases. The use of hormone therapy in patients with breast cancer is becoming more important. Patients with breast cancer treated with tamoxifen show prolonged disease-free and overall survival 10 years after diagnosis; there is more benefit in patients with positive lymph nodes than in women with negative lymph nodes. It appears that the longer the duration of tamoxifen treatment, the greater the benefits. Tamoxifen therapy has been shown to improve cardiac risk factors while reducing rates of myocardial infarction and hospitalizations related to heart disease. Cardiac risk factors in women with a 5-year history of tamoxifen therapy were examined.

Methods.—A total of 140 women who were free of other hormonal agents, lipid-lowering drugs, or nutritional counseling were randomly divided into placebo and tamoxifen (10 mg, given twice daily by mouth) groups. Periodic lipid and bone densitometry measures were taken. After 2 years, decisions as to whether to continue the tamoxifen therapy were

TABLE 2.—Changes at 5 Years in Fasting Levels

Laboratory test	Placebo (n = 32) Mean ± SE	P*	Tamoxifen (n = 30) Mean ± SE	P*	P for differences between two groups†
Total cholesterol mmol/L (mg/dL)	−0.12 ± 0.10 (−4.7 ± 3.8)	.23	−0.73 ± 0.13 (−28.0 ± 5.1)	<.001	.001
HDL cholesterol, mmol/L (mg/dL)	−0.19 ± 0.06 (−7.1 ± 2.1)	.002	−0.17 ± 0.04 (−6.4 ± 1.5)	<.001	NS
LDL cholesterol mmol/L (mg/dL)‡	−0.06 ± 0.10 (−2.3 ± 3.8)	.55	−0.80 ± 0.12 (−30.8 ± 4.6)	<.001	.0001
Triglycerides, mmol/L (mg/dL)	0.27 ± 0.11 (23.8 ± 9.4)	.02	0.52 ± 0.11 (45.6 ± 10.0)	<.001	.12
Apolipoprotein A1, mg/dL	3.6 ± 4.0	.37	16.6 ± 2.9	<.001	.01
Apolipoprotein B, mg/dL	22.3 ± 1.8	<.001	14.9 ± 2.5	<.001	.02
Lipoprotein (a), mg/dL§	−1	.3	>−3.5	.001	.001
Fibrinogen, mg/L	−14.2 ± 14.9	.35	−50.6 ± 14.1	.001	.08
Glucose, mg/dL	13.7 ± 2.6	<.001	22.1 ± 5.0	<.001	NS
Platelets, 10⁹/L	−43.5 ± 6.2	<.001	−55.5 ± 8.7	<.001	NS

* Paired *t*-test, for differences from baseline values.
† Two-sample *t*-test on paired differences.
‡ Estimated from the equation of Friedwald WT, Levy RI, Fredrickson DS: *Clin Chem* 18:499–502, 1992.
§ Changes in median values; for changes from baseline, P value from a one-sample Wilcoxon test; for comparison of changes between two groups, a two-sample Wilcoxon test P value is given.
Abbreviation: NS, not significant.
(Courtesy of Love RR, Wiebe DA, Feyzi JM, et al: Effects of tamoxifen on cardiovascular risk factors in postmenopausal women after 5 years of treatment. *J Natl Cancer Inst* 86:1534–1539, 1994.)

made with the patients' oncologist. All patients were contacted 3 years later, approximately 5 years from the start of the project. Sixty-two of the original 140 patients were reexamined. There were 30 long-term tamoxifen patients and 32 long-term placebo patients. Total lipids and fractions, lipoproteins, glucose, platelets, and fibrinogen were determined on serial blood samples. After 5 years, total cholesterol, low-density lipoprotein cholesterol, and lipoprotein A were significantly lower in the tamoxifen group than the placebo group (Table 2). Apolipoprotein B increased to a greater extent in the placebo group. Of borderline statistical significance were the decrease in fibrinogen and increases in triglyceride in the tamoxifen group. High-density lipoprotein cholesterol did not change in either group.

Conclusion.—There were favorable changes in cardiac risk factors in postmenopausal women undergoing tamoxifen therapy for 5 years. The degree of changes seen is similar to what has been reported in women treated with estrogen. Further research on the risk factors in ethnic groups is needed to determine the importance of tamoxifen treatment in reducing the incidence of heart disease.

▶ Adjuvant hormonal therapy plays an important role in the treatment of postmenopausal women with breast cancer. The meta-analysis of the Early Breast Cancer Trialists' Collaborative Group suggested that this benefit from tamoxifen was experienced in both the estrogen receptor–positive and the estrogen receptor–negative subgroups. Furthermore, there was a reduction in contralateral breast cancers. Early data suggested that tamoxifen would have a *beneficial* effect on cardiovascular risk factors as well.

Love et al. provide long-term data on potential cardiovascular risk factors. Comparing subjects who received placebo or tamoxifen based on random assignment, statistically significant reductions in total cholesterol, low-density lipoprotein cholesterol, and lipoprotein A were observed in the tamoxifen group. After 5 years, fibrinogen levels decreased, as did the serum glucose level and platelet count. These data support the notion that tamoxifen reduces cardiovascular risk factors (see Table 2).

Any interpretation of this study must be regarded cautiously. The study identified only the subgroup of women who had not had a major illness during the follow-up of the original cohort of patients who were randomly allocated to receive either placebo or tamoxifen. Therefore, selection bias is a possible confounding issue. Despite this, the differences observed in total and LDL cholesterol, fibrinogen levels, glucose, and platelet count are most likely the result of tamoxifen. Further follow-up will be required to determine whether these changes in biochemical parameters translate into a reduction of cardiovascular events.

G.J. Bosl, M.D.

19 Novel Therapy

Three-Dimensional Treatment Planning and Conformal Radiation Therapy: Preliminary Evaluation
Perez CA, Purdy JA, Harms W, Gerber R, Graham MV, Matthews JW, Bosch W, Drzymala R, Emami B, Fox S, Klein E, Lee HK, Michalski JM, Simpson JR (Mallinckrodt Inst of Radiology, Washington Univ, St Louis, Mo)
Radiother Oncol 36:32–43, 1995   19–1

Introduction.—The evolution of 3-dimensional radiation treatment planning (3-D RTP) has enabled improvements in the recognition of the spatial relationship between tumor and normal tissues, definition of the target volume, and distribution of the irradiation dose in the target volume. These developments allow better application of complex treatment planning in patients with cancer. The design and application of a fully integrated system of 3-dimensional treatment planning, delivery, and verification were described.

Methods.—A fully integrated, networked 3-D RTP and conformal radiation therapy system was developed; the system allows real-time display manipulations, high-performance computational speed, room-view beam setup display, and room-view dose surface display with concurrent beam's-eye view display, and it has both treatment plan evaluation and treatment plan verification tools. During a 2-year period, the 3-D approach was used to plan treatment for more than 300 patients, of whom 209 were treated with conformal radiation therapy according to the plan. The patients had various malignancies, including brain, head and neck, lung, hepatobiliary-pancreatic, and prostate tumors; 5 were pediatric patients. The time and effort involved in each step of planning and treatment were recorded for each patient. The patients were followed for a median of 12 months.

Results.—The average times for the various steps in CT volumetric simulation were as follows: 74 minutes without and 84 minutes with contrast material, including 36 minutes for contouring the tumor tissue and 44 minutes for contouring normal tissue; 78 minutes for treatment planning; 53 minutes for plan evaluation-optimization; and 58 minutes for verification simulation. The complexity of contouring varied substantially with different anatomical sites, although the time required for plan preparation, documentation, and the physical simulation varied little.

The average daily treatment times were similar with 3-D conformal (11.8–14 minutes) and standard (11.2–12.1) therapy in patients with brain, head and neck, thoracic, and hepatobiliary tumors. The median treatment time for prostate cancer was 19 minutes with 3-D conformal technique and Cerrobend blocks; that time was reduced to 14 minutes with multileaf collimation, whereas standard techniques in these patients required a median treatment time of 9.8 minutes.

With follow-up of 4 months to 3 years, survivors include 10 of 12 patients with brain tumors (5 are disease-free), 40 of 41 patients with head and neck tumors (35 are disease-free), 47% of the patients with local control of lung tumors, 45% of the patients with hepatobiliary-pancreatic tumors, and all of the patients with prostate tumors. Among the patients with prostate tumors, those treated with conformal techniques had fewer complications than did those treated with standard techniques.

Discussion.—The cost, time, and effort required for 3-D RTP and conformal irradiation may vary in tumors with different anatomical sites, but they are reasonable. Because these techniques achieve better tumor target delineation than standard techniques, they may result in better tumor control and disease-free survival and, possibly, in reduced distant metastasis and improved overall survival. Prospective randomized studies are needed to assess the long-term benefits of this treatment strategy.

▶ It is interesting to see the evolution of a technical field such as radiation therapy. These days, a great deal of touting goes on about the benefits of 3-D RTP and conformal radiation therapy. These developments have some potential, but at the moment, conformal aspects of radiation therapy use the multileaf collimators simply to shape the fields as glorified blocks. The 3-dimensional aspect of the treatment planning is all based on a stack of 2-dimensional images, with no new information, merely a better "picture."

Frankly, it is hard for me to see how this is actually going to change the bottom line in terms of outcome. The fundamental problem is still how to identify precisely where the tumor is, and I do not see these innovations as being terribly helpful in that regard. As far as the multileaf collimation is concerned, when a computer program is available to control the leaves throughout the entire course of treatment, when the beam is arcing around the patient and moving (and the leaves themselves move as well), perhaps then this really will be a step forward. It remains to be seen. In the meantime, work continues, but it is hard to see how this is going to be paid for in the brave new world of managed care. After all, we have prospectively randomized data dealing with lung cancer, breast cancer, and rectal cancer, all of which show that postoperative radiation therapy significantly improves local control anywhere from 20 to 60 percentage points. That is not translated, however, into significant gains in survival, presumably because of the presence of micrometastatic disease that, at present, eludes our ability to detect it.

If these developments were not so expensive, I would be much more enthusiastic. The cost of these technologies, along with a significant increase in manpower needed to carry out these treatments, raises serious questions in my mind as to just what the risk/benefit ratio is. The authors are correct that this kind of treatment is still in its infancy, and it will require efforts to include dose escalation studies to obtain the answers. It is not clear to me just how much the improvements of increasing dose will be able to buy in terms of improvements of local control, i.e., the improvement in outcome will depend on the true steepness of a dose-response curve. In addition, if we really do not improve the survival of patients, what will happen to this kind of research? In today's changing world, with the overwhelming emphasis on cost containment, I think research will be in trouble. To expect third-party carriers to pay for it, this area desperately requires prospective data that establish clear superiority over traditional approaches.

E. Glatstein, M.D.

A 10-Year Experience of Pediatric Brachytherapy

Healey EA, Shamberger RC, Grier HE, Loeffler JS, Tarbell NJ (Joint Ctr for Radiation Therapy, Boston; Harvard Med School, Boston)
Int J Radiat Oncol Biol Phys 32:451–455, 1995   19–2

Objective.—Brachytherapy in children delivers high doses of radiation to localized tumors while minimizing the exposure of nearby normal tissues. A 10-year experience with pediatric brachytherapy at the Joint Center for Radiation Therapy Children's Hospital Division was evaluated.

Methods.—After surgery, 18 children aged 6 months to 23 years received 19 implants. Fifteen patients also received external beam therapy. Permanent interstitial implants of iodine-125 were given to 15 children; temporary high-activity ^{125}I implants were given to 3; a temporary pelvic iridium-192 implant was given to 1; and a temporary high-activity ^{125}I brain implant, followed 3 years later by a permanent ^{125}I brain implant, was given to 1. Diagnoses included 5 primary brain tumors, 1 germ cell tumor metastatic to the brain, 2 parameningeal rhabdomyosarcomas, 2 soft tissue sarcomas, 2 primitive neuroectodermal tumor/Ewing's sarcomas, 1 suprarenal neuroblastoma, 1 hepatoblastoma, and 1 pancreatic adenocarcinoma.

Results.—Patients were followed for a median of 31 months. The median follow-up for patients still alive is 55 months. Three of 8 patients receiving implants as part of primary surgery are still alive, as is 1 patient who underwent resection followed by a permanent ^{125}I implant for locally recurrent cerebral primitive neuroectodermal tumor. One patient died after surgery, and the remaining 13 died of their disease. In 13 of 17 patients available for evaluation, disease was controlled in the area of the implant. One of 2 patients with treatment-related morbidity died of sepsis. The other recovered from an Adriamycin recall reaction.

Conclusion.—Adjunctive brachytherapy offers good local control and low overall morbidity in selected pediatric patients with carcinoma.

► Brachytherapy has fallen into disuse in a variety of centers, and these days its use is especially infrequent among children. Nonetheless, as the authors of this paper emphasize, there are still individual cases for which this kind of treatment makes a great deal of sense, even for children. This series consists of 18 children who received a total of 19 implants at the Joint Center for Radiotherapy in Boston. Fourteen of the implants were ^{125}I implants given by permanent implant technique. The point of the study is that the majority of the patients remain alive out to 119 months. The authors have carefully chosen their patients, which is no crime; it makes sense to be selective. Obviously, these investigators have skills and talents that are not commonly in use any more. The authors make a true case that this type of treatment still plays a major role in selected patients.

E. Glatstein, M.D.

20 Complications of Therapy

Risk Factors for Infection of Adult Patients With Cancer Who Have Tunnelled Central Venous Catheters
Howell PB, Walters PE, Donowitz GR, Farr BM (Univ of Virginia, Charlottesville)
Cancer 75:1367–1375, 1995
20–1

Objective.—In patients with cancer, long-term central venous catheters provide reliable access for infusion of chemotherapeutic agents, blood transfusions, parenteral nutrition, and antibiotics. However, they can also result in serious bloodstream infection. Although the incidence of these infections has been well studied, the potential risk factors for them have not. Furthermore, no studies have examined the effect of neutropenia on the incidence of catheter-related infection. Neutropenia and other variables were evaluated as potential risk factors for infection related to long-dwelling tunneled central venous catheters in patients with cancer.

Methods.—The study cohort comprised 71 adult patients with cancer who had tunneled central venous catheters. The patients were followed until catheter removal, death, or the end of the 7-month study, for a total of 12,410 catheter days. Fifteen demographic, catheter, and laboratory variables were assessed for possible association with catheter-related infections or sepsis of unknown origin.

Results.—Catheter-related infection occurred in 18% of patients at a rate of 1 infection/1,000 catheter days. Thirty-two percent of patients had sepsis of unknown origin. Neutropenia was a significant risk factor for catheter-related infection (relative risk, 15.1) and for sepsis of unknown origin (relative risk, 10.3) (Table 5). Other factors associated with sepsis of unknown origin were inpatient status, acute leukemia, and cytosine arabinoside therapy; however, these lost significance after adjustment for neutropenia.

Conclusion.—In adult patients with cancer, only neutropenia is identified as an independent risk factor for infection related to long-dwelling tunneled central venous catheters and for sepsis of unknown origin. Randomized trials are needed to determine whether growth factor administration or other prophylactic measures can reduce the risk of catheter-

TABLE 5.—Potential Risk Factors for Catheter Infection and Sepsis of Unknown Origin

Risk factor*		No. of infections/ days exposed to factor	No. of infections/ days unexposed to factor	Relative risk	95% Confidence interval	P value
Inpatient (vs. outpatient)	CRI	6/2732 IP	7/4100 OP	1.3	0.4–3.8	0.91
	SUO	30/2732 IP	4/4100 OP	11.1	4.9–25.5	<0.0001
Neutropenia	CRI	6/1259 N	0/1473 non-N	15.1	2.6–86.5	0.018
	SUO	27/1259 N	3/1473 non-N	10.3	4.0–26.8	<0.0001
New catheter (vs. old)†	CRI	3/1118 NC	3/1614 non-NC	1.4	0.3–7.1	0.94
	SUO	13/1118 NC	17/1614 non-NC	1.1	0.5–2.3	0.94
Parenteral nutrition‡	CRI	0/499 PN	3/1525 non-PN	0.4	0.0–69.4	0.85
	SUO	7/499 PN	17/1525 non-PN	1.3	0.5–3.0	0.75
ARA-C chemotherapy	CRI	3/981 AC	0/378 non-AC	2.7	0.9–8.3	0.76
	SUO	20/981 AC	1/378 non-AC	7.6	1.4–41.0	0.01
Bone marrow transplant	CRI	3/708 BMT	3/2024 non-BMT	2.9	0.6–13.1	0.37
	SUO	6/708 BMT	24/2024 non-BMT	0.7	0.3–1.7	0.61

* All calculations in this table used prospectively observed inpatient catheter days, except for the first factor in the table (i.e., inpatient status as compared with outpatient status).

† New catheter represents catheter inserted during, or within 14 days before, current admission.

‡ Patients undergoing bone marrow transplantation were not included in this calculation, because data were unavailable.

Abbreviations: CRI, catheter-related infection; *SUO*, sepsis of unknown origin; *IP*, inpatient days; *OP*, outpatient days; *N*, neutropenic days; *NC*, days of admissions in which new catheter was inserted at admission or in the 2 weeks before admission; *PN*, days from onset to end of course of parenteral nutrition; *AC*, all days of hospital stays that involved ARA-C treatment; *non-AC*, all days of hospital stays that did not involve ARA-C therapy (patients with bone marrow transplant were not included as controls for this comparison); *BMT*, bone marrow transplantation.

(Courtesy of Howell PB, Walters PE, Donowitz GR, et al: Risk factors for infection of adult patients with cancer who have tunnelled central venous catheters. *Cancer* 75:1367–1375, Copyright © 1995. Reprinted by permission of Wiley-Liss, Inc., a division of John Wiley & Sons, Inc.)

related infection. No risk factors for catheter-related infections among outpatients—who do not usually have neutropenia—are identified.

▶ Indwelling central venous catheters have become part of the standard care of patients with malignancy. Catheters may be placed in many ways, and they may either be subcutaneous and semipermanent or temporary. These catheters occasionally become infected and require prolonged antibiotic therapy or removal for proper management. Tunneled central venous catheters are frequently used in patients requiring prolonged venous access; such patients would include those undergoing bone marrow transplantation. The risk factors for catheter-related infections have not been carefully studied. Howell and colleagues evaluated 71 patients who were followed for more than 12,000 "catheter days." These 71 patients had 87 catheters for evaluation. Forty-six patients had hematologic neoplasms.

Thirteen catheter-related infections were identified during the 7 months of study; 12 of these were associated with documented septicemia, 4 patients had tunnel infections, and 7 had exit-site infections. Despite administration of antibiotics, 5 catheters were removed for persistent infection. Eventually, 9 of 13 infected catheters required removal. Neutropenia was the most prominent statistically significant risk factor for catheter infection (see Table 5). If infection occurred, it nearly always occurred during the first week of neutropenia. Surprisingly, the duration of neutropenia was *not* associated with an increased incidence of catheter-related infections. Nearly as important as neutropenia was inpatient therapy, particularly as a risk factor for septicemia of unknown origin. An association between septicemia of unknown origin and administration of cytosine arabinoside suggests that treatment for hematologic neoplasms increases the risk. This may be simply because the treatment of most solid tumors does not cause prolonged neutropenia and the diseases themselves do not cause bone marrow dysfunction.

Catheter infections are an important cause of morbidity among patients receiving chemotherapy that causes significant neutropenia. Perhaps this risk can be decreased by the administration of hematopoietic growth factors; however, such a notion requires study. The risk factors identified in this study should be carefully weighed by those who regularly use these devices in the care of their patients.

G.J. Bosl, M.D.

The Incidence of First Hickman Catheter-Related Infection and Predictors of Catheter Removal in Cancer Patients

Rotstein C, Brock L, Roberts RS (McMaster Univ, Hamilton, Ont, Canada)
Infect Control Hosp Epidemiol 16:451–458, 1995   20–2

Background.—Infections have been reported in 4% to 56% of patients with cancer in whom Hickman catheters (HC) are used for vascular access. Although HC removal appears to be unnecessary in most patients with such infection, removal may be indicated in some patient subgroups. The incidence of and time to first Hickman catheter-related infection (HCRI) in patients with malignancies were investigated at 1 center, along with the patient characteristics and pathogens predicting HC removal.

Methods and Findings.—Three hundred sixteen consecutive adults with cancer who had Hickman catheters placed between 1986 and 1990 at a regional oncology center were reviewed retrospectively. First HCRI occurred at an incidence of 5.98 per 1,000 catheter days. Forty-nine percent of the patients had their first HCRI before catheter removal. The median time to HCRI was 90 days. The significant risk factors for HCRI in a univariate analysis were male sex and hematologic malignancy. In a Cox model, these factors were again associated with an increased risk of HCRI. Infections occurred at the exit site in 23%, in the tunnel and exit site in 2%, in the bloodstream in 51%, and in the bloodstream and exit site in 24%. The incidence of bloodstream infection was 3.05 per 1,000 catheter days. There were more gram-positive pathogens isolated than gram-negative organisms or fungi. *Staphylococcus epidermidis* was the most common. Thirty-two percent of HCRIs necessitated removal of the catheter. In the univariate analysis, bloodstream infection and pathogen type predicted catheter removal. The most important factor predicting catheter removal in the multiple regression analysis was the presence of a gram-negative or fungal pathogen.

Conclusions.—First HCRIs are more common in men with hematologic malignancies than in patients with solid tumors. The causative pathogen probably predicts catheter removal in oncology patients, but further research is needed to confirm this.

▶ Hickman catheters are widely used to provide convenient, prolonged venous access in patients with cancer. They are used to draw blood, infuse antibiotics and blood products, and to administer systemic chemotherapy. They are, however, fundamentally external devices. A predictable proportion of patients will have infectious complications, including exit site infections, tunnel infections, and intraluminal catheter contamination. This series supports some prior observations: first, 60+% of Hickman-type catheters will result in an infection; second, hematologic malignancies are associated with a greater likelihood of infection, with an incidence approaching 80% or more. For unexplained reasons, catheter-related infections occurred more frequently in men than in women. Not surprisingly, gram-negative and fungal infections more frequently resulted in catheter removal than did gram-positive infections.

In my practice, I recommend implantable, subcutaneous ports for administration of routine chemotherapy in patients with solid tumors. The implantable port is easier to use and requires less maintenance by the patient or family. Hickman-type catheters are required in the management of patients undergoing any form of dose-intensive therapy that will result in profound neutropenia and the likelihood of hospitalization for neutropenic septicemia. Double- or triple-lumen catheters permit blood drawing and administration of blood product, antibiotic, and chemotherapy through different lines. Strict attention must be paid to cutaneous hygiene, and the catheter should be left in place for as short a time as possible. Early catheter removal in the face of infections unlikely to be controlled by antimicrobial agents, particularly gram-negative and fungal infections, is often required.

G.J. Bosl, M.D.

Opportunistic Pulmonary Infections With Fludarabine in Previously Treated Patients With Low-Grade Lymphoid Malignancies: A Role for *Pneumocystis Carinii* Pneumonia Prophylaxis
Byrd JC, Hargis JB, Kester KE, Hospenthal DR, Knutson SW, Diehl LF (Walter Reed Army Med Ctr, Washington, DC)
Am J Hematol 49:135–142, 1995   20–3

Background.—Patients with low-grade lymphoid malignancies who have alkylator-resistant chronic lymphocytic leukemia have been treated with fludarabine, a new antimetabolite, with some success. In such patients treated at Walter Reed Army Medical Center (WRAMC), a high rate of pulmonary infection with opportunistic organisms was observed. In a literature review, the incidence of these infections, the types of organisms responsible, and the best methods for prevention and treatment were determined.

Methods.—From 1990 to 1994, 21 patients at WRAMC were noted to have pulmonary infiltrates secondary to fludarabine treatment. They underwent procedures such as fiberoptic bronchoscopy with bronchoalveolar lavage and transbronchial biopsy to establish a diagnosis. The organisms that were cultured included *Pneumocystis carinii, Aspergillus, Nocardia,* cytomegalovirus, and others. Comparisons were made between patients with these infections and those without, using χ^2 and t tests.

Results.—According to the medical literature, 2,269 patients with low-grade lymphoid malignancies received fludarabine during the time specified. Pneumonia caused by *Pneumocystis carinii* was the most common sequela of fludarabine treatment reported in this group. Of patients who received this treatment, an opportunistic infection developed in 3.2%. The overwhelming majority (97%) had been previously treated with alkylating agents or corticosteroids. It appears that there is a synergistic effect between these agents and the development of an opportunistic infection. Other infections with a high incidence were meningitis caused by *Listeria monocytogenes* and systemic fungal infection. Prophylactic treatment with trimethoprim/sulfamethoxazole was the only effective method of forestalling opportunistic infection.

Discussion.—Opportunistic infections occurring after treatment with fludarabine may be prevented by prophylaxis with trimethoprim/sulfamethoxazole. Patients with other indolent lymphoproliferative disorders may benefit from this treatment as well. They should be worked up aggressively to prevent development of pulmonary involvement.

▶ Lymphoproliferative disorders, including chronic lymphocytic leukemia and low-grade non-Hodgkin's lymphomas, are common malignancies that are generally considered incurable. The standard therapy in the past has been alkylating agents with or without corticosteroids. The purine nucleoside analogues, including fludarabine, are antimetabolites with unique mechanisms of action and have recently been added to the therapeutic armamentarium for these disorders. In particular, the use of fludarabine in patients with previously untreated chronic lymphocytic leukemia has generated excitement because of a very high response rate, including a significant percentage of complete remissions in patients with previously untreated chronic lymphocytic leukemia. This is an achievement not commonly associated with alkylating agents.

All 3 of the purine nucleoside analogues in clinical use are associated with both myelosuppression and immunosuppression. Increasingly, opportunistic infections have been reported as more patients have been treated. A depression in the level of CB4 and CB8 cells is believed to contribute to the emergence of such infections in this setting. In addition, it has been suggested that the use of purine nucleoside analogues together with prednisone may contribute to an increased risk of opportunistic infections.

In this study, investigators at the WRAMC analyzed their own experience in patients receiving fludarabine and also reviewed the literature of patients reported to have had exposure to fludarabine during the 11 years ending in 1994. Seventy-three (3.2%) of 2,269 patients with low-grade lymphoid malignancies who were identified in the literature as receiving fludarabine sustained opportunistic infections. Seventy-one (97%) of such infections occurred in patients previously exposed to alkylating agents or corticosteroids. The high incidence (28%) of opportunistic pulmonary infections observed at the WRAMC in patients who had previously been exposed to alkylating agents and corticosteroids suggests that corticosteroid use before, during, or after fludarabine exposure will have a synergistic effect leading to opportunistic infections. In the literature, the majority (97%) of opportunistic infections described in fludarabine-treated patients with low-grade lymphoid malignancies occurred in patients with a history of both alkylating agent and corticosteroid exposure. These investigators also report that the risk of opportunistic pulmonary infections developing in this setting persists long after treatment with fludarabine has been completed.

A review of the literature indicated that *P. carinii* pneumonia was by far the most common fludarabine-associated pulmonary infection. Systemic fungal infection and *Listeria* meningitis were the 2 most common fludarabine-associated extrapulmonary opportunistic infections among patients reported in the literature. Prophylaxis with trimethoprim/sulfamethoxazole or aerosolized pentamidine appears to be the only prognostic factor accounting for a significant difference between patients with opportunistic infections and those without.

This paper is important because it further documents the significant potential for opportunistic infections, particularly *P. carinii* pneumonia, in patients with indolent lymphoproliferative disorders previously treated with fludarabine with additional exposure to corticosteroids. Prophylactic therapy with trimethoprim/sulfamethoxazole appears to reduce the incidence of *P. carinii* pneumonia and may offer prophylaxis against other bacterial pathogens, including *Listeria monocytogenes*. These same observations may apply to patients exposed to the newer purine nucleoside analogue, 2-chlorodeoxyadenosine, recently approved by the Food and Drug Administration for patients with hairy cell leukemia and now also used with increasing frequency for the treatment of patients with other indolent lymphoproliferative disorders.

M.S. Tallman, M.D.

Magnetic Resonance Imaging in Brachial Plexopathy of Cancer
Thyagarajan D, Cascino T, Harms G (Mayo Clinic, Rochester, Minn)
Neurology 45:421–427, 1995   20–4

Background.—Brachial plexopathy in patients with cancer most commonly results from tumor infiltration. However, several types of plexopathy occur with radiation therapy to the plexus. The use of MRI to investigate brachial plexopathies in patients with cancer was reported.

Methods.—The clinical records of all 71 patients with cancer and brachial plexopathy who had an MRI of the brachial plexus between 1984 and 1993 were reviewed. The MR images were reassessed in a blinded fashion.

Findings.—The presence of a mass adjacent to the brachial plexus on an MR image strongly predicted tumor infiltration as determined by clinicopathologic criteria. It was also the most useful characteristic for distinguishing radiation plexopathy from tumor infiltration. An increased T2 signal in or near the brachial plexus was common in both groups and was therefore unhelpful in distinguishing radiation plexopathy from tumor infiltration.

Conclusions.—Magnetic resonance imaging was very sensitive for indicating brachial plexus abnormalities in these patients. A limited comparison with CT suggests that MRI is better than CT as an imaging modality. However, a prospective comparison of the cost-effectiveness and clinical usefulness of these 2 imaging modalities is warranted.

▶ Once someone has been irradiated for cancer, they are subject to problems secondary to such treatment. The differential diagnosis of brachial plexopathy is a major problem. Is the plexopathy caused by treatment or is it caused by recurrent tumor in the vicinity of the brachial plexus? Computed tomography scanning has not been as helpful in this area as one might have thought, but MRI appears to be much better for this particular problem. This paper deals with a series of 71 patients from the Mayo Clinic, and the problem is beautifully illustrated by carefully chosen MR images. The quality of the pictures is excellent, and the data appear to speak for themselves. One of the advantages that MRI appears to have is the ability to image the patient in a variety of different planes, whereas the CT images in any plane other than the transverse plane appear to be less than ideal.

E. Glatstein, M.D.

Prospective Controlled Survey of Viral Infections in Children With Acute Lymphoblastic Leukemia During Chemotherapy

Möttönen M, Uhari M, Lanning M, Tuokko H (Univ of Oulu, Finland)
Cancer 75:1712–1717, 1995　　　　　　　　　　　　　　　　　　20–5

Introduction.—Although current combination chemotherapy for the treatment of childhood acute lymphoblastic leukemia (ALL) has improved survival, it also is associated with severe immune deficiency. The incidence of common viral infections was assessed in children with ALL and age-matched controls, and the spread of viral infections in their families was investigated.

Methods.—Fifteen children with ALL being treated with chemotherapy (13 in their first remission and 2 in their second remission) and their families and 26 control families, matched for number, ages, and sex of the children, were monitored for the occurrence of infections during a 2-year period. Stool specimens were obtained for virus culture every 2 weeks, and blood samples were obtained for antiviral antibody analysis every 3 months from all family members. Nasopharyngeal specimens were obtained during respiratory illnesses. The numbers of infection episodes were calculated per person per year. An illness occurring in another family member within 13 days of onset in the original member was presumed to be attributable to within-family spread of infection.

Results.—Children with ALL had 6.6 episodes of infection per year, whereas their healthy control counterparts had 5.1 episodes per year. Of the infections with identified etiology, children with ALL had 47 viral infections and controls had 22. The most common viral agents in both groups were parainfluenza viruses, enteroviruses, and adenoviruses. Among family members, the rate of infection was 4.2 episodes per year for siblings of patients with ALL, 5 episodes per year for siblings of controls, 1.7 episodes per year for parents of patients with ALL, and 2.2 episodes per year for parents of controls. The most common viral agents in both family groups were parainfluenza viruses, influenza viruses, adenoviruses, and enteroviruses. No children with ALL required discontinuation of chemotherapy, but doses of 6-mercaptopurine and methotrexate were decreased as required in response to the number of leukocytes during acute infection.

Discussion.—The children with ALL had significantly more common viral infections than did healthy control children but recovered well from these respiratory infections. The incidence of infection in other family members was comparable in the index and control families, indicating no increased spread of infection among the parents and siblings of children with ALL.

▶ Pediatric oncologists are often asked whether their patients are more susceptible to ordinary infections during therapy and whether they handle them normally in the face of multiagent chemotherapy. This neat prospective study tries to answer those questions. Children with ALL had about twice as many episodes of viral infection as did matched controls. However, they handled the infections as well as the controls, and there was no increased spread of the infections among their family members. This is one of those studies that is very handy when talking to parents of children receiving chemotherapy. It is a small pearl to be revealed on rounds with house staff.

J.V. Simone, M.D.

Mucocutaneous and Soft Tissue Infections Caused by *Xanthomonas maltophilia:* **A New Spectrum**
Vartivarian SE, Papadakis KA, Palacios JA, Manning JT Jr, Anaissie EJ (Univ of Texas MD Anderson Cancer Ctr, Houston)
Ann Intern Med 121:969–973, 1994   20–6

Introduction.—*Xanthomonas maltophilia* can cause bacteremia and other serious infections and has become an important cause of morbidity and mortality among hospitalized patients. Most previous reports of skin and soft-tissue infections have focused on wound infections; few have addressed primary and metastatic *X. maltophilia* cellulitis. In a 15-month review, mucocutaneous and soft-tissue infections caused by *X. maltophilia* among patients with cancer were identified.

Methods.—Clinical microbiology records of an academic, referral-based cancer center for a 15-month period were reviewed to identify all cultures positive for *X. maltophilia.* This organism was isolated from 237 patients, all sites included. Of these, 114 patients were judged to have true *X. maltophilia* infection. The analysis was restricted to patients with mucocutaneous and soft tissue infections.

Findings.—Mucocutaneous and soft-tissue infections were identified in 17 of the 114 patients. Metastatic cellulitis was present in 6 patients; primary cellulitis, which is usually associated with catheterization, in 5; and infected mucocutaneous ulcers in 6 (Table 1). Some of the manifestations of metastatic cellulitis were previously undescribed: 5 patients had multiple, hard, tender nodules with surrounding distant cellulitis; the other patient had ecthyma gangrenosum. The infection led to death in 4 patients. The patients identified as having metastatic cellulitis and mucocutaneous infections were hospitalized neutropenic patients who were receiving broad-spectrum antibiotics such as β-lactams or quinolones. These agents commonly showed in vitro activity against the infecting organisms. The factors usually associated with response included recovery from myelosuppression and administration of trimethoprim-sulfamethoxazle, with or without ticarcillin-clavulanate. In primary cellulitis, catheter removal contributed to treatment response.

Discussion.—Patients with cancer are not infrequently found to have mucocutaneous and soft-tissue infections with *X. maltophilia,* which can cause metastatic nodular skin lesions that mimic disseminated fungal infections. Morbidity and mortality may be high in patients with metastatic skin nodules. In patients receiving broad-spectrum β-lactam or quinolone antibiotics, superinfection may develop. For patients with catheter-associated cellulitis without bacteremia, catheter removal may aid outcome. When mucocutaneous or soft-tissue *X. maltophilia* infection is proven by culture, the treatment of choice is trimethoprim-sulfamethoxazle, with or without ticarcillin-clavulanate. However, early empiric therapy may enhance outcome.

TABLE 1.—Clinical Features of 17 Patients with Mucocutaneous and Soft Tissue Infections Caused by *Xanthomonas maltophilia*

Infection[†]	Median Age, y	M/F, n/n	Underlying Malignancy[†]	Previous Antibiotic Therapy[†‡]	Neutropenia, n/n[§]	Relevant Clinical Data[†]	Diagnostic Method[†]	Therapy and Outcome[†‖] (Responders/Total Patients)
Metastatic cellulitis (6)	38	2/4	ALL (4) AML (1) CLL (1)	ciprofloxacin (4) imipenem (2) ceftazidime (2) aztreonam (1) gentamicin (1)	6/6 (2)	Multiple skin lesions; nodular with surrounding cellulitis plus distal cellulitis (5) Ecthyma gangrenosum (1)	Cultures from blood and skin lesions (4) Blood alone (1) Skin lesion (1)	TMP-SMX plus TC (1/3) TMP-SMX plus ceftazidime (1/1) aztreonam (0/1) ceftazidime (0/1)
Primary cellulitis (5)	28	4/1	Solid tumor (4) Lymphoma (1)	None	2/5 (2)	Cellulitis around CVC (2), J-tube (1), suprapubic catheter (1), and neck mass (1)	Culture from catheter site (4) Neck mass (1)	TMP-SMX plus removal of CVC or neck mass (2/2) Removal of J-tube or CVC (2/2) cefoperazone plus removal of suprapubic catheter (1/1)
Mucocutaneous (6)	43	2/4	AML (4) ALL (1) Solid tumor (1)	ciprofloxacin (3) imipenem (3) aztreonam (2) ceftazidime (1) TC (1)	5/6 (2)	Infected ulcers of the gingiva (2), lip (1), and buccal mucosa (3)	Pure cultures from infected ulcers (6)	TMP-SMX (2/2) TMP-SMX plus TC (1/1) ciprofloxacin (0/1) None (0/2)

† Numbers in *parentheses* are the number of patients.
‡ Some patients received more than one antibiotic.
§ Numbers in *parentheses* are the number of patients with subsequent recovery.
‖ Six of the 7 neutropenic patients who responded to treatment also recovered from myelosuppression.
Abbreviations: ALL, acute lymphocytic leukemia; *AML,* acute myelogenous leukemia; *CLL,* chorionic lymphocytic leukemia; *CVC,* central venous catheter; *J-tube,* jejunostomy tube; *M/F,* male/female; *TC,* ticarcillin-clavulanate; *TMP-SMX,* trimethoprim-sulfamethoxazole.
(Courtesy of Vartivarian SE, Papadakis KA, Palacios JA, et al: Mucocutaneous and soft tissue infections caused by *Xanthomonas maltophilia:* A new spectrum. *Ann Intern Med* 121:969–973, 1994.)

▶ Opportunistic infections are often deadly complications in patients with cancer who have received immunosuppressive and myelosuppressive treatment. *Xanthomonas maltophilia* (previously called *Pseudomonas maltophilia*) is a nosocomial pathogen. It usually develops in patients with advanced hematologic disorders who have received extended courses of broad spectrum antibiotics. This manuscript describes mucocutaneous and soft tissue infections caused by this organism. Of 114 patients who had documented *X. maltophilia* infections, 17 (15%) had infections involving mucocutaneous and soft-tissue sites of infection. Three scenarios were observed: primary cellulitis, metastatic cellulitis, and mucocutaneous presentations. Each occurred with approximately equal frequency.

Although a history of broad-spectrum antibiotics is common in patients seen with this infection, those seen with primary cellulitis had *not* received previous antibiotic therapy, and 4 of them had nonhematologic malignancies. Three of these infections appeared in patients with indwelling catheters (central venous access catheter or a J-tube). The removal of these tubes appeared to be important in the control of primary cellulitis along with treatment with trimethoprim-sulfamethoxazole. Patients with metastatic cellulitis and mucocutaneous infections nearly all had advanced hematologic malignancies, were neutropenic, and had received antibiotic therapy. Patients with metastatic cellulitis were seen with multiple skin lesions with cellulitis and erythematous nodules. In patients with both metastatic cellulitis and mucocutaneous infections, resolution of the infection required the use of trimethoprim-sulfamethoxazole with or without ticarcillin-clavulanate.

G.J. Bosl, M.D.

Invasive Fungal Disease in Adults Undergoing Remission-Induction Therapy for Acute Myeloid Leukemia: The Pathogenetic Role of the Antileukemic Regimen

Bow EJ, Loewen R, Cheang MS, Schacter B (Univ of Manitoba, Winnipeg, Canada; Manitoba Cancer Treatment and Research Found, Winnipeg, Canada)
Clin Infect Dis 21:361–369, 1995   20–7

Background.—Patients who are receiving cytotoxic therapy for acute leukemia or bone marrow transplantation and experiencing prolonged, severe neutropenia are at risk for invasive fungal disease, which is associated with high mortality. Anecdotal evidence has suggested that the remission-induction regimen may be a risk factor for invasive fungal disease. This hypothesis was explored in a retrospective study of adults undergoing remission-induction therapy for acute myeloid leukemia (AML), in which the relationships among cytotoxic regimen, intestinal mucosal damage, and fungal colonization were studied.

Methods.—Under study were 138 patients who underwent 1 of 3 remission-induction protocols for untreated AML: cytarabine/daunorubicin (AML-84), high-dose cytarabine/etoposide/daunorubicin (AML-87), and mitoxantrone/etoposide (AML-88). Febrile neutropenic patients were treated empirically with antibacterial agents covering gram-negative organisms. After 7 days of fever treatment with broad-spectrum antibacterial therapy, amphotericin B was given for suspected fungal infections. Cultures were performed with nasopharyngeal, oropharyngeal, rectal, and urinary samples twice weekly until bone marrow recovery was achieved. Gastrointestinal epithelial status was evaluated with the D-xylose absorption test.

Results.—The remission rates were similar with the 3 protocols, but patients undergoing the AML-84 protocol had more prolonged severe neutropenia than the other treatment groups. Invasive fungal disease was documented in 17 patients, including 12 following protocol AML-87 (36.4%), 4 following protocol AML-84 (6%), and 1 following protocol AML-88 (2.6%). Univariate analysis revealed that invasive fungal disease was related to AML subtypes M0, M1, and M2; bacteremic infections, particularly with gram-positive organisms; and rectal yeast colonization. Bacteremia was associated with antibacterial chemoprophylaxis, duration of prophylaxis, and prolonged fever. Multivariate analysis revealed that invasive fungal infection was most strongly related to protocol AML-87, followed by AML subtype, prolonged severe neutropenia, and fungal colonization of multiple sites. In addition, invasive fungal disease was significantly related to serum levels of D-xylose, which were primarily related to treatment with protocol AML-87.

Conclusion.—The cytotoxic regimen for the treatment of AML has a strong influence on the risk of invasive fungal disease, which is independent of other prognostic factors. Cytotoxic therapy–induced gut epithelial damage plays an important role in the pathogenesis of invasive fungal disease. The AML subtype emerged as another independent risk factor.

▶ Although the majority of patients with newly diagnosed AML now achieve complete remission with conventional induction chemotherapy, prolonged neutropenia places some patients at risk for invasive fungal infection, which is associated with a high mortality rate. Although several variables with prognostic importance have been identified—including the duration of chemotherapy, the duration of neutropenia, and the institution of antibiotic therapy—few studies have addressed the crucial role of the particular cytotoxic regimen. This study addresses this issue in a retrospective analysis of 138 adults undergoing remission-induction therapy for previously untreated AML with 3 nonrandomized protocols, which included high-dose cytosine arabinoside, etoposide, and daunorubicin, and mitoxantrone plus etoposide.

Patients receiving standard doses of cytosine arabinoside and daunorubicin were treated between 1984 and 1988. Patients treated with high-dose cytosine arabinoside, etoposide, and daunorubicin were treated between 1988 and 1991 and were all younger than 60 years of age. During the same period (1988–1991), patients between the ages of 60 and 80 years were treated with mitoxantrone and etoposide. The majority of patients (107 of 138, or 77.5%) received a regimen of oral antibacterial chemoprophylaxis that included trimethoprim-sulfamethoxazole, nalidixic acid, norfloxacin, ciprofloxacin, or ofloxacin with or without rifampin. Antifungal prophylaxis was not administered. Febrile neutropenic patients were given empirical antibacterial antibiotics to adequately cover aerobic gram-negative bacteria, although vancomycin was not routinely administered. Empirical therapy with amphotericin was given for suspected fungal infections in neurotropenic patients after 7 days of persistent fever despite broad-spectrum antibiotic therapy.

Invasive fungal infections were defined as pathogenic yeast or filamentous fungus in cultures of blood or tissue specimens. In addition, the diagnosis of an invasive fungal disease could be established by histologic demonstration of a fungus in stain preparations of material obtained by tissue biopsy. Alternatively, fungal colonization was defined as isolation of a particular species of fungus from a defined specimen site for surveillance cultures on at least 2 consecutive occasions. The mean age in years among patients receiving conventional induction chemotherapy was 50.8: 41.1 among patients receiving high-dose cytosine arabinoside, etoposide, and daunorubicin and 67.1 among patients receiving mitoxantrone and etoposide ($P = 0.0001$). The incidence of invasive fungal disease was 6% among patients receiving conventional induction chemotherapy; 36.4% among patients receiving high-dose cytosine arabinoside, daunorubicin, and etoposide; and 2.6% among patients receiving mitoxantrone and etoposide ($P = 0.0001$).

Acute myeloid leukemia subtypes M with the least maturation—including M0, M1, and M2—were associated with a higher incidence of invasive fungal infection than were other AML subtypes. Bacterial infections, particularly with gram-positive organisms, were more common in patients who had invasive fungal infections than in those who did not. The incidence of bacteremia caused by gram-positive organisms was greater among patients who received antibacterial prophylaxis than among patients who did not. Bacteremia caused by gram-positive organisms was associated with antibacterial prophylaxis, the duration of prophylaxis, and prolonged duration of fever, but not with fungal colonization. There was a trend noted between invasive fungal infections and the number of sites of colonization, but only rectal colonization was significantly associated with invasive fungal disease. In a univariate analysis, the variables most strongly associated with invasive fungal disease were receiving high-dose cytosine arabinoside, daunorubicin, and etoposide; the acute myeloid leukemia subtype; prolonged severe neutropenia; and fungal colonization in multiple sites. The incidence of fungal infection was also associated with the degree of intestinal epithelial damage as measured by D-xylose malabsorption.

This report is important because it indicates that the choice of antileukemic chemotherapeutic regimen appears to play an important role in the risk for invasive fungal disease—one that may be independent of other previously reported prognostic factors. In addition, it suggests that patients with a particular subtype of AML may be at increased risk. However, it was also shown that patients with AML subtypes M0, M1, and M2 had longer durations of neutropenia than did patients of other subtypes and that this effect was independent of the particular chemotherapeutic regimen. As might have been expected, the results reported in this study suggest that the pathogenesis of invasive fungal disease is linked to chemotherapy-induced injury of the gut epithelium. The authors have also observed that earlier, more frequent modifications of antibiotic regimens may exert selective pressures on the endogenous intestinal microflora and enhance the risk for fungal colonization of invasive fungal disease.

Several limitations of this study include the lack of hematopoietic growth factor use, which has become a more common practice despite the fact that hematopoietic growth factors have not been approved for this use as yet. In addition, the practice of administering empirical therapy with amphotericin B was instituted after 7 days of persistent fever, despite broad-spectrum antibiotics, which may be a longer waiting period than has become routine in many institutions. However, despite its limitations, this report indicates that as we improve our potentially curative strategies of antileukemic approaches, the chemotherapy regimen itself may be an important consideration with respect to the development of life-threatening invasive fungal disease.

M.S. Tallman, M.D.

Experience With Liposomal Amphotericin-B in 60 Patients Undergoing High-Dose Therapy and Bone Marrow or Peripheral Blood Stem Cell Transplantation

Krüger W, Stockschläder M, Rüssmann B, Berger C, Hoffknecht M, Sobottka I, Kohlschütter B, Kroschke G, Kröger N, Horstmann M, Kabisch H, Zander AR (Univ Hosp Eppendorf, Hamburg, Germany)
Br J Haematol 91:684–690, 1995   20–8

Background.—Patients requiring myeloablative treatment have a high risk of systemic fungal infection developing while they are neutropenic. Intravenous amphotericin B has been the preferred treatment for suspected invasive mycosis or fungal sepsis, but it may cause a number of serious side effects, including renal tubular damage. An alternative is to dilute the drug in a lipid emulsion or encapsulate it within liposomes.

Objective.—The efficacy of liposomal amphotericin B was reviewed in 60 patients receiving high-dose chemotherapy and allogeneic or autologous bone marrow or stem-cell transplantation. Most patients had underlying leukemia or lymphoma. Thirty-four of the 60 patients had previously received conventional amphotericin B treatment. In half of them, a serum creatinine exceeding 1.4 mg/dL had developed. Others had a smaller increase in creatinine or clinical side effects.

Management.—The patients were nursed in isolation and usually received fluconazole as antimycotic prophylaxis. Three patients received amphotericin B orally, and 3 others received the drug by nebulization. Liposomal amphotericin B was given to patients who were febrile or had pulmonary signs on chest radiography and had failed to respond to antibiotic therapy. Thirty patients had serologic evidence of invasive mycosis.

Twenty-six patients received liposomal treatment as the primary antifungal measure. The median dose of liposomally administered drug was 2.9 mg/kg.

Efficacy.—Twenty-seven of the 50 evaluable patients had a clinical response to liposomal amphotericin B therapy. Fungal infection caused 7 deaths. Pulmonary infiltrates resolved during treatment in 9 of 17 patients, but 6 patients failed to respond and died of culture-confirmed mycosis. Eight of 9 patients with a history of *Aspergillus* pneumonia had no evidence of recurrent disease.

Side Effects.—In 2 patients, fever, headache, or abdominal pain developed during and after drug infusion, but 57 patients had no clinical side effects. The median serum creatinine level increased from 1.0 to 1.3 mg/dL. Eight patients, including 3 who had had renal impairment when treated conventionally, had a decrease in the serum creatinine level during liposomal therapy.

Conclusion.—Liposomal amphotericin B may safely be given to patients undergoing bone marrow transplantation for hematologic malignancy, but its effectiveness remains to be established.

▶ Patients undergoing high-dose chemotherapy with bone marrow or peripheral blood stem-cell transplantation are at significant risk for fungal stomach infection. The therapy of choice for patients in whom invasive fungal infections develop is amphotericin B. This agent is commonly administered prophylactically to patients with suspected fungal infection. In an effort to diminish the significant nephrotoxicity associated with this agent, microsomal encapsulation of amphotericin B has been developed; this may result in a higher therapeutic index of the drug and diminish side effects.

In this report, 60 patients undergoing bone marrow or stem-cell transplantation received liposomal amphotericin B for either suspected or documented deep-seated fungal infection. Seven of the 50 evaluable patients had the diagnosis established by culture of fungi. *Candida* antigen was detected in the blood of 28 patients, and *Aspergillus* antigen was detected in the blood of 1 patient; 1 patient's blood was positive for blood *Candida* and *Aspergillus* antigen. Unfortunately, 6 of the 7 culture-positive patients died of their fungal infection, whereas a seventh patient completely recovered. One *Aspergillus* antigen–positive patient and the 28 *Candida* antigen–positive patients were successfully treated. Six of the 7 patients with culture-proven deep-seated fungal infections were at high risk as a result of grade III or IV graft-vs.-host disease and high-dose corticosteroid use, prolonged aplasia, or a history of fungal infection.

Because of other side effects of transplantation and complications such as veno-occlusive disease of the liver and graft-vs.-hose disease, it was difficult in this study to evaluate the impact of the liposomal amphotericin on serum creatinine and bilirubin. However, there was no case of rising creatinine or liver studies that were attributable to the liposomal amphotericin. The drug required discontinuation in only 1 patient because of chills.

Although this study does not clearly prove a benefit of liposomal amphotericin over conventional amphotericin B and has failed to eradicate deep-seated fungal infection in 6 of 7 patients with culture-proven disease, it suggests that the drug is well tolerated. Furthermore, it provides a further basis for studying this agent in a careful, well-designed, phase III randomized trial. Its primary importance is to make physicians aware that such an agent is available and that studies are ongoing to determine its role in patients undergoing high-dose chemotherapy and bone marrow or stem-cell transplantation. Hopefully, liposomal amphotericin B will constitute another therapeutic advance in the supportive care of patients undergoing this intensive therapy.

M.S. Tallman, M.D.

Endometrial Carcinoma and Tamoxifen: Clearing Up a Controversy
Jordan VC, Assikis VJ (Northwestern Univ, Chicago)
Clin Cancer Res 1:467–472, 1995   20–9

Background.—Tamoxifen, which is clearly of beneficial use in the breast cancer therapy, may be associated with an increased incidence of endometrial carcinoma because of its estrogen-like activity in some tissues. Both the relationship of tamoxifen therapy to endometrial carcinoma and the grade and prognosis of such tumors were studied.

Method.—A total of 209 cases of tamoxifen-associated endometrial carcinoma were identified. Data were collected on the menopausal status of each patient, the dosage and duration of tamoxifen therapy, and the grade and stage of the endometrial carcinoma.

Results.—There was no significant difference in the incidence of endometrial carcinoma, regardless of whether the patients received tamoxifen therapy for their breast cancer. There was a modest increase in the occurrence of endometrial carcinoma with long-term tamoxifen therapy: from 1 in 1,000 (in the general population) to about 2 in 1,000. The fraction of tumors in stage I (82%) and stages II–V (18%) was similar to that in a large cohort of patients with primary endometrial carcinoma (74% and 26%, respectively). Grade 1 or 2 tumors were 80% and grade 3 tumors were 20% of the tamoxifen group compared with 79% and 21%, respectively, in the large cohort.

Conclusion.—Although physicians and patients must be alert to any suspicious spotting or bleeding, the benefits of using tamoxifen therapy for breast cancer greatly outweigh the small increased risk of endometrial carcinoma. The majority of endometrial tumors associated with tamoxifen therapy are early stage and low grade.

▶ The clinical and preclinical evidence supporting the use of tamoxifen as a preventive agent against breast cancer in high-risk women was most compelling. Mammary carcinogenesis was inhibited in vivo, bone density was increased in patients, myocardial infarctions were decreased, and contralateral breast cancers were reduced. Almost 20,000 women volunteers have enrolled in worldwide preventive trials. However, these important trials were threatened by reports of endometrial cancer developing in women receiving tamoxifen. This important review critically evaluates the risks and benefits of tamoxifen therapy and is useful reading not only for physicians, but also for women considering entering preventive trials with tamoxifen. In my mind, there is little doubt that the small risk of endometrial cancer is outweighed by the significant benefit that may result from tamoxifen therapy.

R.F. Ozols, M.D., Ph.D.

Leukemogenic Potential of Adjuvant Chemotherapy for Early-Stage Breast Cancer: The Eastern Cooperative Oncology Group Experience
Tallman MS, Gray R, Bennett JM, Variakojis D, Robert N, Wood WC, Rowe JM, Wiernik PH (Northwestern Univ, Chicago; Dana-Farber Cancer Inst, Boston; Univ of Rochester, NY; et al)
J Clin Oncol 13:1557–1563, 1995   20–10

Introduction.—For many patients with early-stage breast cancer, treatment includes adjuvant chemotherapy with cyclophosphamide. This is a known leukemogenic agent, so it is essential to identify the associated risk of secondary acute myeloid leukemia (AML) and myelodysplastic syndrome (MDS). Data from 6 Eastern Cooperative Oncology Group (ECOG) trials were used to assess the risk of secondary acute leukemia among patients with breast cancer receiving adjuvant cyclophosphamide-containing chemotherapy.

Methods.—The trials, conducted from 1978 to 1987, included 2,638 patients with previously untreated primary operable breast cancer. The mean patient age was 51 years. The mean follow-up was 7.3 years, for a total of 19,200 person-years of follow-up. Flow sheets submitted to the ECOG Data Management Office were reviewed to identify all cases of AML or MDS developing in the study patients.

Results.—Myelodysplastic syndrome developed in 3 patients, 2 of whom had a characteristic cytogenetic abnormality. Acute leukemia developed in 2 patients: 1 had adult T-cell leukemia related to human T-lymphotrophic virus type 1, and the other had AML after receiving further cyclophosphamide for breast cancer metastasis. The estimated incidence rate for MDS was 16 per 100,000 person-years of follow-up, with a 95% confidence interval of 3–46 per 100,000 person-years. For MDS and acute leukemia together, the estimated incidence rate was 26 per 100,000 person-years, with a 95% confidence interval of 8–61 per 100,000 person-years.

Conclusion.—For patients who receive standard-dose adjuvant cyclophosphamide-based chemotherapy for early breast cancer, the risk of secondary AML or MDS appears to be similar to that of the general population. However, it cannot be stated for certain that cyclophosphamide does not increase the risk of leukemia. The risk of secondary AML may be greatest in patients receiving higher doses of both alkylating agents and anthracyclines.

▶ Adjuvant chemotherapy for early-stage breast cancer is the current state-of-the-art treatment for most women with node-negative and node-positive breast cancer. The leukemogenicity of alkylating agents is well established, and the possibility that anthracyclines are leukemogenic has been suggested.

In the breast cancer clinical trial database of the ECOG, only 5 of 2,638 patients (0.19%) who received adjuvant chemotherapy based on cyclophosphamide had MDS or acute leukemia. One of the leukemias was an adult T-cell leukemia, which is probably not related to administration of chemotherapy. Therefore, the risk of secondary AML appears to be very low and is equal to or, at worst, minimally greater than that of the general population when cyclophosphamide-based therapy is administered. These data differ from those of adjuvant therapy based on the use of melphalan.[1] With melphalan-based adjuvant chemotherapy, 27 cases of leukemia and 7 of MPS were reported among 5,299 women. Therefore, the leukemic potential of cyclophosphamide-based adjuvant chemotherapy appears to be low. Nonetheless, the benefits of adjuvant chemotherapy far outweigh the risk of secondary leukemia from alkylating agents. Anthracyline-based and dose-intense therapies are more commonly used today in the adjuvant setting, particularly in high-risk patients. Given the recent report of secondary leukemia in the NSABP B-25 trial in which doxorubicin is combined with 1 of 3 schedules of cyclophosphamide,[2] vigilance and study remain critical.

G.J. Bosl, M.D.

References

1. Fisher B, Rockette H, Fisher ER, et al: Leukemia in breast cancer patients following adjuvant chemotherapy or postoperative radiation: The NSABP experience. *J Clin Oncol* 3:1640–1658, 1985.
2. DeCillis A, Anderson S, Wickerham DL, et al: Acute myeloid leukemia (AML) in NSABP B-25. *Proceedings of the 31st Annual Meeting of the American Society of Clinical Oncology* p 98, 1995.

Bladder and Kidney Cancer Following Cyclophosphamide Therapy for Non-Hodgkin's Lymphoma
Travis LB, Curtis RE, Glimelius B, Holoway EJ, Van Leeuwen FE, Lynch CF, Hagenbeck A, Stovall M, Banks PM, Adams J, Gospadarowicz MK, Wacholder S, Inskip PD, Tucker MA, Boice JD Jr (Natl Cancer Inst, Bethesda, Md; Univ Hosp, Uppsala, Sweden; The Ontario Ctr Treatment and Research Found, Toronto, Canada; et al)
J Natl Cancer Inst 87:524–530, 1995   20–11

Objective.—Cyclophosphamide is known to be a carcinogen for the bladder, but the largest study reported to date comprised only 7 cases. For

TABLE 3.—Risk of Bladder Cancer According to All Treatment Administered for Non-Hodgkin's Lymphoma (NHL)

Treatment group	No. of case subjects	No. of control subjects	Matched RR†	95% CI
No radiotherapy, no cyclophosphamide	6	42	1.0	—
Radiotherapy, no cyclophosphamide	6	16	2.8	0.7–11.1
Cyclophosphamide with or without radiotherapy	18	30	4.5‡	1.5–13.6
Other§	1	1	2.5	0.2–40

Note: Treatment groups are mutually exclusive and reflect all therapy administered for NHL within the matched time interval. Exposure was defined as treatment with cyclophosphamide for more than 1 month or radiotherapy that resulted in a dose of .5 Gy or more to the bladder. Cyclophosphamide was usually given in combination with other drugs.

† The referent group consists of 6 case subjects and 42 control subjects who did not meet exposure criteria.

‡ $P < .05$.

§ Includes 1 case subject and 1 control subject for whom radiotherapy status was unknown.

(Courtesy of Travis LB, Curtis RE, Glimelius B, et al: Bladder and kidney cancer following cyclophosphamide therapy for non-Hodgkin's lymphoma. *J Natl Cancer Inst* 87:524–530, 1995.)

this reason, the risk of bladder/kidney cancer in recipients of cyclophosphamide was estimated in 6,171 adult patients with non-Hodgkin's lymphoma (NHL) who lived for 2 years or longer after treatment. The 48 patients with urinary tract cancers—31 with transitional cell carcinoma of the bladder and 17 with renal cell carcinoma—were matched with 136 NHL patients who did not have a second malignancy develop.

Findings.—Cyclophosphamide was given to 58% of the patients with secondary bladder cancer and to 34% of the matched control subjects. Radiotherapy alone was given to 19% and 18% of patients, respectively. The median dose was 20.4 Gy for controls and 12.9 Gy for cases. Among patients not given radiotherapy, the median cumulative dose of cyclophosphamide was about threefold greater for case subjects than for controls.

TABLE 4.—Risk of Bladder Cancer According to Cumulative Dose and Duration of Cyclophosphamide Therapy

Cyclophosphamide	Median dose or duration*	No. of cases	No. of controls	Matched RR†	95% CI
Cumulative dose, g					
<20‡	10.0 g	8	22	2.4	0.7–8.4
20–49	34.0 g	5	6	6.3§	1.3–29
≥50	87.7 g	5	2	14.5§,¶	2.3–94
Duration of therapy, y					
<1	6 mo	8	20	2.5	0.7–9.0
1–2	18 mo	3	6	3.7	0.6–22
≥2	51 mo	7	4	11.8§,¶	2.3–61

* Median cumulative dose of cyclophosphamide or median duration of therapy among all patients within the specified category.

† The referent group consists of 6 case subjects and 42 control subjects who did not meet exposure criteria. The multivariate model also included terms for patients who received radiotherapy without cyclophosphamide (6 case subjects and 16 control subjects) or for whom radiotherapy status was unknown (1 case subject and 1 control subject).

‡ The minimum cumulative dose of cyclophosphamide in this group was 2.1 g.

§ $P < .05$.

¶ P for trend $< .005$.

(Courtesy of Travis LB, Curtis RE, Glimelius B, et al: Bladder and kidney cancer following cyclophosphamide therapy for non-Hodgkin's lymphoma. *J Natl Cancer Inst* 87:524–530, 1995.)

The drug typically was given in combination with vincristine and prednisone. Cyclophosphamide alone was associated with a significant risk of secondary bladder cancer, but radiotherapy alone was not (Table 3). The risk increased with the cumulative dose of cyclophosphamide (Table 4). Neither cyclophosphamide nor radiotherapy increased the risk of kidney cancer.

Discussion.—Three excessive bladder cancers may be expected in 100 patients with NHL who received a total of 20 to 50 g of cyclophosphamide and are followed for 15 years. The risk must be weighed against the expected therapeutic gain.

▶ Anecdotal reports linking the administration of cyclophosphamide with the development of urothelial malignancies has been reported for many years. However, the largest number of cases in any one report is less than 10. In this report by Travis et al., more than 6,000 two-year survivors of NHL were evaluated for secondary malignancies of the genitourinary tract. Forty-eight patients with secondary malignancies in the urinary tract were compared with a matched group of 136 control patients in whom a secondary malignancy did not develop. Bladder cancer accounted for the majority of cases ($n = 31$) compared with renal cell carcinoma ($n = 17$). No transitional cell carcinomas of the renal pelvis or ureter were observed. The latency period was greater than 5 years in more than 85% of the patients having secondary malignancies develop. The relative risk of bladder cancer developing was 2.8 for patients receiving radiotherapy and no cyclophosphamide, and 4.5 for those receiving a cyclophosphamide but no radiotherapy (see Table 3). The relative risk was highest in patients receiving a cumulative cyclophosphamide dose of 50 g or more (see Table 4). The relative risk of kidney cancer developing was minimally increased, if it was increased at all; when all doses of cyclophosphamide were considered, the relative risk was 1.2, whereas the relative risk was 2.6 for those receiving a cumulative cyclophosphamide dose of 20 g or more.

These data establish that cyclophosphamide is associated with the development of subsequent bladder cancer, whereas a similar risk probably does not exist for renal cell carcinoma. This risk must be balanced against the importance of cyclophosphamide in combination chemotherapy regimens used to treat patients with NHL. Cyclophosphamide should be used as necessary, but exposure should be limited to achieve maximum therapeutic gain. Perhaps this study has its greatest importance in the treatment of those patients who do not have malignant disorders; long-term cumulative drug exposure should be minimized, and if the disease requires protracted administration, the physician should counsel the patient about the risk and should evaluate urinary tract symptoms carefully.

G.J. Bosl, M.D.

Radiation Retinopathy in Patients With Both Diabetes Mellitus and Ophthalmic Graves' Disease

Polak BC, Wijngaarde R (The Rotterdam Eye Hosp, The Netherlands)
Orbit 14:71–74, 1995   20–12

Background.—Local or external beam irradiation of the head and neck may be followed by posterior eye segment complications. Ocular signs and symptoms may not develop for many years after radiation therapy. These complications are more likely in patients receiving simultaneous chemotherapy and in those with diabetes mellitus. In the latter group, the radiation-related changes may mimic those of diabetic retinopathy. Radiation retinopathy developed in 3 patients with diabetes mellitus and ophthalmic Graves' disease (OGD).

Patients.—Twelve patients with ocular symptoms developing after radiation therapy were reviewed. The patients received radiation dosages of 14–70 Gy for various diseases of the head and neck region (Table 1). There were 3 patients with OGD and diabetes mellitus, as well as 2 other patients with diabetes who were treated for carcinomas of the maxillary sinuses. The diabetes had been recognized between 2 and 40 years earlier in all

TABLE 1.—Survey of Patients With Retinopathy and/or Neuropathy After Irradiation Therapy for Various Intraocular or Retrobulbar Diseases and Lesions in the Head and Neck Region, in Relation to the Used Total Radiation Dosage and Fractions, the Latency Period, and Eventual Ocular Therapy

	Sex	Age	Tumor/disease (diabetes mellitus)	Radium dosage in Gy (and fractions)	Latency	OD/OS	Retinopathy/neuropathy	Treatment
1	male	30	retinoblastoma	45 (15)	1	OD	retinopathy	prednisone + argon laser + vitrectomy
2	female	68	orbital lymphoma	40 (16)	2,5	OD	retinopathy	
3	female	68	ophthalmic Graves' disease (diabetes mellitus)	20 (10)		ODS	retinopathy	argon laser
4	female	74	ophthalmic Graves' disease (diabetes mellitus)	20 (10)	2	ODS	retinopathy + neuropathy	
5	female	74	ophthalmic Graves' disease (diabetes mellitus)	20 (10)	3	ODS	retinopathy	
6	female	68	intraocular metastasis	50 (25)	1	OD	retinopathy	argon laser
7	male	34	nasopharynx	64 (29)	11	ODS	retinopathy	
8	female	54	sinus maxillaris	64 (32)	5	OS	retinopathy	argon laser
9	female	64	sinus maxillaris (diabetes mellitus)	14 (7)	1/2	ODS	neuropathy	
10	female	65	sinus maxillaris (diabetes mellius)	14 (7)	1	ODS	retinopathy	
11	female	66	sinus maxillaris	70 (31)	8/15	ODS	neuropathy	
12	female	76	septum nasi	68	10	OD	retinopathy	

Note: Three patients with ophthalmic Graves' disease (cases 3, 4, and 5) and 2 other patients (cases 9 and 10) were known to have diabetes mellitus.

(Courtesy of Polak BC, Wijngaarde R: Radiation retinopathy in patients with both diabetes mellitus and ophthalmic Graves' disease. *Orbit* 14:71–74, 1995. Published with permission of the journal *Orbit*. Copyright Æolus Press.)

patients, none of whom had retinal vasculopathy before receiving radiation therapy. Hypertension and other internal or hematologic disorders were excluded.

The other 7 patients, who did not have diabetes mellitus, had radiation retinopathy in 1 or both eyes 1–15 years after undergoing local or external beam radiation therapy. Three patients without diabetes and 1 patient with diabetes underwent argon laser therapy. One patient without diabetes underwent argon laser therapy combined with corticosteroid treatment; this patient also had vitrectomy. The radiation retinopathy was self-limiting in the rest of the patients.

Discussion.—Radiation retinopathy may occur after a low irradiation dosage in patients with OGD and diabetes mellitus. Ocular radiation therapy should therefore be avoided in these patients, if possible. The physician should ask specifically about previous radiation therapy, because most patients who underwent irradiation a long time ago will not spontaneously provide information about their disease.

▶ This is an interesting report of 3 patients that had Graves' exophthalmopathy as well as diabetes mellitus. Patients were generally treated with modest doses of radiation in the 20- to 40-Gy range. Nonetheless, these 3 patients ultimately had radiation retinopathy, generally occurring a few years after treatment.

I must say I have never recognized this problem, and I have treated my share of eyes for Graves' exophthalmopathy. In general, radiation therapy to doses of around 2,400 rad or so is really pretty effective if it is used to deal with the problem early. Unfortunately, many patients have been receiving steroids for several months—and even years—before anyone thinks of using radiation therapy for the problem. The patient who has been receiving steroids for more than 6 months has a relatively modest chance of benefiting from radiation, whereas the patient who is treated fairly early in the game frequently can achieve remarkable benefit.

As noted previously, I have not recognized radiation retinopathy in any of those patients. Perhaps it is because I have generally stopped at a relatively modest dose. Some of the retinopathy included in the authors' table (see Table 1) reflects high doses because of overt neoplastic disease either in the eye or in the adjacent orbital region. I believe this report is worth examining, and the information should then be carried back to the clinic to determine whether other people see this problem with any significant regularity. Obviously, the report is provocative, but it seriously needs confirmation.

E. Glatstein, M.D.

Cytotoxic Drug-Induced Pulmonary Disease in Infants and Children
Fauroux B, Meyer-Milsztain A, Boccon-Gibod L, Leverger G, Clément A, Biour M, Tournier G (Hôpital d'Enfants Armand Trousseau, Paris; Hôpital Saint Antoine, Paris)
Pediatr Pulmonol 18:347–355, 1994   20–13

Background.—The increased survival rate from malignant diseases as a result of more aggressive treatment contributes to the occurrence of drug-induced pulmonary disease (DIPD). The occurrence and severity of DIPD in infants and children treated with cytotoxic drugs were retrospectively reviewed.

Patients and Findings.—Fifteen children with a DIPD were studied. The mean patient age was 9 years, with a range of 1 to 17 years. Fourteen patients had an underlying malignant disease (9 leukemias). Acute hypersensitivity lung disease caused by methotrexate (6 patients) or azathioprine (1 patient) was observed. In these patients, bronchoalveolar lavage (BAL) showed alveolar-interstitial infiltrate with a hypercellularity (mean, 714,286 cells/mL) and increased lymphocyte counts (mean, 39%) with predominantly CD8-suppressor/cytotoxic lymphocytes.

Inhibition of leukocyte migration or leukocyte aggregation in the presence of low drug concentrations was positive in 5 patients who were tested. A restrictive pattern was noted on lung function tests, and the outcome of DIPD was always favorable. Chronic pneumonitis/fibrosis was noted in 6 patients who received a variable association of cyclophosphamide (3 patients), bleomycin (2 patients), bischloroethylnitrosourea (2 patients) and melphalan (1 patient). Progressive symptoms of an alveolar-interstitial pneumonitis were observed. On BAL, a moderate increase in total cell numbers (mean, 495,000 cells/mL) was seen. Restrictive patterns were observed on lung function tests. Although corticosteroid therapy was administered to 4 children, 1 died after bleomycin lung injury, and 2 had functional lung impairment. Noncardiogenic pulmonary edema occurred in 2 patients with leukemia undergoing treatment with recombinant interleukin II. Hypercellularity was shown on BAL, and the outcome was rapidly favorable.

Conclusion.—Three typical patterns emerged from this analysis: hypersensitivity lung disease, chronic pneumonitis, and noncardiogenic pulmonary edema. Inefficiencies in systematic lung evaluation may result in underdiagnosis of DIPD in children treated with cytotoxic drugs.

▶ This paper is included as a cautionary tale indicating that pulmonary side effects of chemotherapy occur in children as well as in adults. The authors report on a group of 15 children in whom DIPD developed after chemotherapy. Some of the occurrences became chronic, and, at least in 1 case the disease was fatal. Chronic fibrosis was seen mainly with alkylating agents, as one would expect. However, the authors also remind us that there are acute pulmonary conditions that can occur with biological as well as chemotherapeutic agents. Because the authors do not indicate the size of the population from which these patients were drawn, we have no information on the frequency of these side effects. In my experience, they are relatively uncommon but can be, at least, a nuisance and, at most, a fatal complication.

J.V. Simone, M.D.

Bone Marrow Transplant-Associated Thrombotic Microangiopathy: A Case Series
Zeigler ZR, Shadduck RK, Nemunaitis J, Andrews DF, Rosenfeld CS
(Western Pennsylvania Cancer Inst, Pittsburgh)
Bone Marrow Transplant 15:247–253, 1995   20–14

Introduction.—Bone marrow transplant (BMT) can be a curative treatment for patients with benign and malignant diseases. However, several complications can develop, including thrombotic microangiopathy (TM). Reported mortality rates associated with thrombotic microangiopathy have ranged from 0% to 100%. The experience with BMT-TM in 1 regional institution was evaluated.

Methods.—During a 7-month period, 52 allogeneic and 65 autologous BMTs were performed. All patients with increased lactate dehydrogenase (LD) levels had blood smears examined for fragmented erythrocytes. Data collected for these patients included the time to development of BMT-TM, the treatment and treatment response, other complications, and the clinical outcome. Clinical parameters were also measured in 17 controls who received allogeneic BMT and had no clinical evidence of BMT-TM. A grading system, ranging from grade 0 to grade 4, was used to classify the LD level and percentage of fragmented cells, which were used to interpret BMT-TM severity.

Results.—Of the 17 controls, 10 had grade 0 BMT-TM and 7 had grade 1 BMT-TM, which was found at a median of 61 days after they underwent allogeneic BMT. Grade ≥ 2 BMT-TM developed in 22 patients, with higher grades associated significantly with male sex and with the cyclophosphamide/total body irradiation preparative regimen. Patients with BMT-TM with grades higher than 1 were identified at a median of 36 days after BMT. Among the clinical parameters measured, the LD/platelet count ratio increased in association with the grade of BMT-TM, and serum creatinine values increased significantly only in patients with grade 4 severity. The severity of BMT-TM generally correlated positively with the severity of acute graft-vs.-host disease and negatively with survival. Bone-marrow transplant-thrombotic microangiopathy was manifested clinically in various symptoms, including hypertension, edema, neurologic symptoms, hemorrhagic cystitis, fever, and diarrhea. Complete resolution was seen in 7 patients with grade 2 BMT-TM (spontaneous in 5 and after discontinuation of cyclosporine in 2), but in none of the patients with grade 3 or 4 BMT-TM. Exchange with cryosupernatant produced a greater (though partial) response in patients with grade 4 BMT-TM than did exchange with fresh frozen plasma.

Conclusion.—Thrombotic microangiopathy is a common complication of BMT, particularly in patients who receive allogeneic BMT with cyclosporine prophylaxis. The grade of the disorder varies considerably and correlates with survival and response rate, suggesting that the percentage of fragmented cells is a significant prognostic indicator. Patients with grade 3–4 may improve with exchange using cryosupernatant and/or protein A immunoadsorption.

▶ Bone marrow transplantation is curative treatment for many patients with a variety of malignant diseases. However, this intensive approach is associated with a variety of complications that may limit the benefits. Although much has been written about graft-vs.-host disease, veno-occlusive disease, and interstitial pneumonitis, TM is one complication that has received less attention and may be underrecognized.

This study by Zeigler and colleagues is important because it continues to draw our attention to this often fatal complication. In addition, the authors establish a system for the grading and diagnosis of this complication. Somewhat surprisingly, the authors found that evidence of TM was present in 42% of patients undergoing allogeneic BMT. The authors propose that the elevated LD level in association with increased fragmented cells establishes the diagnosis and grade of TM.

There has been a suggestion that cyclosporine may play a role in the pathogenesis of this complication; however, in this particular study, discontinuing the use of cyclosporine did not correlate with the grade of TM. The therapeutic results achieved with fresh-frozen plasma exchange were disappointing. Other possible therapeutic maneuvers included exchange transfusion with cryosupernatant and protein A immunoadsorption. It is apparent that this syndrome represents endothelial cell damage which may be a delayed toxicity of chemoradiotherapy administered as part of the preparatory regimen. The disorder may range from a subtle self-limited complication to a fatal one. Physicians caring for patients undergoing high-dose chemotherapy with BMT must be aware of this often overlooked complication.

M.S. Tallman, M.D.

Malignancy-Related Pericardial Effusion: 127 Cases From the Roswell Park Cancer Institute
Wilkes JD, Fidias P, Vaickus L, Perez RP (Roswell Park Cancer Inst, Buffalo, NY)
Cancer 76:1377–1387, 1995
20–15

Background.—Malignant pericardial effusion is a common, potentially life-threatening complication of malignancy. Because it often has an insidious onset and nonspecific clinical manifestations, it can be difficult to diagnose. Its management is controversial. However, clinical experience suggests that early recognition and treatment can prolong life in many of these patients. A 26-year experience with malignancy-related pericardial effusions at a tertiary care cancer center was reviewed to elucidate the clinical signs and symptoms, diagnosis, therapy, and survival determinants.

Methods.—The medical records of 127 patients who underwent an invasive surgical procedure involving the pericardium and who had a diagnosis or history of malignancy were reviewed.

Results.—Of the patients with cytologically or histologically documented malignant effusions, 81% had diagnoses of lung cancer, breast cancer, non-Hodgkin's lymphoma, or Hodgkin's disease. The most common symptom was dyspnea, occurring in 81%. Chest discomfort and orthopnea were other fairly common symptoms. The most common sign was an abnormal pulsus paradoxus, occurring in 32% of patients. Other common signs included diminished breath sounds, tachycardia, edema, increased jugular venous pressure, and hypotension.

Chest radiographs showed cardiomegaly in 76% and demonstrated pleural effusion in 42%. Echocardiographic findings included a diminished principal deflection in echocardiogram amplitude, sinus tachycardia, and pericarditis. Echocardiography detected pericardial effusion in 76 of 79 patients and pericardial tamponade in 9 patients. Diagnostic sensitivities were 90% with cytology, 56% with biopsy, and 94% with combined cytology and biopsy.

The initial therapeutic intervention was subxyphoid pericardiotomy in 85 patients, pericardiocentesis in 26 patients, and anterior thoracotomy with pleuropericardial window in 7 patients. Pleuropericardial window formation was indicated in patients with large pleural effusions. The therapeutic failure rates were 47% for pericardiocentesis, 6% for subxyphoid pericardiotomy, and 0% for pleuropericardial window formation.

The major complication rate was 5% with subxyphoid pericardiotomy and 11% with pericardiocentesis. The median survival was 73 days (range, 0–5,538 days), but the 1-year survival rate was more than 25%. Hematologic malignancies and breast cancer were the predominant diagnoses among long-term survivors. There were no significant survival differences between patients with malignant effusions and patients with idiopathic, infectious, radiation, or other nonmalignant causes.

Conclusion.—Pericardial disease should be suspected in any patient with a malignancy who demonstrates unexplained dyspnea, tachycardia, arrhythmia, or symptoms of heart failure. These patients should undergo echocardiography, which has a diagnostic accuracy of nearly 100%. Subxyphoid pericardiotomy is safe and effective in patients requiring invasive intervention.

▶ Pericardial effusions are a frequent complication of malignant disease. The development of symptoms of heart failure or unexplained dyspnea, tachycardia, or arrhythmia in a patient with a malignancy should lead to an echocardiogram, which can detect pericardial effusions with almost 100% accuracy. The appropriate management for these patients is reviewed in this extensive experience from Roswell Park Cancer Institute. Although a malignancy-related pericardial effusion is associated with widespread metastatic disease and a poor prognosis in most situations (median survival in this series was a little more than 2 months), approximately 25% of the patients can have a rate of survival greater than 1 year.

Most of these patients have breast cancer, leukemia, or lymphoma with some degree of sensitivity to radiation or chemotherapy. Consequently, these treatment modalities can be used in selected patients who have pericardial effusion without surgical intervention. However, this study demonstrates that a subxyphoid pericardiotomy is a safe and effective intervention that can relieve pericardial effusions in almost 100% of cases. The rate of recurrence is low, and the complications of the procedures are acceptable.

R.F. Ozols, M.D., Ph.D.

Primary Hypothyroidism as a Consequence of 131-I-Metaiodobenzylguanidine Treatment for Children With Neuroblastoma

Picco P, Garaventa A, Claudiani F, Gattorno M, De Bernardi B, Borrone C (G Gaslini Inst for Children, Genoa, Italy; Galliera Hosp, Genoa, Italy)
Cancer 76:1662–1664, 1995   20–16

Introduction.—Cure rates are high in infants and children with localized operable neuroblastoma who are treated with surgery, often without adjuvant therapy. However, patients with disseminated neuroblastoma have a poor prognosis. Preliminary studies have shown promising results of treatment with ^{131}I-metaiodobenzylguanidine (^{131}I-MIBG) in patients with disseminated neuroblastoma. However, there is little information regarding the effects of this treatment on the thyroid gland. Therefore, thyroid function was studied prospectively in children with disseminated neuroblastoma treated with ^{131}I-MIBG.

Methods.—Over 7 years, 58 children with unresectable or disseminated neuroblastoma that either did not respond to chemotherapy or had relapsed, were treated with ^{131}I-MIBG in doses ranging from 2.5 to 5.5 gigabecquerels (GBq). Patients were also given oral iodide for 7 days before and 7 days after ^{131}I-MIBG was administered to inhibit thyroid uptake of radioiodine. The patients were followed up every 3–6 months, with assessments of height, weight, and pubertal stage done. Before and 6, 12, and 24 months after treatment, serum concentrations of thyroid hormones and thyroid-stimulating hormone were measured.

Results.—The 2-years' follow-up in 14 survivors showed decreased thyroid function in 12 patients. Thyroid dysfunction developed within 6 months in 5 patients, with 2 of these patients having overt hypothyroidism. Eight of the 14 patients demonstrated overt primary hypothyroidism at 2 years. These patients were treated with L-tiroxine, which resolved the hypothyroidism-related symptoms and signs. The cumulative dose of ^{131}I-MIBG ranged from 0.25 to 1.2 GBq/kg in patients with overt hypothyroidism and from 0.15 to 0.87 GBq/kg in patients with compensated hypothyroidism.

Conclusion.—Infants and children treated with ^{131}I-MIBG for neuro-blastoma must be closely monitored for thyroid function. In order to more effectively inhibit thyroid uptake of radioiodine, it may be necessary to increase the oral iodide doses, prolong administration of iodide doses, and/or investigate alternative methods.

▶ The authors report a very high incidence of hypothyroidism among children given ^{131}I-MIBG for the treatment of neuroblastoma. The effect was marked and rapid, becoming apparent in less than a year of completion of the therapy. The hypothyroidism occurred in 12 of the 14 patients, despite the administration of iodine in the form of Lugol's solution for 1 week before and 1 week after administration of the radioisotope.

Interpretation of the study is somewhat complicated by the fact that 3 of the patients also received total body irradiation before autologous bone marrow transplantation. The latter fact raises concern about the possibility of thyroid carcinoma in any survivors. Previous investigators have reported a relatively low incidence of hypothyroidism after this form of treatment; therefore, one wonders whether others have not searched adequately or whether there was something unique about this trial. Radiolabeled MIBG is certainly not curative treatment, but it appears to play some role in palliation of neuroblastoma. If, however, ^{131}I-MIBG became part of a regimen given to patients with a reasonable likelihood of cure, this late effect and the thus-far-unrealized possibility of thyroid carcinoma would give one pause with regard to including it.

J.V. Simone, M.D.

Oral Ondansetron for the Control of Cisplatin-Induced Delayed Emesis: A Large, Multicenter, Double-Blind, Randomized Comparative Trial of Ondansetron Versus Placebo

Navari RM, Madajewicz S, Anderson N, Tchekmedyian NS, Whaley W, Garewal H, Beck TM, Chang AY, Greenberg B, Caldwell KC, Huffman DH, Gould JR, Carron G, Ossi M, Anderson EM (Simon Williamson Clinic, Birmingham, Ala; State Univ of New York, Stony Brook; Univ of Rochester Cancer Ctr, New York; et al)

J Clin Oncol 13:2408–2416, 1995   20–17

Objective.—Cisplatin administration is associated with a biphasic pattern of emesis: an acute phase, which peaks 6–8 hours after administration, and a delayed phase, which begins after 24 hours. The delayed phase is less severe than the acute phase, but its management and pathophysiology are less well understood. The 5-hydroxytryptamine (5-HT$_3$) receptor antagonist ondansetron was evaluated for use in the treatment of delayed cisplatin-induced emesis.

Methods.—The multicenter, randomized, double-blind, placebo-controlled study included 538 chemotherapy-naive patients with cancer who were receiving cisplatin chemotherapy in a dose of at least 70 mg/m^2.

Patients who required rescue antiemetic therapy for acute emesis were excluded from the study. The patients were randomly assigned to receive 1 of 3 oral regimens for the control of delayed emesis. Those in group I received placebo on days 2–6; those in group II received ondansetron, 8 mg twice daily, on days 2–3 and placebo on days 4–6; and those in group III received ondansetron on days 2–6. On day 1, all patients received IV ondansetron, 0.15 mg/kg every 4 hours for 3 doses, for control of acute emesis. The main outcome measure was number of episodes of emesis on days 2 and 3, when delayed emesis is expected to be worst.

Results.—On days 2 through 5, patients receiving ondansetron had significantly fewer episodes of emesis than did those receiving placebo. Furthermore, a complete plus major response—defined as 2 or fewer emetic episodes—occurred on days 2 and 3 in 56% of patients receiving ondansetron vs. 37% of those receiving placebo. The rates of complete plus major responses were 94% vs. 85% on day 4 and 98% vs. 88% on day 5. Compared with day-1 nausea scores, significantly less nausea was experienced on days 2 and 3 by patients receiving ondansetron. By day 5, this difference was no longer significant. The overall incidence of adverse effects was greater for the patients receiving ondansetron, but the 3 groups were not significantly different in terms of laboratory indices of safety.

Conclusions.—For patients who do not require rescue therapy for acute emesis, oral ondansetron appears to be effective in controlling delayed emesis after cisplatin chemotherapy. The benefits of ondansetron in controlling delayed nausea and vomiting are most apparent in the first 2 days after cisplatin administration. The difference between treatment arms narrows thereafter, raising questions about the clinical application of oral ondansetron after day 3.

▶ Acute emesis associated with cisplatin-based chemotherapy can be controlled by 5-HT$_3$ receptor antagonists. However, management of delayed emesis associated with cisplatin-based therapy has been less effective. Typically, delayed emesis begins 2–3 days after the administration of cisplatin and can last for as long as 1 week. The delayed nausea and vomiting leads to anorexia, weight loss, and a general decrease in the quality of life for patients undergoing treatment with cisplatin.

This study demonstrates that oral ondansetron has a significant effect in the control of cisplatin-induced delayed emesis. This effect was particularly noted in patients who had excellent control of acute emesis. However, there still was a substantial delayed emesis in a large number of patients, particularly on days 2 and 3. Additional studies are needed to evaluate the potential benefit of combining oral ondansetron with dexamethasone. Also, the optimum time when oral ondansetron should be initiated requires further study.

R.F. Ozols, M.D., Ph.D.

Obesity After Successful Treatment of Acute Lymphoblastic Leukemia in Childhood

Van Dongen-Melman JEWM, Hokken-Koelega ACS, Hählen K, De Groot A, Tromp CG, Egeler RM (Erasmus Univ, Rotterdam, The Netherlands)
Pediatr Res 38:86–90, 1995

20–18

Background.—Many survivors of childhood acute lymphoblastic leukemia are overweight or obese. Excessive weight gain has been documented in particular during the first year after antileukemic treatment is completed. Although most authorities believe that this weight gain is the result of cranial irradiation, others think that corticosteroid medication may be an important factor.

Methods.—One hundred thirteen children treated for acute lymphoblastic leukemia were assessed up to 10 years after the completion of treatment with or without cranial irradiation and with different modes of corticosteroid medication. The patients were 58 boys and 55 girls aged 6 months to 15 years at diagnosis. The criteria for inclusion were complete first remission for 2 years or more after treatment cessation and no evidence of CNS or constitutional chromosomal abnormality. Corticosteroid therapy was included in all treatment regimens. Fifty-two patients received cranial irradiation as well.

Findings.—The prevalence of overweight was increased after treatment. This increase persisted over time. Weight gain did not differ between patients treated with or without cranial irradiation, demonstrating that corticosteroid therapy rather than cranial irradiation may explain weight gain in these children. Dexamethasone was associated with significantly increased weight after treatment completion. Forty-four percent of the children receiving combined prednisone and dexamethasone had obesity as a late effect, which was the highest prevalence in the study. Sex and age at diagnosis were unassociated with increases in weight.

Conclusion.—Protocols with cranial irradiation are not associated with more weight gain than protocols without cranial irradiation. The highest prevalence of obesity after completion of treatment occurred in children treated with corticosteroids and without irradiation. The use of corticosteroids may, therefore, have a greater effect on weight gain than irradiation-induced pituitary dysfunction.

▶ It has long been known by pediatric oncologists that children treated for acute lymphoblastic leukemia often become obese. The key observation in this study of 113 children was that obesity developed with the same frequency regardless of whether patients received cranial radiation. The authors point the finger at corticosteroid therapy. Because they had 6 groups to look at, they demonstrated that the greatest frequency of obesity occurred in the population that received 35 weeks of dexamethasone medication without cranial radiation and the least obesity was associated with a 5-week course of prednisone with cranial radiation. However, 5 to 7 years after diagnosis, long after treatment had been discontinued, the mean body mass index for all groups was above the normal average. Because there no longer is any reason to administer extended courses of steroids to children with leukemia, the frequency of this side effect should be reduced in future studies. However, even in the groups that received shorter courses of steroids, obesity was still a problem. Therefore, I am not convinced that the entire story lies with steroids, which may be an aggravating factor but not the sole cause.

J.V. Simone, M.D.

Growth and Puberty After Growth Hormone Treatment After Irradiation for Brain Tumours

Ogilvy-Stuart AL, Shalet SM (Christie Hosp, Manchester, England)
Arch Dis Child 73:141–146, 1995   20–19

Background.—Cranial irradiation of 27 Gy or more to the hypothalamic-pituitary axis is known to produce growth hormone deficiency and impair growth in children with intracranial malignancies. Chemotherapy also appears to affect growth adversely in such patients. The value of growth hormone therapy after treatment for a brain tumor distant from the hypothalamic-pituitary axis was investigated.

Methods.—Final height, segmental growth during puberty, and duration of puberty were determined in 29 children who had had cranial or craniospinal irradiation with or without cytotoxic chemotherapy. Growth hormone therapy had been given to all children for radiation-induced growth hormone deficiency.

Findings.—Craniospinal irradiation and chemotherapy significantly and equally reduced the final height of these children. This effect was additive in children undergoing both treatment modalities. The degree of height loss was associated with age at irradiation. The most marked effect on final height was documented in the youngest children undergoing radiation therapy. The mean duration of puberty did not differ significantly from the norm.

Conclusions.—Although growth hormone acclerates growth in children with radiation-induced growth hormone deficiency, final height is still significantly less than midparental height (Fig 1). Spinal irradiation and chemotherapy in the initial treatment of brain tumors markedly affect growth. Poor growth is also partly attributable to early puberty of normal duration.

▶ This study of children treated for brain tumors reiterates some well-known observations and reports new information. The observation that irradiation of the craniospinal axis and the administration of multiagent chemotherapy limits the growth of many children is well known. It is also well known that the younger the child is when treatment is administered, the more profound the reduction in expected height. What the authors have added to the literature is a description of the limitations of the use of growth

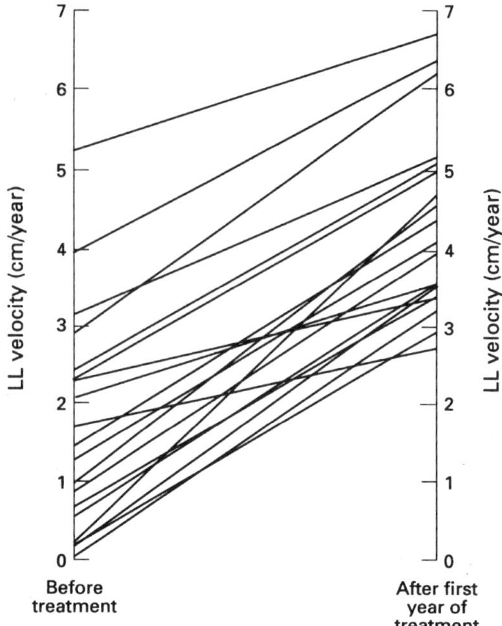

FIGURE 1.—Subischial leg length (*LL*) velocities before and after first year of growth hormone treatment. (Courtesy of Ogilvy-Stuart Al, Shalet SM: Growth and puberty after growth hormone treatment after irradiation for brain tumours. *Arch Dis Child* 73:141–146, 1995.)

hormone in attempting to overcome growth impairment in these children. Irradiation of the spine in particular appears to severely restrict any increase in growth that might be obtained with the use of growth hormone. This is not surprising, because the effect is directly on the growth centers of the spinal column, which are responsible for a large proportion of growth that the child undergoes. The more indirect effect of chemotherapy and cranial irradiation can be partly overcome by using growth hormone, although none of the children so treated achieved midparental adult height.

Is it reasonable to administer growth hormone, which is expensive and a nuisance to give? The mean pretreatment leg length growth velocity was 2 cm per year before treatment and 4.3 cm per year after treatment, for an average gain of 1.3 cm, or about a half inch. Because the average loss in final height compared to that of a normal child in the 50th percentile was substantial regardless of treatment group (ranging from 24 to 34 cm), one would think that growth hormone should be seriously considered.

The authors discuss a change in their own criteria over the years. They state that all children, irrespective of age, will be considered for growth hormone treatment if they are growth hormone deficient 2 years from diagnosis and radiotherapy. Although the velocity of growth has been improved by this treatment, the follow-up is too short to know what the effect will be on ultimate height. One would expect the children to be closer to the normal range for peers than they would be without growth hormone. One can only conclude that this treatment must be seriously considered in young children who have a reasonable chance of cure.

J.V. Simone, M.D.

Cognitive Sequelae of Treatment in Childhood Acute Lymphoblastic Leukemia: Cranial Radiation Requires an Accomplice
Waber DP, Tarbell NJ, Fairclough D, Atmore K, Castro R, Isquith P, Lussier F, Romero I, Carpenter PJ, Schiller M, Sallan SE (Children's Hosp, Boston; Harvard Med School, Boston; Dana-Farber Cancer Inst, Boston; et al)
J Clin Oncol 13:2490–2496, 1995   20–20

Background.—Cranial radiation (CRT) has been shown to prevent CNS relapse in children with acute lymphoblastic leukemia (ALL), but it has also been associated with a risk for adverse cognitive outcomes. However, patients undergoing CNS treatment without CRT can also experience similar cognitive outcomes. Intelligence quotient (IQ) and academic achievement were evaluated in ALL survivors who had been treated with conventional or high-dose methotrexate (HD-MTX) with or without CRT to evaluate the impact of CRT on cognitive outcomes.

Methods.—Between 1987 and 1991, children with ALL were randomly assigned to receive either conventional-dose methotrexate (CD-MTX), 40 mg/m², or a single IV dose of HD-MTX, 4 g/m², with leucovorin rescue. High-risk patients also received CRT (18 Gy). Between 1992 and 1993, 66 survivors in continuous complete remission between the ages of 6 and 16 years and without a preexisting risk for neurobehavioral impairment were studied with neuropsychological evaluations. The relationships between treatment effects and cognitive outcomes were analyzed.

Results.—Overall, there were no significant differences in IQ between patients treated with CD-MTX and those treated with HD-MTX, or between patients treated with and without CRT. Girls who were treated with both HD-MTX and CRT had statistically significantly lower IQ scores than all other treatment groups. All subgroups demonstrated significant reductions in the Digit Span subtest, compared with other IQ subtests, and in the spelling test, compared with other achievement subtests.

Conclusion.—The cognitive outcomes associated with treatment for childhood ALL were influenced by sex, dose levels, and agent combinations together. Cranial radiation was not, in itself, a risk factor for cognitive decline. Its toxicity appears to be related to its therapeutic context.

▶ This is the latest in a long series of studies of the effect of CRT on neuropsychological function in children with leukemia. It is generally accepted that irradiation of the brain, particularly in children younger than 6 years of age, has negative consequences. The authors maintain, however, that systemic and intrathecal chemotherapy without irradiation may have the same effect and that the radiation effect requires such prior exposure.

Others have reported that in the context of multiple-agent aggressive chemotherapy, children given 18-Gy, 24-Gy, or no cranial radiation had similar changes in neuropsychological function. Still others dispute this finding, claiming that CRT alone is responsible for the negative effects often observed (based in part on observations in patients with brain tumor, who usually receive much higher doses).

It is my own view that too much blame has been placed on CRT as being solely responsible for declines in neuropsychological function. It is clear that chemotherapy and CNS involvement of the meninges can also be factors, as demonstrated by the far greater likelihood of side effects in those who have overt CNS leukemia. However, any form of therapy that can safely be eliminated, particularly radiation in a growing child, should be left out. Most investigators restrict the use of CNS irradiation in children with leukemia to those at high risk for treatment failure. Nonetheless, this article and others remind us that leukemia infiltration of the meninges and aggressive chemotherapy also may have an impact on neuropsychological function.

J.V. Simone, M.D.

Biphasic Patterns of Memory Deficits Following Moderate-Dose Partial-Brain Irradiation: Neuropsychologic Outcome and Proposed Mechanisms
Armstrong C, Ruffer J, Corn B, DeVries K, Mollman J (Univ of Pennsylvania, Philadelphia; Jefferson Univ, Philadelphia)
J Clin Oncol 13:2263–2271, 1995   20–21

Background.—Radiation therapy is a mainstay of treatment for patients with brain tumors. There are few data on the neurocognitive sequelae in these patients, but 2 phases of posttreatment injury have been identified: early, temporary neurocognitive symptoms, and the late changes associated with progressive dementia and characterized by leukoencephalopathy. The neuropsychological effects of radiotherapy were assessed in a prospective, longitudinal study.

Methods.—Twelve patients with supratentorial brain tumors with favorable histology who were treated with radiotherapy were studied. Treatment consisted of total radiation doses of 46–63 Gy given in fraction sizes of either 1.8 or 2 Gy, over 4.5–7 weeks. The 12 patients and their healthy controls underwent testing of 10 neuropsychological domains at baseline (after surgery and immediately before radiotherapy). Testing was repeated in the patients at 3-month intervals for the first year, semiannually for the second year, and then annually.

Results.—At baseline, the patients and controls demonstrated equivalent long-term memory retrieval and had no significant differences in any other cognitive measures. At 1.5 months after the completion of radiotherapy, the patients demonstrated a decline in retrieval from verbal long-term memory, which improved by the next follow-up and had returned to baseline by 1 year. There was also a slope of improvement in the speed of processing information during the first year. There was a significant decline in long-term memory retrieval in all 6 patients evaluated at 2 years, which remained unchanged in the 4 patients evaluated at 3 years. There were no other short-term or long-term neurocognitive changes.

Discussion.—The early, transient effects on memory retrieval and improvements in processing speed during the first year suggest that disruption of myelin synthesis, and not edema, is the pathophysiologic mechanism involved in the early-delayed effects. The decline in long-term memory retrieval occurring more than 1 year after treatment and after a rebound from the early decline suggests that the late effects are mediated by multiphasic pathophysiologic processes involving cerebrovascular changes, demyelination, and autoimmune-mediated injury. It is suggested that neuropsychological testing be incorporated into national collaborative trials to further elucidate the mechanisms involved in early and late sequelae of radiotherapy in patients with brain tumors.

▶ There has long been a controversy concerning the effects of radiation on the brain. In general, most radiation oncologists believe that partial brain radiation therapy is very well tolerated. This study included patients in whom there were baseline measurements, and subjects served as their own controls. Even with partial-volume radiation, these patients showed a significant long-term memory deficit. Unfortunately, one cannot tell from this paper if a specific size of volume or specific location (e.g., hypothalamus or midbrain) is especially critical. Larger studies of this type are clearly needed.

E. Glatstein, M.D.

Evaluation of Reproductive Capacity in Germ Cell Tumor Patients Following Treatment With Cisplatin, Etoposide, and Bleomycin
Stephenson WT, Poirier SM, Rubin L, Einhorn LH (Indiana Univ, Indianapolis; Univ of Utah, Salt Lake City)
J Clin Oncol 13:2278–2280, 1995   20–22

Background.—First-line chemotherapy with cisplatin, etoposide (VP-16), and bleomycin ($PVP_{16}B$) has been found to be less toxic and may be more effective than cisplatin, vinblastine, and bleomycin (PVB) in patients with advanced germ cell tumors. However, the incidence of infertility after $PVP_{16}B$ chemotherapy has not been thoroughly investigated.

Methods.—Thirty patients who had had chemotherapy with 2–4 cycles of $PVP_{16}B$ underwent a single semen analysis 24–78 months after chemotherapy was begun. All the patients were continuously free of disease. Eight had also had nerve-sparing retroperitoneal lymph node dissection.

Findings.—The patients had a median sperm concentration of 33.9×10^6. The median volume was 3.2 mL and the median total sperm count, 86.4×10^6. Forty-three percent of the patients had oligospermia, and 6 of those 13 patients (20%) were azoospermic. The incidence of morphologically abnormal sperm was high. Only 1 patient had more than 50%

normal spermatozoa. Only 43% of the patients had sperm motility exceeding 50%. Semen antisperm immunoglobulin G (IgG) was positive in 5 patients. Nonetheless, 8 patients, including 3 with documented oligospermia, fathered children.

Conclusions.—A substantial risk for persistent semen abnormalities is associated with $PVP_{16}B$ chemotherapy in patients with germ cell tumors. However, some patients with oligospermia seem to recover slowly, and others are still able to father children despite continued oligospermia.

▶ Late toxicities are important in patients who have been cured of malignancy. In men with germ cell tumors, persistent renal and gonadal dysfunction and peripheral neuropathy are well known. Long-term effects on reproductive capacity are not well studied. Reduction in sperm count, diminished sperm motility, and abnormal sperm forms are known to exist before chemotherapy. Whether this is an effect of the disease or an altered fertility status that is somehow related to the disease has never been convincingly demonstrated. However, metastatic germ cell tumors are now cured with chemotherapy, and questions about fertility frequently arise. This study documents frequent reduction in sperm concentration and sperm count, along with a high incidence of abnormal sperm forms after treatment with VP-16, bleomycin, and cisplatin. It certainly provides evidence for reduced semen quality after chemotherapy. Unfortunately, this study is flawed by the absence of pretreatment semen studies. The contribution of chemotherapy to the abnormal sperm counts is unknown. A prior study by this group suggested that sperm quality 2 years after completing chemotherapy was similar to that before chemotherapy.

In my practice, fertility issues frequently arise as these men marry and begin to consider raising a family. I recommend sperm banking in every patient undergoing first therapy, regardless of initial semen quality (providing that aspermia is not present). I refer all patients who have undergone a retroperitoneal lymph node dissection and who have retrograde ejaculation to fertility specialists to determine the best method for obtaining sperm. For those patients who have not undergone a node dissection or whose ejaculatory status is normal, I recommend semen analysis at the time they express an interest or concern regarding fathering children. First, I reassure them that children fathered under these circumstances are likely to be normal, whether they use their banked sperm or sperm that have regenerated after chemotherapy. There is no evidence of an increased frequency of birth defects. Second, I reestablish that impairment of fertility may accompany testicular cancer and that postchemotherapy semen analysis may not be much better than that done before chemotherapy. A realistic expectation of the likelihood of fatherhood is important for these patients, and reassurance, support, and proper consultations are imperative.

G.J. Bosl, M.D.

Systems Analysis of Adverse Drug Events
Leape LL, for the ADE Prevention Study Group (Harvard School of Public Health, Boston)
JAMA 274:35–43, 1995   20–23

Background.—Up to two thirds of unintended injuries resulting from medical therapy may be caused by management errors. Adverse drug events (ADEs) causing injury commonly occur in hospitals. Many medical injuries may result from systems failures, in which an accident is the end result of a chain of events caused by a faulty system design that either induces errors or makes them difficult to detect. Systems analysis methods were used to evaluate the systems failures underlying ADEs and potential ADEs.

Methods.—The analysis included all admissions to 11 medical and surgical units in 2 tertiary care hospitals during a 6-month period. Information on actual and potential drug-related injuries was solicited from unit personnel and by record review. All ADEs and potential ADEs were classified as to whether they were preventable and the type of the causative error. The events were ascribed to various stages in the drug ordering-delivery system by a multidisciplinary panel of physicians, nurses, pharmacists, and systems analysts. The proximal cause, or apparent reason, for the error was classified and the underlying systems failures were identified. Ideas were then generated as to how systems could be redesigned to reduce failures.

Results.—Two hundred sixty-four preventable and potential ADEs were identified as arising from 334 errors. Nearly 80% of the errors occurred in the physician ordering and nurse administration stages. Dosing errors were by far the most common type. Although proximal errors often cut across multiple stages in the drug ordering-delivery system, lack of knowledge regarding the drug was the most common cause.

The underlying causes of the errors were 16 major systems failures. Dissemination of drug knowledge, especially to physicians, was the most common of these, accounting for 29% of errors. Eighteen percent of the errors involved the unavailability of patient information, such as laboratory results. These and 5 other systems failures—dose and identity checking, order transcription, the allergy defense system, medication order tracking, and interservice communication—were responsible for 78% of errors. All of these systems failures could have been prevented by better information systems.

Conclusion.—The types of systems failures underlying ADEs in the hospital were identified. Hospital staff willingly participated in the detection and investigation of such errors. The most frequent types of systems failures were those involving the dissemination of drug knowledge and the availability of drug and patient information. The chances of drug errors will be reduced by systems changes to improve the dissemination and display of drug and patient information.

► Antineoplastic drugs invariably have a narrow therapeutic window. Their systemic toxicities and vesicant attributes are fearsome to the patient and the trainee, but they are often taken for granted by the experienced oncologist. The recent tragic chemotherapy errors recorded in the media regarding drug overdoses in a patient with breast cancer in Boston and a patient with testicular cancer in Chicago should make us pause and consider preventable chemotherapy errors. Leape et al. examined the actual and potential ADEs among adult patients at Brigham and Women's Hospital and Massachusetts General Hospital over 6 months in 1993. Although the events were derived from a general hospital population, the lessons are applicable to the administration of cytotoxic chemotherapy. Most disconcerting was the observation that physician ordering and nurse administration were approximately equally frequent and accounted for almost 77% of the recorded errors.

The denominator of drug orders written is not given, but I think it is irrelevant. We need to ask ourselves: How can the risk of error be minimized? Given the drugs that we use, the calculations that must be performed to determine correct drug dose, and the multitude of physiologic factors that must be considered (e.g., renal function), I suggest the following:

1. Maximize the use of generic drug names and avoid abbreviations; "MTX" may mean methotrexate or mitoxantrone, and "mg" and "µg" cannot be misinterpreted if "milligram" and "microgram" are spelled out.

2. Write legibly.

3. Avoid the "trailing" 0; 10.0 mg cannot, therefore, be misinterpreted as 100 mg.

4. Encourage nurses and pharmacists to call with *any* question regarding a patient's drug dose; the less experienced the intermediary, the more likely the probability of error.

5. Always double-check dose and body surface area calculations.

6. Set pharmacy guidelines for maximum drug orders so that they cannot be exceeded by accident.

The potential for iatrogenic injury with antineoplastic agents is great because of the narrow therapeutic window. We cannot become too comfortable with the use of cytotoxic agents. Human errors will continue to occur, and it is our responsibility to prevent as many as we can.

G.J. Bosl, M.D.

Burnout and Psychiatric Disorder Among Cancer Clinicians
Ramirez AJ, Graham J, Richards MA, Cull A, Gregory WM, Leaning MS, Snashall DC, Timothy AR (Guy's Hosp, London; Western Gen Hosp, Edinburgh, Scotland; Univ College London; et al)
Br J Cancer 71:1263–1269, 1995   20–24

Background.—Physicians and other health care professionals are believed to be at risk for "burnout," a syndrome of work-related distress. Because of the frequent exposure to death and dying, cancer medicine is thought to be inherently stressful. There is also a conflict between curative and palliative goals in management of cancer. The prevalence of burnout and psychiatric disorder among senior oncologists and palliative care specialists in the United Kingdom was determined.

TABLE 3.—Factors Describing the Main Sources of Work-Related Stress

Factor (questionnaire items)	Percentage of consultants describing each item as contributing "quite a bit" or "a lot" to overall job stress	Mean percentage of items in factor rated as contributing "quite a bit" or "a lot" to overall job stress
1 Feeling overloaded and its effect on home life		
Having conflicting demands on your time*	68	55
Having too great an overall volume of work	65	
Disruption of your home life through long working hours	50	
Disruption of your home life through taking paperwork home	38	
2 Having organisational responsibilities/conflicts		
Having conflicting demands on your time*	68	42
Feeling under pressure to meet deadlines	48	
Having a conflict of responsibilities	44	
Having to take on more managerial responsibilities	42	
Uncertainty over the future funding of your unit/institution	35	
Being responsible for the welfare of other staff	15	
3 Dealing with patients' suffering		
Being involved with the emotional distress of patients	36	24
Being involved with the physical suffering of patients	31	
Having to break bad news to patients and relatives	26	
Being unable to control patients' symptoms	20	
Being involved with fatal illness and death	17	
Being unable to cure patients	16	
4 Being involved with treatment toxicity and errors		
Having to make treatment decisions where mistakes can have severe consequences	26	21
Feeling responsible for toxicity caused by treatment you prescribe	21	
Dealing with the threat of being sued for malpractice	15	

* This item contributed to 2 factors.

(Courtesy of Ramirez AJ, Graham J, Richards MA, et al: Burnout and psychiatric disorder among cancer clinicians. *Br J Cancer* 71:1263–1269, 1995.)

Methods.—Questionnaires were mailed to 69 medical oncologists, 253 radiotherapists, and 154 palliative care specialists. Psychiatric disorder was determined by the 12-item General Health Questionnaire, and the Maslach Burnout Inventory was used to investigate the 3 components of burnout—emotional exhaustion, depersonalization, and low personal accomplishment.

Findings.—The response rate was 83%. The prevalence of psychiatric disorder among cancer clinicians was estimated to be 28%. Burnout was more common among radiotherapists than among medical oncologists and palliative care specialists. Independent correlates of psychiatric disorder included the stress of feeling overloaded, dealing with treatment toxicity and errors, and obtaining little satisfaction from professional status. These factors were also associated with burnout, which was also related to high stress and low satisfaction from dealing with patients and with low satisfaction with adequate resources. Levels of distress were significantly higher among clinicians who believed their training in communication and management skills was inadequate compared with clinicians who believed they were sufficiently trained (Tables 3 and 5).

Conclusion.—Contrary to popular belief, the distress levels of cancer clinicians apparently are not greater than those of other medical professionals. Of all cancer clinicians, radiotherapists seem to have the most work-related distress. This is associated with high stress and low satisfaction from work-related sources. However, radiotherapists are not at greater risk for psychiatric disorder than medical oncologists or palliative care specialists.

TABLE 5.—Factors Describing the Main Sources of Work-Related Satisfaction

Factor (questionnaire items)	Percentage of consultants describing each item as contributing "quite a bit" or "a lot" to overall job satisfaction	Mean percentage of items in factor rated as contributing "quite a bit" or "a lot" to overall job satisfaction
1 Dealing well with patients and relatives		
Having good relationships with patients	97	85
Helping patients through controlling their symptoms	93	
Feeling you deal well with relatives	79	
Feeling you manage death and dying well for patients	71	
2 Having professional status/esteem		
Being perceived to do your job well by colleagues	81	72
Having a high level of responsibility	80	
Having a high level of autonomy	66	
Being able to bring about positive change in your unit/institution	62	
3 Deriving intellectual stimulation		
Deriving intellectual stimulation from teaching	53	44
Being involved in activities which contribute to the development of your profession	49	
Deriving intellectual stimulation from research	38	
Having opportunities for personal learning (developing clinical/research/management skills)	38	
4 Having adequate resources		
Feeling you have the staff necessary to do a good job	54	43
Feeling you have adequate facilities to do a good job	45	
Feeling you have adequate financial resources to do a good job	34	

(Courtesy of Ramierez AJ, Graham J, Richards MA, et al: Burnout and psychiatric disorder among cancer clinicians. *Br J Cancer* 71:1263–1269, 1995.)

▶ This important paper from Britain serves as a reminder of the personal difficulties incurred among those who treat patients with cancer. The study used questionnaires that were sent to oncologists and palliative care specialists. As shown in Table 3, there are a number of sources of work-related stress, but they are predominantly concerned with feeling overloaded and facing the conflicting demands on time that impinge on home life.

Interestingly, although dealing with the patients' suffering, treatment, toxicity, and errors provided sources of stress, those factors did not loom as large as sheer workload, conflicting demands on time, and administrative responsibilities. In fact, only 16% to 17% of those who responded described involvement with fatal illness and death or an inability to cure patients as contributing substantially to overall job stress. Therefore, one might safely predict that in the United States, burnout among oncologists is likely to increase as health care reform forces greater constraints on oncologists' time.

There was, however, a bright spot in the survey, as shown in Table 5. The factor that most contributed to overall job satisfaction was dealing well with patients and their relatives. Respondents generally liked having a high level of responsibility and being perceived by colleagues as doing their job well. Only one third to one half cited some form of intellectual stimulation as contributing substantially to their job satisfaction; one suspects that the degree of academic involvement may have a great deal to do with this.

All in all, this study once again raises the flag of caution concerning the psychological risks of the practice of oncology. If one looks simultaneously at Tables 3 and 5, one might anticipate an expansion of those factors that contribute to dissatisfaction or stress and an erosion of those factors that contribute to job satisfaction by trends toward making medical care a commodity managed by measures of economic productivity.

J.V. Simone, M.D.

21 Supportive Care

Reconstitution of Hematopoiesis After High-Dose Chemotherapy by Autologous Progenitor Cells Generated Ex Vivo
Brugger W, Heimfeld S, Berenson RJ, Mertelsmann R, Kanz L (Albert Ludwigs Univ, Freiburg, Germany; CellPro Corp, Bothell, Wash)
N Engl J Med 333:283–287, 1995   21–1

Background.—In patients with solid tumors or hematologic malignancies, giving autologous peripheral blood progenitor cells can restore the formation of blood after high-dose chemotherapy. However, a large volume of blood must be taken by leukapheresis for the collection of peripheral blood progenitor cells. To minimize contamination of these collections by tumor cells, a method of growing progenitor cells ex vivo from a relatively small blood volume was developed. The ability of ex vivo–generated peripheral blood progenitor cells to restore hematopoiesis after high-dose chemotherapy was investigated.

Methods.—The study included 10 patients who had received high-dose chemotherapy before transplantation with ex vivo–generated autologous progenitor cells. The starting population for cell growth was 11 million CD34+ hematopoietic progenitor cells, which represented less than 10% of the typical preparation of peripheral blood CD34+ mononuclear cells used in leukapheresis. The growth medium for these cells included autologous plasma, recombinant human stem-cell factor, interleukin-1β, interleukin-3, interleukin-6, and erythropoietin.

Results.—Transplantation of the ex vivo–generated cells carried no toxic effects. When given after high-dose chemotherapy with etoposide, 1,500 mg/m²; ifosfamide, 12 g/m²; carboplatin, 750 mg/m²; and epirubicin, 150 mg/m², the cells promoted a rapid and sustained hematopoietic recovery. Compared with historical controls treated with unseparated mononuclear cells or positively selected CD34+ cells, patients treated with ex vivo–generated cells had an identical pattern of hematopoietic reconstitution.

Conclusion.—Transplantation with ex vivo–generated peripheral blood CD34+ cells can supply a population of hematopoietic precursors capable of restoring blood formation after high-dose chemotherapy. For the ex vivo method, only a small amount of the patient's blood is required. In addition, the method may reduce the chances of tumor cell contamination, avoid the need for leukapheresis, and permit repeated cycles of a high-dose chemotherapy.

▶ A major problem associated with high-dose chemotherapy that requires hematologic support has been the cost and inconvenience associated with autologous bone marrow transplantations or harvesting of circulating stem cells by leukapheresis. This study demonstrates that it may be possible to reconstitute bone marrow using transplants of autologous progenitor cells that have been grown ex vivo from peripheral blood CD34+ cells, thereby obviating the need for extended leukapheresis or collection of autologous bone marrow cells. Although the reconstitution of hematopoiesis after high-dose chemotherapy has become easier with peripheral stem cell transfusions, the fundamental question of the importance of high-dose chemotherapy, however, has not been answered. The downside of facilitating hematopoietic recovery using cytokines and transplants is that it facilitates the routine use of very high-dose chemotherapy, which has not yet been established as being beneficial in the case of most solid tumors. Before high-dose chemotherapy with transplantation can be recommended in any solid tumor, it must be established as being beneficial on the basis of a prospective, randomized trial.

R.F. Ozols, M.D., Ph.D.

Dexamethasone, Granisetron, or Both for the Prevention of Nausea and Vomiting During Chemotherapy for Cancer
Roila F, for the Italian Group for Antiemetic Research (Policlinico Hosp, Perugia, Italy)
N Engl J Med 332:1–5, 1995   21–2

Purpose.—In patients receiving moderately emetogenic chemotherapy, the serotonin-receptor (5-HT_3) antagonists appear to be as effective as corticosteroids in preventing emesis. However, it is unclear whether high-dose corticosteroids offer an advantage over any single 5-HT_3 antagonist, or whether the combination of a 5-HT_3 antagonist plus dexamethasone can improve the control of acute and delayed nausea and vomiting. The antiemetic effect of granisetron plus dexamethasone was compared with that of each drug administered alone in a prospective, randomized, double-blind study.

Methods.—The sample was comprised of 428 consecutive patients scheduled to receive their first treatment with moderately emetogenic chemotherapy. This consisted of 1 or more of the following: cyclophosphamide, 600 to 1,000 mg/m²; doxorubicin, 50 mg/m² or more; epirubicin, 75 mg/m² or more; or carboplatin, 300 mg/m² or more. The patients were randomized to receive either dexamethasone, 8 mg, given intravenously (IV) given before chemotherapy, followed by 4 mg given orally just before chemotherapy and then every 6 hours for a total of 4 doses; granisetron,

3 mg, given IV before chemotherapy; or a combination of the 2 in the same doses.

Results.—The final analysis included 408 patients. Complete protection against vomiting in the first 24 hours after chemotherapy was achieved in 71% of patients receiving dexamethasone alone, in 72% of those receiving granisetron alone, and in 93% of those receiving the combination. Complete protection against nausea was achieved in 55% for patients receiving dexamethasone, 48% for patients receiving granisetron, and 72% for patients receiving the combination. The 3 regimens were equally well tolerated. Protection against delayed nausea and vomiting was significantly less in patients receiving granisetron alone vs. those receiving either dexamethasone alone or the combination regimen.

Conclusions.—In patients receiving moderately emetogenic chemotherapy, the combination of granisetron and dexamethasone appears to be the most effective regimen for prevention of emesis. This regimen provides protection against delayed vomiting as well, even though treatment is restricted to the first 24 hours. Dexamethasone alone may be a satisfactory treatment that is less expensive than the combination regimen.

▶ This large, well-designed trial established an advantage for using the combination of dexamethasone plus granisetron for the treatment of chemotherapy-induced nausea and vomiting, compared with single-agent treatment. It is of interest that dexamethasone alone was superior to granisetron and was, in fact, a highly effective regimen in moderate emetogenic regimens: the combination increased effectiveness by 20%. Both dexamethasone and the combination treatment were effective against delayed nausea and vomiting and were superior to granisetron. Although the combination is statistically superior because of the marked efficacy of the more economical dexamethasone, the selection of an antiemetogen regimen for the treatment of nausea and vomiting associated with moderately emetogenic chemotherapy may be based, in part, on cost-effective analyses.

R.F. Ozols, M.D., Ph.D.

Comparative Clinical Trial of Granisetron and Ondansetron in the Prophylaxis of Cisplatin-Induced Emesis
Navari R, on behalf of the Granisetron Study Group (Simon-Williamson Clinic, Birmingham, Ala)
J Clin Oncol 13:1242–1248, 1995   21–3

Introduction.—Cisplatin is the gold standard against which new antiemetic agents should be tested, and it was the antiemetic challenge in a recent trial. Almost 100% of patients receiving high-dose cisplatin without the use of antiemetics will experience severe nausea and vomiting. The efficacy and safety of a single IV dose of granisetron or 3 doses of ondansetron were compared for efficacy and safety in a multicenter, double-blind, parallel-group study.

Methods.—A total of 987 patients were randomly assigned to receive either a single IV infusion of granisetron, 10 or 40 µg/kg, 30 minutes before the start of chemotherapy, or ondansetron in 3 doses of 0.15 mg/kg each 30 minutes before and 4 and 8 hours after the start of chemotherapy. A placebo of 0.9% saline was administered in both granisetron groups at 4 and 8 hours after the start of chemotherapy to maintain blind status. Cisplatin was administered IV over 3 hours with or without the use of other chemotherapy agents. Concomitant use of dexamethasone or other antiemetics was not allowed. Rescue antiemetics were used at the discretion of the investigator for breakthrough emesis or significant nausea. All adverse experiences were recorded throughout a 5- to 11-day follow-up.

Results.—The percentages of patients receiving other cytotoxic agents were comparable across treatment groups. The mean dose of cisplatin was 81.5 mg/m^2. Cisplatin doses $\geq$100 mg/m^2 were readministered to 267 patients who were analyzed within the total patient population and as a separate group. Total control rates (no nausea, vomiting, or use of rescue antiemetics) for patients receiving granisetron, 10 or 40 µg/kg, or ondansetron were 38%, 41%, and 39%, respectively; they were 28%, 33%, and 25%, respectively, for patients receiving high-dose cisplatin.

No emesis rates (no vomiting, retching, or use of rescue antiemetics) for patients receiving granisetron, 10 or 40 µg/kg, or ondansetron were 47%, 48%, and 51%, respectively; they were 38%, 37%, and 35%, respectively, for patients receiving high-dose cisplatin. No nausea rates (no use of rescue antiemetics) for patients receiving either granisetron, 10 or 40 µg/kg, or ondansetron were 39%, 42%, and 40%, respectively; they were 28%, 36%, and 28% for patients receiving high-dose cisplatin. No emesis, no nausea, and total control rates were higher for men than women in both the high-dose cisplatin and overall patient groups.

Conclusion.—The efficacies of the 3 antiemetics investigated were comparable. Men generally responded better than women to antiemetic therapy while receiving cisplatin for the treatment of cancer.

▶ Granisetron and ondansetron are both 5-HT$_3$ receptor antagonists that have been used as antiemetic agents. This important prospective, randomized trial demonstrates equivalency with regard to granisetron compared with ondansetron in the prevention of nausea and vomiting induced by cisplatin chemotherapy. Patients were randomized to receive either a single dose of granisetron or 3 separate doses of ondansetron. An important aspect of the study design was the prohibition of dexamethasone use in all patients who received the 5-HT$_3$ receptor antagonists, because steroids can potentiate the antiemetic effects of these agents. Because both agents are equally effective in the treatment of cisplatin-induced emesis, the choice of which agent to use will likely be dictated by economic considerations.

R.F. Ozols, M.D., Ph.D.

Randomized Placebo-Controlled Multicenter Evaluation of Diethyldithiocarbamate for Chemoprotection Against Cisplatin-Induced Toxicities

Gandara DR, Nahhas WA, Adelson MD, Lichtman SM, Podczaski ES, Yanovich S, Homesley HD, Braly P, Ritch PS, Weisberg SR, Williams L, Diasio RB, Perez EA, Karp D, Reich SD, McCarroll K, Hoff JV (Univ of California, Davis; Wright State Univ, Dayton, Ohio; State Univ of New York Health Sciences Ctr, Syracuse; et al)

J Clin Oncol 13:490–496, 1995   21–4

Introduction.—Cisplatin is a very effective antineoplastic agent, but it also has dose-limiting toxic effects. One strategy to allow maximal therapeutic dosing is to concurrently administer chemoprotective agents. The chemoprotective properties of diethyldithiocarbamate (DDTC) were evaluated in a randomized, placebo-controlled trial in patients with cancer treated with cisplatin.

Methods.—Over 2 years, 221 patients with either small-cell lung cancer, non–small-cell lung cancer, or ovarian cancer were randomly assigned to receive chemotherapy with either DDTC or placebo. The chemotherapeutic agents used were cisplatin with cyclophosphamide for patients with ovarian cancer and cisplatin with etoposide for patients with the lung cancers. Six cycles were planned. The patients were assessed for completion of all cycles, nephrotoxicity, ototoxicity, neuropathy, relative response rates, cisplatin dose intensity, and cumulative dosing.

Results.—The trial was suspended at the time of interim analysis. In the placebo group, 28.3% had completed 6 cycles of therapy, 31.3% were receiving ongoing therapy, and 40.4% had withdrawn, most commonly because of progressive disease (22%), chemotherapy toxicity (9%), or patient request (6%). In the DDTC group, 6.3% had completed 6 cycles, 19.8% were ongoing, and 74% had withdrawn early, most commonly because of chemotherapy toxicity (23%), patient request (13.5%), or adverse effects (12.5%). The patients in the DDTC group had significantly higher serum creatinine concentrations, and acute renal failure occurred in 3 DDTC-treated patients and in none of the patients taking placebo. The 2 groups had a similar clinical hearing loss and incidence of clinical peripheral neuropathy, leukopenia and thrombocytopenia, and vomiting. The DDTC-treated patients experienced a greater incidence of transient hypertension, hyperglycemia, dehydration, and taste alteration. Patients in both groups received cisplatin in the same dose intensities, but DDTC-treated patients received a lower mean cumulative dose of cisplatin as a result of the higher early withdrawal rate. The overall response rate was 49% in the DDTC group and 43% in the placebo group, which is not a statistically significant difference.

Conclusion.—It appears that DDTC failed to protect against cisplatin-related toxicities, and, in fact, resulted in even earlier withdrawal for chemotherapy-induced side effects. In addition, DDTC itself was associated with several adverse effects. Therefore, DDTC cannot be considered as a rescue agent in patients undergoing chemotherapy with cisplatin.

▶ For chemoprotective agents to be clinically useful, they must simultaneously protect against toxicity to normal tissues while not decreasing any antitumor effects. Furthermore, they must themselves have an acceptable toxicity profile. Although many chemoprotective agents have been identified in preclinical studies, there are few, if any, that have widespread application for alkylating agents and platinum drugs. It seems that a more productive way to decrease the toxicity of some drugs is to develop less toxic analogues. Most cisplatin-based toxicities can be eliminated by using carboplatin in its place. Testicular cancer is the notable exception, in which carboplatin has less efficacy than cisplatin. In most common tumors, the toxicity of platinum compounds can be decreased by using carboplatin, particularly when area-under-the-curve dosing is used.

R.F. Ozols, M.D.

Opioid Rotation for Toxicity Reduction in Terminal Cancer Patients
de Stoutz ND, Bruera E, Suarez-Almazor M (Innere Medizin, Klinik C, Kantonspital, St Gallen, Switzerland; Edmonton Gen Hosp, Alberta, Canada; Univ of Alberta, Edmonton, Canada)
J Pain Symptom Manage 10:378–384, 1995   21–5

Background.—Metabolites may underlie the development of dose-limiting toxicity in patients receiving long-term opioid treatment for cancer pain. Changing opioids may permit metabolite clearance while maintaining or improving pain control in such patients. One experience with opioid rotation (OR) was analyzed to determine its efficacy in relieving opioid toxicity.

Methods.—Of 191 patients consecutively admitted to the palliative care unit of 1 hospital, 80 underwent OR. The indications were cognitive failure, hallucinations, myoclonus, nausea and vomiting, local toxicity, and persistent pain. In 90% of the opioid changes, morphine, hydromorphone, and methadone were used. Diamorphine and fentanyl were used occasionally (Table 2).

Findings.—Relief of the leading symptoms improved in 73% of the patients. Pain control, as indicated on a 10-cm visual analogue scale, improved from a mean of 4.4 to 3.6 at an opioid dose significantly lower than that judged to be equianalgesic. The mean doses were 577 mg before OR and 336 mg after the opioid change.

Conclusions.—Symptoms of opioid toxicity can be alleviated by OR. A choice of 2 or 3 different opioids is needed for satisfactory long-term pain control. Morphine, hydromorphone, and methadone should be included in the standard armamentarium. Additional research is now needed to establish reliable conversion factors, particularly for chronic methadone use.

TABLE 2.—Types of Opioid Rotation (First Opioid Rotation of Each Patient)

| | From | | | | |
To	Morphine	Hydromorphone	Methadone	Diamorphine	Fentanyl
Morphine		7	1	0	0
Hydromorphone	53		1	0	1
Methadone	2	8		2	0
Diamorphine	4	1	0		0
Fentanyl	0	0	0	0	

(Reprinted by permission of Elsevier Science, Inc., from de Stoutz ND, Bruera E, Suarez-Almazor M: Opioid rotation for toxicity reduction in terminal cancer patients. *J Pain Symptom Manage* 10:378–384, Copyright 1995 by the U.S. Cancer Pain Relief Committee.)

▶ These authors have done a very nice job of attempting to reduce the side effects of opioid treatment in their palliative care unit. Their plan was simply to rotate different agents in an attempt to avoid or reduce the severity of the side effects. They also achieved satisfactory pain control but concluded that 2 or, even better, 3 opioids were necessary to obtain satisfactory long-term pain control.

Several comments should be made about this study. Patients who were particularly difficult pain management problems were selected for the OR. Therefore, the 73% success rate for improving symptoms is substantial. Also, at the time of OR, 16 of the 80 patients had biochemically defined renal failure, which limited the ability to give pain-controlling doses. Typical ORs are shown in Table 2. The most common rotation was from morphine to hydromorphone.

Because the purpose of palliative care is to provide comfort in the last days or weeks of a patient's life, being able to relieve the side effects of opioids, such as myoclonus, nausea and vomiting, delirium, hallucinations, and uncontrolled pain, the latter presumably the result of tolerance, should be a high priority. These are all unacceptable side effects, and a regimen that may reduce or eliminate them should be a welcome addition to any oncologist's armamentarium.

J.V. Simone, M.D.

Aminophylline for Methotrexate-Induced Neurotoxicity
Bernini JC, Fort DW, Griener JC, Kane BJ, Chappell WB, Kamen BA (Univ of Texas Southwestern Med Ctr, Dallas; Children's Med Ctr of Dallas, Tex)
Lancet 345:544–547, 1995   21–6

Introduction.—Methotrexate, which is used to treat patients with acute lymphoblastic leukemia (ALL) and other autoimmune diseases, has several neurotoxic effects. It has been proposed that these effects are produced when methotrexate polyglutamates or partially reduced folate polyglutamates cause the inhibition of purine synthesis, allowing an exaggerated adenosine response in the CNS. It was hypothesized that an adenosine antagonist, by displacing adenosine from its receptor, could reduce the neurotoxic effects.

Methods.—Six patients with ALL or lymphoma and refractory acute methotrexate neurotoxicity were treated with 2.5 mg of aminophylline per kg of body weight. Their responses were noted. In addition, the CSF adenosine concentrations were analyzed from 11 patients receiving systemic methotrexate, 8 patients with newly diagnosed leukemia or lymphoma, and 12 patients at least 1 week after methotrexate treatment.

Results.—The symptoms of neurotoxicity began within 24 hours infusion of methotrexate and were completely resolved within 30 minutes infusion of aminophylline in 4 of the 6 patients. The other 2 had improvements in some symptoms but persistent nausea. Patients who had never received methotrexate or had not received it for at least a week demonstrated similar CSF adenosine concentrations, which were significantly lower than those demonstrated by the 11 patients completing a course of methotrexate.

Discussion.—The increased adenosine concentrations found in the CSF of children receiving systemic methotrexate and the complete resolution of neurotoxic symptoms in 4 of 6 patients after treatment with aminophylline support the hypothesized mechanism for methotrexate neurotoxicity. Before a theophylline is routinely used to prevent methotrexate neurotoxicity, its effects on the cytotoxicity of methotrexate require investigation.

▶ Not everybody reads *The Lancet,* so I thought it was important to include this very interesting paper. Through some slick chemical detective work, the authors predicted that aminophylline would be a potentially important antagonist to methotrexate toxicity. This is based on the observation that the inhibition of purine synthesis by methotrexate may cause the release of adenosine, which is a CNS depressant. The authors tested this hypothesis in 6 patients with toxicity. They found a dramatic response to aminophylline in 4 and improvement of all symptoms but nausea in the remaining 2. This pearl should be filed away in one's head; it is guaranteed to impress one's colleagues on rounds.

J.B. Simone, M.D.

Need for Hospital Care and Palliative Treatment for Prostate Cancer Treated With Noncurative Intent
Aus G, Hugosson J, Norlén L (Göteborg Univ, Sweden)
J Urol 154:466–469, 1995

21–7

Introduction.—For men with stage M0 prostate cancer, deferred treatment offers a 10-year survival rate nearly as good as that associated with more aggressive treatments, i.e., radical prostatectomy or radiation therapy. There are no reliable long-term follow-up studies of patients treated with noncurative intent and few data on the need for hospital care and palliative treatment in patients with different stages of prostate cancer. The demands for palliative treatments and hospital care among patients with prostate cancer treated with noncurative intent were assessed.

Methods.—The retrospective study included 514 patients with a known diagnosis of prostate cancer who died between 1988 and 1990. Patients with no metastases on bone scan or skeletal x-ray studies, including at least the pelvis and columna, were classified as having stage M0 disease. Those with metastases other than regional nodes were classified as having stage M1 disease, and those in whom relevant staging was not performed were classified as having stage Mx. The patients' needs for hospital care and various palliative measures were analyzed in terms of stage at diagnosis and cause of death.

Findings.—Thirty percent of the patients had metastases at diagnosis. Thirty-six percent had primary deferred treatment, defined as active treatment, that was postponed 6 months or longer. Sixty-four percent received hormonal therapies, i.e., surgical castration or estrogens. Other second-line therapies included hormonal treatment in 18% of patients, cytotoxic drugs in 10%, and cortisone in 9%. Fifty-three percent of the patients died of causes directly related to prostate cancer; 9% of causes to which prostate cancer contributed; and 38% of unrelated causes. Deaths from prostate cancer increased with increasing observation time (Table 2).

The patients spent a mean of 27 days in the hospital on an average of 2.8 occasions. One hundred eight-five patients underwent 271 transurethral resections of the prostate. A total of 103 received palliative radiation therapy, and 55 had upper urinary tract procedures (Table 3). Sixty-one percent of the patients who died of prostate cancer required some type of palliative therapy compared with 29% of those who died of unrelated causes.

Conclusion.—Patients receiving deferred treatment for prostate cancer consume considerable health care resources before they die. Resource consumption is greatest among patients who die as a direct or indirect result of their prostate cancer, especially those who are without metastases at diagnosis. Studies of the results of treatment for prostate cancer should

---

TABLE 2.—Cause of Death of Patients with Stage M0 Prostate Cancer Divided into 5-Year Periods

Yrs.	Ca Death (No. pts.)	Other Causes (No. pts.)	% Risk of Ca Death
0 to 5	51	80	39
5 to 10	57	48	54
10 to 15	21	16	57
15 to 20	15	6	71
20+	5	2	71
Total No. (%)	149(50)	152(50)	

(Courtesy of Aus G, Hugosson J, Norlén L: Need for hospital care and palliative treatment for prostate cancer treated with noncurative intent. *J Urol* 154:466–469, 1995.)

TABLE 3.—Palliative Treatments and Cause of Death in 514 Patients

	Death From Prostate Ca (319 pts.)	Death From Other Causes (195 pts.)	p Value
Days hospital care	37	10	<0.0001
Mean occasions/pt.	3.7	1.5	<0.0001
No. pts. undergoing transurethral prostatic resection (%)	131 (41)	54 (28)	0.0018
No. transurethral prostatic resections	212	59	0.003
No. pts. receiving palliative radiation (%)	98 (31)	5 (3)	<0.0001
No. pts. undergoing upper urinary tract procedure (%)	53 (17)	2 (1)	<0.0001

(Courtesy of Aus G, Hugosson J, Norlén L: Need for hospital care and palliative treatment for prostate cancer treated with noncurative intent. *J Urol* 154:466–469, 1995.)

include data on cause of death and the need for palliative therapy. The impact of the disease on patients is not sufficiently described by differences in survival only.

▶ The national shift in attention to the economics of medical care has drawn attention to so-called "futile care," i.e., treatment that has no chance of cure and yet is of considerable expense. In the world of cancer research, the use of chemotherapy, radiation, or surgery that has no chance of cure has come under criticism because of its cost. What has been lost sight of by many is that the 50% of patients with cancer in whom we cannot achieve a cure still require palliative medical care even if, from the beginning, one cannot treat with curative intent.

The study reported in this abstract is important because of the long-term follow-up, the good records that were available to these Swedish investigators, and careful analysis. The authors point out that even when patients are undergoing a treatment course in which they receive only palliative care for prostate cancer, a substantial proportion of them will require significant hospital stays and intervention by either surgery or radiotherapy. The palliative measures are predictable and include transurethral resection for urinary obstruction, urinary diversion by other means, and palliative radiation for bony metastases.

National data, as well as those obtained at our own institution, indicate that the vast majority of hospital costs incurred by patients with cancer are amassed in the last 6 months of life. In a sense, this is a self-fulfilling revelation because the last 6 months is when recurrent or progressive disease often requires hospitalization and major palliative measures, as shown in this study. However, we should be extremely careful in this era of managed care to recognize that these palliative treatments may be necessary for the comfort of the patient, even when cure is not an option. After all, that is a major part of our role as cancer physicians: to cure when possible and to provide comfort in all cases.

J.V. Simone, M.D.

Subcutaneous Urinary Diversions for Palliative Treatment of Pelvic Malignancies
Desgrandchamps F, Cussenot O, Meria P, Cortesse A, Teillac P, Le Duc A
(Saint-Louis Hosp, Paris)
J Urol 154:367–370, 1995   21–8

Background.—Palliative urinary diversion for patients with advanced pelvic malignancies poses difficult challenges in maintaining quality of life. Percutaneous nephrostomy causes problems because of the posterior location of the tube, which prevents the patient from reclining comfortably and requires assistance during dressing changes; mechanical complications are also a risk. Pyelovesical bypass and anterior cutaneous nephrostomy were reported as alternative procedures for patients undergoing permanent palliative percutaneous nephrostomy.

Methods.—The experience included 21 patients undergoing permanent subcutaneous urinary diversion because of advanced pelvic tumors that were invading or compressing the urinary tract. The percutaneous nephrostomy tube was replaced by a self-retaining expanded polytetrafluoro-ethylene-silicone tube tunneled beneath the skin. Thirteen patients under-

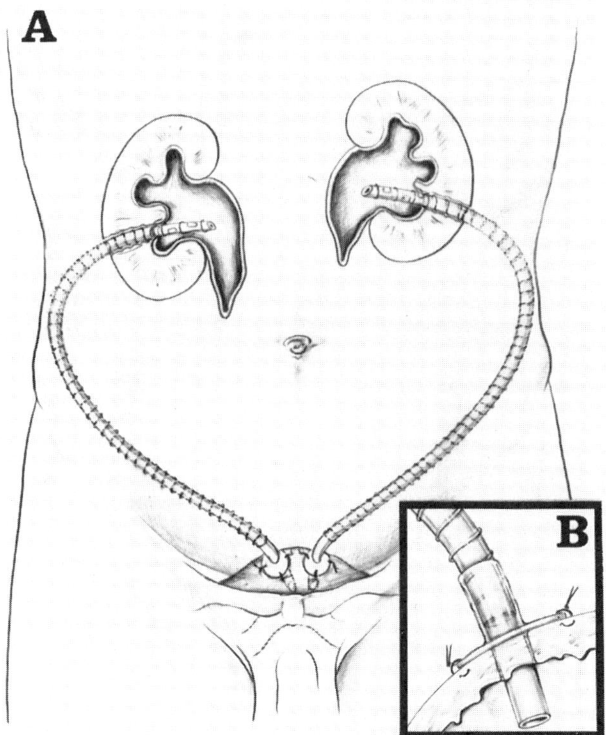

FIGURE 1.—**A,** subcutaneous pyelovesical bypass. **B,** detail of vesical extremity. (Courtesy of Desgrandchamps F, Cussenot O, Meria P, et al: Subcutaneous urinary diversions for palliative treatment of pelvic malignancies. *J Urol* 154:367–370, 1995.)

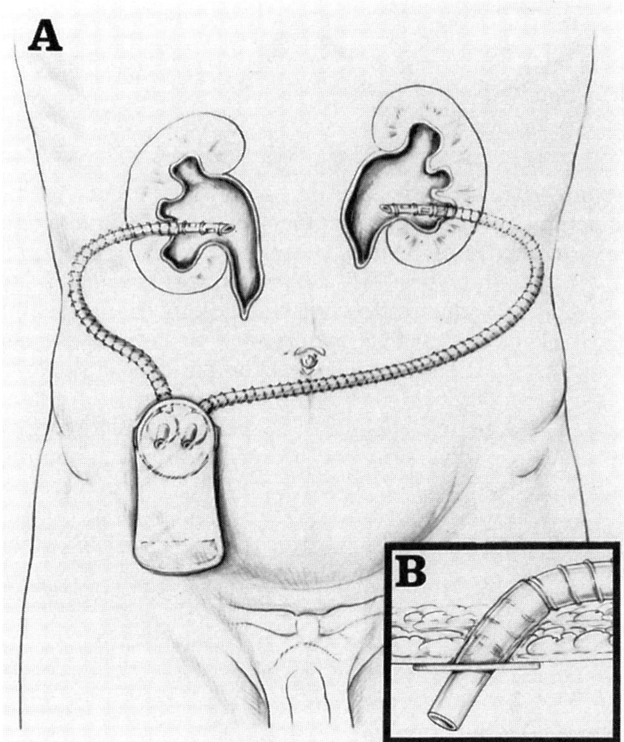

FIGURE 2.—**A,** anterior cutaneous nephrostomy. **B,** detail of cutaneous extremity. (Courtesy of Desgrandchamps F, Cussenot O, Meria P, et al: Subcutaneous urinary diversions for palliative treatment of pelvic malignancies. *J Urol* 154:367–370, 1995.)

went a total of 19 pyelovesical bypass procedures, in which the distal extremity of the tube was introduced into the bladder (Fig 1). This was always done after failure of Double-J stent diversion. Eight patients whose lower urinary tract precluded use of the bladder underwent a total of 13 anterior cutaneous nephrostomy procedures, in which the distal extremity of the tube is brought out directly through a cutaneous orifice (Fig 2).

Results.—Secondary complications occurred in 2 of 31 evaluable subcutaneous diversions: 1 case of delayed healing with exposure of the graft and 1 case of obstruction by an intrarenal nodule. Thus, 1 patient in each group required removal of the prosthesis and replacement with a standard nephrostomy tube. There were no instances of tube dislodgement, and none of the tubes became blocked by incrustation or angulation. All patients emphasized the improvement in quality of life offered by these procedures, and all were able to continue adjuvant therapy for their underlying disease.

Conclusion.—Pyelovesical bypass and anterior cutaneous nephrostomy are useful alternatives to a permanent palliative percutaneous nephrostomy tube. Pyelovesical bypass avoids the need for external drainage in patients with a functional bladder. For those with a nonfunctional bladder, anterior cutaneous nephrostomy produces a single, easily dressed anterior stoma. Because of the risk of long-term graft incrustation, these 2 procedures are currently recommended only for patients with limited life expectancy.

▶ These authors report 2 approaches to urinary diversion in the treatment of patients with pelvic malignancies. The techniques proposed— subcutaneous pyelovesical bypass (see Fig 1) and anterior cutaneous nephrostomy (see Fig 2)—are more comfortable types of diversion than the traditional percutaneous nephrostomy, and patient acceptance has been better. They certainly are easier for the patient to manage, because the outlets are anterior. The authors caution that these procedures should be used only in patients who have a limited life expectancy because of the risk of graft incrustation in long-term placement.

I include this article because I sometimes worry that we do not spend enough time and energy addressing comfort issues for patients in whom we cannot cure cancer. As I tell the young trainees at our institution, you do not become a real cancer physician until you manage patients for whom you have no specific curative therapy with the same care and diligence as you treat those who have a chance for cure.

J.V. Simone, M.D.

Social Support and Survival Among Women With Breast Cancer
Maunsell E, Brisson J, Deschênes L (Université Laval, Québec, Canada; Hôpital du St Sacrement, Québec, Canada)
Cancer 76:631–637, 1995   21–9

Background.—The impact of social support on the survival of women with localized or regional breast cancer has not been thoroughly studied. The association between social support indicators and overall survival in the first 7 years after the diagnosis of breast cancer was investigated.

Methods.—Two hundred twenty-four patients with newly diagnosed, surgically treated, localized or regional breast cancer at 7 hospitals in Quebec City in 1994 participated in the study. The patients were interviewed at home 3 months after surgery. The patients' medical records were searched for pertinent information on disease and treatment characteristics.

Findings.—After adjustment for age, presence of invaded axillary lymph nodes, adjuvant radiotherapy, and adjuvant systemic treatment, women who had at least one confidant had a 7-year hazard ratio of 0.61 compared with women who talked with no confidants in the 3 months after surgery. Women talking with 2 or more types of confidants had a hazard ratio of 0.54. Women whose confidants included a physician or nurse had a 0.51 hazard ratio (Fig 1).

Conclusions.—Social support seems to merit serious consideration as a factor that may favorably affect survival in women with breast cancer. The

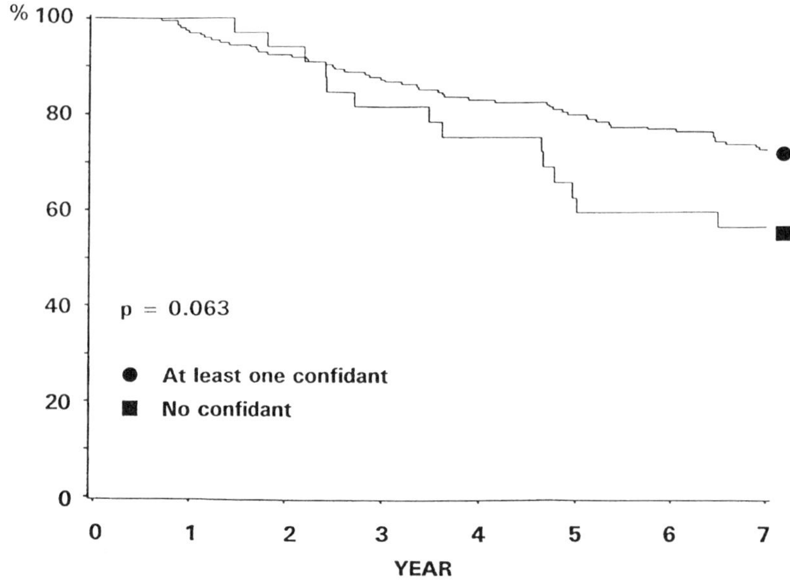

FIGURE 1.—Overall survival according to use of confidants in the 3 months after surgery. (Courtesy of Maunsell E, Brisson J, Deschênes L: Social support and survival among women with breast cancer. *Cancer* 76:631–637, copyright © 1995. Reprinted by Wiley-Liss, Inc., a division of John Wiley & Sons, Inc.)

relative differences found in 7-year survival rates in this study are equal to or greater than those considered medically significant in studies of adjuvant hormone therapy or chemotherapy in patients with breast cancer.

▶ This is the kind of paper that reinforces the common view among laymen that a positive mental attitude improves the outcome of cancer treatment. This study describes a variant of that belief—that a social support system has the same effect. The authors define social support as the presence of a confidant for the patient in the 3 months after surgery for breast cancer. The authors trot out the usual theories to explain this effect; for example, the reduction of stress, which might, in turn, improve immune function; better compliance with treatment; or better health behavior associated with better overall physical condition. None of these issues was studied by the authors, however, and although they went to great lengths to adjust for known prognostic factors in this population, it is still possible that other uncontrolled factors might contribute to the difference observed.

However, the authors may have lost sight of the most important issue. Although not everyone would agree and not all studies would confirm that a stronger social support system improves the *duration* of survival from cancer, almost any reasonable person would agree that the *quality* of life of the patient with cancer would be better in the presence of a strong social support. Loneliness is a serious danger for patients with cancer, as it is for all chronically ill patients. Thus, even if the duration of survival is not improved, a better quality of whatever time the patient has left is certainly a worthy objective.

J.V. Simone, M.D.

Scalp Cooling Has No Place in the Prevention of Alopecia in Adjuvant Chemotherapy for Breast Cancer
Tollenaar RAEM, Liefers GJ, van Driel OJR, van de Velde CJH (Univ Hosp Leiden, The Netherlands; Diaconessenhuis Eindhoven, The Netherlands)
Eur J Cancer 30A:1448–1453, 1994   21–10

Background.—Alopecia is among the most distressing side effects of chemotherapy in patients with cancer. The use of scalp hypothermia to prevent alopecia was reviewed.

Methods.—Thirty-five women younger than 70 years with operable breast cancer were studied. The newly developed Theracool cooling machine was used to induce scalp hypothermia. The chemotherapeutic regimen consisted of doxorubicin, 50 mg/m^2; cyclophosphamide, 600 mg/m^2; and 5-fluorouracil, 600 mg/m^2, given as a single course perioperatively.

Findings.—Only 11% of the patients had acceptable hair preservation, with no or minor alopecia. Thirty-four percent of the patients had moderate alopecia, all of whom needed a wig. Complete alopecia occurred in 54%. There were no scalp metastases after scalp cooling.

Findings.—Scalp hypothermia to prevent alopecia may be effective only in a cytotoxic regimen in which anthracycline is the sole alopecia-inducing agent. Scalp hypothermia has no place in current adjuvant chemotherapy for breast cancer in which a combination of cyclophosphamide and an anthracycline is often used.

▶ Alopecia is an important morbidity for patients requiring chemotherapy. Reassurance that the effect is temporary does not alleviate their concerns. Many patients and physicians have requested or advocated various techniques to reduce the likelihood of scalp alopecia. These include scalp cooling and scalp tourniquets. Theoretically, these methods could reduce blood flow to the scalp and predispose to scalp metastases because of the failure of chemotherapy to reach circulating tumor cells trapped by the reduced scalp circulation. Is there any truth to any of this? Tollenaar and colleagues attempted to study this issue prospectively. Thirty-five patients randomized to receive cyclophosphamide, doxorubicin, and 5-fluorouracil (CAF) on the first postoperative day underwent scalp hypothermia. The scalp was cooled from 30 minutes before to 240 minutes after drug therapy. The scalp temperature stayed below 22°C throughout the postinfusion period. No complications of scalp cooling were observed. However, only 4 patients had no or minor alopecia; 54% had grade 3 (complete) alopecia. In no patient did scalp metastasis develop with a mean follow-up of 46 months.

Using the technique of Tollenaar et al., scalp hypothermia does not reduce scalp alopecia caused by CAF chemotherapy. Whether scalp cooling can reduce alopecia in single-drug regimens or in the use of other drugs cannot be determined from this study. However, routine use of the scalp hypothermia device does not appear warranted and provides false hope to the patient.

G.J. Bosl, M.D.

Euthanasia: A Personal Experience in Gynecologic Oncology
Heintz APM (Univ Hosp Utrecht, The Netherlands)
Int J Gynecol Cancer 5:71–75, 1995   21–11

Background.—The term *euthanasia* comes from the Greek work meaning "good death." It refers to actively, through a medical act, causing the death of a seriously ill patient who is expected to die. Simply not instituting treatment or stopping treatment does not constitute euthanasia, nor does performing a medical act that is necessary to relieve serious suffering and is intended for this purpose.

Ethical Aspects.—So-called "mercy killing" has always been controversial. Many physicians have undertaken euthanasia to relieve unbearable suffering but have not spoken of it. Today euthanasia is discussed more openly, and patient requests that it be carried out are accepted. In some situations, not directly rejecting the possibility of euthanasia may give the patient a sense of peace and confidence.

Legal Status.—All countries have forbidden euthanasia by law. It remains illegal in The Netherlands, but physicians who commit euthanasia are assured of not being prosecuted. The purpose is to avoid situations where the wish of a patient to die brings the physician who wishes to fulfill his or her duty to help the patient into conflict with the law.

The Process.—When deciding on euthanasia, the relevant factors are whether the doctor and patient have communicated effectively regarding the patient's clinical status and wishes; the family's view; and the opinion of the attending team. The team must be adequately informed by the patient's physician. A number of methods are available. On the author's service the patient is given IV diazepam to induce sleep, followed by thiopental and Pavulon.

▶ Dr. Heintz is a world-renowned expert in the treatment of gynecologic cancers. In this thought-provoking article, Dr. Heintz describes in analytical detail his personal involvement in euthanasia in patients with cancer in The Netherlands. He makes it unequivocally clear that euthanasia is an active process in which the physician deliberately administers agents that will shorten the life of a seriously ill patient because of the expressed wish of the patient that they die without suffering. Euthanasia, as practiced by Dr. Heintz, is a process that requires an extraordinary doctor-patient relationship and must meet several established criteria. Even though euthanasia is forbidden by law in The Netherlands, "guidelines" that will not lead to prosecution of physicians performing assisted suicides have been officially approved.

Euthanasia is an emotional, ethical issue that is currently being legally challenged in the courts in the United States. If it works in The Netherlands, will it work in the United States? This is an unanswered question, but Dr. Heintz's description of both the process and its emotional toll on caregivers should be considered. By describing his experiences and his thoughts in an international journal, Dr. Heintz has elevated the debate regarding euthanasia to a new level. Regardless of whether one agrees with his position, Dr. Heintz's personal perspective on euthanasia is worth reading and discussing.

R.F. Ozols, M.D., Ph.D.

A Prospective Study of the Psychological Adjustment of Children With Cancer

Sawyer MG, Antoniou G, Nguyen A-MT, Toogood I, Rice M, Baghurst P
(Women's and Children's Hosp, South Australia, Australia)
Am J Pediatr Hematol Oncol 17:39–45, 1995   21–12

Introduction.—There have been conflicting reports of the psychological and social adjustment of children successfully treated for cancer. The differences in the results may reflect differences in the ages of the children, the length of time since diagnosis, the methods of assessment, and the stages of treatment and recovery. The prevalence of emotional and behavioral problems was studied prospectively in children with cancer at diagnosis and 1 year later and was compared with the prevalence of these problems among a comparison group of healthy children.

Methods.—Forty children, aged 4–16 years, who were given a diagnosis of cancer (excluding those with brain tumors) and 44 randomly chosen control children who were matched for age and sex, were assessed at diagnosis and after 1 year of treatment. The assessment instruments were the Child Behavior Checklist (CBCL), which was completed by the mothers, and the Youth Self Report (YSR), completed by the children. Both instruments were used to assess children aged 11–16 years; only the CBCL was used to assess children aged 4–10 years. The data were analyzed separately for the 2 age groups.

Results.—At diagnosis, the patients with cancer in the 4- to 10-year age group had higher scores than did the control children for the behavior scales measuring internalization of problems, withdrawn, and anxious/depressed; they had lower scores on the competency scales of total competence and activity. However, these scores had improved significantly at the 1-year follow-up, with little difference in the behavior problems and competencies between cancer and control patients. In the older children, there were no statistically significant differences between the cancer and control groups at either time point, but there was a trend toward fewer externalizing problems among the children with cancer than in their healthy counterparts.

Discussion.—Although the younger patients with cancer exhibited more withdrawn, depressed, and anxious behavior than did the control children, the differences were not great and had largely disappeared 1 year after diagnosis. The greater likelihood of internalizing problems in younger patients with cancer may be explained by the greater distress caused by separation from their parents and the greater difficulty they have in understanding why they must be subjected to painful and unpleasant assessments and treatments. The results show the importance of both analysis by age and longitudinal assessment in evaluating the psychosocial adjustment of children to cancer and survival.

▶ I include this study because it supports my own experience, which up until now has been only an anecdotal bias. The authors compared the adjustment of children with cancer at diagnosis and 1 year later with matched controls from the community. The major conclusion is that children aged 4–10 years had adapted emotionally and behaviorally much better after a year of therapy than those between the ages of 11 and 16 years. This has certainly been my experience. Adolescents and teenagers have a much harder time adjusting to the difficulties of having cancer and dealing with its treatment. This study also pointed out, however, that the younger children had more difficulty in the immediate period after diagnosis and initial treatment. Furthermore, they found that the older children with cancer did not appear to have more problems than children in the community who did not have cancer and were of the same age. This probably speaks to the fact that adolescents have a difficult time regardless of whether they have cancer. Any parent who has had adolescent children can sympathize with that finding.

J.V. Simone, M.D.

Current Lifestyle of Young Adults Treated for Cancer in Childhood
Evans SE, Radford M (Univ of Southampton, England)
Arch Dis Child 72:423–426, 1995   21–13

Introduction.—The psychosocial impact of surviving cancer in childhood has been minimally researched. The lifestyle and psychosocial problems of young adult survivors of childhood cancer were analyzed in 48 survivors and 38 control siblings.

Methods.—The survivors were between ages 16 and 30 years. The mean survivor age was 20 years. The mean sibling age was 21 years. Survivors and siblings were interviewed using 2 questionnaires and an unstructured interview.

Results.—Survivors included 8 patients with CNS tumors, 7 with acute lymphoblastic leukemia, 1 with acute myeloblastic leukemia, and 32 with various solid tumors. There was an interval of more than 5 years between completion of treatment and interview in 32 cases and an interval of less than 5 years in 16 cases.

Academic achievements were comparable between survivors and siblings, and they were actually higher than the national average. However, survivors were significantly less likely than their siblings to seek higher education. Twelve survivors (25%) and 18 siblings (48%) received higher education compared with a national average of 17.3%. The majority of survivors thought that re-entry into school after treatment was problematic because of lack of communication between teachers, parents, and medical staff. Thirty-two survivors (67%) and 4 siblings (10%) thought their education had been compromised because of their or their sibling's illness. There was no significant difference between survivors, siblings, and the national average in receiving a driver's license, participation in competitive sports, marital status, qualifying for a mortgage, employment status, or salary earned. However, 8 survivors (17%) reported being denied life or health insurance or having to pay higher premiums because of their medical history.

Three survivors reported that they had been turned down from job applications because they revealed that they had been treated for childhood cancer. Seventeen survivors (36%) reported that their appearance had changed because of illness or treatment, and 8 reported that they had a residual mobility problem. Using the Oxford Psychologist Press adult self-esteem questionnaire, 30 survivors (63%) and 23 siblings (61%) were found to have high self-esteem.

Conclusion.—Academic achievement, self-esteem, and employment histories were similar for survivors and their siblings. However, survivors were less likely to pursue higher education than were siblings. In addition, 36% of survivors reported that their appearance had changed and 22% noted problems with physical mobility. It is possible that the low number of survivors with CNS tumors was too small to make firm conclusions about their lifestyles.

▶ For at least 20 years, pediatric oncologists have been interested in the issue of the social adaptation of patients cured of their cancers. Some patients, unfortunately, have serious physical maladies; however, the majority do not, and many studies have shown a remarkable degree of adaptation and resumption of a normal social life. This study demonstrates that, by and large, children who were cured of cancer coped reasonably well in adult life, although some specific problems had been identified.

Probably the most remarkable findings were that, compared with the general population, cured patients were equally employable and were earning similar salaries, and they were also equally active socially and equally likely to partake in competitive sports. This is reassuring; however, as the authors point out in their discussion, the sample contained a small number of patients with CNS tumors, a population that might be expected to have more difficulty in adulthood. In fact, the authors do not elaborate on the cancer diagnoses of the patients; this is a weakness of the study, as there are major differences in the expected late complications among various diagnostic groups.

J.V. Simone, M.D.

Family Cohesion and Expressiveness Promote Resilience to the Stress of Pediatric Bone Marrow Transplant: A Preliminary Report
Phipps S, Mulhern RK (St Jude Children's Research Hosp, Memphis; Univ of Tennessee, Memphis)
J Dev Behav Pediatr 16:257–263, 1995   21–14

Background.—Some children respond to significant life stress with development of behavioral or psychological problems, whereas others adjust positively, despite difficult life circumstances. To better understand this paradox, the field of developmental psychopathology has changed its focus from identifying risk factors (such as poverty) that directly lead to psychiatric disturbance to calculating the notion of resilience and protective processes in adjustment and assessing the variables that promote healthy outcomes. The relationship of perceived family conflict, cohesion, and expressiveness to child adjustment was assessed concurrently and longitudinally in children who were about to undergo bone marrow transplantation (BMT).

Methods.—A cohort of 64 patients aged 19 months to 23 years was enrolled. Fifty-two percent were male, and 83% were in social classes II–IV. Seventy-eight percent of the patients were undergoing transplants for leukemia. The 6- to 12-month posttransplant follow-up data were available for 25 patients. Thirty-two patients (50%) had died by this time. The final group of 41 patients studied were aged 4–16 years at the time of pretransplant assessment. The children's social competence, behavioral problems, and self-esteem were measured. Perceived family conflict, cohesion, and expressiveness were also assessed.

Findings.—Post-BMT social competence and overall self-concept scores were significantly decreased. Before BMT, perceptions of family conflict were moderately inversely correlated with patient adjustment. Family cohesion and expressiveness were either uncorrelated or weakly associated with adjustment measures. By contrast, all pre-BMT family environment variables strongly predicted post-BMT adjustment.

Conclusions.—Perceived family cohesion and expressiveness served as protective factors that promote resilience in these children faced with the stresses of BMT. Family conflict was a direct risk factor, adversely affecting adjustment regardless of stress level.

► Those of us who treat children with cancer would support the conclusions of this study. In our experience, children who are under stress from receiving aggressive modern therapy, such as that given for many forms of cancer and during bone marrow transplantation, fare better if they have a strong family unit. This has nothing to do with political correctness and everything to do with consistent and vibrant support systems for children who are undergoing terrible stress and assaults on their sense of well-being and physical integrity.

As one mulls over this report, two thoughts come to mind. First, it is an unsettling sign of the times that such studies are needed to confirm our belief in what should be common sense. Second, once this observation is made, what is one to do about it? Are medical systems capable of repairing a lack of family cohesion and expressiveness? I doubt it. The practical value, I guess, of studies such as this is to alert caregivers to an increased likelihood of trouble in certain family situations, thereby enabling them to bring increased support from nonfamily sources. Whether one can replace the support absent from the fractured family unit is open to some question and is probably the source of an additional study. Nevertheless, common sense should prevail and should motivate us to provide that additional support to those in need.

J.V. Simone, M.D.

A Prospective, Controlled Evaluation of Home Chemotherapy for Children With Cancer
Close P, Burkey E, Kazak A, Danz P, Lange B (Children's Hosp of Philadelphia; Univ of Pennsylvania, Philadelphia)
Pediatrics 95:896–900, 1995   21–15

Introduction.—Previous studies of patients with cancer have shown that home care is cost-effective and well accepted by patients and their families. Limited information is available for pediatric oncology home care. The medical, psychosocial, and financial results of an expanded home care program for infusion chemotherapy in children were reported in a prospective, controlled evaluation.

Methods.—Fourteen families qualified for voluntary home chemotherapy. The criteria for eligibility included electricity, telephone, refrigeration, access to emergency care, and reliable IV access. Parents needed to be present in the home during infusions, and they had to demonstrate competence with infusion pumps and lines. The family was required to be free of any dysfunction within the home that would interfere with compliance and safety. The first 2 chemotherapy sessions were conducted in the hospital, and subsequent courses were administered in the home. Home health nurses and parents were educated in home administration of IV chemotherapy. Families had 24-hour telephone access to nurses, and nurses had 24-hour access to oncology physicians.

Results.—The patients, aged 31 months to 16 years, received 76 courses of home chemotherapy. This avoided 312 days of hospitalization. The mean billed medical expenses per day for the chemotherapy were $2,329 in the hospital and $1,865 at home. Mean out-of-pocket expenses per day were $68 in the hospital and $12 at home. Parental loss of wages per

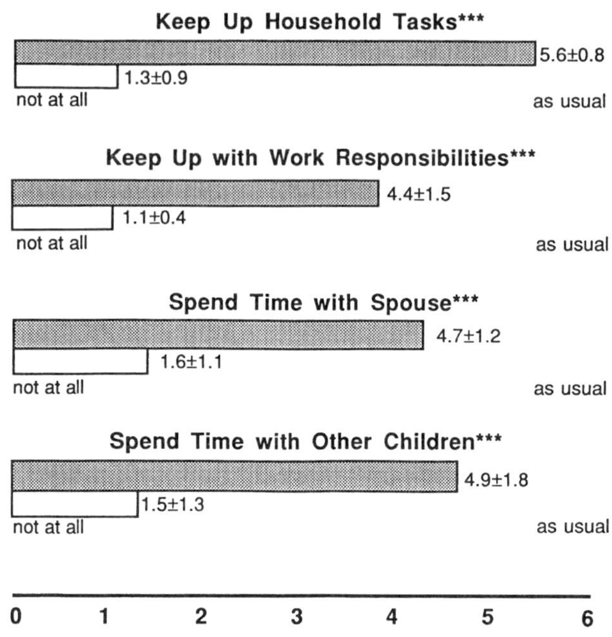

FIGURE 3.—Scale showing the mean and standard deviation for each of 4 variables of quality of parental life, based on 1 course of chemotherapy in the hospital and an identical course of chemotherapy at home. ***$P < .001$. (Courtesy of Close P, Burkey E, Kazak A, et al: A prospective, controlled evaluation of home chemotherapy for children with cancer. Reproduced by permission of *Pediatrics* 95:896–900, Copyright 1995.)

chemotherapy course was $265 in the hospital and $107 in the home. Parents reported that their children had significantly greater well-being, better appetite, more independence, greater contentment, and greater ability to keep up with schoolwork when they were at home instead of in the hospital (Fig 3). No significant differences were reported between the 2 environments with regard to the amount of time the children were out of bed or slept at night. In the home, parents were significantly more able to keep up with household tasks, maintain their jobs, and spend time with each other and other children at home.

Conclusion.—Charges for chemotherapy at home were 17% less per day than hospital charges. Home chemotherapy is a cost-effective means of delivering care, and it preserves a more normal family life compared with hospital care. However, it is important to remember that some families are not able to provide home care. Adequate provisions must be made to protect families from depleting the lifetime reimbursable major medical portion of their insurance with a multifaceted home infusion program.

▶ Pediatric oncologists have historically been at the forefront in trying to reduce the inpatient hospital stays of their patients. The reasons are obvious: Children are not independent and require a parent's presence during their treatment; parents are usually young and need to work; and there often are other children at home who require care. In addition, recent changes in the health care environment have created pressure to move patients not only out of the inpatient environment but, also, out of the hospital environment altogether.

This study demonstrates a process of providing home chemotherapy for children with cancer. It demonstrates very well that, under controlled circumstances, it is feasible, has extremely positive effects on family life, and certainly reduces the overall cost of care. This trend in pediatric oncology is also occurring in adult oncology to some extent, and it demonstrates that some good things will come out of the era of managed care.

J.V. Simone, M.D.

Someone to Live For: Social Well-Being, Parenthood Status, and Decision-Making in Oncology
Yellen SB, Cella DF (Rush-Presbyterian-St Luke's Med Ctr, Chicago)
J Clin Oncol 13:1255–1264, 1995   21–16

Background.—Social support plays a very important role in the diagnosis and treatment of cancer, affecting illness outcomes, health behaviors, survival, coping, and neuroendocrine function. Family ties appear to be a particularly important determinant of the response to acute and chronic illness. However, there are few data concerning the influence of social and family factors on treatment preferences, including the desire for aggressive cancer therapy. The subjective and objective social factors affecting patient preferences for cancer treatment were assessed.

Methods.—The study sample comprised 296 patients who had cancer with various diagnoses and in various disease stages. Each subject read sets of hypothetical vignettes regarding patients with early and advanced cancer. After reading the first set of vignettes, the patients were asked to decide whether they would accept treatments with varying levels of increasing cure or extending survival. The second set of vignettes assessed the point at which the patients' preferences shifted from mild to severe treatment to improve the chances of 1-year survival (switch points). Various factors were assessed for their influence on treatment preferences and switch points, including the quality-of-life domains of the Functional Assessment of Cancer Therapy-General (FACT-G), having children, marital status, and living arrangements.

Results.—For the vignettes describing patients with advanced cancer, the Social Well-Being subscale of the FACT-G predicted both treatment acceptance and switch point; patients with lower Social Well-Being scores preferred less aggressive treatments. Having children at home was associated with more aggressive intent in terms of treatment preferences in the advanced-disease vignettes and in terms of switch points in the early- and advanced-disease vignettes. Patients who lived with others also had more aggressive intent in the advanced-disease vignettes. Treatment acceptance and switch point were not predicted by marital status.

Conclusion.—Patients with cancer and positive social well-being and those with children living at home are more likely to accept aggressive treatments. Acceptance of more aggressive treatment may account for or mediate the previously reported benefits of social support on the outcomes of cancer. Oncologists should be aware of the subjective and objective indices of social support that may affect patients' willingness to accept various treatments.

▶ This paper reveals a different twist on the public's perception that a "positive attitude" improves the outcome of treatment of patients with cancer or other diseases. In this paper, a different question was asked, i.e., whether positive social well-being influences the treatment choices of patients with cancer. The basic finding was that positive social well-being and a tight family structure predicted patients' willingness to accept aggressive treatment. This raises the fascinating question of whether the better outcomes observed among patients with positive social well-being are the result of either the psychological effects or the differences in treatment that the patients are willing to undergo.

My own experience among children and young adults with cancer has led me to conclude that a positive mental attitude has had little influence on the outcome of treatment. Conversely, a negative attitude toward treatment, hospitals, and doctors—particularly among adolescents—has not foreordained a negative outcome. This paper suggests one reason for the observation. In pediatric oncology, with rare exceptions, patients all receive the same aggressive treatment. There have been estimates that 80% of children with cancer are treated by a modern protocol. If this impression were sustained, it would provide support for the suggestion made by the authors in this paper that the difference in outcome among those patients with a positive social environment may be the result of their treatment choices rather than any psychological effect on the interaction of treatment and cancer.

J.V. Simone, M.D.

A Controlled Trial to Improve Care for Seriously Ill Hospitalized Patients: The Study to Understand Prognoses and Preferences for Outcomes and Risks of Treatments (SUPPORT)
The SUPPORT Principal Investigators (Univ of Virginia, Charlottesville)
JAMA 274:1591–1598, 1995   21–17

Introduction.—There is a new focus on obtaining realistic predictions of the results of life-sustaining treatments and on improving patient-physician communication regarding end-of-life decisions. Increased communi-

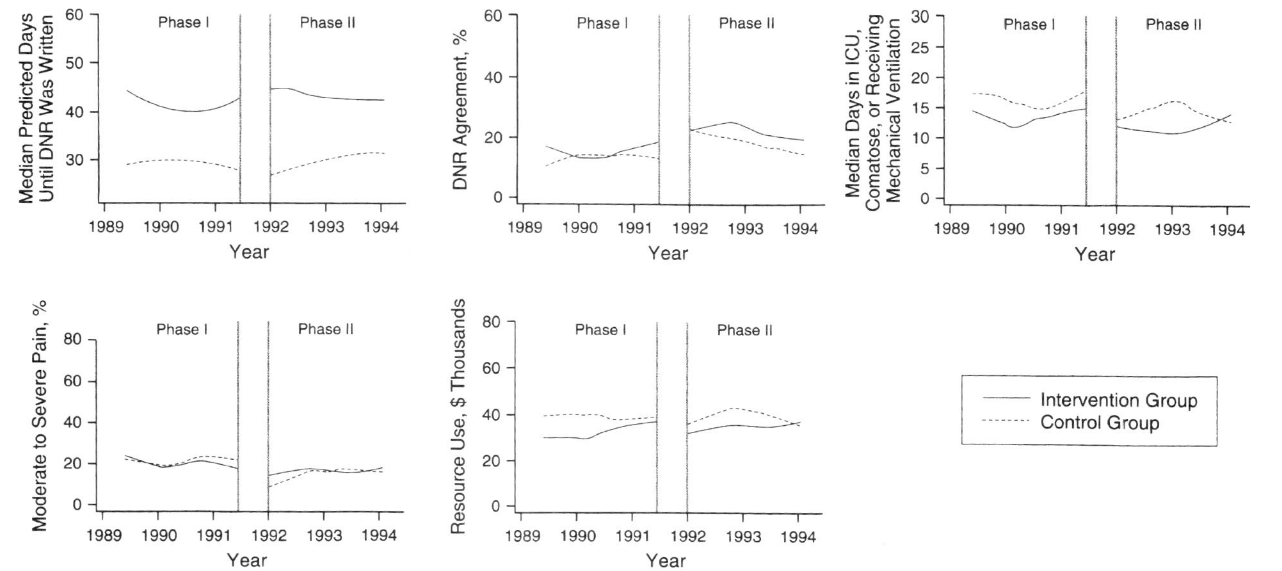

FIGURE 2.—Secular trends in 5 patient outcomes in the SUPPORT intervention. The horizontal axes represent the years of SUPPORT (1989–1994). The time between phase I and phase II is represented by a space. The intervention and control lines have been smoothed nonparametrically. The phase II results represent the actual impact of the trial, and the phase I results are the baseline or historical differences. (Courtesy of The SUPPORT Principal Investigators: A controlled trial to improve care for seriously ill hospitalized patients: The study to understand prognoses and preferences for outcomes and risks of treatments (SUPPORT). *JAMA* 274:1591–1598, 1995. Copyright 1995, American Medical Association.)

cation and better understanding of prognoses and patient preferences could reduce the time needed to make treatment decisions, time spent in undesirable states before death, and resource utilization. This hypothesis was tested in the Study to Understand Prognoses and Preferences for Outcomes and Risks of Treatments (SUPPORT).

Methods.—A phase I, prospective observational study of 4,301 seriously ill hospitalized patients confirmed the presence of barriers to optimal patient management and deficits in patient-physician communication. Therefore, a phase II study was performed to determine whether the SUPPORT interventions were able to improve the decision-making process and to reduce the frequency of the mechanically supported, prolonged process of dying. A total of 4,804 patients and their physicians were randomized by specialty group into intervention and control groups. In the intervention group, physicians received estimates of the likelihood of 6-month survival, the outcomes of CPR, and functional disability at 2 months. Patient preferences were assessed by a trained research nurse who had multiple contacts with the patient and family, as well as with the physician and hospital staff. The nurse also sought to enhance understanding of outcomes, attention to pain control, advance care planning, and patient-physician communication.

Results.—In the phase I study, less than half of physicians knew the situations in which their patients preferred to avoid CPR. Approximately half of the do-not-resuscitate (DNR) orders were not written until 2 days before the patient died. Thirty-eight percent of the deaths occurred after at least 10 days in the ICU, and half of the conscious patients had moderate-to-severe pain at least half the time before they died, according to family reports.

In the phase II study, the SUPPORT interventions made no improvement in patient-physician communication. For example, approximately 60% of both groups failed to discuss their CPR preferences. Nor was there any improvement in the incidence or timing of DNR orders; physician knowledge of patients' resuscitation preferences; number of days in the ICU or percentage of patients receiving mechanical ventilation or becoming comatose before death; or reported level of pain (Fig 2). Utilization of hospital resources was also unaffected by the interventions.

Conclusion.—There are ongoing problems with the care provided to seriously ill patients in the hospital. No improvements in care or patient outcomes were noted with implementation of the SUPPORT interventions. The results suggest that increased patient-physician communication may be insufficient to alter usual practice surrounding end-of-life decisions. Progress in this area may require increased commitment on the part of individuals and society, as well as more aggressive interventions.

▶ This major and revealing study was aimed at finding ways to improve end-of-life decisions and to reduce the frequency of a painful and prolonged process of dying. It consisted of 2 phases: a study phase and an intervention phase. The intervention phase consisted of attempts to improve patient-physician communication and to attain a better understanding of the desires of the patient regarding DNR orders, CPR preferences, and the level of reported pain. As shown in Figure 2, there was no improvement in any of the measurable factors as a result of the intervention. Furthermore, there were no secular trends toward improvement in the control or intervention for patients during the 5 years of the data collection.

As the authors point out, these results raise fundamental questions regarding the premises on which this type of intervention is based. For a study as large and as carefully done as this one, it is instructive to learn the validity of the claim that pouring additional resources into collaborative decision-making between the physician and the patient will improve communication and end-of-life decisions. It is possible that there was no movement toward what we empirically believe to be better practice because all participants were comfortable with the current situation. Upon questioning, most patients and families indicated that they were satisfied with the process no matter what happened to them. Physicians, of course, have long-established patterns of care and, despite intervention by SUPPORT nurses, physician behavior was unchanged. It appeared that the physician and the patient found a mutually acceptable adaptation to their particular circumstances.

This is an important study for helping us to understand end-of-life issues and how care might be improved. The medical profession is often deservedly criticized—sometimes by me—for not being more sensitive to patients' wishes in the terminal phase of disease. However, patients and families come to that crossroad with a unique set of cultural and psychological experiences and expectations. Perhaps we expect too much from both parties during that difficult period. Each party protects itself and adapts as best it can to those circumstances. Perhaps we should have a little more respect for the common sense of both parties.

J.V. Simone, M.D.

Health Values of the Seriously Ill
Tsevat J, for the SUPPORT Investigators (Harvard Med School, Boston)
Ann Intern Med 122:514–520, 1995   21–18

Objective.—Time-tradeoff utilities, defined as a quantification of a person's preference for quality, rather than quantity, of life, were used to assess the health values of seriously ill hospitalized patients, their surrogate decision-makers, and their physicians. The determinants of health values, changes in health values over time, and health ratings were also evaluated.

Participants and Methods.—A total of 1,438 seriously ill patients with at least 1 of 9 diseases who had a projected overall 6-month mortality rate of 50% were included in this prospective, longitudinal, multicenter study. Patients' surrogates and their physicians also participated. Patients and surrogates were independently asked how much of the patients' life expectancy, if any, would be exchanged for a shorter life in excellent health.

An overall health rating scale, in which respondents rated the patients' current state of health on a scale anchored by 0 (death) and 100 (perfect health), was also completed.

Results.—At study day 3, patients had a mean time-tradeoff utility of 0.73. This indicated that patients equated living 1 year in their current state of health with living 8.8 months in excellent health. Scores were, however, widely varied: 34.8% of the patients were unwilling to exchange any time in their current state of health for a shorter life in excellent health, and 9% were willing to live 2 weeks or less in excellent health as opposed to 1 year in their current state of health. Little variation in mean time-tradeoff scores was noted across disease categories, although large inter-patient variation was seen in scores within disease categories. Patients' mean trade-off scores also exceeded that of their 1,041 paired surrogates. Health rating scores of patients averaged 57.8 on day 3, with patients rating their state of health higher than surrogates and physicians. Time-tradeoff scores were associated with psychosocial well-being, health ratings, desire for resuscitation, and extension of life rather than relief of pain and discomfort, degree of willingness to live with constant pain, and perceived prognosis for survival and independent functioning. Scores of surviving patients were found to increase by an average of 0.06 after 2 months and 0.08 after 6 months.

Conclusion.—Health values of seriously ill patients vary widely, are higher than surrogates suspect, are associated with few other preferences and health status measures, and increase over time. Another finding with potential clinical significance is that utilities correlate inversely, though modestly, with depression. Thus, treating depression may have an effect on how patients value their state of health.

▶ It is worth your time to try to understand this complex study. The goal of this study is to understand the choices that patients make about their subsequent course when they are seriously ill. The authors asked patients how much of their life, given their current state of health, they would be willing to exchange for living in excellent health. It turned out that, on average, patients were willing to exchange about one quarter of their remaining life for enjoying excellent health in the time they had left.

Of course, the reason for doing the study is not that one can practically make that exchange in so mathematical a manner. It was done to try to understand and convey to patients the meaning of undertaking certain forms of treatment that influence the quality of life vs. alternative treatments or no treatment. The authors carefully and wisely studied whether patients were depressed at the time the question was asked and, also, whether their assessment changed when the question was asked 2 and 6 months later. Not surprisingly, depressed patients were willing to trade away more time. When asked later in the course of disease, patients were willing to trade less time.

Perhaps the most important finding in this study was the great variability from patient to patient, regardless of diagnosis and regardless of the acuity of disease. This certainly has been my experience. I have been unable to predict, based on the objective facts, whether a family or a patient would choose aggressive therapy at all costs or make the quality of their remaining life a higher priority. Studies like these are probably the only way we are going to be able to understand how to involve patients and families in the difficult decisions necessary in an environment of cost containment of health care.

J.V. Simone, M.D.

Patients' Perspectives on Dying and on the Care of Dying Patients
McCormick TR, Conley BJ (Univ of Washington, Seattle)
West J Med 163:236–243, 1995

21–19

Objective.—Death is a part of life, so caring for dying individuals is an important part of medical care. However, during their medical education, physicians do not learn the attitudes and skills they need to care for dying patients. Much has been written about physicians' attitudes toward and practices regarding dying patients, but little research has addressed the patients' viewpoints on communication during a life-threatening illness or their perceptions of support from the patient-physician relationship. The patient and/or physician may be the source of barriers to effective communication about death and dying. Patients' perspectives on dying, including the findings of a small qualitative study, were discussed.

Disclosure.—Discussions with 6 patients suggested that the patients' experience from diagnosis to death consisted of 4 periods (Fig 3). The first was disclosure of the original diagnosis, which was always a critical event. The acute crisis was lessened by the belief that caregivers had a strong interest in helping. If the proposed treatment was described as potentially curative, the patients assumed that they would be cured. This permitted a positive outlook on the future, which lessened patient anxiety.

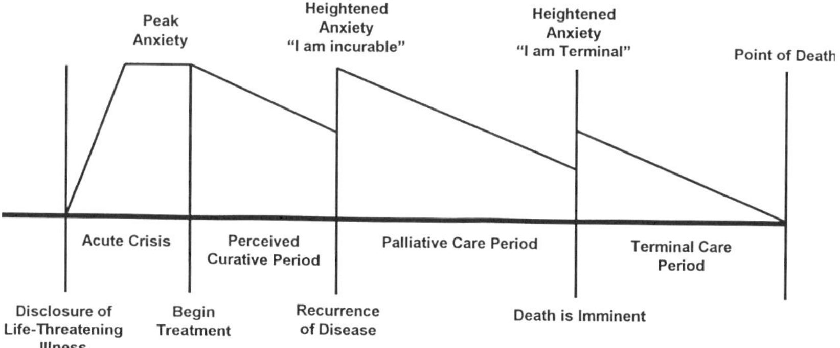

FIGURE 3.—This diagram from the patients' perspective shows heightened anxiety at the time of diagnosis, when the disease recurs, and when it appears that death is imminent. (Courtesy of McCormick TR, Conley BJ: Patients' perspectives on dying and on the care of dying patients. *West J Med* 163:236–243, 1995.)

Curative Care.—For all patients, the period of curative care marked the end of the acute crisis of facing a life-threatening illness. They thought of themselves as cured, even though their physicians might have better described them as currently free of any signs of cancer. The disparity raised the difficult question of how explicit the physician should be regarding the chances of recurrence—a question that is answered differently in different cultures. When their cancer recurred, the patients varied in terms of how and when they became aware that they were entering the palliative period. Some found out that they were in the palliative phase at about the same time their physicians did. Others thought the treatment they received for their recurrence was curative; only later did they learn that it was palliative. One patient refused a radical operation because it would leave him with an unacceptable level of functioning, and another received a single course of chemotherapy before starting palliative care.

Palliative Care.—The patients associated the early palliative care period with the term "incurable" and the late palliative care period with the term "terminal." One defined "incurable" as meaning that she was going to die at some indeterminate point in the future and "terminal" as meaning that she had to prepare herself to die. All 6 patients described the point at which they understood that death was imminent as the most important time in their illness. All could point to a single conversation with a health care professional after which they knew that death was near. Three were given this information in an explicit manner, e.g., being told by a nurse or being enrolled in a hospice program. The patients found their nurses to be more comfortable than physicians in terms of talking about death. Some expressed appreciation at knowing they only had so much time to take care of "practical business," such as spending time with family and friends.

Discussion.—Some of the greatest suffering among patients with cancer may be related to fears and anxieties that they do not discuss with their physicians. Physical and psychological pain both decrease when physicians use good communication skills, show sensitivity to the patient's viewpoint, and work to eliminate the barriers to mutual understanding.

▶ This study is based on the conventional view that physicians and their patients who are dying do not communicate well and that, therefore, the patients' preferences for palliative rather than life-prolonging care are not recognized or honored. This paper is based on the general experience of the investigators and is illustrated by a small study of 6 patients with cancer who they interviewed. They divide the periods of anxiety as shown in Figure 3, with the patients' understanding and expectations listed at each point during the course of disease.

The most important part of the interviews was the patients' understanding of what it meant to be either "incurable" or "terminal." It is interesting to me, as a physician, that patients separated these 2 terms, but it makes sense. To 1 patient, being incurable meant that she would have to live with the disease, knew that she would die, but could regard death as something in the future. Thus, the focus was on living as much as she could during the time available and on facing the process of dying only in the same sense that everyone else does, that is, "everybody dies." Of course, the situation was different when the patient came to the realization that she was "terminal." In this study, the physicians often very poorly conveyed this news to the patients and, sad to say, often did so indirectly through a nurse or through notification that hospice care was being arranged.

Although this study reports on only 6 patients in detail and has all the failings of a small sample, I found it useful because it was personalized and included direct quotations from the patient interviews. I recognize, however, that simply raising the sensitivity of physicians and other health care providers does not necessarily solve the problem. Dealing with dying patients is very difficult; there is no other way to describe it. Each of us has to find the best way to help the patient and family while retaining our ability to continue to function as a professional.

J.V. Simone, M.D.

Multicentre Study of Cancer Pain and Its Treatment in France
Larue F, Colleau SM, Brasseur L, Cleeland CS (Université de Paris; Univ of Wisconsin, Madison; Hôpital Ambroise Paré, Boulogne, France)
BMJ 310:1034–1037, 1995   21–20

Purpose.—American studies of cancer pain suggest that this pain is often undertreated. In France, where there is new emphasis on the treatment of pain, there are no data on the prevalence, severity, and treatment of pain in patients with cancer. The treatment of cancer pain in France and the predictive factors for inadequate pain management were assessed in a cross-sectional survey.

Methods.—The study sample included 605 patients with cancer at 20 treatment centers, including cancer centers, university and state hospitals, private clinics, and a home care setting. All patients were asked to rate their prevalence and severity of pain and any functional impairment resulting from pain. Their physicians were asked about the patients' cancer characteristics, performance status, pain severity, and analgesic drugs ordered.

Results.—Fifty-seven percent of the patients reported cancer-related pain. Of these, 69% said that their worst pain was severe enough to impair their functional ability. Thirty percent said they were receiving no medication for their pain. Treatment information was available for 270 of the patients in pain. Of these, 51% were not receiving adequate pain relief as assessed by the World Health Organization guidelines. The physicians tended to underestimate the severity of their patients' pain. Undertreatment of pain was more likely for younger patients, those without metastatic disease, those with better performance status, and those who rated their pain as more severe than their physician did.

Conclusion.—The assessment and treatment of pain in French patients with cancer are inadequate. More than half of the patients with cancer have pain; more than two thirds of these have pain that impairs their ability to function, and half do not receive adequate treatment for their pain. The data from this survey will help in establishing a national program for the control of cancer pain.

▶ Readers of the YEAR BOOK may recall that I have commented rather bitterly on the generally inadequate pain control for patients with cancer in the United States. This stems from a combination of unreasonable fears of addiction, ignorance of the medical and nursing professions, and an often unexpressed attitutde that taking pain medication is a sign of weakness. Unfortunately, we are not alone. This study from France indicates that at least one half the patients with cancer pain received inadequate pain relief. French physicians were found to underestimate the severity of their patients' pain. Sadly, younger patients were among those who were least likely to receive adequate pain control. Children cannot articulate symptoms as well as adults, and an unfortunate assumption is often made that a lack of complaint means a lack of pain.

The other finding in this study was that a much higher proportion of patients with cancer were found to have significant pain than had been previously realized. The bottom line is that the French do no better than Americans in controlling cancer pain, and I suspect that this is a problem all over the world—an international scandal.

J.V. Simone, M.D.

Special Issues in Pain Control During Terminal Illness
Librach SL (Univ of Toronto)
Can Fam Physician 41:415–419, 1995   21–21

Background.—The basics of pain management have been well documented in the literature. Special issues of pain management were reviewed for family physicians.

Blocks to Effective Pain Management.—There are many enduring hindrances to effective pain management in terminally ill patients. The first is lack of education. In many family medicine programs, education on basic pain physiology, assessment, and management is still deficient. Failure to assess pain properly is another important block. Such failure includes problems in obtaining an adequate pain history and in trusting patients' reports of pain. There is also a continuing bias against opioids because many physicians still fear addiction, despite evidence that such addiction is not that prevalent, even in patients with chronic pain. Failure to use adjuncts properly is another hindrance to effective pain management (Table 1). Patient-related factors are also important. A recent survey found that many patients still feared addiction and side effects. The idea that "good" patients do not complain about pain was prevalent. Effective pain management can also be compromised by clinicians' failure to consider total pain. Pain is a complex biopsychosocial phenomenon with cofactors,

TABLE 1.—Adjunct Analgesic Drugs and Therapies

Therapy	Example	Dosage	Cautions	SS	DS	V	N
					Pain Type		
No Consultation Required							
Corticosteroids	Prednisone	10–60 mg/d	Long-term use associated with multiple problems	√	√	√	√
Nonsteroidal anti-inflammatory drugs	Dexamethasone Acetaminophen	4–32 mg/d 650–1000 mg/4 h	Liver failure	√	√	√	√
	Naproxen Diclofenac Piroxicam	375 mg bid 50 mg bid 20 mg/d	Monitor for GI bleeding, GI distress, renal failure	?	?	?	√
Tricyclic antidepressants	Amitriptyline Imipramine	For both, gradually increase to 100–150 mg/d	Adds to many opioid side effects				√
Anticonvulsants	Valproic acid	Begin with 250 mg at bedtime, increase to maximum100 mg	Check blood levels. Drowsiness a problem				√
	Carbamazepine	200 mg bid increasing to 800–1000 mg total/d	Might add to bone marrow suppression. Monitor blood levels. Possible toxicity if used with TCAs				√
Consultation Required							
Membrane stabilizing drugs	Mexiletine	100 mg bid, increase to 400 mg/d	CNS toxicity, cannot be used with TCAs				√

(Continued)

TABLE 1 (cont.)

Bisphosphonates	Pamidronate		Limited to bone metastases (usually from breast cancer) response with other tumors. More limited. More research required		√		
Radiotherapy		Can be given as a single fraction. Use of radiopharmaceuticals (ie, strontium) might increase	Radiotherapists will require bone scan or other investigations to localize tumor	√	√	√	?
Chemotherapy			Toxicity might limit use in advanced disease		√	√	?
Nerve blocks	Regional blocks, plexus blocks, spinal blocks		Mixed results in studies. Possible nerve damage leading to weakness and bladder or bowel dysfunction		?	√	√
Complementary therapies	Acupuncture, hypnosis, therapeutic touch, relaxation therapy		Dose-response studies lacking. Practitioner qualifications need to be examined. Often limited response. None well studied in palliative care setting	√	√	√	?

Abbreviatons: SS, superficial somatic pain; *DS*, deep somatic pain; *V*, visceral pain; *N*, neuropathic pain; *GI*, gastrointestinal; *TCA*, tricyclic antidepressants.
(Courtesy of Librach SL: Special issues in pain control during terminal illness. *Can Fam Physician* 41:415–419, 1995. Reprinted with permission from Canadian Family Physician.)

including emotional state, personality, and family issues, as well as physical causes.

Conclusion.—Family physicians play an important role in managing pain in terminally ill patients. Necessary knowledge includes the basics of pain physiology, pain assessment, and pain management.

▶ I included this brief review of methods of pain control in terminal illness because it is very well done and can be highly recommended. It also provides an opportunity to publish Table 9, which outlines the potential agents that may be used and the type of pain for which they appear to be most effective. Dr. Librach does a nice job of outlining the obstacles that prevent effective pain management in terminally ill patients. These obstacles range from lack of education to a continuing bias against opioids, to a failure to understand the causes of pain. Our inability to adequately manage pain in terminally ill patients continues to be a vexing and embarrassing fact of life.

J.V. Simone, M.D.

Prediction of Survival of Patients Terminally Ill With Cancer: Results of an Italian Prospective Multicentric Study
Maltoni M, Pirovano M, Scarpi E, Marinari M, Indelli M, Arnoldi E, Gallucci M, Frontini L, Piva L, Amadori D (Ospedale Pierantoni, Forli, Italy; Ospedale S Carlo Borromeo, Milano, Italy; Istituto Oncologico Romagnolo, Forli, Italy; et al)
Cancer 75:2613–2622, 1995   21–22

Background.—Treatment planning for different patient subgroups is facilitated by the use of individualized prognostic variables in the various stages of cancer. The clinical factors previously reported to predict survival in retrospective studies done at single centers were verified in a prospective, multicenter study.

Methods.—Five hundred forty terminally ill patients with solid tumors in the disseminated stage were enrolled. The patients were examined for 23 clinical parameters at study entry and again every 4 weeks thereafter. The median survival among 530 evaluable patients was 32 days.

Findings.—Fifteen factors significantly predicted prognosis. Thirteen factors indicated worse survival in a univariate analysis: age older than 65 years, palliative corticosteroid therapy, anorexia, dry mouth, dysphagia, hospitalization, transfusion, weight loss of 10% or more, dyspnea, pain, increasing amounts of painkiller treatment, increasing number of symptoms, and a worse clinical prediction of survival. The factors indicating better survival were palliative progestin therapy and a higher Karnofsky performance status. A multivariate analysis indicated that the only independent survival predictors were clinical prediction of survival, anorexia,

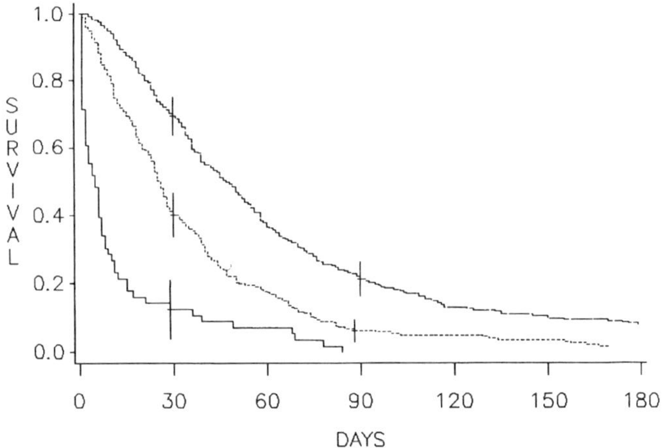

FIGURE 3.—Overall survival by Karnofsky Performance Status (*KPS*). *Vertical bars* represent 95% confidence interval, log rank = 148.67 (2df), *P* < 0.001; *solid line*, KPS of 10–20 (*n* = 56); *short-dashed line*, KPS of 30–40 (*n* = 221); *long-dashed line*, KPS of 50 or greater (*n* = 253). (Courtesy of Maltoni M, Pirovano M, Scarpi E, et al: Prediction of survival of patients terminally ill with cancer: Results of an Italian prospective multicentric study. *Cancer* 75:2613–2622, 1995. Reprinted by permission of Wiley-Liss, Inc., a division of John Wiley & Sons, Inc.)

dyspnea, palliative steroidal therapy, Karnofsky performance status, and hospitalization (Fig 3).

Conclusion.—The importance of certain clinical parameters as prognostic indicators for terminally ill patients with cancer was confirmed, and the importance of other possible factors, such as corticosteroid treatment and hospitalization, was suggested. These may prove useful in making treatment decisions.

▶ I include this paper for an unusual reason. I was attracted to the title because I had hoped it would provide some objective and useful measures of when one might confidently separate patients into groups representing those receiving palliative care only and those that might receive futile specific therapy, such as chemotherapy. This is a major issue in the world of cancer treatment, not only because of its newly important financial implications, but also because in most Western societies the system is expected to provide hope to patients at all costs, and hope is usually interpreted to mean some form of anticancer therapy, regardless of its likelihood of success.

This paper falls short of providing such useful guidelines, but it does demonstrate that it is possible to begin to tease apart some factors that can be useful among groups and institutions in developing a policy. As shown in Figure 3, the overall survival by Karnofsky performance status is what one might expect. The key in the graph, however, is not that a poor Karnofsky score results in a shorter survival; it is that the difference in median survival between those patients with a good Karnofsky score and a poor score is less than 2 months. Whether one needs an elaborate performance score to predict survival is open to question, because most seasoned medical oncologists can provide a reasonably accurate estimate for populations of patients. The difficulty is that no one can predict the outcome and duration of survival for any one patient. Decisions are usually being made at the bedside with an individual patient and the patient's family; this is, in a sense, the wrong place to make the decision.

It is far better to develop policies, based on experience, that have some flexibility but provide institution-wide guidelines, conveyed early to the patient, on what is reasonable to undertake at various times during the disease. I am not kidding myself that these guidelines are easy to apply. Nevertheless, even if one did not consider the financial implications of doing otherwise, I think it is in the best interest of both the patient and the profession to move in that direction.

J.V. Simone, M.D.

Insurance Adjudication Favoring Prophylactic Surgery in Hereditary Breast-Ovarian Cancer Syndrome

Lynch HT, Severin MJ, Mooney MJ, Lynch J (Creighton Univ, Omaha, Neb; Gross and Welch Law Firm, Omaha, Neb)
Gynecol Oncol 57:23–26, 1995   21–23

Background.—Sometimes patients at very high risk for hereditary cancer are denied insurance coverage to cover the cost of prophylactic surgery. One patient who met the criteria for prophylactic surgery based on an estimated 50% cancer risk in a hereditary breast–ovarian cancer (HBOC) pedigree was denied insurance payment to cover the cost of prophylactic oophorectomy.

Case Report.—Woman, 43, was from an HBOC family with linkage to *BRCA1*. This patient was at inordinately high risk for cancer. Despite strong recommendations by her gynecologist and a cancer geneticist–medical oncologist, the patient's insurance company (Blue Cross/Blue Shield) denied coverage for a prophylactic oophorectomy. The company stated that the surgery was not medically necessary because hereditary cancer predisposition was not a disease. A summary judgment issued by a county district court in Nebraska ruled in favor of the company's denial. However, the case was taken to the Nebraska Supreme Court, which concluded that the patient did need this surgery. The district court's decision for insurance denial was overruled.

Conclusion.—This litigation may provide a precedent for insurance coverage for patients at high risk for hereditary forms of cancer. The Nebraska Supreme Court concluded that this plaintiff did indeed have a bodily disorder or disease as defined by her insurance policy.

▶ Genetic screening for the HBOC syndrome is now a reality with the identification and cloning of the *BRCA1* gene. This screening procedure can be used to identify women who are at an inordinately high risk for the development of either breast or ovarian cancer. For women who are carrying the *BRCA1* gene, a prophylactic oophorectomy is routinely recommended after childbearing is completed and after the age of 35. Henry Lynch, a pioneer in the study of HBOC, describes a case in which an insurance company initially refused to cover the cost of prophylactic surgery in a woman at high risk for hereditary cancer.

Screening for the *BRCA1* gene is likely to represent just one of many genetic screening tests that will soon be available. However, numerous medicolegal questions remain as to how our society will deal with the information obtained by such molecular screening techniques. The rights of the patient and confidentiality issues need to be defined. How will this information be used by employers and insurance companies? Who has the right to this information? What are the obligations of the physician in this regard? These issues must be addressed in a timely manner, because genetic screening will become ever more prevalent in the coming months and years.

R.F. Ozols, M.D., Ph.D.

The Cost Effectiveness of Preoperative Autologous Blood Donations
Etchason J, Petz L, Keeler E, Calhoun L, Kleinman S, Snider C, Fink A, Brook R (West Los Angeles Veterans Affairs Med Ctr, Calif; UCLA Ctr for Health Sciences, Los Angeles)
N Engl J Med 332:719–724, 1995   21–24

Background.—The AIDS epidemic has led to much concern regarding the risk of transmitting infection through blood; it has renewed interest in autologous transfusion. Autologous transfusion is a more labor-intensive and more expensive process than allogeneic transfusion, in part because most blood centers in this country do not keep unused autologous units for use in other patients.

Objective.—Decision analysis was done to determine the cost-effectiveness of donating autologous blood for 4 surgical procedures: total hip replacement, coronary bypass grafting, abdominal hysterectomy, and transurethral prostatectomy.

Methods.—Cost data were taken from monitoring of transfusion practices at the University of California, Los Angeles, in 1992. Estimates of the risk of transfusion-related disease and the cost of treating it were taken from the relevant medical literature. Cost-effectiveness was measured as dollars per quality-adjusted year of life saved.

Results.—The direct cost of producing an autologous unit of blood was estimated as being $48 more than that for a unit of allogeneic blood, but the added cost of substituting an autologous unit for an allogeneic one ranged from $68 to as high as $4,783. The added cost resulted mainly from discarding donated units that were not transfused, and from the greater amount of work involved in autologous donation. The highest estimate of expected health benefit from substituting autologous for allogeneic blood was 0.00044 per quality-adjusted year of life saved. Cost effectiveness values ranged from $235,000 to more than $23 million per quality-adjusted year of life saved. Even for younger patients having operations, where as few as 15% of donated units are discarded, the cost-effectiveness of the procedure was at least $105,000 per year of life saved.

Conclusion.—In view of the fact that allogeneic transfusions are safer today, the added protection gained from using autologous blood is limited and may not justify the considerable added expense.

▶ There is little doubt that the cost-effectiveness of many accepted practices will be undergoing careful scrutiny in the coming years. Studies such as this one will be used to make decisions regarding whether certain procedures will be reimbursed. The possibility of transmission of AIDS through blood and blood products has led to a marked increase in autologous blood donations. However, the improvements in the safety of the blood supply system have led to an almost negligible effect on survival when autologous blood is substituted for allogeneic blood. However, the cost is far more insignificant, with the upper end of the cost-effectiveness estimate exceeding $23 million per year of life saved by autologous blood transfusion. Patients should be reassured about the safety of the blood supply, and armed with the cost-effectiveness analysis as performed in this study, the physician has a powerful argument with which to diffuse the anxiety of a patient who is facing a surgical procedure that may require a blood transfusion.

R.F. Ozols, M.D., Ph.D.

Subject Index*

A

Abdomen